Psychogenic Movement Disorders and Other Conversion Disorders

Psychogenic Movement Disorders and Other Conversion Disorders

Edited by

Mark Hallett, MD
National Institute of Neurological Disorders and Stroke,
Bethesda, MD, USA

Anthony E. Lang, MD, FRCPC
University of Toronto and Movement Disorders Center,
Toronto Western Hospital, ON, Canada

Joseph Jankovic, MD
Parkinson's Disease Center and Movement Disorders Clinic,
Baylor College of Medicine, Houston, TX, USA

Stanley Fahn, MD
Center for Parkinson's Disease and Other Movement Disorders,
Columbia University, New York, USA

Peter W. Halligan, DSc, FBPS, FMedSci
School of Psychology
Cardiff University, UK

Valerie Voon, MD
Behavioral and Clinical Neuroscience Institute,
University of Cambridge, UK

C. Robert Cloninger, MD
Center for Psychobiology of Personality, Washington University School of Medicine,
St. Louis, MO, USA

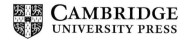

CAMBRIDGE
UNIVERSITY PRESS

CAMBRIDGE UNIVERSITY PRESS
Cambridge, New York, Melbourne, Madrid, Cape Town,
Singapore, São Paulo, Delhi, Tokyo, Mexico City

Cambridge University Press
The Edinburgh Building, Cambridge CB2 8RU, UK

Published in the United States of America by Cambridge University Press, New York

www.cambridge.org
Information on this title: www.cambridge.org/9781107007345

First published 2011

Printed in the United Kingdom at the University Press, Cambridge

A catalogue record for this publication is available from the British Library

Library of Congress Cataloguing in Publication data
Psychogenic movement disorders and other conversion disorders / [edited by]
Mark Hallett ... [et al.].
p. ; cm.
Includes bibliographical references and index.
ISBN 978-1-107-00734-5 (hardback)
1. Conversion disorder.   2. Psychomotor disorders.   I. Hallett, Mark, 1943–
[DNLM: 1. Psychomotor Disorders.   2. Conversion Disorder.   3. Movement Disorders. WM 197]
RC552.S66.P79 2011
616.85′24–dc23   2011028096

ISBN 978-1-107-00734-5 Hardback

Contents

Section 3. Assessment

Section 4. Treatment

Color plates appear between pages 164 and 165.

Contributors

Karen E. Anderson, MD
Clinical Associate Professor of Psychiatry and
Neurology, University of Maryland School of
Medicine, Baltimore, MD, USA

Bonnie Applewhite, MD
Resident Physician, Barnes-Jewish Hospital and
Department of Psychiatry, Washington University, St.
Louis, MO, USA

Selma Aybek, MD
Clinical Researcher and Consultant Neurologist,
Section of Cognitive Neuropsychiatry, Department of
Psychological Medicine, Institute of Psychiatry, King's
College London, UK

Patricia Bakvis, PhD
Clinical Psychologist and Research Fellow, SEIN
(Epilepsy Institute of the Netherlands), Heemstede,
the Netherlands

Arthur J. Barsky, MD
Professor of Psychiatry, Harvard Medical School and
Vice Chair for Psychiatric Research, Brigham and
Women's Hospital, Boston, MA, USA

Christopher Bass, MA, MD, FRCPsych
Department of Psychological Medicine, John Radcliffe
Hospital, Oxford, UK

Vaughan Bell, PhD, DClinPsy
Neuropsychologist, Universidad de Antioquia,
Colombia and Institute of Psychiatry, King's College
London, UK

Teresa Bennett, MD, FRCP(C)
Clinical Scholar, Department of Psychiatry and
Behavioural Neuroscience, McMaster University,
Hamilton, ON, Canada

Alfredo Berardelli, MD
Professor of Neurology, Department of Neurological
Sciences and Neuromedical Institute, Sapienza,
University of Rome, Italy

Elisabeth B. Binder, MD, PhD
Max Planck Institute of Psychiatry, Munich, Germany
and Assistant Professor, Departments of Psychiatry
and Behavioral Sciences and Human Genetics, Emory
University School of Medicine, Atlanta, GA, USA

Kevin J. Black, MD
Departments of Psychiatry, Neurology, Radiology,
and Anatomy and Neurobiology, Washington
University School of Medicine, St. Louis, MO, USA

Bethany Brand, PhD
Department of Psychology, Towson University,
Towson, MD, USA

Christina A. Brezing, MD
Resident, Department of Psychiatry, Massachusetts
General Hospital–McLean Hospital, Boston, MA,
USA

Alan J. Carson, MBChB, MPhil, MD, FRCPsych
Consultant Neuropsychiatrist, NHS Lothian and Part-
Time Senior Lecturer, University of Edinburgh, UK

Robert Chen, MA, MBBChir, MSc, FRCPC
Professor of Medicine (Neurology), University of
Toronto and Toronto Western Research Institute,
Toronto, ON, Canada

C. Robert Cloninger, MD
Wallace Renard Professor of Psychiatry and Director,
Center for Psychobiology of Personality, Department
of Psychiatry, Washington University School of
Medicine, St. Louis, MO, USA

Yann Cojan
Department of Neurology, University Hospital of
Geneva, University of Geneva, Switzerland

Tom K. Craig, PhD, FRCPsych
Professor of Psychiatry, Health Service and Population
Research Department, Institute of Psychiatry, King's
College London, UK

Anthony S. David, MD, MRCP, FRCPsych

Professor of Neuropsychiatry, Section of Cognitive Neuropsychiatry, Department of Psychological Medicine, Institute of Psychiatry, King's College London, UK

Quinton Deeley, MA, MBBS, MRCPsych, PhD

Senior Lecturer in Social Behaviour and Neurodevelopment, Forensic and Neurodevelopmental Sciences, Institute of Psychiatry, King's College London, UK

Floris P. de Lange, PhD

Junior Principal Investigator, Donders Institute for Brain Cognition and Behaviour, Radboud University, Nijmegen, the Netherlands

Nika Dyakina, DO

Assistant Clinical Professor in Psychiatry in Child and Adolescent Psychiatry, Columbia University Medical Center, New York, USA

Alberto J. Espay, MD, MSC

Movement Disorders Center, Department of Neurology, University of Cincinnati College of Medicine, Cincinnati, OH, USA

Stanley Fahn, MD

H. Houston Merritt Professor of Neurology and Director of the Center for Parkinson's Disease and Other Movement Disorders, Columbia University, New York, USA

Joseph M. Ferrara, MD

Division of Movement Disorders, Department of Neurology, University of Louisville, Louisville, KY, USA

Elisa Filevich

PhD Student, Institute of Cognitive Neuroscience, University College London, UK

Prudence Fisher, PhD

Adjunct Assistant Professor, Columbia University School of Social Work, New York, USA

Elizabeth E. Franz, PhD

Associate Professor of Psychology, University of Otago, Dunedin, New Zealand

James Fulton, FRANZCR

Senior Radiologist, Dunedin Hospital, New Zealand

Donald L. Gilbert, MD, MS

Associate Professor of Pediatrics and Neurology and Director of the Movement Disorders and Tourette Syndrome Clinics, Cincinnati Children's Hospital Medical Center, Cincinnati, OH, USA

Christopher G. Goetz, MD

Professor of Neurological Sciences and Pharmacology, Rush University Medical Center, Chicago, IL, USA

Joseph Graber, BA

Patrick Haggard, PhD

Professor, Institute of Cognitive Neuroscience, University College London, UK

Mark Hallett, MD

Chief of the Human Motor Control Section, Medical Neurology Branch, National Institute of Neurological Disorders and Stroke, National Institutes of Health, Bethesda, MD, USA

Peter W. Halligan, DSc, FBPS, FMedSci

Professor of Neuropsychology and Dean of Strategic Futures and Interdisciplinary Studies, School of Psychology, University Cardiff, UK

Graeme D. Hammond-Tooke, MBBCh, PhD, FCP(SA), FRACP

Senior Lecturer in Medicine, University of Otago, New Zealand

Vanessa K. Hinson, MD, PhD

Associate Professor of Neurology, Medical University of South Carolina, Charleston, SC, USA

Christine Hunter, RN

Research Manager of the Parkinson's Disease Center and Movement Disorders Clinic, Baylor College of Medicine, Department of Neurology, Houston, TX, USA

Kelly M. Isaacs, BA

Graduate Student, Department of Clinical Psychology, Xavier University and Cincinnati Children's Hospital Medical Center, Cincinnati, OH, USA

Joseph Jankovic, MD

Professor of Neurology, Distinguished Chair in Movement Disorders, and Director of the Parkinson's Disease Center and Movement Disorders Clinic,

Baylor College of Medicine, Department of Neurology, Houston, TX, USA

Matthew D. Johnson, BS
Medical Student, University of Cincinnati School of Medicine, Cincinnati, OH, USA

Richard A. Kanaan, MD, PhD, MRCPsych
Consultant Neuropsychiatrist, Department of Psychological Medicine, Institute of Psychiatry, King's College London, UK

Erica Kao
Undergraduate Student, Yale University, New Haven, CT, USA

Irving Kirsch, PhD
Professor of Psychology, University of Hull, UK

Torsten Klengel, MD
Resident in Psychiatry, Max Planck Institute of Psychiatry, Munich, Germany

W. Curt LaFrance, Jr. MD, MPH
Director of Neuropsychiatry and Behavioral Neurology, Rhode Island Hospital and Assistant Professor of Psychiatry and Neurology (Research), Brown Medical School, Providence, RI, USA

Anthony E. Lang, MD, FRCPC
Professor and Director of the Division of Neurology and Jack Clark Chair for Parkinson's Disease Research, University of Toronto and Director of the Movement Disorders Center, Toronto Western Hospital, ON, Canada

Ruth A. Lanius, MD, PhD
Department of Psychiatry, University of Western Ontario, London, ON, Canada

Alan D. Legatt, MD, PhD
Departments of Neurology and Neuroscience, Montefiore Medical Center and the Albert Einstein College of Medicine, Bronx, NY, USA

Bonnie E. Levin, PhD
Professor of Neurology and Chief of the Neuropsychology Division, Department of Neurology, University of Miami Miller School of Medicine, Miami, FL, USA

Johan Marinus, PhD
Epidemiologist, Department of Neurology, Leiden University Medical Center, the Netherlands

Michael F. Mazurek, MD, FRCP(C)
Professor of the Departments of Medicine (Neurology), Psychiatry and Behavioural Neuroscience, McMaster University, Hamilton, ON, Canada

Amie Myrick, MS, LCPC
Department of Psychology, Towson University, Towson, MD, USA

Fatta B. Nahab, MD
Assistant Professor of Neurology and Director of Movement Disorders Research, Department of Neurology, University of Miami Miller School of Medicine, Miami, FL, USA

Timothy R. J. Nicholson, MD, MSc, MRCP, MRCPsych
Clinical Researcher and Honorary Specialist Registrar, Section of Cognitive Neuropsychiatry, Department of Psychological Medicine, Institute of Psychiatry, King's College London, UK

David A. Oakley, PhD, BSc, FRSM, FBPsS
Emeritus Professor of Psychology, Division of Psychology and Language Sciences, University College London, UK

José L. Ochoa, MD, PhD, DSc
Clinical Professor of Neurology and Neurosurgery, Oregon Health and Science University and Oregon Nerve Center, Good Samaritan Hospital, Portland, OR, USA

Jill Oliver, MSC
Senior Charge Radiographer, Dunedin Hospital, New Zealand

Fred Ovsiew, MD
Professor of Clinical Psychiatry and Behavioral Sciences, Feinberg School of Medicine, Northwestern University, Chicago, IL, USA

Karin Roelofs, PhD
Professor of Experimental Psychopathology, Behavioral Science Institute and Donders Institute For Brain Cognition and Behavior, Radboud University, Nijmegen, the Netherlands

Richard Rogers, PhD, ABPP
Professor of Psychology, University of North Texas, Denton, TX, USA

Patricia I. Rosebush, MScN, MD, FRCP(C)

Professor, Department of Psychiatry and Behavioural Neuroscience, McMaster University, Hamilton, ON, Canada

John C. Rothwell, MA, PhD

Professor of Human Neuropsychiatry, Institute of Neurology, University College London, UK

Vedat Sar, MD

Professor, Department of Psychiatry, Istanbul Faculty of Medicine, Istanbul University, Turkey

Alexandra Sebastian

Department of Psychology, University of Ontago, Dunedin, New Zealand

Michel C. F. Shamy, MD

Chief Neurology Resident, University of Toronto, ON, Canada

Michael Sharpe, MA, MBBS, MD, FRCP, FRCPsych

Professor of Psychological Medicine and Symptoms Research, University of Edinburgh, UK

Lisa M. Shulman, MD

Professor, Department of Neurology, University of Maryland School of Medicine, Baltimore, MD, USA

Jon Stone, MBChB, PhD, FRCP

Consultant Neurologist and Honorary Senior Lecturer, NHS Lothian and University of Edinburgh, UK

Philip D. Thompson, MB, BS, PhD, FRACP

Professor of Neurology, University of Adelaide and Royal Adelaide Hospital, Australia

Ivan Toni, PhD

Principal Investigator, Donders Institute for Brain Cognition and Behaviour, Radboud University, Nijmegen, the Netherlands

Jacobus J. van Hilten, MD, PhD

Professor, Department of Neurology, Leiden University Medical Center, the Netherlands

Valerie Voon, MD

Clinical Research Associate, Behavioral and Clinical Neuroscience Institute, Department of Psychiatry, University of Cambridge, UK

Patrik Vuilleumier

Department of Neurology, University Hospital of Geneva, University of Geneva, Switzerland

Richard Watts, BSc, DPhil

Senior Lecturer and Director of MR Research, University of Canterbury and Van der Veer Institute for Parkinson's and Brain Research, Christchurch, New Zealand

Daniel T. Williams, MD

Attending Psychiatrist, Columbia University Medical Center, New York, USA

Chelsea Wooley, MS

Doctoral Student in Clinical Psychology, University of North Texas, Denton, TX, USA

Fernando Zelaya, PhD

Reader in Neuroimaging, Department of Neuroimaging, King's College London, UK

Preface

Psychogenic movement disorders and other conversion disorders are common. All physicians encounter patients with conversion symptoms. Neurologists often see patients with psychogenic movement disorders, psychogenic seizures, and a variety of other unexplained neurological problems that eventually are thought to have a psychological basis. However, these patients are rarely referred to psychiatrists, partly because of a failure to recognize the underlying psychological basis, partly because of the various obstacles in accessing appropriate and competent psychiatric care – and many other reasons. These patients are falling through the cracks of our medical system. Such patients utilize a large fraction of healthcare resources, estimated at 16% of dollars in the USA. Despite the impact these symptoms have on productivity and quality of life, there is a paucity of research and evidence-based reports on the mechanisms and treatment of these disorders.

This book is an outcome of the *Second International Conference on Psychogenic Movement Disorders and Other Conversion Disorders*, held in Washington, DC, in April 2009, and sponsored by the Movement Disorder Society, the National Institute of Neurological Disorders and Stroke, and the National Institute of Mental Health. It is our hope that the book will increase awareness and knowledge of these conditions and serve as an educational and scientific resource for physicians and other healthcare providers in different specialties to improve their diagnostic acumen and plan therapeutic strategies tailored to patient's individual needs.

In the absence of a definitive biomedical diagnosis, the poor understanding of psychogenic disorders has led to misconceptions within the medical community, and the mere mention of the topic continues to generate a great deal of controversy. These misconceptions begin with the name used to describe the disorder. Psychogenic movement disorders are essentially defined as involuntary movement disorders presumed to be of psychological/psychiatric origin. The basic idea of conversion, advocated by Freud, is that

a psychological symptom is converted to a somatic symptom as a means of dealing with the psychological symptom. While many patients with psychogenic movement disorders do indeed report considerable stress (past and/or present), anxiety, and/or depression, some do not because of denial, because of an inability to connect the stress with the onset of the movement disorder, or for other reasons. Even for those that do, there is a real possibility that the stress/anxiety is an understandable response to the specific conversion outcome. Does this mean that a psychological etiology is not always present or that the psychological underpinnings are not fully recognized by the physician or the patient? While endorsing psychological accounts, many neurologists do not understand their patients in such terms. This is further complicated by the natural resistance of many patients to accept the proposition of a psychological origin. Such patients, if told that they have a psychological or psychiatric condition, will just move to another doctor and often undergo treatments and procedures that may make their overall condition worse.

The traditional view of a relationship between a psychogenic presentation and demonstrable psychopathology has changed, and many clinicians use the term "functional" to describe the condition. This approach does not deny or mitigate the reality of illness but rather provides a rationale whereby a dysfunction rather than a structural problem explains the condition: a "software problem, not a hardware problem". Other clinicians use the term "functional" for a different reason – they believe that there is a psychological etiology but are afraid to confront the patient and family with that message. A problem with the term "functional" is that it might imply normal function rather than dysfunction and contradicts the notion that the treating physician wants and should convey to the patient about the "cause" of the psychogenic disorder. Some physicians find it helpful to explain to the patient that the body reacts in different ways to stress, whether the stress is consciously perceived or not, for example by raising blood pressure or by causing involuntary movements, such as tremors, and other motor abnormalities we refer to as "psychogenic movement disorders." Acute or chronic stressors, while not always initially identifiable by the patient or the physician, probably do play an important role in most, but not necessarily all, cases. It may be helpful to let the patients know that it may take more than one visit with the neurologists and/or psychiatrists to identify all potential stress factors. This may be important in order to better understand which, if any, experiences in the past have contributed to the onset and maintenance of the movement disorder.

Neurologists and not psychiatrists must make the diagnosis of a psychogenic movement disorder. Neurologists are trained in movement disorders and their differential diagnosis. However, psychiatrists have an important role in further exploring the possible psychodynamic and stress-related factors and, in collaboration with a neurologist, planning a therapeutic strategy. Clearly, neurologists and psychiatrists need to work together in understanding and treating the patient. An additional conclusion is that since psychiatrists cannot always identify a psychiatric etiology, neurologists (and others) need to keep an open mind about the fundamental etiology.

The aim of this book is to provide a balanced multidisciplinary review of the scientific basis of psychogenic movement disorders, explore the role of psychological, social, and biological factors, and also provide a practical guide to the diagnosis and treatment of this group of challenging disorders. Uniquely, the book is supplemented by numerous video segments illustrating many facets of the disorder. The video library by itself is extremely valuable since the diagnosis of psychogenic movement disorders not only requires a detailed history but also a careful observation and assessment of phenomenology. In many cases of paroxysmal or intermittent movement disorders, the physician must rely on the description of the phenomenology by the patient and other observers, but the increased accessibility to video technology, such as the video capability of many cell phones, enables the relevant movements to be recorded and used to aid in the diagnosis.

In addition to discussion of neurological and movement disorder aspects of psychogenic movement disorders, we have also tried to review the various psychiatric mechanisms that might underlie conversion in general. How is conversion considered? What might be the role of anxiety and depression, dissociation and hypochondriasis? And should one consider a biopsychosocial model? There is likely an underlying biology for psychogenic movement disorders, as there is for other psychiatric disorders. The role of genetics, childhood trauma, and stress, and their interactions, is considered together with the social/cultural context, in particular the patient beliefs in which the symptoms arise and are managed.

The underlying physiology for conversion is also explored in greater detail. The clinical neurophysiology is important, and a number of neuroimaging studies are showing how the brain may be malfunctioning in the setting of psychogenic disorders. Is the limbic system malfunctioning? Perhaps this physiology will ultimately displace the Freudian analogies, many of which are increasingly being challenged even by psychoanalysts. There are many unanswered questions, but the two that are particularly crucial to our understanding are what systems produce the involuntary movements and why the movements are not considered to be voluntary. Several chapters in this book attempt to address these important questions.

Treatment and management issues are also carefully considered. There is a long way to go in this area and clinical trials are sorely needed. However, some practical advice can be provided even now. The difficult issue of placebo, both for diagnosis and treatment is reviewed. Can it be used? If so, when would it be appropriate? The patients are often highly suggestible. What does that tell us about the biology, and does it suggest that there should be a role for placebo or hypnosis in the diagnosis and treatment?

While this volume is a second book in a "series," it is not a second edition. All the chapters are new, and there is less attention to phenomenology and more to biology and etiology. Psychogenic movement disorders in children are considered. After the first book, many readers told us that a video was needed, and we have been responsive to that. We hope that this book will be widely read by neurologists, psychiatrists and others interested in this important topic. Our patients depend on better dissemination of knowledge about this group of disorders.

Mark Hallett, Anthony E. Lang,
Joseph Jankovic, Stanley Fahn, Peter W. Halligan,
Valerie Voon, and C. Robert Cloninger

Introduction to the psychiatry of conversion disorders

Fred Ovsiew

Here is a description of a psychogenic movement disorder from the clinical literature.

> A 34-year-old woman fell down a flight of stairs some two weeks prior to the reported examination. No serious injury was evident. However, immediately thereafter she developed dystonia of the left lower extremity. The limb was described as rigid with no voluntary movement; passive movement was equally impossible. The thigh and lower leg were held straight out and the foot was plantar flexed at the ankle, so that the three segments of the extremity were held in a straight line "like a rigid bar." The extremity was internally rotated so that the patella and foot pointed inward. Additionally present was a left hemianesthesia involving limbs, trunk, and face.
>
> This patient had a history of epilepsy, with nocturnal convulsions featuring incontinence and biting of the tongue occurring up to weekly and showing a catamenial predominance. In addition, she had a history of psychogenic nonepileptic seizures, which had been almost completely in remission for about 5 years. Frequently, the nonepileptic seizures had been followed by a right lower extremity dystonia and right hemianesthesia lasting weeks. Nothing was reported regarding her mental or social state beyond her living in a residential facility.

What should we call this disorder, the condition in which factors other than organic disease of the nervous system lead to symptoms that mimic those produced by nervous system disease? Many terms have been used, and each new proposal has been superseded, perhaps because the proposals for new names rested on "the, surely vain, hope that old confusions were but word deep" (Porter, 1993 [1], p. 230). The term "psychogenic," used widely and in the title of this book, was reviewed by Lewis, who found its philosophical underpinnings confused and referred to the "shimmering, unfocused quality" that made it "speciously attractive." He thought it should be "given a decent burial" (Lewis, 1972 [2],

p. 214). The current official term is conversion disorder (CD), which derives from a now-rejected early Freudian theory about "conversion" of affect into somatic form. The framers of DSM-III preferred that term to its older and more capacious rival "hysteria" [3]. The concept of hysteria was deliberately "split asunder" [4] in the formulation of DSM-III, with the somatic symptoms placed into the somatoform disorders category and the mental elements considered as aspects of personality disorders (notably histrionic personality disorder) or dissociative disorders. More recently, symptoms such as those shown by the patient described above have been called "functional" or "medically unexplained."

Whatever term we use, patients such as the one described are still with us, widespread psychiatric opinion to the contrary notwithstanding. They are often complicated and difficult patients both diagnostically and therapeutically, and an improved understanding of the basis of their psychopathology and of its manifestations will be welcome. They are difficult diagnostically partly because confident distinction of CD from the organic conditions it mimics is required. Fortunately, the differential diagnosis can be adequately made, as Stone and his colleagues showed and as is discussed elsewhere in this volume [5].

The patients are diagnostically complicated as well because they often have other psychopathology. For example, Lieb and colleagues showed that adolescents and young adults with CD were far more likely than their peers to have a variety of psychiatric disorders (see Table 1.1) [6]. Patients with CD are also more likely than comparison subjects to have dissociative symptoms or to meet criteria for a dissociative disorder [7]. The disproportions are so marked that we may wonder whether "splitting asunder" the category of hysteria is genuinely cutting nature at the joints. Perhaps the

Psychogenic Movement Disorders and Other Conversion Disorders, ed. Mark Hallett, Anthony E. Lang, Joseph Jankovic, Stanley Fahn, Peter W. Halligan, Valerie Voon, and C. Robert Cloninger. Published by Cambridge University Press. © Cambridge University Press 2011.

Table 1.1 Odds ratios for additional diagnoses in patients with conversio disorder in a population sample of adolescents and young adults

Disorder	Odds ratio (all significant)
Substance dependence	8.19
Dysthymia	11.69
Generalized anxiety disorder	11.81
Any eating disorder	29.44
Any psychiatric disorder	5.23
Two or more disorders	6.48
Source: adapted from Lieb *et al.*, 2000 [6].	

patients can be understood properly only by taking other psychopathology into account.

Patients presenting with a conversion symptom are likely to have other non-organic somatic symptoms. Followed over the long-term, patients with CD are likely to show multiple medically unexplained symptoms in multiple organ systems [8]. Clinicians must particularly keep this in mind because of the low accuracy of the history provided by the patient at the point in the course when a given clinician happens to see the patient. Schrag *et al.* compared the accounts of patients with non-organic neurological symptoms with the records of their primary-care physicians. Only 22% of self-reported diagnoses were confirmed [9]. Simon *et al.* found that 61% of medically unexplained symptoms and 43% of all symptoms reported at a first interview were not reported on inventories of "lifetime" symptoms on a second interview one year later [10]. Consequently, a comprehensive view, over time and with adequate medical records, may show that patients with CD make more extensive use of somatization than is initially apparent.

Two other non-organic conditions need to be considered in the differential diagnosis of CD: factitious disorder (FD) and malingering. These two diagnostic groups comprise patients whose non-organic symptoms are voluntarily produced, in contrast to the definitional involuntary nature of symptom production in CD. By definition, in FD the goal of producing these symptoms is the assumption of the sick role; in malingering, by contrast, although the symptoms are equally under voluntary control, the goal of their display is an external incentive, such as monetary gain. Although it is likely that these three domains – CD (with involuntary production of symptoms), FD (with voluntary

production of symptoms for the purpose of assuming the sick role), and malingering (with voluntary production of symptoms for an external, practical goal) – broadly capture separable phenomena, it might well be doubted that the dividing lines between them are bright and that doctors are reliably capable of recognizing what is going on in patients' minds. The varieties of deception may form a continuum, on which the deceptions seen in patients with malingering and FD lie at various positions in regard to the degree and nature of self-deception involved [11]. The self-deception central to CD can be particularly puzzling: how could they possibly *not* know what they're doing, we may wonder. Symonds [12] (p. 408) quoted the London psychiatrist Birley as posing the issue in this way: the self-deception of the hysteric is a particular kind of mental deficiency.

Kanaan and Wessely reviewed neurological presentations of FD [13]. They suggested that neurologists' diagnosis of FD and perhaps patients' choice of which symptoms to manufacture are affected by the available border with CD. Patients may avoid production of symptoms that could be diagnosed not only as genuine neurological disease, with the attendant gain of sympathy and care, but also as hysteria, with its attendant opprobrium. Doctors, by comparison, perhaps partly for fear of litigation, are especially reluctant to diagnose deliberate production of symptoms in the absence of observational proof (such as seeing the patient heat the thermometer to produce factitious fever) when the diagnosis of CD is easily at hand as an alternative.

The distinction of malingering from unconscious simulation or from conscious simulation for purposes other than practical gain is often problematic. Observational proof that neurological impairment is malingered – for example from video recordings of behavior inconsistent with the claimed impairment – is usually unavailable and is obtained by lawyers, almost never by doctors [14]. Kaanan *et al.* showed that neurologists in the UK, while aware of the distinction between malingering and CD, do not consider it within their purview to make this distinction [15]. A large neuropsychological literature has grown up on identifying exaggerated cognitive impairment. The combination of findings inconsistent with brain disease and the presence of an external incentive is recognized to be common, but some neuropsychologists doubt that they can objectively attribute the excessive impairment to an internal state that is hard to assess [16]. As a "best practices" guideline points out (p. 136), "Although symptom validity tests are commonly referred to as malingering tests, malingering is just one possible cause of invalid performance" [17]. While other clinicians may feel that it is, therefore, up to the psychiatrist to discern the patient's private intentions and secret goals, psychiatrists too lack telepathic powers.

For everyday social interaction, we all confidently believe we can usually distinguish between voluntary actions and involuntary ones, by ourselves or others, and we believe we can usually infer others' goals from their actions or their statements. Social life would be impossible without fair accuracy in these respects. But how well can we do in pathological cases at recognizing whether symptom creation is "deliberate" or "voluntary," or has one thing or another as its goal? Indeed how well do concepts such as deliberateness or voluntariness or goal, comfortably used in ordinary language under ordinary circumstances, capture experience in pathological circumstances or in unconscious mentation?

The diagnosis of CD under DSM-IV criteria requires the identification of psychological stressors deemed to be responsible for the symptoms [18]. This identification, the criteria say, is confirmed by the temporal sequence, symptoms following stressor. Some psychiatrists insist that the diagnosis of CD should be made only on the basis of "positive psychiatric findings," such as *la belle indifférence* or the presence of a symbolic meaning for the symptom [19]. Can these modes of inference genuinely validate the assignment of symptoms to a conversion reaction caused by a particular psychological stressor? Can clinicians reliably and validly confirm that a patient meets this diagnostic criterion?

Few data support an affirmative answer to these questions [20,21]. Perusal of case reports of incorrect diagnoses of CD suggests that undue diagnostic reliance on presumed psychological stressors is a frequent cause of error [22]. Stress, like meaning, is simply too easy to find, irrespective of the medical diagnosis. Here is an example of the appeal of psychodynamic explanations.

> Mrs. N., a woman of about 40, was left to raise two daughters after her husband died of a stroke early in the marriage. Deaths of family members ran through her history: of her 13 sibs, only four were still alive; she had memories from ages seven and nine of seeing her sister and then her aunt in their coffins. She had symptoms of anxiety and depression, and she suffered phobias and vivid

> pseudohallucinations. It was possible in a detailed way to trace these symptoms to her experiences.

> She had motor symptoms as well. These included "spastic interruptions" of her speech, "ceaseless agitation" of her fingers, and "frequent convulsive *tic*-like movements of her face and the muscles of her neck, during which some of them, especially the right sterno-cleido-mastoid, stood out prominently. Furthermore, she frequently interrupted her remarks by producing a curious 'clacking' sound from her mouth."

Many clinicians today would be likely to consider that Mrs. N. had Gilles de la Tourette syndrome. As it happens, the clinician who described this case knew Gilles de la Tourette well and surely was familiar with the syndrome he described [23]. The point here is not that Sigmund Freud – for it was he who described the case of Frau Emmy von N. ([24] (quotations from p. 49)– misdiagnosed a case of Tourette syndrome as hysteria. The boundaries between the two have shifted over time, and Freud's diagnostic thinking was appropriate to his time [23]. The point is that psychodynamic explanations – that is, explanations of symptoms in terms of their meanings to patients based on the patients' life experiences – can be magnetically attractive, irrespective of diagnosis [25]. If the diagnosis is indeed of symptom-causation by such psychological mechanisms, then recognition of the meanings of the symptom to the patient forms the core of psychological treatment. A necessary servant, but a treacherous master, is psychodynamic thinking.

Patients themselves may use psychological explanations to deny medical illness [26]. I vividly recall the patient who at the point of admission for workup of dysphagia explained to me how the symptom arose from the stresses in his life. He had motor neuron disease.

Non-physiological neurological signs, such as giveway weakness or asymmetric vibratory sensation on the sternum, also can be misleading [27,28]. The exception is when the non-physiological finding directly reflects the abnormality that is the patient's complaint. For example, when the Hoover sign is present in a patient who complains of leg weakness, the complaint is shown to be non-physiological. Even here, false positives can occur because of limitation of effort by pain or because of a mixture of organic and non-organic weakness [29]. But when a patient complaining of abnormal movements shows non-physiological sensory abnormalities on examination, all that has been demonstrated is the patient's suggestibility. Suggestibility is widespread in the normal population and lacks diagnostic validity as a marker of CD.

The author of the case reported at the beginning of this chapter used the term "hysteria," but he knew no better because he was writing at the dawn of the modern age of the study of hysteria. In fact, he can lay claim to having initiated the modern age. Jean-Martin Charcot, who provided the case description [30] (p. 35) that was recast here, inherited a diagnostic category with carefully catalogued symptoms but no satisfactorily understood pathophysiology. Charcot believed that the disorder arose from a hereditary disturbance of the functional state of the nervous system, what he referred to as a "dynamic lesion." As the historian Toby Gelfand put it, "He believed that he had captured hysteria for the specialty of neurology" [31]. (How dismayed Charcot would be that his *Clinical Lectures on Diseases of the Nervous System* was reissued in the series of Tavistock Classics in the History of Psychiatry! [30].) Although Charcot (p. 210 [30]) insisted that he believed that "the psychic element plays a very important part in most of the cases" of hysteria, perusal of his case descriptions yields the impression that he interested himself but little in the emotional or mental state of his hysterical patients. Indeed, he appears to have had little conversation with them, as this description [32] of a clinical examination suggests:

> He sits down at a bare table and at once calls for the patient. The intern reads the history while the master listens attentively. Then, there is a long silence during which he looks and looks at the patient while drumming his fingers on the table… All the while, Charcot says nothing. Finally, he orders the patient to make a special movement, makes him talk, asks for his reflexes to be tested, his sensory system to be explored. And again a mysterious silence.

Freud, Charcot's acolyte from the time of his visit to the Salpêtrière in 1885, took the crucial steps of abandoning the search for a brain lesion and instead listening to the patient: no more the "mysterious silence" between doctor and hysterical patient. These steps played a large role in determining the future shape of the specialty of psychiatry, arguably not entirely for the better. However, what we have learned subsequently about hysteria, notwithstanding new information about the brain state that corresponds to it [33], has put us on a path toward a developmentally based, psychological understanding of somatization in relation to trauma, dissociation, and self-awareness [34–38]. These advances confirm that Freud's hesitant

steps in this direction were necessary for the understanding of patients with non-organic symptoms [24] (pp. 160–161):

> Like other neuropathologists, I was trained to employ local diagnoses and electro-prognosis, and it still strikes me myself as strange that the case histories I write should read like short stories and that, as one might say, they lack the serious stamp of science… The fact is that local diagnosis and electrical reactions lead nowhere in the study of hysteria, whereas a detailed description of mental processes…enables me…to obtain at least some kind of insight into the course of that affection.

References

1. Porter R. The body and the mind, the doctor and the patient. In Gilman SL, King H, Porter R, Rousseau GS, Showalter E, eds. *Hysteria Beyond Freud.* Berkeley, CA: University of California Press, 1993:225–285.

2. Lewis A. "Psychogenic": a word and its mutations. *Psychol Med* 1972;**2**:209–215.

3. American Psychiatric Association. *Diagnostic and Statistical Manual of Mental Disorders*, 3rd edn. Washington, DC: American Psychiatric Press, 1980.

4. Hyler SE, Spitzer RL. Hysteria split asunder. *Am J Psychiatry* 1978;**135**:1500–1504.

5. Stone J, Carson A, Duncan R, *et al.* Symptoms "unexplained by organic disease" in 1144 new neurology out-patients: how often does the diagnosis change at follow-up? *Brain* 2009;**132**:2878–2888.

6. Lieb R, Pfister H, Mastaler M, Wittchen HU. Somatoform syndromes and disorders in a representative population sample of adolescents and young adults: prevalence, comorbidity and impairments. *Acta Psychiatr Scand* 2000;**101**:194–208.

7. Brown RJ, Cardeña E, Nijenhuis E, Şar V, van der Hart O. Should conversion disorder be reclassified as a dissociative disorder in DSM V? *Psychosomatics* 2007;**48**:369–378.

8. Mace CJ, Trimble MR. Ten-year prognosis of conversion disorder. *Br J Psychiatry* 1996;**169**:282–288.

9. Schrag A, Brown RJ, Trimble MR. Reliability of self-reported diagnoses in patients with neurologically unexplained symptoms. *J Neurol Neurosurg Psychiatry* 2004;**75**:608–611.

10. Simon GE, Gureje O. Stability of somatization disorder and somatization symptoms among primary care patients. *Arch Gen Psychiatry* 1999;**56**:90–95.

11. Ekman P, O' Sullivan M. From flawed self-assessment to blatant whoppers: the utility of voluntary and involuntary behavior in detecting deception. *Behav Sci Law* 2006;**24**:673–686.

12. Symonds C. Hysteria. In Merskey H, ed. *The Analysis of Hysteria: Understanding Conversion and Dissociation.* London: Gaskell, 1995 [1970]:407–413.

13. Kanaan RA, Wessely SC. Factitious disorders in neurology: an analysis of reported cases. *Psychosomatics* 2010;**51**:47–54.

14. Ochoa JL, Verdugo RJ. Neuropathic pain syndrome displayed by malingerers. *J Neuropsychiatry Clin Neurosci* 2010;**22**:278–286.

15. Kanaan R, Armstrong D, Barnes P, Wessely S. In the psychiatrist's chair: how neurologists understand conversion disorder. *Brain* 2009;**132**:2889–2896.

16. Delis DC, Wetter SR. Cogniform disorder and cogniform condition: proposed diagnoses for excessive cognitive symptoms. *Arch Clin Neuropsychol* 2007;**22**:589–604.

17. Ruff R. Best practice guidelines for forensic neuropsychological examinations of patients with traumatic brain injury. *J Head Trauma Rehabil* 2009;**24**:131–140.

18. American Psychiatric Association. *Diagnostic and Statistical Manual of Mental Disorders*, 4th edn. Washington, DC: American Psychiatric Press, 1994.

19. Rosenbaum M, McCarty T. The misdiagnosis of conversion disorder in a psychiatric emergency service. *Gen Hosp Psychiatry* 1992;**14**:145–148.

20. Ford CV, Folks DG. Conversion disorders: an overview. *Psychosomatics* 1985;**26**:371–374,380–373.

21. Cloninger CR. Diagnosis of somatoform disorders: a critique of DSM-III. In Tischler GL, ed. *Diagnosis and Classification in Psychiatry: A Critical Appraisal of DSM-III.* Cambridge, UK: Cambridge University Press, 1987:243–259.

22. Fishbain DA, Goldberg M. The misdiagnosis of conversion disorder in a psychiatric emergency service. *Gen Hosp Psychiatry* 1991;**13**:177–181.

23. Kushner HI. Freud and the diagnosis of Gilles de la Tourette's illness. *Hist Psychiatry* 1998;**9**:1–25.

24. Freud S. Studies on hysteria. In Strachey J, ed. *Standard Edition of the Complete Psychological Works of Sigmund Freud.* London: Hogarth Press, 1893–1895:1–305.

25. Pappenheim E. Freud and Gilles de la Tourette. Diagnostic speculations on 'Frau Emmy von N.'. *Int Rev Psychoanalysis* 1980;**7**:265–277.

26. Weddington WW, Jr. Psychogenic explanation of symptoms as a denial of physical illness. *Psychosomatics* 1980;**21**:805–807, 811–803.

27. Fishbain DA, Cole B, Cutler RB, *et al.* A structured evidence-based review on the meaning of nonorganic physical signs: Waddell signs. *Pain Med* 2003;**4**:141–181.

28. Gould R, Miller BL, Goldberg MA, Benson DF. The validity of hysterical signs and symptoms. *J Nerv Ment Dis* 1986;**174**:593–597.

29. Stone J, Zeman A, Sharpe M. Functional weakness and sensory disturbance. *J Neurol Neurosurg Psychiatry* 2002;**73**:241–245.

30. Charcot JM, Harris R. *Clinical Lectures on Diseases of the Nervous System.* London: Tavistock/Routledge, 1991.

31. Gelfand T. Neurologist or psychiatrist? The public and private domains of Jean-Martin Charcot. *J Hist Behav Sci* 2000;**36**:215–229.

32. Goetz CG, Bonduelle M, Gelfand T. *Charcot: Constructing Neurology.* New York: Oxford, 1995:1137 [quoting Souques A, Meige H. Jean-Martin Charcot. *Les Biographies Médicales* 1939:321–336, 337–352].

33. Nowak DA, Fink GR. Psychogenic movement disorders: aetiology, phenomenology, neuroanatomical correlates and therapeutic approaches. *Neuroimage* 2009;**47**:1015–1025.

34. Lyons-Ruth K. Contributions of the mother–infant relationship to dissociative, borderline, and conduct symptoms in young adulthood. *Infant Ment Health J* 2008;**29**:203–218.

35. Ovsiew F. An overview of the psychiatric approach to conversion disorder. In Hallett M, Fahn S, Jankovic J, *et al.*, eds. *Psychogenic Movement Disorders: Neurology and Neuropsychiatry.* Philadelphia, PA: Lippincott Williams & Wilkins, 2006:115–121.

36. Subic-Wrana C, Beutel ME, Knebel A, Lane RD. Theory of mind and emotional awareness deficits in patients with somatoform disorders. *Psychosom Med* 2010;**72**:404–411.

37. Craig TK, Bialas I, Hodson S, Cox AD. Intergenerational transmission of somatization behaviour: 2. Observations of joint attention and bids for attention. *Psychol Med* 2004;**34**:199–209.

38. Craig TK, Cox AD, Klein K. Intergenerational transmission of somatization behaviour: a study of chronic somatizers and their children. *Psychol Med* 2002;**32**:805–816.

Chapter

2

Phenomenology of psychogenic movement disorders

Anthony E. Lang

This brief chapter will highlight the phenomenology of psychogenic movement disorders and will serve as a springboard for the review of the accompanying DVD. There are a large number of reviews describing the clinical aspects of psychogenic movement disorders including their phenomenological features (e.g., [1–5]). Psychogenic movement disorders largely overlap with conversion disorders (see Chapter 1 for diagnostic criteria) although there are differences, including the less common possibility of malingering and factitious disorders causing psychogenic movement disorders. Psychogenic movement disorders are common in neurological practice and particularly in subspecialty clinics. One of the earliest surveys by Factor *et al.* estimated that these patients accounted for 3.3% of consecutive movement disorder cases seen over a 71-month period [6]. It has been the experience of many movement disorder specialists working in tertiary referral clinics that the prevalence of these disorders is greater in recent years, presumably because of better recognition.

Psychogenic counterparts may be seen for all types of movement disorder. Table 2.1 provides an estimate of the relative frequencies of the different types of psychogenic movement disorder phenotype. Tremor and dystonia are the commonest phenotypes. Probably one of the least common of these is typical chorea; indeed, this author has only seen one or two such cases over the past 25 years. One patient with strong family history of Huntington's disease and psychogenic chorea was recently described [8]. Surveys of movement disorder clinics provide quite variable figures for the relative frequencies of the different types of psychogenic movement disorder, in part related to differing ascertainment methods (some emphasizing only the dominant movement disorder and others all movement disorder types

Table 2.1 Relative frequencies of psychogenic movement disorder phenotypes

Psychogenic movement disorder	Approximate percentages (range)[a]
Tremor	40 (14–56)
Dystonia	31 (24–54)
Myoclonus	13 (0–19)
Gait disorder	10 (0–50)
Parkinsonism	5 (0–12)
Tics	2 (0–7)
Other	5 (0.4–30)

[a] Methods of classification and designation varied from center to center contributing to these figures (e.g., listing only the dominant movement disorder versus all movement disorders). Referral bias also plays a role in some centers' classifications.
Source: Lang 2006 [7].

seen in an individual patient) or referral bias (some clinics emphasizing dystonia or parkinsonism).

The classification of psychogenic movement disorders has generally followed the original approach described by Fahn and Williams in their initial report on psychogenic dystonia [9]. There have been a small number of further attempts to provide newer diagnostic criteria. For example, Shill and Gerber developed a scheme involving primary and secondary criteria [10]; however, the application of these is problematic [11]. Recently a revision of the Fahn/Williams criteria has been proposed, emphasizing the ability to establish a diagnosis based on the presence of definitive clinical features alone ("clinically established minus other features") and the importance of adding a category of "laboratory supported definite" [12]. Table 2.2

Psychogenic Movement Disorders and Other Conversion Disorders, ed. Mark Hallett, Anthony E. Lang, Joseph Jankovic, Stanley Fahn, Peter W. Halligan, Valerie Voon, and C. Robert Cloninger. Published by Cambridge University Press. © Cambridge University Press 2011.

Table 2.2 Diagnostic classification of psychogenic movement disorders

	Traditional classification of degrees of certainty in diagnosis[a]	**Proposed revision of classification of degrees of certainty in diagnosis**[b]
1. Documented	Remittance with suggestion, physiotherapy, psychotherapy, placebos, "while unobserved"	As in original
2. Clinically established	Inconsistent over time/Incongruent with clinical condition plus other manifestations: other "false" signs, multiple somatizations, obvious psychiatric disturbance	(a) Clinically established plus other features, as in original (b) Clinically established minus other features: unequivocal clinical features incompatible with organic disease with no psychiatric problems
Clinically definite	Documented and clinically established as above [13]	Documented and clinically established as above (2a + 2b)
Laboratory-supported definite	–	Electrophysiological evidence proving a psychogenic movement disorder (primarily in cases of psychogenic tremor and psychogenic myoclonus)
Probable	(a) Inconsistent/incongruent: no other features (b) Consistent/congruent + "false" neurological signs[c] (c) Consistent/congruent + multiple somatizations[c]	
Possible[d]	Consistent/congruent + obvious emotional disturbance	–

[a] From Fahn and Williams [9].
[b] From Gupta and Lang [12].
[c] It has been proposed to reclassify these patients under "possible" [12].
[d] The utility of retaining the "possible" category is questioned since this generally represents patients with organic movement disorders with additional psychiatric problems rather than a true "possible psychogenic movement disorder" [12].

outlines the original Fahn/Williams criteria as well as the proposed revision of Gupta and Lang [12].

There are a variety of clues that may assist in the diagnosis of psychogenic movement disorders. These can be subdivided under those obtained in the patient's history and those evident on the clinical examination. Tables 2.3 and 2.4, respectively, outline the more important historical and clinical clues. It should be emphasized that all of the points listed are no more than clues, and exceptions to each of them can be found in patients with organic neurological dysfunction. Importantly, a detailed history may require obtaining extensive records involving previous assessments, hospitalizations, and so on. Patients may not volunteer the full details of their previous assessments or may report inaccurate or inexact information related to these [14,15]. In some patients where the clinical features are uncertain or questionable, repeated assessments may need to be conducted over several visits. Video surveillance has been used to document the absence of the movement disorder [16], but, of course, this approach has to be used carefully. Where available and appropriate, the electrophysiological laboratory may be extremely helpful in confirming the diagnostic suspicion [17,18], although occasionally it can provide somewhat misleading information [19].

A detailed description of each of the psychogenic movement disorder phenotypes is beyond the scope of this introductory chapter (see Hallett *et al.* [20]). Tables 2.5–2.9 summarize most of the important clinical characteristics of the commonest psychogenic movement disorders and, where possible, contrast these features with the abnormalities seen in patients with their organic counterparts. Possibly two of the most important descriptors that apply to psychogenic movement disorders are their inconsistency and their incongruency. The abnormal movements are generally inconsistent over various time frames (either over the course of an individual examination or at different times on repeated assessments). Equally important

Table 2.3 Historical clues suggesting that a movement disorder may be psychogenic

Common historical clues	Exceptions/caveats
Abrupt onset often triggered by minor injury	Slow onset occasionally seen; "organic" movement disorders occasionally begin abruptly
Static course, early development of maximal or near maximal severity	Progressive course sometimes seen, possibly more often in psychogenic parkinsonism than others
Spontaneous remissions (inconsistency over time)	Spontaneous remissions occasionally seen in "organic" movement disorders such as cervical dystonia
Obvious psychiatric disturbance	Caution: overt psychiatric disturbances may not be evident and psychiatric problems are not uncommonly present with "organic" movement disorders
Multiple somatizations	
Employed in health profession	Obviously does not exclude the possibility of an "organic" movement disorder
Pending litigation or compensation	As above, i.e., does not exclude an organic disorder by any means
Presence of secondary gain	May not be evident
Young female	Psychogenic movement disorders may be seen at all ages in both genders

Table 2.4 General clinical clues suggesting that a movement disorder may be psychogenic

1. Inconsistent character of the movements (amplitude, frequency, distribution)
2. Movements increase with attention or decrease with distraction
3. Inconsistencies between performance on examination (often movements are most prominent) and times when the patient is not actively being examined (e.g., while giving a history or observed surreptitiously)
4. Selective disabilities not typical of "organic" task-specific movement disorders
5. Ability to trigger or relieve the abnormal movements with unusual or non-physiological interventions implying suggestibility (e.g., trigger points on the body, tuning fork; encouraging spread of movements to unaffected regions while restricting movement in the originally affected area [i.e., immobilizing])
6. Paroxysmal movement disorder[a]
7. Deliberate slowness of movements; performance of requested movements may appear to require extreme effort (often with excessive sighing or hyperventilation); commonly there is a major dissociation between this performance (on examination) and spontaneous performance of movements at other times (e.g., when not formally being examined)
8. Suffering or strained facial expression (particularly when asked to perform various tasks on physical examination)
9. Active resistance to passive movements (particularly with dystonic postures; also may account for "pseudorigidity" in psychogenic parkinsonism)
10. Movement abnormality that is bizarre, multiple, or difficult to classify
11. Functional disability out of proportion to examination findings
12. False weakness
13. False sensory complaints
14. Self-inflicted injuries[b]
15. Response to placebo, psychotherapy, isolated physiotherapy

[a] Must consider organic paroxysmal movement disorders.
[b] This may be seen in some "organic" movement disorders including tic disorders and neuroacanthocytosis.

Table 2.5 Clinical features of psychogenic versus "organic" tremors

Psychogenic tremor	Organic tremor
Often rest = posture = action; sometimes posture = action without a rest component	Variable depending on cause; rest tremor of Parkinson's disease diminishes/abates with action (may re-emerge in the new position); typically in other disorders rest < posture < action
Often marked variability in direction, joint and muscle involvement	Generally consistent but may vary depending on posture and activity
Variability in frequency; irregular	Frequencies generally consistent, usually regular; dystonic tremors may be irregular
Fingers uncommonly involved particularly in isolation	Fingers not infrequently involved
Often subsides or becomes more irregular with stressful tasks (e.g., mental arithmetic)	Amplitude frequently increases with stress while frequency remains constant
Complex physical tasks often cause tremor to subside (distractibility) or become more irregular (changing frequency); repetitive rhythmical task (e.g., tapping to a constant frequency using a metronome) may entrain the tremor to the new frequency or simply change the original frequency. Slow, side to side movements of the tongue may be associated with two possible outcomes: distractibility with changes in the frequency of the tremor or persistence of the tremor but extremely poor performance of the tongue movements in the absence of any dysarthria or other disturbances of orolingual function	Frequency remains relatively constant while amplitude often increases
Common features of the tremor: absent isolated finger tremor; flapping movements with variable direction; tremor often at physiological clonus frequency (distractibility and entrainability may be less in this circumstance) Leg tremors: foot plantar flexed with heel lifted slightly from the floor; leg partially flexed at knee with tremor in the thigh causing flexion/extension movements below the knee. May appreciate the "co-contraction sign" in evaluating tone	

Table 2.6 Clinical features of psychogenic versus "organic" dystonia

Psychogenic dystonia	Organic dystonia
Inconsistent/variable	Consistent and relatively stereotyped; may be action specific or largely action induced
Fixed dystonic postures common and often early in the course	With certain exceptions, dystonia is usually "mobile" and often purely action specific or action induced initially
Response to sensory tricks exceedingly rare	Response to sensory tricks (gestes antagoniste) common particularly early in the course (more typical of idiopathic than symptomatic dystonias)
Pattern usually inconsistent with organic counterparts	Recognized patterns of dystonia typical in different age groups (e.g., generalized and segmental forms more common in children while focal involvement [most often cranial, cervical, upper limb] more common in adults)
Pain may be a prominent feature, often associated with profound tenderness	Often painless (the main exception is cervical dystonia)
Often associated with marked resistance to passive movement even giving the sense of actively resisting the examiner	Tone may be normal or increased at times that the dystonic postures are most evident (dystonic rigidity)
Common features of dystonia: fixed dystonia at onset; leg involvement beginning in adult life (no evidence of additional neurological deficit such as parkinsonism); tonic downward pull of the mouth (unilateral or bilateral)	
Tonic posturing often persists despite attempted distracting maneuvers (i.e., distractibility is far less common in psychogenic dystonia than in more "mobile" psychogenic movement disorders such as tremor or myoclonus)	

Table 2.7 Clinical features of psychogenic versus "organic" myoclonus

Psychogenic myoclonus	Organic myoclonus
Often variable in distribution	Apart from multifocal myoclonus, distribution is more consistent
Distractibility, suggestibility	No influence of these maneuvers
If movements are stimulus induced (including excessive response to startle), the latency may be obviously long or quite variable (formal electrophysiology testing may be required to confirm this); jerks may be triggered by the threat of stimulus (e.g., following repeated taps with the reflex hammer a subsequent tap may be held up before touching the patient)	Consistent short latency evident
Characteristic features of myoclonus: large amplitude synchronous flailing of the arms from the sides or crossing the chest; pronounced trunk flexion (caution – organic propriospinal myoclonus); pelvic thrusts	
Electrophysiological characteristics: latency within voluntary reaction time, variable duration of bursts (usually > 300 ms), varying patterns of muscle involvement); activity may be preceded by a Bereitschaftspotential in the trace	

Table 2.8 Classification of gait disorders: clinical features of "organic" and psychogenic gaits

Type	Features
Lower level gait disorders	Peripheral skeleto-motor problems: antalgic/arthritic gait, myopathic gait (waddling), peripheral motor neuropathic gait (steppage)
	Peripheral sensory neuropathy (sensory ataxia)
Middle level gait disorders	Hemiplegic, diplegic
	Cerebellar ataxia
	Spastic ataxia
	Parkinsonism
	Hyperkinetic (chorea, dystonia, myoclonus, tics [including obsessive-compulsive behaviors]): sometimes "bizarre" and confused with psychogenic (these are better classified as "higher level gait disorders")
Higher level gait disorders	Frontal gait disorders: "march-a-petit pas," lower body parkinsonism
	Cortical-subcortical gait disorders: gait initiation failure, magnetic gait, "slipping clutch" apraxia
	Subcortical disequilibrium: tottering, astasia-abasia, "pusher syndrome," thalamic astasia
	Cautious gait/elderly gait (fear of falling): this may accompany other disorders such as orthostatic tremor
Psychogenic gait disorders	Variable and mixed patterns including hemiparetic (often with leg dragging), paraparetic (including dragging of both feet), ataxic, trembling (including vertical shaking), dystonic (including camptocormia), myoclonic.
	Other common features (see also Table 2.4): stiff-legged (robot), slapping (tabetic), appearance of walking on ice, hesitation with every step, uneconomic postures with waste of muscle energy, sudden buckling (with or without falls, sometimes dramatic falls), astasia, tightrope walking (assumes tandem gait), bizarre gait with flailing of arms and legs, waddling gait

Table 2.9 Clinical features of psychogenic versus "organic" parkinsonism

Feature	Psychogenic parkinsonism	Organic parkinsonism
Bradykinesia	Extreme slowness on performing rapid repetitive and alternating movements; no clear fatiguing of speed/amplitude, may be irregular; true arrests in ongoing movement uncommon, accompanied by apparent great effort including sighing; may have normal speed when not being examined. If facial expression is masked there is often underlying depression accounting for this	Fatiguing with slowing of movements and reduced amplitude; arrests in ongoing movement
Tremor (see Table 2.5)	Reduces or changes with distraction; often remains the same or worsens with movement while being examined; typically, rest = posture = action	Typically worsens with distracting maneuvers and decreases with goal directed movement
Rigidity	Gives the impression of voluntary resistance; may decrease with distraction; no true cogwheeling (may appreciate the co-contraction sign if psychogenic tremor persists but usually resistance "breaks" periodically giving the appreciation of underlying normal tone)	Increases with slow passive movement, worsens with activating maneuvers; often has cogwheeling superimposed

Table 2.9 (*Cont.*)

Feature	Psychogenic parkinsonism	Organic parkinsonism
Posture and gait	Tends to be upright with little flexion; gait is often very slow and laborious, antalgic if pain associated; when limb involvement is unilateral (or very asymmetrical), the arm may be held extended and unmoving at the side with little or no change in this position on running; may have considerable difficulty with tandem gait; arm tremor when persistent is often a flexion/extension or rotation movement at the wrist with the fingers held extended	Early in the course, stride and turns are often normal; affected upper limb is usually more flexed at the elbow, with reduced or absent arm swing, but running typically results in the arm flexing in front of the body and swinging more normally; typical resting tremor (fingers often involved) is commonly evident on walking
Postural stability (response to "pull test")	Often exaggerated and bizarre response to minimal postural displacements; arms may flail from the sides (this may occur rapidly and very symmetrically in otherwise very slow patients who have pronounced asymmetries of upper limb involvement)	Normal early in the course of Parkinson's disease (may be abnormal in atypical parkinsonism), impaired in moderate to advanced disease; initially patient may demonstrate retropulsion but later may show no protective reflex response; arms often move minimally in response to a posterior postural perturbation
Speech	Unusual stuttering with repetition of multiple syllables; bizarre dysarthria	Hypophonia, sometimes stuttering; tachyphemia

is the fact that the movement disorders are generally incongruent with the organic counterparts. It should be emphasized that this latter criterion obviously requires that the physician making the diagnosis has considerable experience and expertise in the assessment and care of all types of organic movement disorder. The tables highlight these and other features that characterize psychogenic movement disorders and help to differentiate them from non-psychogenic movement disorders.

References

1. Sa DS, Galvez-Jimenez N, Lang AE. Psychogenic movement disorders. In Watts R, Obeso JA, Standaert D, eds. *Movement Disorders*. New York: McGraw-Hill, 2010:in press.

2. Hinson VK, Haren WB. Psychogenic movement disorders. *Lancet Neurol* 2006;**5**:695–700.

3. Peckham EL, Hallett M. Psychogenic movement disorders. *Neurol Clin* 2009;**27**:801.

4. Thomas M, Jankovic J. Psychogenic movement disorder: diagnosis and management. *CNS Drugs* 2008;**18**:437–452.

5. Schrag A, Lang AE. Psychogenic movement disorders. *Curr Opin Neurol* 2005;**18**:399–404.

6. Factor SA, Podskalny GD, Molho ES. Psychogenic movement disorders: frequency, clinical profile, and characteristics. *J Neurol Neurosurg Psychiatry* 1995;**59**:406–412.

7. Lang AE. General overview of psychogenic movement disorders: epidemiology, diagnosis, and prognosis. In Hallet M, Fahn S, Jankovic J, et al., eds. *Psychogenic Movement Disorders:Neurology and Neuropsychiatry*. Philadelphia, PA: Lippincott Williams & Wilkins, 2006:35–41.

8. Fekete R, Jankovic J. Psychogenic chorea associated with family history of Huntington disease. *Movement Disord* 2010;**25**:503–504.

9. Fahn S, Williams PJ. Psychogenic dystonia. *Adv Neurol* 1988;**50**:431–455.

10. Shill H, Gerber P. Evaluation of clinical diagnostic criteria for psychogenic movement disorders. *Mov Disord* 2006;**21**:1163–1168.

11. Voon V, Lang AE, Hallett M. Diagnosing psychogenic movement disorders: which criteria should be used in clinical practice? *Nat Clin Pract Neurol* 2007;**3**:134–135.

12. Gupta A, Lang AE. Psychogenic movement disorders. *Curr Opin Neurol* 2009;**22**:430–436.

13. Williams DT, Ford B, Fahn S. Phenomenology and psychopathology related to psychogenic movement disorders. In Weiner WJ, Lang AE, eds. *Behavioural Neurology in Movement Disorders*. New York: Raven Press, 1994:231–257.

14. Schrag A, Brown RJ, Trimble MR. Reliability of self-reported diagnoses in patients with neurologically

unexplained symptoms. *J Neurol Neurosurg Psychiatry* 2004;**75**:608–611.

15. Schrag A, Trimble M, Quinn N, Bhatia K. The syndrome of fixed dystonia: an evaluation of 103 patients. *Brain* 2004;**127**:2360–2372.

16. Kurlan R, Brin MF, Fahn S. Movement disorder in reflex sympathetic dystrophy: a case proven to be psychogenic by surveillance video monitoring. *Mov Disord* 1997;**12**:243–245.

17. Brown P, Thompson PD. Electrophysiological aids to the diagnosis of psychogenic jerks, spasms, and tremor. *Mov Disord* 2001;**16**:595–599.

18. Deuschl G, Raethjen J, Kopper F, Govindan RB. The diagnosis and physiology of psychogenic tremor. In

Hallet M, Fahn S, Jankovic J, *et al.*, eds. *Psychogenic Movement Disorders: Neurology and Neuropsychiatry*. Philadelphia, PA: Lippincott Williams & Wilkins, 2006:265–273.

19. Hung SW-S, Molnar GF, Ashby P, Chen R, Voon V, Lang AE. Electrophysiologic testing in psychogenic tremor: does it always help? In Hallet M, Fahn S, Jankovic J, *et al.*, eds. *Psychogenic Movement Disorders: Neurology and Neuropsychiatry*. Philadelphia, PA: Lippincott Williams & Wilkins, 2010:334–335.

20. Hallet M, Fahn S, Jankovic J, *et al.* (eds.). *Psychogenic Movement Disorders: Neurology and Neuropsychiatry*. Philadelphia, PA: Lippincott Williams & Wilkins, 2006.

Psychogenic parkinsonism

Joseph Jankovic and Christine Hunter

Introduction

Psychogenic movement disorders (PMDs) are a group of heterogeneous disturbances of motor function that are not explained by organic conditions and often occur in association with underlying psychiatric disease [1]. Although different psychiatric diagnoses have been proposed, most patients with PMDs are categorized as suffering from a somatoform disorder. The true prevalence of psychogenic parkinsonism (PP) is not known, but it is thought to be relatively uncommon, representing only approximately 10% (range, 1.7–25) of all PMDs in the various series [2–6]. In the absence of a reliable diagnostic marker, the differentiation between PD and PP depends on an interpretation of signs by a clinician experienced in movement disorders and on historical and clinical features consistent with PP. In some cases, the use of imaging techniques, such as demonstration of reduced fluorodopa uptake on positron emission tomography (PET) or reduced dopamine transporter density by single photon emission computed tomography (SPECT) is helpful in differentiating PD from PP [7–12]. Whether 3.0 tesla MRI and high-resolution diffusion tensor imaging, recently reported to differentiate between early PD and healthy controls [13], can be used to differentiate between PD and PP remains to be determined. In a study that we have recently conducted, we characterize the clinical features of PP and explore the usefulness of placebo as an ancillary technique in supporting the diagnosis of PP.

In order to characterize our population of patients with PP, we collected relevant data from a chart review of all patients diagnosed with documented or clinically established PP [14] at the Baylor College of Medicine Parkinson Disease and Movement Disorders Clinic between 1978 and 2009. The presence of at least five of the following characteristic features (one of which

had to be 1 or 2) was used in arriving at the diagnosis of PP [5].

1. Slow, deliberate, effortful (associated with grimacing or sighing) rapid succession movements without decrementing amplitude, but normal speed of movement when distracted.
2. Abnormal response to postural stability testing; patients may have exaggerated, bizarre responses to minimal perturbations on testing of postural instability, which may include the flailing of arms and reeling backwards without falling.
3. Tremor of an abrupt onset, typically involving the dominant hand.
4. Tremor with a variable frequency, direction, and anatomical distribution and reduced amplitude or speed with distraction.
5. Tremor that spreads to other body parts when the affected limb is immobilized.
6. Active resistance against passive movement; true "cogwheel" rigidity could not be present and if present would decrease with distraction.
7. Stuttering, whispering, gibberish speech.
8. Other psychogenic features, such as "give-way" weakness, non-anatomical sensory loss, and other PMDs.

In most patients, the diagnosis of PP could be established on the basis of clinical history and examination, but those patients in whom the diagnosis was in some doubt or could not be fully confirmed by standard assessment were challenged with a placebo (carbidopa, serial saline injections, or the application of a tuning fork with a suggestion that the particular sign will change as a result of the vibration) [15]. The patients challenged with placebo were told that in order to better understand their condition, we wished to assess

Psychogenic Movement Disorders and Other Conversion Disorders, ed. Mark Hallett, Anthony E. Lang, Joseph Jankovic, Stanley Fahn, Peter W. Halligan, Valerie Voon, and C. Robert Cloninger. Published by Cambridge University Press. © Cambridge University Press 2011.

how they responded to an "active" or an "inactive" treatment. The suggestion that accompanied the administration of the placebo (e.g., carbidopa or a tuning fork) was "customized" to the patient's particular sign. For example, if the patient exhibited predominantly right-hand tremor, we would apply the tuning fork to the affected limb along with the suggestion that the vibration should stop the tremor. Alternatively, if the patient provided a history that he or she had tremor in the foot, but the tremor was not present at the time of the examination, the application of the vibrating tuning fork to the "affected" foot, along with suggestion that the vibration may precipitate the tremor, would often cause the patient to exhibit the tremor. After the placebo test, all patients were told that they had received an inactive drug and that their response helped us confirm the diagnosis of stress-induced or psychogenic parkinsonism. After signing a consent form, approved by the Baylor College of Medicine Institutional Review Board, the pre- and post-placebo examination was videotaped. The video segments were edited, randomized, and rated by a movement disorder specialist who was "blinded" to the pre- or post-treatment sequence using the following criteria: 1, marked improvement; 2, moderate improvement; 3, mild improvement; 4, no response; and 5, worsening of symptoms.

There were 32 patients, 17 (53%) women, with a mean age at diagnosis of 48 years (±8.6) and mean duration of symptoms 5.24 years (±1.2). A precipitating event was identified in 56% of our patients and included job-related stress in 11 (34%), personal life stress in 4 (13%), physical trauma in 4 (13%); 13 (41%) had a combination of multiple stressors. A majority of our patients (56%) had a history of comorbid psychiatric disorder, with depression being most common. The mean educational level was 14 years (±2.5) and 13% were employed in the healthcare field. Twenty one (66%) of the patients were married, 20 (63%) were on disability, and 7 (22%) had pending litigation. A family history of tremor or parkinsonism was present in nine (28%) patients.

Sixteen of the PP patients underwent a placebo challenge: 12 with carbidopa, 2 with a tuning fork, and 2 with saline injections. The pre- and postexaminations were videotaped in 10 of these patients. The improvement after placebo, based on a "blinded" review of videos, was rated as 1 or 2 (marked or moderate improvement) in four (40%) patients and 3 (mild

improvement) in six (60%). None of the patients had a neutral or negative response to placebo (Table 3.1).

After a thorough evaluation focusing on the neurological aspects of the patients' symptoms and on the underlying psychodynamic issues, as well as a discussion of the placebo effect and various treatment options, all 32 patients accepted the possibility of PP, although some expressed doubt about the diagnosis to a variable degree. At follow-up, 3–6 months after the diagnosis, six of the ten videotaped patients had had a complete resolution of their symptoms.

This study, which includes the largest reported series of PP, highlights the typical features of this psychogenic disorder, including slight female preponderance (in contrast to typical male preponderance in organic PD), frequent precipitating events and psychiatric comorbidities, early disability, and atypical features on examination that were incongruous with organic PD. In contrast to tremor in patients with organic PD, the tremor in PP usually does not disappear with movement of the limb. Furthermore, similar to psychogenic tremor without parkinsonism [15], in additional to marked distractibility, the frequency of tremor in PP varies in rhythmicity and direction of oscillation. Rigidity, if present, is often associated with active resistance against passive movement and there is usually no cogwheeling. While slowness of movement (bradykinesia) is present in almost all patients with PP, there is usually no decrementing amplitude on rapid succession movements, which is typically seen in PD. Patients with PP often demonstrate slow and deliberate movement when asked to perform a particular task but are able to function normally when distracted or when they do not think they are being observed; they can dress and perform other activities of daily living without any perceptible slowness. The handwriting is often labored and irregular but without the typical micrographia. On a pull test, the patient has minimal displacement without retropulsion or propulsion. When asked to walk fast or to run, the gait often becomes stiffer and the short stride is maintained, but there is no freezing. Speech in a patient with PP often becomes stuttering, "baby-like," or demonstrating a foreign accent. If the patient has "levodopa-related dyskinesia," the hyperkinetic movement is often bizarre and incongruous with typical levodopa-induced stereotypy, chorea, or dystonia.

Table 3.2 summarizes the literature on PP.

Table 3.1 Clinical summary of videotaped subjects

Patient	Age (years)/ sex	Fahn class	Duration (months)	Identified potential for patient gain	Precipitating event	Video rating[a]
1[b]	40/F	Documented	24	Disability	Daughter abusive relationship; brother-in-law murdered, job stresses	1
2[b]	46/F	Probable	72	Disability	Job loss, two motor vehicle accidents	3
3[b]	44/M	Probable	24	Early retirement	Forced retirement, cardiac illness, depression	3
4	57/F	Probable	24	Disability	Abusive spouse, separated twice	2
5	60/F	Probable	36	Disability	Work injury, forced disability	3
6	22/F	Probable	60	Litigation	Abusive adoptive parents, prior conversion disorder	3
7	32/M	Probable	60	Disability	Family stresses, near-fall out of attic	3
8	50/F	Documented	30	Disability	Pulmonary embolus on vacation in England, hospitalization > 1 month in England alone	1
9	42/F	Probable	18	Disability, spousal attention	Father exposed to "agent orange," severe arthritic changes in knees	3
10	55/M	Probable	48	Disability	Spouse's infidelity, job loss	2

[a] Video rating: 1, marked improvement; 2, moderate improvement; 3, mild improvement; 4, no response; 5, worsening of symptoms.
[b] Videotape included.

Table 3.2 Review of the literature on psychogenic parkinsonism

Reference	Number of subjects	Mean age (years)	Mean duration (years)	Movement onset abrupt (%)	Female: male
Lang *et al.* 1995 [2]	14	48	5.3	79	7:7
Factor *et al.* 1998 [3]	2	53.5	6.0	100	1:1
Booij *et al.* 2001 [8]	4	51	NA	NA	NA
Gaig *et al.* 2006 [9]	8	53.7	6.1	55	5:4
Benaderette *et al.* 2006 [10]	9	49.9	4.7	44	4:5
Felicio *et al.* 2010 [12]	15	37.4	3.9	NA	9:6
Current study	32	48	5.2	84	17:15

NA, not available.

As the confidence of general neurologists in accurately diagnosing movement disorders has been gradually improving, more and more atypical disorders, many of which are PMDs, are referred to specialty clinics, partly accounting for the rising incidence of PMDs in movement disorders clinics [16]. The evaluation and therapy of these disorders is often quite challenging and the long-term prognosis is usually poor

[17,18]. The adverse impact of PMD, including PP, on patients' functioning and quality of life is similar to that of organic, neurodegenerative PD [19]. Patients with PMD utilize healthcare resources at high rates, including numerous consultations, demands for technologically sophisticated testing, and unnecessary surgical interventions. Some authors have referred to this group of disorders as a "crisis for neurology" [20]. While the diagnosis of PP may be difficult, a thorough clinical history and detailed physical examination by an experienced clinician, designed not only to exclude organic parkinsonism but also to elicit features supporting a psychogenic etiology, are critical [2,4,6,16,21,22].

Our study suggests that the response to placebo may be helpful in differentiating between organic parkinsonism and PP. While in the past we have used intramuscular injections of saline as a placebo in selected patients, we have gradually transitioned to other methods such as the use of a tuning fork accompanied by a suggestion that the vibration will change the observed sign [15]. In the case of parkinsonism, we have utilized carbidopa as a placebo since many patients are familiar with levodopa/carbidopa as a treatment for PD and, in the low dosages used, we believe that carbidopa acts as an inert substance (placebo). We have reasoned that the patients' improvement after carbidopa, which does not cross the blood–brain barrier and provides no independent benefit in idiopathic PD, is supportive evidence of the diagnosis of PP.

We acknowledge that there are several limitations of our study. Since our patients did not undergo functional imaging of the dopaminergic system, we cannot exclude the possibility that some of our patients also had underlying mild organic PD. We did not perform formal neuropsychological testing and thus the frequency of depression and other psychiatric comorbidities was based on clinical impression. We also recognize that using a suggestion along with the tuning fork to trigger a tremor indicates that the patient is suggestible and that the induced tremor is psychogenic, but it does not necessarily prove that the presenting tremor is psychogenic. As in many studies with PMD, long-term follow-up is difficult, but all our patients were evaluated at least one time, 3–6 months after the initial evaluation. Despite these limitations, however, we feel that our study provides insight into the evaluation and clinical manifestations of PP.

The biochemical basis of the effects of placebo on motor function are still not well understood, but the growing interest in the neurobiology of placebos has provided new insights into the mechanism of the behavioral response to placebos and its potential utility in the diagnosis and treatment of various psychiatric, neurological and medical disorders [23,24]. Several studies have provided evidence that placebos and sham surgeries may not necessarily be physiologically inert [7,25–27]. For example, PET studies have shown that dopamine is released in response to a placebo and that the placebo effect may be related to reward mechanisms, now documented to be partly under the control of the nigrostriatal system [28,29]. The placebo-induced changes in striatal raclopride binding in patients with idiopathic PD were of similar magnitude to those obtained after therapeutic doses of levodopa or apomorphine [29]. Furthermore, the estimated amount of dopamine release was greater in those who *perceived* the placebo effect than those who did not. The authors postulated that the placebo effect in PD was triggered by the expectation of reward. The perception of clinical benefit must be rewarding, thereby suggesting that the dopamine released within the ventral striatum is more related to the expectation of reward rather than to the reward itself.

For many years, placebos have been used in clinical practice and in research as their administration can help to establish a diagnosis, determine the magnitude of a therapeutic benefit, over the expected effect, or obviate the need for a potentially dangerous drug. With the introduction of the scientific method into clinical research and the adoption of double-blind randomized placebo-controlled trials as the standard methodology for evidence-based medicine, placebos have become an indispensable research tool [30–32]. The clinical response to placebo interventions may be influenced by a number of factors, including the psychological state of the patient and the attitude of the investigator. To our knowledge, there are no published data on the acute response to placebo, accompanied by a powerful verbal suggestion by the investigator, in patients with idiopathic PD. In a study of intravenous flumazenil, conducted in our center, the drug reduced the total Unified Parkinson's Disease Rating Scale (UPDRS) score by 3.44 ± 5.82, whereas intravenous administration of placebo produced only 1.25 ± 5.11 point reduction in the total UPDRS score [33]. Although the study does not prove that the placebo response is less robust in PD than in PP, it suggests that PD is less likely to improve with acutely administered placebo. We did not perform UPDRS ratings in our patients with PP, partly because of atypical findings and many associated physical and psychological features that would be difficult to rate.

Although the use of placebos in clinical research is a well accepted and standard practice, the utilization of placebos as therapy has raised some ethical concerns [23,34]. A recent survey by Tilburt *et al.* [35] showed that about half of the 679 internists and rheumatologists who responded reported prescribing placebo treatments on a regular basis. Types of "placebos" used were saline (3%), sugar pills (2%), over-the-counter analgesics (41%), and vitamins (38%). A small but notable proportion of physicians used antibiotics (13%) and sedatives (13%) as placebo treatments. Of this group, only rarely did they explicitly describe these treatments as placebos (5%) to their patients, but, most commonly (68%) described them as potentially beneficial medicines and treatments not typically used for their condition. The authors concluded that physicians may not be totally transparent about the use of placebos and might have mixed motivations for the recommendation of such treatments. Although some physicians have justified the use of placebos as possible mood elevators, effective placebo treatment induces changes in brain function that are distinct from those associated with antidepressant medication. Using quantitative electroencephalographic techniques, prefrontal neurophysiological changes have been found in patients administered placebo, and these changes may be predictive of subsequent response to antidepressant medications [36].

When a patient meets the criteria of PMD and the diagnosis is clear, then appropriate treatment can be instituted [37]. However, when the diagnosis is in doubt, additional information such as the response to placebo may be useful. In the case of PP, if an inactive placebo, such as carbidopa, produces robust improvement in the parkinsonian and other symptoms, the disclosure of the observation to the patient often frames the discussion of the diagnosis and this may avoid the use of potentially harmful pharmacotherapy. We, therefore, believe that the use of placebo, as long as it is fully transparent, is potentially beneficial in the management of patients with PMDs, not just PP. This view is also increasingly accepted by neurological community. In a recent review on the role of placebos or suggestion in PMD, the author concluded that suggestion is "ethically justifiable" for patients with PMD and that "When issues of choice, consent, deceit, disclosure, and decision-making are analyzed from the perspective of an ethics of care, we see that suggestion may enhance patient autonomy and does not violate the trust between doctors and their patients" [38].

Acknowledgements
We thank Octavian Adam, MD for his blinded review of videos and Cathy Jankovic for her technical assistance.

References
1. Thomas M, Jankovic J. Psychogenic movement disorders. In Fahn S, Lang A, Schapira A, eds. *Movement Disorders* 4. Edinburgh: Elsevier, 2010:630–650.

2. Lang AE, Koller WC, Fahn S. Psychogenic parkinsonism. *Arch Neurol* 1995;**52**:802–810.

3. Factor SA, Podskalny GD, Molho ES. Psychogenic movement disorders: frequency, clinical profile, and characteristics. *J Neurol Neurosurg Psychiatry* 1995;**59**:406–412.

4. Hinson VK, Haren WB. Psychogenic movement disorders. *Lancet Neurol* 2006;**5**:695–700.

5. Jankovic J. Psychogenic parkinsonism. *J Neurol Neurosurg Psychiatry* 2011; in press.

6. Ferrara J, Jankovic J. Psychogenic movement disorders in children. *Mov Disord* 2008;**23**:1875–1881.

7. de la Fuente-Fernandez R, Ruth TJ, Sossi V, *et al.* Expectation and dopamine release: mechanism of the placebo effect in Parkinson's disease. *Science* 2001;**293**(5532):1164–1166.

8. Booij J, Speelman JD, Horstink MW, Wolters EC. The clinical benefit of imaging striatal dopamine transporters with [123I]FP-CIT SPECT in differentiating patients with presynaptic parkinsonism from those with other forms of parkinsonism. *Eur J Nucl Med* 2001;**28**:266–272.

9. Gaig C, Martí MJ, Tolosa E, Valldeoriola F, Paredes P, Lomeña FJ, Nakamae F. ^{123}I-ioflupane SPECT in the diagnosis of suspected psychogenic parkinsonism. *Mov Disord* 2006;**21**:1994–1998.

10. Benaderette S, Zanotti Fregonara P, Apartis E, *et al.* Psychogenic parkinsonism: a combination of clinical, electrophysiological, and [(123)I]-FP-CIT SPECT scan explorations improves diagnostic accuracy. *Mov Disord* 2006;**21**:310–317.

11. Scherfler C, Schwarz J, Antonini A, *et al.* Role of DAT-SPECT in the diagnostic work up of parkinsonism. *Mov Disord* 2007;**22**:1229–1238.

12. Felicio AC, Godeiro-Junior C, Moriyama TS, *et al.* Degenerative parkinsonism in patients with

psychogenic parkinsonism: a dopamine transporter imaging study. *Clin Neurol Neurosurg* 2010 **112**:282–285.

13. Vaillancourt DE, Spraker MB, Prodoehl J, *et al*. High-resolution diffusion tensor imaging in the substantia nigra of de novo Parkinson disease. *Neurology* 2009;**72**:1378–1384.

14. Williams DT, Ford B, Fahn S. Phenomenology and psychopathology related to psychogenic movement disorders. *Adv Neurol* 1995;**65**:231–257.

15. Kenney C, Diamond A, Mejia N, Davidson A, Hunter C, Jankovic J. Distinguishing psychogenic and essential tremor. *J Neurol Sci* 2007;**263**:94–99.

16. Thomas M, Jankovic J. Psychogenic movement disorders: diagnosis and management. *CNS Drugs* 2004;**18**:437–452.

17. Jankovic J, Vuong KD, Thomas M: Psychogenic tremor: long-term outcome. *CNS Spectrums* 2006;**11**:501–508.

18. McKeon A, Ahlskog JE, Bower JH, Josephs KA, Matsumoto JY. Psychogenic tremor: long term prognosis in patients with electrophysiologically-confirmed disease. *Mov Disord* 2009:**24**:72–76.

19. Anderson KE, Gruber-Baldini AL, Vaughan CG, *et al*. Impact of psychogenic movement disorders versus Parkinson's on disability, quality of life, and psychopathology. *Mov Disord* 2007;**22**:2204–2209.

20. Hallett M. Psychogenic movement disorders: a crisis for neurology. *Curr Neurol Neurosci Rep* 2006;**6**:269–271.

21. Miyasaki JM, Sa DS, Galvez-Jimenez N, Lang AE. Psychogenic movement disorders. *Can J Neurol Sci* 2003;**30**(Suppl 1):S94–S100.

22. Shill H, Gerber P. Evaluation of clinical diagnostic criteria for psychogenic movement disorders. *Mov Disord* 2006;**21**:1163–1168.

23. Biller-Adorno N. The use of placebo effect in clinical medicine: ethical blunder or ethical imperative? *Sci Eng Ethics* 2004;**10**:43–50.

24. Pollo A, Benedetti F. Placebo response: relevance to the rheumatic diseases. *Rheum Dis Clin North Am* 2008;**34**:331–349.

25. Benedetti F, Mayberg HS, Wager TD, *et al*. Neurobiological mechanisms of the placebo effect. *J Neurosci* 2005;**25**:10390–10402.

26. Lim ECH, Ong BKC, Seet RCS. Is there a place for placebo in management of psychogenic movement disorders? *Ann Acad Med Singapore* 2007;**36**:208–210.

27. Zaghloul KA, Blanco JA, Weidemann CT, *et al*. Human substantia nigra neurons encode unexpected financial rewards. *Science* 2009;**323**:1496–1499.

28. de la Fuente-Fernandez R, Stoessl AJ. The biochemical bases of reward: implications for the placebo effect. *Eval Health Prof* 2002;**25**:387–398.

29. Lidstone SC, Schulzer M, Dinelle K, *et al*. Effects of expectation on placebo-induced dopamine release in Parkinson disease. *Arch Gen Psychiatry* 2010;**67**:857–865.

30. Shapiro A, Shapiro E. *The powerful placebo*. Baltimore, MD: Johns Hopkins Press, 1997.

31. Frenkel O. A phenomenology of the "placebo effect": Taking meaning from the mind to the body. *J Med Phil* 2008;**33**:58–79.

32. Goetz CG, Wuu J, McDermott MP, *et al*. Placebo response in Parkinson's disease: comparisons among 11 trials covering medical and surgical interventions. *Mov Disord* 2008;**23**:690–699.

33. Ondo WG, Silay YS. Intravenous flumazenil for Parkinson's disease: a single dose, double blind, placebo controlled, cross-over trial. *Mov Disord* 2006;**21**:1614–1617.

34. Finniss DG, Kaptchuk TJ, Miller F, Benedetti F. Biological, clinical, and ethical advances of placebo effects. *Lancet* 2010;**375**:686–695.

35. Tilburt JC, Emanuel EJ, Kaptchuk TJ, Curlin FA, Miller FG. Prescribing "placebo treatments": results of national survey of US internists and rheumatologists. *BMJ* 2008;**337**:1938.

36. Hunter AM, Ravikumar S, Cook IA, Leuchter AF. Brain functional changes during placebo lead-in and changes in specific symptoms during pharmacotherapy for major depression. *Acta Psychiatr Scand* 2009;**119**:266–273.

37. Jankovic J, Cloninger CR, Fahn S, Hallett M, Lang AE, Williams DT. Therapeutic approaches to psychogenic movement disorders. In Hallett M, Fahn S, Jankovic J, *et al*., eds. *Psychogenic Movement Disorders: Neurology and Neuropsychiatry*. Philadelphia, PA: Lippincott Williams & Wilkins, 2006:323–328.

38. Shamy MC. The treatment of psychogenic movement disorders with suggestion is ethically justified. *Mov Disord* 2010;**25**:260–264.

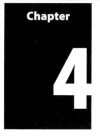

Epidemiology and clinical impact of psychogenic movement disorders

Alan J. Carson, Jon Stone, and Michael Sharpe

Introduction

Epidemiological studies of psychogenic movement disorder (PMD) in particular, and conversion disorder in general, are bedevilled by the twin problems of case definition and case ascertainment.

Barriers to epidemiology

Miyasaki and colleagues [1] suggested that "perhaps the most elegant descriptions of psychogenic movement disorders belongs to Sir Henry Head. In 1922, he wrote the following description of psychogenic dystonia '… any attempt to break down a spasm of this kind, to open the closed hand, or to straighten the flexed knee, meets with intense resistance… resistance may be experienced not only in pushing the head towards the normal shoulder, but also in moving it farther in the direction of the affected side' "[2]. Examination of such patients led Head to conclude that "hysteria is sometimes said to imitate organic affections; but this is a highly misleading statement. The mimicry can only deceive an observer ignorant of the signs of hysteria or content with perfunctory examination."

The description was indeed elegant but Head's belief in the ease with which the distinction could be made may have said more about his clinical acumen than his awareness of his colleagues' skills; for many clinicians, this is an area fraught with difficulty. Making the diagnosis is usually dependent on clinical assessment, and those without neurological training often feel hopelessly bewildered. Even amongst neurologists, there can often be considerable lack of confidence in diagnosing a PMD and it is perhaps only among those who specialize exclusively in movement disorders that confidence in making the diagnosis comes close to that of Head. The consequence of this is that any meaningful epidemiological studies will be limited by the availability of clinicians actually able to assess the patients. Furthermore, such diagnostic skills allow the clinician to separate those with neurological disease from those without. They do not allow any interpretation of what may be the even more vexed question of distinguishing those with genuine PMDs from those who are simply malingering – a task with which even Head may have struggled!

The need for highly specialized clinicians to conduct diagnostic assessments renders the possibility of true community-based incidence and prevalence studies unlikely if not impossible. In reality, most epidemiological estimates will come from hospital-based clinic samples, often in tertiary centers, with all the problems of sample bias this may bring. Although there are no data to support the notion, it seems reasonable to assume that some forms of PMD may be more likely to be reviewed in such settings than others. One might hypothesize that the more dramatic presentations such as psychogenic "parkinsonism" and gait disorders may be overrepresented while the more "everyday" symptomatology of tremor may be underrepresented.

As to how many patients with PMD are actually genuine we can only ever guess, as it seems unlikely that ethical permission or funding for widespread covert surveillance would ever be granted. Neuroimaging studies are beginning to attempt to make this separation but are still a long way from being able to do so clinically [3].

There are further problems with case definition even after the neurological diagnosis is made. Some patients may only be classified as having a PMD; others may have been classified psychiatrically as conversion disorder and others still may be classified as somatization disorder (which "trumps" conversion disorder in DSM-IV). The widely used definition of

Psychogenic Movement Disorders and Other Conversion Disorders, ed. Mark Hallett, Anthony E. Lang, Joseph Jankovic, Stanley Fahn, Peter W. Halligan, Valerie Voon, and C. Robert Cloninger. Published by Cambridge University Press. © Cambridge University Press 2011.

PMD by Williams *et al.* [4] puts considerable weight on psychological factors, and the DSM-IV criteria for conversion disorder [5] stipulates: "psychological factors are judged to be associated with the symptom or deficit because the initiation or exacerbation of the symptom or deficit is preceded by conflicts or other stressors." By contrast a recent survey of 519 neurologists by the Movement Disorders Society [6] indicated that only 18% regarded emotional disturbance as relevant to diagnosis. Studies looking for a formal somatoform disorder such as "conversion disorder" in patients with a PMD generally only find it in a subset of those patients (for example only 7 of 67 [11%] patients with fixed dystonia had clear evidence of conversion disorder) [7]. Future plans to remove the need for psychological stressors in the DSM-V revision of conversion disorder should, if carried through, make this aspect of epidemiology a little easier [8,9].

Even after all this, there are yet more difficulties about case definition of what is essentially a symptom. How does one classify the clearly psychogenic movement disorder found in a patient with complex regional pain syndrome type 1 (Chapter 13)?

Incidence

We are unaware of any incidence studies of PMD. High quality studies of the incidence of conversion disorder are generally lacking and accurate case ascertainment and definition is again the major barrier. Nonetheless, there is some consistency of results, despite different methodologies and geographical settings; reported annual rates of "conversion disorder" are between 4–12 per 100 000 population [10–13]. Our own study of functional weakness in Scotland [12] and a similar study in Sweden [11] both found an estimated minimum annual incidence of 4–5 per 100 000 for motor conversion symptoms. By way of comparison these conservative estimates are broadly equivalent to the incidence of multiple sclerosis.

Studies of psychogenic non-epileptic seizures (PNES) have estimated annual incidence of 1.5–3 per 100 000 population for video electroencephalographic (EEG)-confirmed cases [14,15], but it is acknowledged that many more cases will not have been subject to this degree of scrutiny, and so this is likely to be an underestimate.

Prevalence

We are unaware of any reliable estimates of the community prevalence of PMD. Accepting these limitations, the lower estimates of community prevalence of conversion disorder, extracted from population-based case registers, are approximately 50/100 000 population [16]. The prevalence of PNES has been estimated at between 2 and 33 per 100 000 [17]. The figure rises depending on the definition studied, in particular how the overlap with other somatoform symptoms is considered and the time frame of sampling, with annual prevalence figures being roughly double that of point prevalence figures.

Frequency in neurology settings

There are more reports of prevalence figures from neurology clinic settings, reflecting the ease of case ascertainment. However, they are liable to a range of potential biases depending on the clinic sampled.

Studies in general neurology outpatient clinics have found that approximately one-third have symptoms rated as unexplained by disease [18–20], although taking out patients with headache and patients with "functional overlay" leaves about one sixth with a purely "functional/psychogenic" diagnosis [21]. In general neurology clinics, the only data that we are aware of regarding PMD are from our own Scottish Neurological Symptoms Study (SNSS), which found a prevalence of 11 patients with PMD (including two with functional gait disorders) out of 3781 consecutive new attenders at neurology clinics across Scotland (0.3%). The frequency was 5.6% for all conversion disorders with non-epileptic attacks; sensory disturbance and weakness all being more common than PMD (see Chapter 5).

In movement disorder clinics, the reported frequency of PMD is typically 3–6% according to center, the type of movement in question, and when the diagnoses were being made [22–24]. We suspect that the more generalizable figures are estimates of less than 1% in general neurology clinics and approximately 5% in specialist movement disorder clinics. Of particular note, a study in Houston, USA, found a rising frequency of PMD from 0 to 6% of new referrals between 1982 and 2002, reflecting increasing confidence in making the diagnosis [23]. Another analysis in Toronto suggested that certain symptoms in movement disorder clinics, such as dystonia, may be more likely to be diagnosed as psychogenic than others (such as myoclonus)[24].

With respect to symptoms, tremor appears to be the most common symptom, usually accounting for approximately half of presentations, followed by

Table 4.1 The percentage of psychogenic movement disorder patients presenting with each symptom, showing the relative frequency of each symptom within a series on a gray scale

	Relative frequency								
Symptom	**Albany clinic**	**Toronto**	**New York**	**Florida**	**Paris**	**Spain[a]**	**Baylor College, Houston[a]**	**Chicago[a]**	**Turkey [25]**
Tremor	47	45	14	32	29	48	56	48	44
Dystonia	24	27	54	25	27	29	39	28	24
Myoclonus	13	19	7	7	0	17	13	12	6
Parkinsonism	9	5	2	0	12	6	3	14	8
Tics	2	0	1	4	1	50	7	7	4
Gait	0	2	9	2	25	47	3	47	12

[a] The studies in Spain, Baylor College, and Chicago recorded more than one symptom in some patients.
Source: Adapted and extended from Lang 2006 [24] (with permission of Lippincott, Williams & Wilkins).

dystonia then myoclonus, with parkinsonism, tics, and gait disorders notably rarer (Table 4.1). The unusual "peak" of psychogenic tics in the Spanish cohort highlights that there are significant differences in diagnostic thresholds for some symptoms in different countries.

Age and sex

There is uniformity in cited studies that PMD and conversion disorders are more frequent in woman, with estimates tending to be approximately 60–75% female [4,25–30]. There was similar consistency with regards to age, with onset tending to be between 35 and 50 years of age [28,30,31], but clinicians should note that one message coming from reported cases series is that incident cases are reported in all ages, from young children to the elderly.

Geographical and historical epidemiology

Most studies of conversion disorder have been conducted in industrialized countries. It has generally been accepted in academic textbooks that rates are higher in non-industrialized countries and that the prevalence has dramatically decreased in the industrialized nations during the twentieth century. A number of extravagant anthropological explanations have been provided for this. However, the theories do seem to have run ahead of the data, which are notably absent. There have been a small number of high-quality international studies in somatoform disorders in general, and they have concluded very similar rates internationally [32]. Historical comparators are equally hard to achieve; however, where available, they are notably in keeping with modern figures. Sydenham suggested that a third of the patients he was seeing with neurological symptoms had "the vapours" (the equivalent of functional symptoms) [33], a figure strikingly close to modern data. Charcot's assistant Guinon reported a frequency of 8% for hysteria in 3168 consultations [34], again a figure very in keeping with current estimates. Interpretation of such historical data is fraught with complication but does at least suggest we should be highly sceptical of historically revisionist claims that hysteria was once frequent and is now rare [35].

Onset

There is agreement that it is difficult and unreliable to use historical factors alone to differentiate a PMD from an "organic" movement disorder. Nonetheless a sudden onset is often seen in PMD, with a frequency of 54–92% [22,25,26,28,31]. Physical injury or pain at onset is particularly typical in sudden-onset cases. The injury, as in patients with complex regional pain syndrome type 1 (discussed in Chapter 13) is often relatively trivial. In Schrag's series of patients with fixed dystonia, physical injury occurred in 63% of 103 patients [7]. In a systematic review of 132 studies (n = 869) looking at physical injury in motor and sensory conversion disorder, we found that physical injury was reported in 121 of 357 cases of PMD (34%; the overall rate for all symptoms was 37%) [36]. The methodology of this analysis has limitations but the frequency of physical injury is striking.

A frequency of litigation of 15–30% in PMD [7,22,26,28,37] has been commented on by several studies. Although this must raise suspicion of malingering in some cases, it could also simply reflect a close relationship between physical injury and PMD.

Physical symptom and disease comorbidity

PMDs do not usually present as an isolated physical symptom. Pain, fatigue, psychogenic patterns of weakness and sensory disturbance, and an additional type of PMD are all very common [28,30,38]. Neurological disease is also more common than would be expected by chance [37]. For example 12 of one series of 70 patients with psychogenic tremor (17%) had a coexistent organic movement disorder [28].

Disability

Descriptions of disability in PMD and conversion disorder are infrequent but fairly consistent in their findings. In general, and perhaps not surprisingly, physical measures of disability tend to describe a clinical impact of roughly similar severity to the equivalent "organic" neurological disorder but substantially increased rates of total symptom burden and mental distress [39,40]. This work reports self-rated disability. However, it seems unlikely that observer-derived disability scores would lead to different conclusions; if a patient with a substantive motor conversion disorder in the form of the typical "dragging" leg rates themselves as having difficulty climbing stairs on the physical function subscale of the SF36, an observer-rated scale such as the Rankin or Barthel will come to the same conclusion if applied in the setting of a clinic or home visit. However, while one might reasonably assume some consistency in such a score following a stroke, or other structural lesion, that same assumption cannot be made in association with conversion disorder. Gaining evidence about the degree of fluctuation of disability in conversion disorder is a priority in this field.

Psychological comorbidity

Psychological comorbidity, is also consistent with rates of depression between 20 and 40% [26,37] and anxiety probably somewhat higher. In the study of Feinstein *et al.* [26], the frequency of a current anxiety disorder was 38%. Our own experience is that, particularly with tremor and other hyperkinetic movement disorders, anxiety is very common but it may not present overtly. The interpretation of standard diagnostic structured interviews can be problematic as the question "do you feel anxious?" will get a very different response from "do your symptoms make you feel anxious?" Overall, around two-thirds to three-quarters of patients with PMD will have some kind of axis 1 emotional disorder. By contrast patients with equivalent disability from neurological disease tend to report rates of approximately half that of the corresponding conversion disorder [12].

There are serious problems with using standard methodologies for diagnosis of psychiatric disorder in this group of patients, particularly questionnaires. Patients with PMD and other conversion disorders often may go to some effort to try to persuade the examining doctor (and sometimes themself in the process) that they do not have any difficulties with anxiety or low mood [12].

Studies of personality are limited in PMD. Although a high rate of personality disorder (42%) was found in one study, caution is warranted as this group of patients was seen in a specialist tertiary clinic with chronic symptoms. In our experience (writing as neurologists and psychiatrists), the patients referred to psychiatry from neurology often have increased rates of personality disorder. Furthermore, although most clinicians believe there is some form of relationship between PMD and personality, from an epidemiological perspective the diagnosis of personality disorder is fraught with issues of validity and reliability.

Outcome

Misdiagnosis

Misdiagnosis is often a significant clinical fear and a number of respected authorities have commented on concerns of high rates of misdiagnosis [25]. However, more recent evidence does not support the apparent degree of worry. In a systematic review of 27 studies of conversion symptoms ($n = 1466$), we found the reported frequency of misdiagnosis has been consistently approximately 4% since 1970 [41]. This figure was unaffected by the widespread introduction of clinical imaging. We concluded that the higher rates of misdiagnosis reported in earlier studies (Fig. 4.1) largely reflected poor case definition and study methodology rather than recently enhanced diagnostic skills.

In the SNSS we found, at baseline, that 1144 of 3781 patients had neurological symptoms that were either "not at all" or only "somewhat" explained by

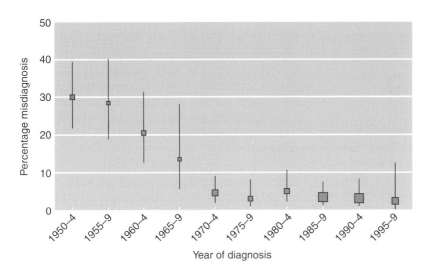

Fig. 4.1. Misdiagnosis of conversion symptoms and hysteria (mean with bars indicating 95% confidence intervals; random effects) plotted at the midpoints of 5-year intervals according to when patients were diagnosed. Size of each point is proportional to the number of subjects at each time point (total 1466). (Reprinted with permission from Stone *et al.*, 2005, BMJ publications [41].).

neurological disease. At 12-month follow-up, we had diagnostic outcome data on 1030 of these 1144 patients (90%) and there had been nine deaths. We realized that the analysis of misdiagnosis was not straightforward; in particular clinical error leading to misdiagnosis was only one of a number of explanations for diagnostic revision in an outcome study. We operationalized criteria for describing diagnostic revision according to criteria described in Table 4.2.

This led to 45 diagnostic revisions, but only 4 of these were category 1 misdiagnoses, the others being differential diagnostic change (12), diagnostic refinement (22), de novo development of disease (1) and disagreement between doctors (6) [18].

These data should not lead to complacency. Our personal experience is that non-neurologists remain poor at distinguishing between psychogenic and "organic" neurological diagnoses. Too often they are swayed by the factors we found to be associated with misdiagnosis: the presence of obvious psychiatric or personality factors or apparent "bizarreness" of symptoms, especially in gait or movement disorders. Studies of misdiagnosis will need to continue, particularly as the diagnosis is made more often. Recognizing that different kinds of diagnostic change occur will be useful for any such studies.

Clinical outcome

In studies of PMD, variable rates of poor outcome have been cited although studies have varied in whether they report complete resolution or improvement in symptoms [4,22,26,27,29,31,37,38,42,43] (Table 4.3).

The proportion with symptoms the same or worse at follow-up ranges from 30 to 77%. Fixed dystonia appears to be associated with a particularly poor prognosis, with Ibrahim and colleagues [42] reporting only 6% of patients in a large well-defined series going into remission and only 23% showing any improvement.

It is likely that factors leading to referral influence these figures considerably.

In keeping with these findings, studies of conversion disorder in general [46–48] and paralysis [49], despite a disparate range of symptoms and populations under study, commonly report rates of lack of recovery for between a half and two-thirds of patients [50]. In SNSS, a study of a wide range of functional symptoms in less-severely affected outpatients, patient rated follow-up data were available on 716 of 1144 patients at 12 months. A poor outcome (clinical global improvement of "unchanged," "worse," or "much worse") was reported by 67% of these patients [51].

Prognostic factors

Table 4.3 gives some prognostic factors found in studies of PMD. These are similar to frequently cited good prognostic factors in conversion disorder, including a shorter duration of symptoms, young age at onset, and change in marital circumstances. By contrast, personality disorder, anger at the diagnosis of a "'non-organic'" disorder, delayed diagnosis, multiple other physical symptoms/somatization disorder, concurrent organic disease, sexual abuse, receipt of financial benefits, and litigation are often cited as negative prognostic factors.

Table 4.2 A new classification for diagnostic revision used in the Scottish Neurological Symptoms Study

Type of diagnostic revision	Example	Degree of clinician error
Diagnostic error	Patient presented with symptoms that were plausibly caused by MS but the diagnosis of MS was not considered and was unexpected at follow-up	Minor–major
Differential diagnostic change	Patient presented with symptoms that were plausibly related to a number of conditions; doctor suggested chronic fatigue syndrome as most likely but considered MS as a possible diagnosis; appropriate investigations and follow-up confirmed MS	None–minor
Diagnostic refinement	Doctor diagnosed epilepsy but at follow-up the diagnosis was refined to juvenile myoclonic epilepsy	Minor
Comorbid diagnostic change	Doctor correctly identified the presence of both epilepsy and non-epileptic seizures in the same patient; at follow-up, one of the disorders was remitted	None
Prodromal diagnostic change	Patient presented with an anxiety state but at follow-up had developed dementia; with hindsight, anxiety was a prodromal symptom of dementia but the diagnosis could not have been made at the initial consultation as the dementia symptoms (or findings on examination/investigation) had not developed	None
De novo development of disease	Patient correctly diagnosed with chronic fatigue syndrome; during the period of follow-up, the patient developed subarachnoid haemorrhage as a new condition	None
Disagreement between doctors, without new information at follow-up	Patient is diagnosed at baseline with chronic fatigue syndrome and at follow-up with chronic Lyme disease by a different doctor even although there is no new information; however, if the two doctors had both met the patient at baseline, they would still have arrived at the same diagnoses and this reflects similar divided opinion among their peers	None
Disagreement between doctors, with new information at follow-up	Patient is diagnosed at baseline with chronic fatigue syndrome and at follow-up by a different doctor with fatigue caused by a Chiari malformation because of new information at follow-up (in this case an MRI scan ordered at the time of the first appointment); however, the first doctor seeing the patient again at follow-up continues to diagnose chronic fatigue syndrome believing the Chiari malformation to be an incidental finding and this too would reflect divided opinion among their peers	None

MS, multiple sclerosis.
Source: Stone *et al.*, 2009 [18].

In SNSS, although many expected variables correlated with outcome in a univariate analysis (e.g., age, physical disability, distress, and number of symptoms), in a multivariate analysis only three strong independent predictors of poor outcome were found [51]: patients' beliefs (expectation of non-recovery) [odds ratio [OR], 2.0; 95% confidence interval [CI], 1.4–3.0), non-attribution of symptoms to psychological factors (OR, 2.2; 95% CI, 1.5–3.3), and the receipt of health-related benefits at the time of initial consultation (OR, 2.3; 95% CI, 1.4–3.9). This suggests that illness beliefs lie at the heart of prognosis and can rightly be seen as an important target for treatment.

Risk factors

Epidemiological studies have highlighted a range of risk factors for the occurrence of PMD and conversion disorder in general. The risk factors are similar to those described for disorders in the neurotic spectrum and include predisposing factors, precipitating factors, and perpetuating factors.

Table 4.3 Prognostic studies of psychogenic movement disorders

References	Size	Population sampled	Mean follow-up (years [% followed up])	Clinical outcome	Prognostic factors
Thomas *et al.*, 2006; Jankovic *et al.*, 2006 [27,44]	2282	Various PMD (56% tremor, 39% dystonia)	3.4 (54%)	57% improvement, 21% same, 22% worse	*Positive*: short duration, perceived effective treatment by physician, elimination of stressors, younger age
McKeon *et al.*, 2009 [45]	333	Tremor	5.1 (53%)	27% improvement, 8% same (mild), 64% moderate or severe	
Ibrahim *et al.*, 2009 [42]	41	Dystonia	7.6 (85%)	6% resolved, 17% improved, 46% same, 31% worse	*Negative*: diagnosis of complex regional pain syndrome
Crimlisk *et al.*, 1998 [37]	64	Weakness (50%), various PMD (50%)	6	50% medically retired or off sick, 7% had died (1 overdose, 1 pneumonia secondary to immobility, 1 cardiac, 2 malignancy)	*Positive*: duration < 1 year, the presence of an axis 1 psychiatric disorder, change in marital circumstances *Negative*: receipt of benefits and litigation
Koller *et al.*, 1989 [38]	24	Tremor	–	25% resolved, 61% fluctuating course, 4% worse	
Monday and Jankovic, 1993 [29]	18	Myoclonus	–	58% improvement, 25% worse	
Deuschl *et al.*, 1998 [31]	25	Tremor	– (76%)	24% resolved, 60% same/ fluctuating, 16% worse; 85% of those employed subsequently retired	*Positive*: young age
Ehrbar and Waespe, 1992 [43]	47	Gait	– (89%)	60% resolved, 30% same/ fluctuating	
Factor *et al.*, 1995 [22]	28	Various PMD	– (71%)	50 % resolved, 50% same/ worse	
Feinstein *et al.*, 2001 [26]	88	Various PMD (62% tremor, 24% dystonia)	3.2 (53%)	9.5% resolved (but half of these had a different somatoform disorder), 33% improved, 24% same, 33% worse	*Poor outcome*: longer duration, gradual onset, number of axis 1 diagnoses *No influence*: age, marital status, education, years of employment, litigation, type of movement disorder
Williams *et al.*, 1995 [4]	21	Various PMD	1.8 (95%)	30% resolved, 35% improvement, 35% same/ worse	*No influence*: age, gender, education, chronicity, type of movement disorder

PMD, psychogenic movement disorder.

Predisposing factors. Female sex, lower social class, adverse childhood experiences (including physical and sexual abuse), abusive events in adult life, difficulties in interpersonal relationships, possible modeling of symptoms on others in some cases, and perceived stress. There is no evidence either in PMD or in other conversion disorders of lower IQ [52].

Precipitating factors. Particular prominence has been given to the issue of life events as a precipitant to conversion disorders, and this is supported within the DSM-IV definition. Little work has been done on this specifically in relation to PMD. Studies in other conversion symptoms do suggest a higher frequency of life events prior to symptom onset [53] but others have found no difference in the number or severity of events [54], although there are certainly many patients where it is not possible to determine a specific life event.

Perpetuating factors. Illness beliefs, avoidance of activity, litigation, financial benefits, anger at diagnosis, or diagnostic uncertainty. There have been no studies of illness beliefs in PMD. People with functional weakness [12] and non-epileptic attacks [55] have been found to have similar illness beliefs to their corresponding disease counterparts except that, paradoxically, they tend to be less likely to attribute their symptoms to stress than patients with disease.

We have already discussed the role of physical injury in PMD. Other research has found a high frequency of panic symptoms in patients with non-epileptic attacks [56]. In line with nineteenth century thinking on the topic, we think there is value in exploring more "proximal" events in the onset of PMD. Our own experience is that an acute panic attack (a "shock" in nineteenth century parlance), a dissociative episode, an episode of sleep paralysis, or general anaesthetic may provide more of a window to understanding the onset of PMD than a thorough exploration of life events and childhood factors.

We do not wish to suggest that life events and other stressors are irrelevant or unimportant but simply that we need more data and better understanding of their role before assumptions about the universality of their etiological role are made, and we welcome their proposed deletion from psychiatric definitions.

Conclusions

Epidemiological studies of PMD, in particular, and conversion disorder in general pose many problems.

Conversion disorders are much more common than many realize, accounting for approximately 1 in 20 neurological presentations. Although PMD is among the rarer forms of the disorder, with a suspected prevalence of less than 1% of neurological presentations, this nonetheless indicates a substantive disease burden and one which has received far less attention than many other disorders of significantly lower prevalence.

References

1. Miyasaki JM, Sa DS, Galvez-Jimenez N, Lang AE. Psychogenic movement disorders. *Can J Neurol Sci* 2003;**30** Suppl 1:S94–100.

2. Head H. The diagnosis of hysteria. *BMJ* 1922;**i**:827–829.

3. Cojan Y, Waber L, Carruzzo A, Vuilleumier P. Motor inhibition in hysterical conversion paralysis. *Neuroimage* 2009;**47**:1026–1037.

4. Williams DT, Ford B, Fahn S. Phenomenology and psychopathology related to psychogenic movement disorders. *Adv Neurol* 1995;**65**:231–257.

5. American Psychiatric Association. *Diagnostic and Statistical Manual of Diseases*, 4th edn, text revision. Washington DC: American Psychiatric Press, 2000.

6. Espay AJ, Goldenhar LM, Voon V, *et al.* Opinions and clinical practices related to diagnosing and managing patients with psychogenic movement disorders: an international survey of Movement Disorder Society members. *Mov Disord* 2009;**24**:1366–1374.

7. Schrag A, Trimble M, Quinn N, Bhatia K. The syndrome of fixed dystonia: an evaluation of 103 patients. *Brain* 2004;**127**:2360–2372.

8. Stone J, LaFrance WC, Levenson JL, Sharpe M. Issues for DSM-5: conversion disorder. *Am J Psychiatry* 2010;**167**:626–627.

9. Kanaan RA, Carson A, Wessely SC, *et al.* What's so special about conversion disorder? A problem and a proposal for diagnostic classification. *Br J Psychiatry* 2010;**196**:427–428.

10. Stefansson JG, Messina JA, Meyerowitz S. Hysterical neurosis, conversion type: clinical and epidemiological considerations. *Acta Psychiatr Scand* 1976;**53**:119–138.

11. Binzer M, Andersen PM, Kullgren G. Clinical characteristics of patients with motor disability due to conversion disorder: a prospective control group study. *J Neurol Neurosurg Psychiatry* 1997;**63**:83–88.

12. Stone J, Warlow C, Sharpe M. The symptom of functional weakness: a controlled study of 107 patients. *Brain* 2010;**133**:1537–1551.

13. Stevens DL. Neurology in Gloucestershire: the clinical workload of an English neurologist. *J Neurol Neurosurg Psychiatry* 1989;**52**:439–446.

14. Szaflarski JP, Ficker DM, Cahill WT, Privitera MD. Four-year incidence of psychogenic nonepileptic seizures in adults in Hamilton County, OH. *Neurology* 2000;**55**:1561–1563.

15. Sigurdardottir KR, Olafsson E. Incidence of psychogenic seizures in adults: a population-based study in Iceland. *Epilepsia* 1998;**39**:749–752.

16. Akagi H, House A. The epidemiology of hysterical conversion. In Halligan PW, Bass C, Marshall JC, eds. *Contemporary Approaches to the Study of Hysteria: Clinical and Theoretical Perspectives*. Oxford: Oxford University Press, 2001:73–87.

17. Benbadis SR, Allen HW. An estimate of the prevalence of psychogenic non-epileptic seizures. *Seizure* 2000;**9**:280–281.

18. Stone J, Carson A, Duncan R, *et al.* Symptoms "unexplained by organic disease" in 1144 new neurology out-patients: how often does the diagnosis change at follow-up? *Brain* 2009;**132**:2878–2888.

19. Fink P, Steen HM, Sondergaard L. Somatoform disorders among first-time referrals to a neurology service. *Psychosomatics* 2005;**46**:540–548.

20. Snijders TJ, de Leeuw FE, Klumpers UM, Kappelle LJ, van Gijn J. Prevalence and predictors of unexplained neurological symptoms in an academic neurology outpatient clinic – an observational study. *J Neurol* 2004;**251**:66–71.

21. Stone J, Carson A, Duncan R, *et al.* Who is referred to neurology clinics? The diagnoses made in 3781 new patients. *Clin Neurol Neurosurg* 2010;**112**:747–751.

22. Factor SA, Podskalny GD, Molho ES. Psychogenic movement disorders: frequency, clinical profile, and characteristics. *J Neurol Neurosurg Psychiatry* 1995;**59**:406–412.

23. Thomas M, Jankovic J. Psychogenic movement disorders: diagnosis and management. *CNS Drugs* 2004;**18**:437–452.

24. Lang AE. General overview of psychogenic movement disorders: epidemiology, diagnosis and prognosis. In Hallett M, Fahn S, Jankovic J, *et al.*, eds. *Psychogenic Movement Disorders: Neurology and Neuropsychiatry*. Philadelphia, PA: Lippincott Williams & Wilkins, 2006:35–41.

25. Ertan S, Uluduz D, Ozekmekci S, *et al.* Clinical characteristics of 49 patients with psychogenic movement disorders in a tertiary clinic in Turkey. *Mov Disord* 2009;**24**:759–762.

26. Feinstein A, Stergiopoulos V, Fine J, Lang AE. Psychiatric outcome in patients with a psychogenic movement disorder: a prospective study. *Neuropsychiatry Neuropsychol Behav Neurol* 2001;**14**:169–176.

27. Thomas M, Vuong KD, Jankovic J. Long-term prognosis of patients with psychogenic movement disorders. *Parkinsonism Relat Disord* 2006;**2**:382–387.

28. Kim YJ, Pakiam AS, Lang AE. Historical and clinical features of psychogenic tremor: a review of 70 cases. *Can J Neurol Sci* 1999;**6**:190–195.

29. Monday K, Jankovic J. Psychogenic myoclonus. *Neurology* 1993;**43**:349–352.

30. Lang AE. Psychogenic dystonia: a review of 18 cases. *Can J Neurol Sci* 1995;**22**:136–143.

31. Deuschl G, Köster B, Lücking CH, Scheidt C. Diagnostic and pathophysiological aspects of psychogenic tremors. *Mov Disord* 1998;**13**:294–302.

32. Simon G, Gater R, Kisely S, Piccinelli M. Somatic symptoms of distress: an international primary care study. *Psychosom Med* 1996;**58**:481–488.

33. Sydenham T. *The Works of Thomas Sydenham* [trans. RG Latham]. London: The Sydenham Society, 1848.

34. Guinon G. *Les Agents Provocateurs de l'Hysterie*. Paris: Delahaye & Lecrosnier, 1889.

35. Stone J, Hewett R, Carson A, Warlow C, Sharpe M. The 'disappearance' of hysteria: historical mystery or illusion? *J R Soc Med* 2008;**101**:12–18.

36. Stone J, Carson A, Aditya H, *et al.* The role of physical injury in motor and sensory conversion symptoms: a systematic and narrative review. *J Psychosom Res* 2009;**66**:383–390.

37. Crimlisk HL, Bhatia K, Cope H, *et al.* Slater revisited: 6 year follow up study of patients with medically unexplained motor symptoms. *BMJ* 1998;**316**:582–586.

38. Koller W, Lang A, Vetere-Overfield B, *et al.* Psychogenic tremors. *Neurology* 1989;**39**:1094–1099.

39. Carson A, Stone J, Hibberd C, *et al.* Disability, distress and unexployment in neurology outpatients with symptoms 'unexplained by disease'. *J Neurol Neurosurg Psychiatry* 2011; Epub ahead of print, PMID 21257981.

40. Anderson KE, Gruber-Baldini AL, Vaughan CG, *et al.* Impact of psychogenic movement disorders versus Parkinson's on disability, quality of life, and psychopathology. *Mov Disord* 2007;**22**:2204–2209.

41. Stone J, Smyth R, Carson A, *et al.* Systematic review of misdiagnosis of conversion symptoms and "hysteria." *BMJ* 2005;**331**:989.

42. Ibrahim NM, Martino D, van de Warrenburg BP, *et al.* The prognosis of fixed dystonia: a follow-up study. *Parkinsonism Relat Disord* 2009;**15**:592–597.

43. Ehrbar R, Waespe W. Funktionelle Gangstörungen. *Schweiz Med Wochenschr* 1992;**122**:833–841.

44. Jankovic J, Vuong KD, Thomas M. Psychogenic tremor: long-term outcome. *CNS Spectr* 2006;**11**:501–508.

45. McKeon A, Ahlskog JE, Bower JH, *et al.* Psychogenic tremor: long-term prognosis in patients with electrophysiologically confirmed disease. *Mov Disord* 2009;**24**:72–76.

46. Couprie W, Wijdicks E-FM, Rooijmans H-GM, van Gijn J. Outcome in conversion disorder: a follow-up study. *J Neurol Neurosurg Psychiatry* 1995;**58**:750–752.

47. Mace CJ, Trimble MR. Ten-year prognosis of conversion disorder. *Br J Psychiatry* 1996;**169**:282–288.

48. Stone J, Sharpe M, Rothwell PM, Warlow CP. The 12 year prognosis of unilateral functional weakness and sensory disturbance. *J Neurol Neurosurg Psychiatry* 2003;**74**:591–596.

49. Stone J, Sharpe M. Functional paralysis and sensory disturbance. In Hallett M, Fahn S, Jankovic J, *et al.*, eds. *Psychogenic Movement Disorders: Neurology and Neuropsychiatry*. Philadelphia, PA: Lippincott Williams & Wilkins, 2006:88–111.

50. Ron M. The prognosis of hysteria / somatisation disorder. In Halligan P, Bass C, Marshall JC, eds. *Contemporary Approaches to the Study of Hysteria: Clinical and Theoretical Perspectives*. Oxford: Oxford University Press, 2001:271–281.

51. Sharpe M, Stone J, Hibberd C, *et al.* Neurology out-patients with symptoms unexplained by disease: illness beliefs and financial benefits predict 1-year outcome. *Psychol Med* 2009;1–10.

52. van Beilen M, Griffioen BT, Leenders KL. Coping strategies and IQ in psychogenic movement disorders and paralysis. *Mov Disord* 2009;**24**:922–925.

53. Stone J, Sharpe M, Binzer M. Motor conversion symptoms and pseudoseizures: a comparison of clinical characteristics. *Psychosomatics* 2004;**45**:492–499.

54. Roelofs K, Spinhoven P, Sandijck P, Moene FC, Hoogduin KA. The impact of early trauma and recent life-events on symptom severity in patients with conversion disorder. *J Nerv Ment Dis* 2005;**193**:508–514.

55. Stone J, Binzer M, Sharpe M. Illness beliefs and locus of control: a comparison of patients with pseudoseizures and epilepsy. *J Psychosom Res* 2004;**57**:541–547.

56. Goldstein LH, Mellers JD. Ictal symptoms of anxiety, avoidance behaviour, and dissociation in patients with dissociative seizures. *J Neurol Neurosurg Psychiatry* 2006;**77**:616–621.

The Scottish Neurological Symptoms Study: diagnoses, characteristics, and prognosis in 1144 new neurology outpatients with symptoms unexplained by disease

Jon Stone, Alan J. Carson, and Michael Sharpe

Introduction

The Scottish Neurological Symptoms Study (SNSS) was a large prospective study of all patients newly referred to neurologists across Scotland, UK over a 1-year period. It involved neurologists from all four regional centers (Edinburgh, Glasgow, Dundee, and Aberdeen). The study aimed to replicate previous studies that have found approximately one-third of new outpatients have symptoms "not at all" or "somewhat" explained by disease [1,2] and to look more carefully at the diagnoses of patients in this group, the diagnostic change over the first 18 months, the global outcome, and prognostic factors. This chapter summarizes the first wave of data published from this study [3–7], with further analyses planned for the future.

Methods

This was a prospective 18-month cohort study of new outpatients to general neurology clinics across Scotland (36 neurologists). All new patients attending participating general neurology clinics were eligible for the study, excluding patients younger than 16 years of age, those who could not read English, and those too cognitively impaired/distressed or ill to consent. Neurologists were asked to give their initial diagnosis and their rating of how explained the symptom was by disease. Patients with no exclusion criteria completed questionnaires at baseline and 12 months including: symptom counts, distress (Hospital Anxiety and Depression Scale [HADS]), illness perception items, illness worry, employment/benefit status, physical disability, and Clinical Global Impression rating. At the 18-month follow-up, the primary care doctors were asked if there had been a change in diagnosis, and any deaths were traced via national databases. Neurologists were contacted to provide additional information in these cases.

Results

Of new neurology outpatients, 4161 were eligible to participate. Of these, 3781 took part (91% recruitment).

Neurologists' diagnoses

In total, 1144 patients (30%) were rated as having symptoms not at all explained (12%) or somewhat explained (18%) by disease. Those with symptoms unexplained by disease were younger and more likely to be female.

These 1144 patients were given the following diagnoses [3]:

- neurological disease but symptoms rated as unexplained: 293 (26%)
- headache diagnoses: 292 (26%)
- conversion symptoms: 209 (18%) (blackouts for 85, sensory for 68, weakness for 45, and movement/gait for 11)
- "functional/non-organic": 107 (9%); no specific symptom specified but patient given diagnoses such as "non-organic" or "not explained by disease"
- primary diagnosis of anxiety/depression: 77 (6.7%)
- pain symptoms: 63 (5.5%)
- dizziness: 32 (2.8%)

Psychogenic Movement Disorders and Other Conversion Disorders, ed. Mark Hallett, Anthony E. Lang, Joseph Jankovic, Stanley Fahn, Peter W. Halligan, Valerie Voon, and C. Robert Cloninger. Published by Cambridge University Press. © Cambridge University Press 2011.

- fatigue: 29 (2.5%)
- cognitive symptoms: 22 (1.9%).

Conversion symptoms ($n = 209$), therefore, accounted for 5% of the whole 3781 new neurology outpatient cohort [5]. This can be contrasted with other major categories of neurological disorder in the 3781 new patients, which included headache (19%), epilepsy (14%), peripheral nerve disorders (11%), miscellaneous (10%), multiple sclerosis/demyelination (7%), spinal disorders (6%), movement disorders (6%), and syncope (4%).

Diagnostic change at follow-up

In only 4 of the 1144 patients with symptoms poorly explained by disease was there clear evidence of misdiagnosis at the initial assessment [3]. Other forms of diagnostic change where no error had occurred were also characterized and enumerated in 19 patients. Most commonly (in 12 patients), a neurologist had made an initial differential diagnosis including both "organic" and "psychogenic" diagnoses and at follow-up the patient had an organic diagnosis. These kinds of "differential diagnostic change" have been incorporated misleadingly into previous studies of misdiagnosis [6]. In addition, there were five deaths in patients with non-epileptic attacks in which the nature of diagnostic change/cause of death were uncertain.

Comorbidity of disease diagnoses and symptoms unexplained by disease

In the study, 293 patients had a diagnosis of a neurological disease such as multiple sclerosis but had been rated as having symptoms "somewhat explained" or "not at all explained" by disease (headache disorders were excluded). This accounted for 12% of patients with a diagnosis of a neurological disease. It has been suggested that some disorders, perhaps CNS disorder such as multiple sclerosis, are more likely to be associated with additional "functional overlay" than patients with other neurological conditions. In this analysis, we did not find any particular disease category that was overrepresented. Only epilepsy appeared a little underrepresented. In these 293 patients, both physical and psychological symptom reporting was higher than in the patients rated as having symptoms explained by their disease [6].

Distress, disability, and employment at baseline

We compared differences between 1144 patients with symptoms unexplained by disease (cases) and 2637 patients with symptoms explained by disease (controls). Cases had worse physical health status (SF-12 score 42 vs 44); and worse mental health status (SF-12 score 43 vs 47). Unemployment was similar in cases and controls (50% vs 50%) but cases were more likely not to be working for health reasons (54% vs 37% (of the 50% not working)), and also more likely to be receiving disability-related state financial benefits (27% vs 22%; odds ratio 1.3; confidence interval, 1.1–1.6). This confirmed earlier findings that patients with symptoms unexplained by disease have just as much (and maybe more) disability, more distress, and more disability-related state financial benefits than patients with symptoms explained by disease [7].

Patient outcome and prognostic factors

Of the 1144 patients with symptoms poorly unexplained by disease, 716 (63%) completed follow-up questionnaires at 12 months [4]. Of these 716 patients, 229 (32%) were better or much better, 344 (48%) were the same, and 136 (19%) were worse or much worse. A univariate analysis of outcome predictors found that older age, physical disability, HADS distress, negative expectation of recovery, "non-psychological" attribution, and receipt of benefits predicted worse outcome. However, in the multivariate analysis, only negative expectation of recovery, "non-psychological" attribution, and receipt of benefits predicted worse outcome (odds ratio ~2.0 for all these). A coefficient of determination (R^2) of only 16% indicated that there must be other important predictive factors.

Discussion

The study has replicated previous smaller studies showing how common symptoms unexplained by disease are in general neurological practice. In addition, it has examined in much more detail the nature of the clinical problem with which patients in this "unexplained" category present. A particularly relevant finding to the topic of this book is that conversion symptoms accounted for 5% of all new neurology outpatients, a comparable number to many other major categories of neurological disorder. Non-epileptic attacks were the most common symptom, movement disorders the least common.

At 18 months follow-up, misdiagnosis was rare in the 1144 patients with symptoms poorly explained by disease, but there was an unexpected mortality in patients with an initial diagnosis of non-epileptic attacks that we cannot fully explain. A systematic review of misdiagnosis in 27 previous studies stretching over 40 years found that misdiagnosis rates have been 4% or less since 1970, similar to other neurological and psychiatric disorder [8] (see Fig. 4.1, p. 24). This study found a much lower rate, perhaps because of the more rigorous way in which diagnostic change was codified. We would expect more diagnostic errors to appear if a longer follow-up and more detailed follow-up methods were used. Diagnostic follow-up studies remain important in the field of conversion disorder because there remains, certainly outside the neurological community, a widespread anxiety that such diagnoses often turn out to be incorrect [9]. This study also shows the importance of classifying diagnostic change carefully.

At 12 months follow-up, two-thirds of the patients with symptoms unexplained by disease were feeling the same or worse than at entry to the study. Patient-rated global outcome was surprisingly not predicted by symptom count, physical disability, emotional distress, or even age in a multivariate analysis. Instead, belief in non-recovery, "non-psychological attribution," and receipt of financial benefits were modestly predictive. Two of these factors are illness beliefs and are potentially modifiable, although it remains to be seen how easily they can be modified and whether modifying them can influence outcome. The data suggest that clinicians should not necessarily be gloomy about prognosis because a patient is old, very disabled, has lots of symptoms, or is very distressed. Instead they should explore carefully and perhaps attempt to modify the patient's beliefs about the potential reversibility of their symptoms and the degree to which the patient may be able to influence that recovery themselves.

Acknowledgements

This chapter was developed from a poster presented at the PMD meeting in April 2009.

The chapter is presented by the authors on behalf of the SNSS collaborators: Alan J. Carson, Michael Sharpe, Jon Stone, Gordon Murray, Jane Walker, Roger Smyth, Charles Warlow, and Roger Cull (Edinburgh); Rod Duncan, Jonathan Cavanagh, Alex McMahon, Tony Pelosi, and Andrew Walker (Glasgow); Richard Coleman and Rainer Goldbeck (Aberdeen); and Richard Roberts and Keith Matthews (Dundee).

References

1. Carson AJ, Ringbauer B, Stone J, *et al*. Do medically unexplained symptoms matter? A prospective cohort study of 300 new referrals to neurology outpatient clinics. *J Neurol Neurosurg Psychiatry* 2000;**68**:207–210.

2. Fink P, Steen HM, Sondergaard L. Somatoform disorders among first-time referrals to a neurology service. *Psychosomatics* 2005;**46**:540–548.

3. Stone J, Carson A, Duncan R, *et al*. Symptoms "unexplained by organic disease" in 1144 new neurology out-patients: how often does the diagnosis change at follow-up? *Brain* 2009;**132**:2878–2888.

4. Sharpe M, Stone J, Hibberd C, *et al*. Neurology outpatients with symptoms unexplained by disease: illness beliefs and financial benefits predict 1-year outcome. *Psychol Med* 2010; **40**: 689–698.

5. Stone J, Carson A, Duncan R, *et al*. Who is referred to neurology clinics? The diagnoses made in 3781 new patients. *Clin Neurol Neurosurg* 2010;**112**:747–751.

6. Carson A, Stone J, Hibberd C, *et al*. Disability, distress and unemployment in neurology outpatients with symptoms "unexplained by organic disease." *J Neurol Neurosurg Psychiatry* 2011; in press.

7. Stone J, Carson A, Duncan R, *et al*. Which neurological diseases are most likely to be associated with "symptoms unexplained by organic disease." *J Neurol* 2011; in press.

8. Stone J, Smyth R, Carson A, *et al*. Systematic review of misdiagnosis of conversion symptoms and "hysteria." *BMJ* 2005;**331**:989.

9. Espay AJ, Goldenhar LM, Voon V, *et al*. Opinions and clinical practices related to diagnosing and managing patients with psychogenic movement disorders: an international survey of Movement Disorder Society members. *Mov Disord* 2009;**24**:1366–1374.

Chapter

6

Predisposition and issues of mixed etiology in psychogenic movement disorders

C. Robert Cloninger

Introduction

The term "psychogenic" is defined in the *New Oxford American Dictionary* as "having a psychological origin or cause, rather than a physical one" [1]. Psychogenic disorders are common in neurology. For example, they are estimated to account for 1–9% of all admissions to neurological units [2]. From 2 to 25% of patients in modern neurological clinics are diagnosed with psychogenic movement disorders (PMDs) [3]. From 10 to 30% of patients treated by neurologists have medically unexplained motor symptoms, that is, symptoms for which there is currently no pathophysiological explanation [4].

The most common psychogenic neurological disorders in one large series were PMDs, such as tremor (55%), dystonia (39%), myoclonus (13%), tics (6%), gait disorder (3%), and parkinsonism (2%) [5]. In another series of medically unexplained motor symptoms, 48% of patients had absence of motor function (e.g., hypokinetic disorders such as hemiplegia) and 52% had abnormal motor activity (e.g., hyperkinetic disorders such as tremor, dystonia, or ataxia) [6].

Given the importance of psychological variables, it is not surprising that PMDs occur together with psychiatric disorders in about 70% of patients, particularly with somatoform disorders (35%) and depressive disorders (14%), and others with financial compensation or litigation issues (21%) [7]. The somatoform disorders include disorders of conversion, somatization, and pain.

Medically unexplained motor symptoms are currently attributed to a variety of psychosocial mechanisms, including autosuggestion, disorders of volition or attention, and poor integration of sensori-motor functioning with personal goals and values, which is characterized by immature coping styles and emotional dysregulation [4]. However, the definition of "psychogenic" as having psychological causes, rather than physical causes, may be questioned because psychological and physical causes often occur together. Among those with PMD, approximately 10–15% are recognized to have underlying organic movement disorders in addition to psychogenic signs and symptoms [8]. In addition, about 4% diagnosed as psychogenic after thorough neurological assessments in recent years can be found to have neurological causes after long-term follow-up [9]. Hence what have been called PMDs may sometimes be truly complex "neuropsychiatric" disorders with a multifactorial mixture of neurobiological and psychosocial contributions, rather than being definable in terms of a dichotomy between psychological and physical causation.

Nevertheless, just because medically explained and unexplained symptoms occur together does not mean that it is not possible to distinguish cases that are predominantly psychogenic from those that are neurophysiologically explained. For example, some patients with epilepsy may also develop pseudoseizures as a way of using their knowledge of seizures to cope with stress or obtain secondary gains. The presence of pseudoseizures does not mean that someone cannot have epilepsy, or vice versa. Therefore, practical tests of the usefulness and accuracy of clinicians in distinguishing among psychosocial and neurobiological causes of symptoms are to contrast the demographic and clinical characteristics of psychogenic movement disorders from other movement disorders and to conduct follow-up and family studies [10].

Psychogenic Movement Disorders and Other Conversion Disorders, ed. Mark Hallett, Anthony E. Lang, Joseph Jankovic, Stanley Fahn, Peter W. Halligan, Valerie Voon, and C. Robert Cloninger. Published by Cambridge University Press. © Cambridge University Press 2011.

Demographics of psychogenic movement disorders

Psychogenic movement disorders are most common in women of low socioeconomic status but can occur in any demographic group [7]. The excess in women can be explained by the high prevalence of somatoform disorders, such as conversion and somatization disorders, in people with PMDs [10,11]. Somatoform disorders are associated with impaired executive functioning, which are characteristic of people diagnosed with PMDs [4,11,12]. Low socioeconomic status is associated with frequent exposure to early developmental stress, social neglect, poor education, and poor neuropsychological performance [13]. The causal impact of low socioeconomic status on risk of somatoform disorders has been demonstrated in adoption studies [14–17]. However, PMDs and somatoform disorders occur in people from all demographic groups.

Clinical characteristics

The diagnosis of PMDs is often through an effort to exclude physical causes or neurophysiological processes [7] or to demonstrate the importance of psychosocial or emotional processes [18]. About 70% of cases of PMD are associated with concurrent psychiatric disorders even though the patients themselves nearly always deny that the cause is psychogenic [6,7,19]. In any case, PMDs are often associated with emotional distress and difficulty in the relief of anxiety [20]. Outcomes with psychogenic seizures are better when people have more education, fewer additional somatoform complaints, less dissociation, and less anxiety and emotional dysregulation [12]. Both PMDs and somatoform disorders are often associated with insecure or disorganized emotional attachments, which are, in turn, associated with early childhood distress, abuse, and neglect [21]. Nevertheless, the associations among personality, emotionality, attachment, and stress vary widely between individuals, and PMDs may occur in usually well-adjusted individuals under acute stress or after injury.

Follow-up studies

Clinicians have often been reluctant to diagnose PMDs in the past because of concerns about the high rate of misdiagnosis in early studies. Likewise, early follow-up studies of conversion disorders revealed a highly variable outcome, with frequent subsequent diagnoses of medical and neurological disorders [10]. However, more recent studies have demonstrated a high reliability and accuracy for the diagnosis of PMD and conversion disorders: few people diagnosed with conversion disorder or PMD are subsequently found to have had a neurophysiological cause in prospective follow-ups [6,9,22,23]. A systematic review of misdiagnosis of conversion disorders revealed a reduction in the frequency of misdiagnosis after 1970 [9]. Misdiagnosis occurred in about 29% of cases diagnosed as psychogenic in studies conducted during the 1950s but in only 4% of cases reported after 1970. The improvement in diagnostic accuracy is attributed to the quality of the studies and the thoroughness of neuropsychiatric assessment, rather than the use of brain imaging [9].

In addition to the absence of diagnosable neurological disease during prospective follow-ups, the prognosis is strongly predicted by psychosocial variables that at least contribute to predisposition, the precipitation of symptoms, and the continuation of symptoms. The presence of personality disorders is particularly common as a risk factor for onset and continuation of PMDs [4], presumably because personality disorders are characterized by immature executive function, whereas improvement is associated with elimination of stressors, positive social life perceptions, a positive therapeutic alliance with the physician, and treatment with a specific medication [23]. Hence, modern follow-up studies clearly document the importance of psychosocial variables in the etiology and course of PMDs and also demonstrate the reliability of neuropsychiatric assessment to detect the presence of psychiatric disorder and the absence of neurological disorders.

Twin and adoption studies

Twin and adoption studies are available only for somatization, anxiety, and personality traits generally, and not specifically for PMDs. Genetic, shared sibling environment, and factors unique to individuals are all important in twin and adoption studies of somatic distress [24,25]. The shared family environment is most important, with associated impaired attachment and sexual abuse [26]. Recent genome-wide association studies show that no common genetic variants are consistently detectable for most complex traits such as personality and emotionality, suggesting that genetic variants relevant to PMDs are rare or of very small effect [27]. Gene–gene and gene–environment interactions are prominent in complex traits [28]. Gene expression is also modified by childhood experience and voluntary choices made by people [29]. As a result, it is impossible to separate nature from nurture or the causes of neurobiological functions from psychosocial functions in the development of complex phenomena [30]. Nevertheless, the interdependence of psychosocial and neurobiological functions does not mean that it is not possible to reliably distinguish people in whom psychosocial processes are prominent from others, as has been demonstrated by follow-up studies.

The genetic epidemiology of somatoform disorders is helpful in understanding the mixed etiology that sometimes occurs in PMD. The psychiatric disorders with the highest risk for conversion disorders are somatization disorder in women and antisocial personality disorder in men [31]. These two disorders frequently occur together in the same individuals and in families [32,33]. The familial association is maintained even in biological relatives separated at birth [15]. Despite marked differences in the clinical features of somatization disorder and antisocial personality disorders, both are strongly associated with cluster-B personality disorders characterized by low self-directedness and high novelty seeking [34]. Consequently, predisposition to conversion disorders, somatization, and PMD is associated with both poor executive functioning and low socioeconomic status; these, in turn, also predispose people to an increased risk of diverse medical disorders [13]. As shown in family and adoption studies, the mixed etiology observed in PMD is likely to be the result of the increased risk of both neurophysiological deficits associated with poor executive functions and the psychosocial deficits associated with low socioeconomic status.

Implications of complex etiology for diagnosis of psychogenic movement disorders

Both neurobiological and psychosocial predispositions are often mixed in the development of PMD, as described above. The nature of the mixture varies widely between individuals and at different times in the same individual. As a result, many people have striven to find algorithms to dichotomize movement disorders as psychogenic or not. Although it is impossible to separate neurophysiological and psychosocial

processes entirely, follow-up studies do demonstrate that psychogenic cases can be reliably distinguished from cases in which neurophysiological processes are predominant. The reliability of the distinction between psychogenic cases from others means that clinicians can focus on variables that have a beneficial impact on outcome. In other words, when psychosocial processes are prominent, they can be treated with appropriate pharmacotherapy and psychotherapy rather than exposing patients to unnecessary and expensive additional workups and referrals for additional opinions [19].

In my opinion, a sound approach is to recognize the potential importance and interaction of both neurobiological and psychosocial influences. In addition, it may be more useful to describe medically unexplained motor symptoms as just that – "medically unexplained motor symptoms" – rather than emphasizing psychogenicity, which patients usually reject or deny. Patients are more likely to accept and comply with a treatment plan if they agree that its objective is useful for them, such as suggesting that it is helpful to treat depression, anxiety, and enhance a person's skill in dealing with stress and attachment issues.

Such an approach recognizes that neither biological nor psychological processes can be entirely separated in the development and course of complex forms of movement disorders. It also recognizes that cases can be reliably distinguished in which psychogenic variables are predominant from those in which they are not. Obviously there are some forms of movement disorder, such as Huntington's chorea, which have relatively simple etiology despite some variability in expression. In the absence of such relatively simple etiology, it may be more useful to enumerate and quantify a range of neurobiological and psychosocial variables that influence risk. Such risk assessment would allow targeted treatment of causes and avoid counterproductive stigmatization of some people as having purely psychogenic symptoms. At the same time, a doctor cannot treat neurophysiological processes that he or she cannot detect. Movement disorder specialists frequently identify people in whom they can demonstrate no abnormal neurophysiology. Such medically unexplained motor symptoms are usually associated with prominent and treatable psychiatric disorders. When both neurophysiological and psychosocial variables are identified, patients are likely to benefit from multimodal treatments that address all contributing pathogenetic influences.

Conclusions

The PMDs are often mixed neuropsychiatric disorders involving both neurobiological and psychosocial dysfunctions. People with PMD are often young women with poor neuropsychological performance and low socioeconomic status, but it can occur in any demographic group. The occurrence of PMD is associated with psychiatric disorders with underlying disorders of personality and emotional regulation, but sometimes PMD occurs in usually well-adjusted individuals under stress or after injury. Histories of early childhood stress and abuse with insecure or disorganized attachments are frequent, but also inconsistent between individuals. Acute psychosocial stress or somatic injuries are also associated with PMD, but these also occur often in neurological or physical disorders generally. Genetic and shared environmental influences are important in some cases of PMD, but variables unique to individuals are also important. In summary, both neurobiological and psychosocial predispositions are important in understanding PMD and vary widely in importance between individuals and in the same individual at different times. As a result, thorough neuropsychiatric assessments are needed of patients suspected to have PMD.

Thorough assessment of both neurological and psychiatric functioning has been shown to allow reliable distinctions between patients in whom psychosocial variables are important in predisposition, precipitation, and continuation of symptoms and those in whom neurophysiological processes are predominant. Mixed etiology does occur, but most patients with PMD do not have identifiable neurophysiological causes. Treatment of psychosocial problems reduces unnecessary referrals and additional workups and improves long-term outcomes.

References

1. Stevenson A, Lindberg CA (eds.). *The New Oxford American Dictionary*, 3rd edn. New York: Oxford University Press, 2010.

2. Factor SA, Podskalny GD, Molho ES. Psychogenic movement disorders: frequency, clinical profile, and characteristics. *J Neurol Neurosurg Psychiatry* 1995;**59:**406–412.

3. Miyaski JM, Sa DS, Galvez-Jimenez N, Lange AE. Psychogenic movement disorders. *Can J Neurol Sci* 2003;**30:**94–100.

4. Reuber M, Mitchell AJ, Howlett SJ, Crimlisk HL, Grunewald RA. Functional symptoms in neurology: questions and answers. *J Neurol Neurosurg Psychiatry* 2005;**76:**307–314.

5. Jankovic JJ, Thomas M. Psychogenic tremor and shaking. In In Hallett M, Fahn S, Jankovic J, *et al.*, eds. *Psychogenic Movement Disorders: Neurology and Neuropsychiatry*. Philadelphia, PA: Lippincott Williams & Wilkins, 2006::42–47.

6. Crimlisk HL, Bhatia K, Cope H, *et al*. Slater revisited: 6 year follow up study of patients with medically unexplained motor symptoms. *BMJ* 1998;**316:**582–586.

7. Bhatia KP, Schneider SA. Psychogenic tremor and related disorders. *J Neurol* 2007;254:569–574.

8. Anderson KE, Lang AE, Weiner WJ (eds.) *Behavioral Neurology of Movement Disorders*, 2nd edn. Philadelphia, PA: Lippincott Williams & Wilkins, 2005.

9. Stone J, Smyth R, Carson A, Lewis S, Prescott R, Warlow C, Sharpe M. Systematic review of misdiagnosis of conversion symptoms and "hysteria." *BMJ* 2005;**331:**989.

10. Boffeli TJ, Guze SB. The simulation of neurologic disease. *Psychiatr Clin North Am* 1992;**15:**301–310.

11. Cloninger CR (1994). Somatoform and dissociative disorders. In Winokur G, Clayton PJ, eds. *The Medical Basis of Psychiatry*. Baltimore, MD: WB Saunders, 1994: 169–192.

12. Reuber M, Pukrop R, Bauer J, *et al*. Outcome in psychogenic nonepileptic seizures: 1 to 10-year follow-up in 164 patients. *Ann Neurol* 2003;**53:**305–311.

13. Wilkinson RG. *The impact of inequality*. New York: New Press, 2005.

14. Sigvardsson S, von Knorring AL, Bohman M, Cloninger CR. An adoption study of somatoform disorders. I. The relationship of somatization to psychiatric disability. *Arch Gen Psychiatry* 1984;**41:**853–859.

15. Sigvardsson S, Bohman M, von Knorring AL, Cloninger CR. Symptom patterns and causes of somatization in men: I. Differentiation of two discrete disorders. *Genet Epidemiol* 1986;**3:**153–169.

16. Cloninger CR, von Knorring AL, Sigvardsson S, Bohman M (1986b). Symptom patterns and causes of somatization in men: Ii. Genetic and environmental independence from somatization in women. *Genet Epidemiol* **3:**171–185.

17. Zoccolillo M, Cloninger CR. Somatization disorder: psychologic symptoms, social disability, and diagnosis. *Compr Psychiatry* 1986;**27:**65–73.

18. Fahn S, Williams PJ. Psychogenic dystonia. *Adv Neurol* 1988;**50:**431–455.

19. Crimlisk HL, Bhatia KP, Cope H, *et al*. Patterns of referral in patients with medically unexplained motor symptoms. *J Psychosom Res* 2000;**49:**217–219.

20. Lawton G, Mayor RJ, Howlett S, Reuber M. Psychogenic nonepileptic seizures and health-related quality of life: the relationship with psychological distress and other physical symptoms. *Epilepsy Behav* 2009;**14**:167–171.

21. Gerval J. Environmental and genetic influences on early attachment. *Child Adolesc Psychiatry Ment Health* 2009;**4**:25.

22. Feinstein A, Stergiopoulos V, Fine J, Lang AE. Psychiatric outcome in patients with a psychogenic movement disorder: a prospective study. *Neuropsychiatry Neuropsychol Behav Neurol* 2001;**14**:169–176.

23. Thomas M, Vuong KD, Jankovic J. Long-term prognosis of patients with psychogenic movement disorders. *Parkinsonism Relat Disord* 2006;**12**:382–387.

24. Cloninger CR, Sigvardsson S, von Knorring AL, Bohman M. An adoption study of somatoform disorders. Ii. Identification of two discrete somatoform disorders. *Arch Gen Psychiatry* 1984;**41**:863–871.

25. Gillespie NA, Zhu G, Heath AC, Hickie IB, Martin NG. The genetic aetiology of somatic distress. *Psychol Med* 2000;**30**:1051–1061.

26. Dinwiddie S, Heath AC, Dunne MP, *et al.* Early sexual abuse and lifetime psychopathology: a co-twin-control study. *Psychol Med* 2000;**30**:41–52.

27. Verweij KJH, Zietsch BP, Medland SE, *et al.* A genome-wide association study of cloninger's temperament scales: Implications for the evolutionary genetics of personality. *Biol Psychol* 2010;**85**:306–317.

28. Keltikangas-Jarvinen L, Jokela M. Nature and nurture in personality. *Focus* 2010;**8**:180–186.

29. Champagne FA. Epigenetic influence of social experiences across the lifespan. *Dev Psychobiol* 2010;**52**:299–311.

30. Cloninger CR. *Feeling Good: The Science of Well-being.* New York: Oxford University Press, 2004.

31. Guze SB, Cloninger CR, Martin RL, Clayton PJ. A follow-up and family study of Briquet's syndrome. *Br J Psychiatry* 1986;**149**:17–23.

32. Cloninger CR, Reich T, Guze SB. The multifactorial model of disease transmission: Iii. Familial relationship between sociopathy and hysteria (Briquet's syndrome). *Br J Psychiatry* 1975;**127**:23–32.

33. Cloninger CR, Martin RL, Guze SB, Clayton PJ. A prospective follow-up and family study of somatization in men and women. *Am J Psychiatry* 1986;**143**:873–878.

34. Cloninger CR. A unified biosocial theory of personality and its role in the development of anxiety states. *Psychiatr Dev* 1986;**4**:167–226.

Chapter 7

Psychogenic movement disorders in children

Joseph M. Ferrara and Joseph Jankovic

Introduction

Most psychogenic movement disorders (PMDs) fall within the spectrum of somatoform disorders, a category of psychiatric illness characterized by bodily complaints that cannot be explained in terms of a physical disorder. Somatoform disorders are distinct from malingering in that patients do not deliberately produce their symptoms, though phenomenologically PMDs may resemble volitional movements. The two subtypes of somatoform disorder that are most relevant to a discussion of PMDs are conversion disorder and somatization disorder, which are defined (as per DSM-IV criteria) in Table 7.1 [1]. About 80–90% of childhood PMDs, the focus of this review, meet criteria for conversion disorder, while the remaining 10% consist largely of somatization disorder, with rare cases of factitious disorder [2]. This distribution is similar to the reported distribution in adults [3].

Psychogenic movement disorders have long been recognized in children. Indeed, Pierre Briquet, one of the first clinicians to rigorously study psychogenic disorders, believed that about one-fifth of somatoform disorders begin during childhood, and that the majority of cases manifested by age 20 years [4,5]. Despite this recognition and data that interpersonal trauma during early life may predict the development of somatoform disorders in adults [6–11], remarkably little had been published regarding PMDs in the pediatric population until the past few years, when our group (Baylor College of Medicine, Houston, TX) and colleagues in the UK, Australia, and Spain reported on the clinical features of a combined 97 children with PMDs [2,12–14]. These publications, along with case reports, have provided the basis of published knowledge about pediatric PMDs reviewed in this chapter. Additional data from centers in Ontario, Canada, and Cincinnati, Ohio, are contained in Chapters 8 and 9 of this volume. The discussion is organized into considerations of epidemiology, clinical manifestations, differential diagnosis, pathophysiology, treatment, and prognosis.

Epidemiology

The population prevalence of PMDs is not known, in children or adults. Considering the frequency with which PMDs are misdiagnosed in clinical practice and the lack of a valid screening questionnaire, the prospect of a community-based prevalence study is untenable. Conversion symptoms in general are estimated to affect 2–5 per 100 000 children [15,16] and account for 2–15% of children attending outpatient pediatric neurology clinics [17–20]. Some studies report significantly higher rates of conversion disorder – in the range of 1 per 1000 children, by the age 17 years [21]. Such data, however, are derived from patient surveys and structured interviews, so methodological problems abound. Potential concerns include recall bias, bias introduced by parental reporting of symptoms, uncertainty whether questions were suitably framed for young children, and issues regarding the validity of diagnosing somatoform symptomatology in the absence of a thorough medical examination.

It is unclear what percentage of children with PMDs reach medical attention, but slightly over 3% of children evaluated in our movement disorder clinic had a PMD, which is similar to the prevalence of PMDs among adults both in our center [22] and in similar subspecialty clinics [23,24]. In two pediatric neurology clinics, PMDs accounted for 2.4 and 2.7% of all diagnoses [12] (see Chapter 8). While at another institution, a striking one-third of prospectively evaluated

Psychogenic Movement Disorders and Other Conversion Disorders, ed. Mark Hallett, Anthony E. Lang, Joseph Jankovic, Stanley Fahn, Peter W. Halligan, Valerie Voon, and C. Robert Cloninger. Published by Cambridge University Press. © Cambridge University Press 2011.

Table 7.1 Diagnostic criteria for conversion and somatization disorder

Diagnosis	Criteria
Conversion disorder	Each of the following criteria must be met: • one or more symptoms or deficits affecting voluntary movement or sensory function that suggests a neurological or general medical condition • the initiation or exacerbation of the symptom is preceded by conflicts or other stressors • the symptom is not intentionally produced or feigned • the symptom cannot, after appropriate investigation, be fully explained by a general medical condition, the direct effects of a substance, or a culturally sanctioned behavior • the symptom causes significant distress, warrants medical evaluation, or results in impairment in function (social, occupational, or otherwise) • the symptom is not limited to pain or sexual dysfunction, does not occur only in the context of somatization disorder, and is not better accounted for by another mental disorder

Somatization disorder	Each of the following criteria must be met:
	• multiple physical complaints, beginning before age 30 years and occurring over a period of several years, which cause significant distress, warrant medical evaluation, or result in impairment in function (social, occupational, or otherwise)
	• symptoms cannot, after appropriate investigation, be fully explained by a general medical condition or, when there is a related general medical condition, the symptoms are in excess of what would be expected from the clinical findings
	• symptoms are not intentionally produced or feigned
	• during the course of the illness patients must experience:
	  – pain related to at least four different sites or functions
	  – two gastrointestinal symptoms
	  – one sexual or reproductive symptom
	  – one pseudoneurological symptom

Source: American Psychiatric Association, 2000 [1].

Table 7.2 Diagnostic criteria for psychogenic movement disorders

Diagnostic confidence[a]	Clinical criteria
Documented	Abnormal movements that are inconsistent over time and incongruent with an organic movement disorder, and which either (1) durably remit following psychotherapy or suggestion or (2) cease when the patient is observed unknowingly
Clinically established	Abnormal movements that are inconsistent over time and incongruent with an organic movement disorder, and which are accompanied by (1) additional deficits that are definitely psychogenic, (2) multiple somatizations, or (3) an obvious psychiatric disturbance
Probable	Abnormal movements that are inconsistent over time and incongruent with an organic movement disorder but are not accompanied by evidence of overt psychiatric disease
Possible	Abnormal movements that are phenotypically congruent with an organic movement disorder but are accompanied by an obvious psychiatric disturbance

[a] The categories of documented and clinically established psychogenic movement disorders (PMD) are sometimes combined into a single category, clinically definite PMD. The category of possible PMD could reasonably be abandoned, owing to its extremely low specificity [3].

children with movement disorders met criteria for a PMD, albeit with varying levels of diagnostic certainty (12% documented, 15% probable, and 6% possible; see Table 7.2 for definitions) [25]. Inpatient and emergency room settings, which treat primarily movement disorders of acute onset are likely to have a higher proportion of psychogenic disease [14]. Longitudinal data from our clinic show that the overall volume of PMD

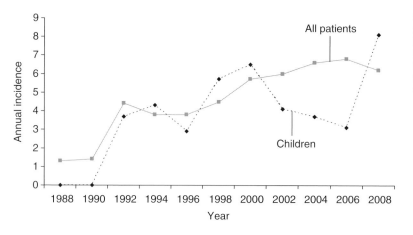

Fig. 7.1. Annual incidence of psychogenic movement disorders at the Movement Disorders Clinic at Baylor College of Medicine, Houston, USA. Percentage of total and pediatric new patient encounters diagnosed with a psychogenic movement disorder from 1988 to 2008.

referrals has increased and that the upsurge includes both adult and pediatric referrals (Fig. 7.1).

Of children (defined as under 18 years of age) within our clinic, the mean age at onset of PMD was 14 years. Fewer than one-fifth of children were under 13 years at symptom onset, and no child was younger than 7. Data from other groups are similar, with the youngest reported patient being younger than 5 years at the time of symptom onset [2,3,12,26]. Other conversion disorder phenotypes have been reported in children as young as 3 years [16], but somatoform disorders are uncommon before age 10 and the diagnosis of a PMD during early childhood should be suspect.

Most children with PMDs are girls, just as most adults with PMDs and other somatoform disorders are women [3,23,26–29]. Pooled data from the four largest published case series of pediatric PMDs demonstrate that girls outnumber boys 3.9:1 [2,12–14]. Only one prospective study (performed through the pediatric clinic of King George Hospital, Essex, UK) provides conflicting data [25]. Of nine children in that series who met criteria for a probable or documented PMD, five were boys, four of whom had psychogenic tics. All five boys were 11 years old or younger, while three of the four girls in this study were 14 years or older. In our PMD cohort, there was no female predominance in children younger than age 13 years, compared with a female-to-male ratio of 5.3:1 in children age 13 years and older. Prior studies have also noted that the apparent female predilection for conversion disorder increases after adolescence [16,30,31], and additional data provided by Bennett and colleagues (Chapter 9) supports this finding, while data from Cincinnati Children's Hospital (Chapter 8) do not.

The basis of the observed gender discrepancy in somatoform disorders is far from clear. Proposed explanations include differences in referral patterns, willingness to admit discomfort, propensity to seek medical attention, sensitivity to bodily sensations, psychiatric comorbidities, and exposure to psychosocial trauma, including sexual abuse [32]. In our clinic population, sexual abuse was recorded in only 6% of children (three girls), but no child with a history of sexual or physical abuse was reported in other case series [2,14]. Unfortunately, the current literature consists of retrospective data, and most reports do not include a formal assessment by a child psychiatrist, so underreporting of abuse seems likely. In Chapter 9, Bennett and colleagues report abuse or neglect in 40% of children with PMDs from their cohort of children referred to psychiatrists.

Clinical manifestations

Phenomenology

When discussing abnormal movements, neurologists customarily classify disorders based upon phenomenology. In regards to organic movement disorders, there is no doubt that this practice serves some utility because phenomenology dictates the differential diagnosis and provides guidance regarding potential therapies. However, the PMDs are by their very nature incongruous with known organic movement disorders and may at times be difficult to categorize. For instance, psychogenic "tremor" may lose its oscillatory nature, "dystonia" may be unpatterned, and "myoclonus" may be slower and more complex than its organic counterpart. Classifying PMDs is also complicated by the fact that patients often exhibit multiple types of abnormal movement, and clinical features may evolve considerably even during the course of a single office visit. Perhaps, an alternative and less specific nomenclature might be preferable in order to avoid muddling our current movement disorder lexicon – for example psychogenic "shaking," "spasms," and "jerking." We have found, however, that many patients (particularly adults) welcome the phenomenological characterization of their PMD, particularly those who present with the complaint that multiple prior doctors "had never seen anything like it before." For this reason, and because traditional movement disorder nomenclature facilitates communication among specialists, we usually retain standard phenomenological terminology in reference to PMDs.

The PMDs may mimic essentially every organic movement disorder phenotype, including less common conditions like "jumpy stump" [33], camptocormia [34], Creutzfeldt–Jakob disease [35], propriospinal myoclonus [36,37], and palatal tremor [38]. The phenomenological variety of PMDs in children broadly resembles that which has been reported in adults [3,23,27,28,39,40]. Hyperkinetic movement disorders predominate, and approximately two-thirds of children have multiple types of abnormal movement. The relative frequency of different PMD phenomenologies varies between studies, with tremor, dystonia and myoclonus being most prevalent (Table 7.3) [2,12–14,26,41]. One series found that psychogenic tics constituted the majority of PMDs (55%), followed by tremor, although this cohort was somewhat atypical: 46% of children with tic phenomenology were found to have a PMD, and boys with PMDs outnumbered girls nearly 2 to 1 [25]. A recent abstract from the Columbia University Movement Disorders Group, which included adult patients whose PMD started during childhood, also found a higher frequency of tics (4 of their 19 patients) [26], and tics were a common PMD phenotype at Cincinnati Children's Hospital (Chapter 8). Potential challenges in establishing the psychogenicity of tics are discussed below.

Perhaps more important than cataloging the phenomenology of PMDs is noting with what frequency various movement disorder phenotypes prove to be psychogenic. In our clinic, approximately one-third of children who presented with myoclonus or tremor had a PMD, while only 10% of dystonia was psychogenic. Even though historically dystonia was

Table 7.3 Relative frequency of different psychogenic movement disorders phenomenologies in children

Feature	Frequency (%)
Tremor	25–65
Dystonia (including fixed dystonia)	35–50
Myoclonus	5–40
Astasia–abasia and other gait disorders	15–30
Speech disorders, tics, convergence spasm, other	0–10

often wrongly attributed to psychological etiologies, mobile dystonia, in contrast to fixed dystonia [42,43], is rarely a form of PMD [44]. Excluding Tourette syndrome, only 1% of children seen in our clinic had an "organic" paroxysmal dyskinesia, yet over 60% of children with PMDs had paroxysmal symptoms. In contrast to nineteenth century literature by Charcot and others, chorea is notably rare in all modern series of PMDs. This disparity, however, likely reflects differences in nomenclature rather than phenomenology, as Charcot included repetitive rhythmic dancing movements within the realm of chorea [45].

Examination features

The same clinical characteristics that favor the diagnosis of a PMD in adults generally hold true in children [40,46]. Examination features indicative of a PMD include: (1) inconsistencies in the type of abnormal movements (e.g., tremor evolving into myoclonus or dystonia); (2) inconsistencies in the character of the abnormal movements (e.g., random fluctuations in the amplitude, frequency, and anatomical distribution of tremor); (3) paroxysmal symptoms (e.g., attacks of tremor punctuating an otherwise normal neurological examination, or unexplained remissions lasting minutes to days); (4) generation or intensification of movements following non-physiological triggers (e.g., eliciting axial dystonia by touching a specific spinous process or emergence of an abnormal movement in a body part not previously affected when the affected body part is forcefully restrained); (5) response to suggestion (e.g., remission following administration of placebo); (6) intensification of movements with attention to the PMD and reduction with distraction (e.g., attenuation of hand tremor when the patient moves his or her tongue side to side or performs calculations); (7) excessive, but delayed, startle or atypical stimulus sensitivity; (8) slow execution of volitional movements; (9) entrainment of tremor frequency to a voluntary repetitive movement on the contralateral side; (10) breath holding [47]; and (11) concomitant psychogenic findings, such as give-way weakness and active resistance to passive movement. Forced eye closure during paroxysms of spasm or shaking also generally indicates a psychogenic etiology [48]. An examination feature that was once commonly purported to be a reliable indicator of conversion disorder, which has been challenged by some as a psychogenic feature, is so-called "la belle indifference"[49].

Physicians' interest in the laterality of conversion symptoms dates back to Briquet, who noted that psychogenic numbness was more pronounced on the left side of the body [4,5]. Subsequent studies have found that in adults psychogenic weakness and numbness are more prominent on the left body, while right-sided symptoms predominate in children [2,13,14,41,50]. Right-sided symptoms may also be more common in hyperkinetic PMDs overall, when compared with psychogenic sensory disturbances and weakness [50]. Why conversion disorder would preferentially affect one side of the body is not known, but some authors have speculated that left-sided symptoms may arise from non-dominant hemisphere dysfunction akin to a form of hemineglect. Interestingly, in a recent study utilizing functional magnetic resonance imaging (fMRI), right temporoparietal junction hypoactivity was noted in adult patients with psychogenic symptoms [51]. Alternatively, the reported asymmetry might reflect observation biases [50]. In our population, PMD symptoms were asymmetric in only 59% of patients at the time of our evaluation; however, in patients whose PMD exhibited clear laterality, the dominant side was preferentially affected in 88%, including six left-handed children. A hemibody distribution (ipsilateral arm and leg with or without face) was found in 19%. In one study of childhood PMDs, a single limb was affected in two-thirds of children at the time of symptom onset, and in 90% of these symptoms began on the dominant side [2]. Clearly, the anatomical location of a movement disorder cannot and should not be used to predict whether it is likely to be psychogenic. Symptom laterality, however, may be of significance in terms of PMD neurobiology and it warrants continued attention.

Historical features

There are several features in the patient's history and in the circumstances surrounding the movement disorder onset that support the diagnosis of a PMD. A PMD starts abruptly in over 90% of children and a precipitating event is found in at least 20% and perhaps up to 70% of patients [2,13,26]. Various psychosocial stressors may precede PMD onset, such as death of a friend or family member, separation from a parent, and birth or adoption of a sibling. Curiously, social stressors account for only one-fifth of PMD triggers, while a physical injury or illness precedes the majority of cases. Physical precipitants are surprisingly minor, and patients may not view such injuries as particularly stressful. Since there is often a latency of several hours before abnormal movements develop, most children do not anticipate the development of abnormal movements or other sequelae prior to their onset.

Following symptom onset, PMDs are often initially progressive and then stabilize. In our series, 80% of PMDs were already static at the time of our initial evaluation. The mean PMD symptom duration preceding evaluation was 11 months, but this was not different in children with stable versus progressive symptoms (11 and 13 months, respectively). A history of prior spontaneous remissions was noted in 13% of our pediatric PMD cohort; this is likely an underestimate given the retrospective design.

Secondary gain (unconscious pursuit of personal attention or release from responsibility) may play an important role in some PMDs. However, appearance of secondary gain has proven ineffective in identifying psychogenic illness in adults [40], and secondary gain may be particularly difficult to assess in children. The presence of selective disability may provide a more objective means to gauge whether release from responsibility is associated with a PMD, and in our cohort, it was noted in approximately 40% of children. When evaluating patients, clinicians must take care not to confuse a task-specific movement disorder with selective disability, as has been the case historically [44,52]. Most task-specific movement disorders begin in adulthood [53]. Task-specific movement disorders are often encountered in patients who depend on the specific task in their occupation or other activities of daily living, for example, professional performers or competitive athletes [54]. Accordingly, "overlearned" tasks such as writing or playing a musical instrument tend to be preferentially affected, as a result of which the disorder is often misdiagnosed as "an overuse" syndrome. In many of the children we have seen with selective disability, the movement disorder tended to occur randomly but remitted during enjoyable events

Table 7.4 Patients with probable psychogenic movement disorder modeling

Phenotype	Reported exposure directly preceding symptom onset
Tremor	Mother's new boyfriend with tremor moved into the home
Dystonia	Volunteered at camp for children with neurological illnesses
Dystonia	Stepbrother with generalized dystonia moved into the home
Dystonia	Mother required a wheelchair because of a chronic neuropathy
Dystonia	Visited aunt who had contractures from multiple sclerosis
Dystonia	Close friend at school developed dystonia (also psychogenic)

or tasks, for example while driving or on vacation. The presence of a gestes antagoniste supports the diagnosis of an organic task-specific dystonia, though it has been reported also in psychogenic dystonia [55].

In some patients with PMDs, the abnormal movements resemble the symptoms of a relative or acquaintance [30,31,56–59], and unconscious modeling has been proposed as one of several clinical diagnostic criterion for PMDs [29]. In our population of children with PMD, 35% had a family member or close friend with a movement disorder, mostly a grandparent with mild tremor, but this contact was felt to be related to the onset of a PMD in only six cases (11%) (Table 7.4). In one patient with dystonia, symptoms resembled a classmate who also had a PMD (dystonia). Additional schoolmates were not affected, although psychogenic disorders can occur in epidemics [60]. Mass psychogenic illness ("mass hysteria") typically occurs in children and arises within schools in about half of instances [61–64]. Historically, movement disorders and convulsions made up the majority of epidemics, but a trend toward a greater proportion of sensory, respiratory, and abdominal symptoms has been observed [61]. How mass psychogenic illness differs from the more common individual variant of conversion disorder is unclear, but the course is often more benign. Most outbreaks resolve within 2 weeks and reassurance with supportive care usually suffice as treatment [61]. Data are not yet available whether children who demonstrate PMD modeling also have a more self-limited disease course.

Most children with PMDs have comorbid somatic complaints, a history of other unexplained medical conditions, or a collection of untenable medical diagnoses. One or more somatic or neurological complaints was present in addition to a PMD in 90% of our cohort, the most common being headaches, fatigue, abdominal discomfort, limb pain, and dizziness. It can be challenging to decipher which non-motor symptoms – if any – are psychogenic in any given patient, particularly when patients have seen multiple healthcare specialists who have offered conflicting opinions. We have found that even when patients (and their parents) accept the diagnosis of a PMD, they often fail to recognize that associated somatic complaints may also be psychogenic. As a consequence, patients may actually attribute the onset of their PMD to stress from a "chronic viral infection," "undifferentiated rheumatological disease," or "multiple chemical sensitivities."

Despite the high frequency of somatic complaints, most children with PMDs are otherwise healthy. Comorbid neurological disorders in our clinic population included possible epileptic seizures in 2 of 50 children (4%) and one child had restless legs syndrome; otherwise PMDs were not associated with organic movement disorders. Other reports indicate a prevalence of coexistent neurological disease as high as 40%, with approximately 20% of children with PMDs having an organic movement disorder, in most cases tics [2]. This is congruent with prior work in adults that has found a coexistent organic movement disorder in 10–25% of patients with PMDs [3,13,28,65].

Psychopathology

In adults with PMDs, anxiety and depression affect approximately 10–60% and 30–70% of patients, respectively [3,13,27,28]. A minority of adults with PMDs have other axis I psychiatric conditions, such as schizophrenia [13], and 40–50% meet criteria for a personality disorder [3,27]. How mood disorders and anxiety symptoms alter the expression and course of PMDs is not known. One study showed that the presence of a coexistent personality disorder may predict a poorer outcome in this population [66].

Available data suggest that, compared with adults, children with conversion disorder (including PMDs) are more likely to have anxiety rather than depression [3,13,16,67,68]. The spectrum and severity of comorbid mental health concerns, however, varies considerably between studies, with emergency room-based surveys showing lower rates of mental health disease compared with clinic-based studies that include children with more persistent symptoms [56,69]. In a small study of adolescents with fixed dystonia (the majority of whom met criteria for a PMD), the authors found psychological features to be overwhelmingly present, including anorexia nervosa in two of four patients [70]. In Schwingenschuh and colleagues' case series of pediatric PMDs, a history of psychiatric disease was documented in less than 15% of children, which is significantly less than the adult rates noted above [2]. We found overt depression or anxiety in half of the children we evaluated, and a history of suicidal ideation in 6%. Many of these children, however, had not previously been evaluated by a mental health practitioner and did not present with an established psychiatric diagnosis. Gauging psychiatric disease in PMD is challenging because somatoform disorders are commonly characterized by a distortion in bodily awareness, which may lead to underreporting of affective symptoms [71]. Other potential barriers include controversy regarding diagnostic criteria for emotional and behavioral disorders in children, particularly prior to adolescence [72]. Finally, it is sometimes unclear whether changes in mood that accompany PMDs preceded the onset of motor symptoms or arise in response to disability imposed by the movement disorder.

We have observed that 48% of girls with PMDs have a history of impeccable academic and extracurricular achievement. These young women were highly self-motivated and perfectionistic, as has been noted in a prior study of young women with conversion disorder [56]. In contrast, none of the 12 boys we evaluated displayed perfectionistic personality traits, and two were previously diagnosed with learning disabilities. We found symptoms of attention-deficit hyperactivity disorder in five children (9%), of which three were boys. This percentage is similar to the population prevalence reported by the Centers for Disease Control and Prevention, although discrepancies in age and gender preclude a direct comparison [73]. Prospective studies that include neuropsychiatric testing are lacking and will be necessary to define the spectrum of psychopathology that accompanies childhood PMDs. One prior study of four children with PMDs included a formal psychometric assessment. This study found a learning disability in all children, comorbid adjustment disorder in two, oppositional defiant disorder in one, and major depression in one [73].

Diagnosis

Investigations

Laboratory testing, neuroimaging, and electrophysiological studies may be required in some children, but the diagnosis of PMDs is largely based upon examination findings. This is unsettling to some physicians, patients, and parents, particularly when patients have examination findings which intuitively seem incompatible with a PMD, for example contractures or persistence of abnormal movements during sleep [57,70,74]. In clinical practice, patients often undergo extensive and unneeded testing before the correct diagnosis is reached [13,26] (except, perhaps, those patients with tremor [2]). The reason that clinicians perform superfluous testing in this population may be in large part because of the widely held misconception that PMDs are diagnosed by exclusion. In fact, PMDs are diagnosed based upon clinical findings, which is not different from most organic movement disorders, such as Tourette syndrome, dystonia, and essential tremor. It is also for this reason that we almost never refer patients to a psychiatrist or psychologist to confirm the diagnosis of a PMD. The diagnosis of PMD should be made by a neurologist skilled in recognition and management of movement disorders.

Neurophysiological testing may serve to distinguish PMDs from their organic counterparts, but electrodiagnostic investigations are neither infallible nor readily available (Table 7.5) [75–82]. Overall, electrodiagnostic examinations are more useful in patients with tremor and myoclonus. Most studies have focused on adult patients, but one recent study found EMG was useful in supporting the clinical diagnosis of PMDs in children [83].

Guidelines and pitfalls

Diagnostic guidelines for psychogenic dystonia were originally proposed by Fahn and Williams over 20 years ago, and have subsequently been applied to the entirety of PMDs (Table 7.2) [3,57]. Although these criteria have been widely adopted, they lack formal validation. An adaptation of the Fahn and William criteria was shown in one study to have reasonable diagnostic sensitivity and specificity (with the opinion of movement disorders experts serving as a "gold standard") [29].

One should emphasize certain pitfalls in the diagnosis of PMDs. Although the aforementioned phenomenological and historical features provide guidance,

Table 7.5 Electrophysiological findings that support and oppose the diagnosis of a psychogenic movement disorder

	Findings
Not supportive	
Myoclonus	EMG bursts of < 50 ms in duration
	Reflex myoclonus with a latency of EMG response < 70 ms
	Highly stereotyped pattern of muscle recruitment (EMG activation)
	Preceded by a time-locked cortical EEG correlate
	Associated with a giant evoke potential correlation following peripheral stimulation
	Not preceded by a bereitschaftspotential
Tremor	Different tremor frequencies in different limbs (low coherence/multiple oscillators)
	Decreased tremor amplitude when the extremity is loaded with added weight
Supportive	
Myoclonus	Long-duration bereitschaftspotential preceding spontaneous myoclonus by > 800 ms
	Reflex myoclonus with a latency of EMG response > 70 ms (exceptions: hyperekplexia and propriospinal myoclonus)
	Highly variable pattern of muscle recruitment (EMG activation)
Tremor	Voluntary ballistic movements with one hand cause a transient interference in tremor (oscillatory EMG activity) in the contralateral hand
	Change in tremor frequency of > 1.5 Hz
	Either (1) the same tremor frequency in different limbs (high coherence/single oscillator) or (2) different tremor frequencies in different limbs, produced by continuous cocontraction of antagonist muscles
	Increased tremor amplitude when the extremity is loaded with added weight

Sources: compiled from Deuschl *et al.*, 1998, 2006 [75,79]; Raethjen *et al.*, 2004 [76]; McAuley and Rothwell, 2004 [77]; Brown, 2006 [78]; Kumru *et al.*, 2007 [80]; Kenney *et al.*, 2007 [81]; McKeon *et al.*, 2009 [176].

none is pathognomic, and shared features unfortunately make several organic childhood-onset movement disorders more vulnerable to misidentification as PMDs.

For example, the paroxysmal dyskinesias, a pathogenically heterogeneous group of movement disorders characterized by episodes of dystonia and choreoathetosis, typically begin during childhood and may be misdiagnosed as a PMD because they are episodic and triggered by specific behaviors or environmental cues [84]. Furthermore, the threshold for attacks may be lowered by anxiety and stress. For similar reasons, episodic ataxias also may be misdiagnosed as PMDs. Various inborn errors of metabolism may present as an intermittent movement disorder and can be precipitated by minor physiological stressors, such as a febrile illness. Examples include non-ketotic hyperglycinemia, pyruvate dehydrogenase deficiency, and mutations of glucose transporter type 1, among others [85–88]. Inherited metabolic disorders are often regarded to be diseases of infancy or early childhood but may present in adolescence or adulthood. Furthermore, several metabolic disorders are amenable to specific disease-

modifying treatments, which makes prompt diagnosis essential [85].

Dopa-responsive dystonia, an inherited disorder of dopamine synthesis, classically manifests during childhood with leg dystonia that is more prominent late in the day. Because diurnal fluctuations may be misinterpreted as an inconsistency over time, or as a form of selective disability, patients with dopa-responsive dystonia also have been misdiagnosed with a PMD [89]. Other features of dystonia may falsely suggest the diagnosis of a PMD, such as task specificity, gestes antagonistes, and the ability of patients with dystonic gait to ambulate normally backwards [52,90–92].

Fluctuations in symptom severity and periods of remission, while found in PMDs, are also typical of Tourette syndrome, which is far more prevalent in children than are PMDs. Furthermore, other features of tics may falsely suggest a psychogenic etiology to the inexperienced clinician, for example their suggestibility, suppressibility, resemblance to voluntary behaviors, complexity, social inappropriateness (e.g., coprophenomena), and coexistence with psychiatric symptoms such as obsessive-compulsive disorder, impulsivity, and self-injurious behaviors [93,94]. The phenomenological spectrum of tics is essentially infinite, and unrecognized Tourette syndrome has been suspected even in cases diagnosed as psychogenic tremor [95]. Our current diagnostic criteria, devised for the whole of PMDs (Table 7.2), seem particularly ill-suited for tourettism, and literature on purportedly psychogenic tics invariably fuels queries and disagreements [96–104]. Some clinicians have attempted to utilize suggestion and placebo challenges as a means of confirming a psychogenic etiology in such patients [105]. However, the use of placebo in PMD remains controversial (despite a recent defense) [106]. Distractibility and entrainability, two features commonly associated with PMDs, have also not been systematically studied in Tourette syndrome, and their relevance remains uncertain. Habit reversal therapy, in which patients learn to apply antagonistic movements to inhibit the occurrence of tics, is successful in some patients with Tourette syndrome, although it is highly demanding on the patient, family, and the therapist [107,108]. The beneficial effects of this form of behavioral therapy may be unfortunately misinterpreted by some as evidence of psychogenicity in Tourette syndrome. In addition to Tourette syndrome, psychiatric comorbidity is common in many pediatric movement disorders (e.g., juvenile Huntington's disease, Sydenham chorea, myoclonus-dystonia, etc.) and may create diagnostic confusion, particularly in diseases which produce multiple phenomenologies [109–111].

Abrupt symptom onset is unusual for organic movement disorders, but some conditions, such as rapid-onset dystonia–parkinsonism, usually present precipitously during adolescence. Also, rapid-onset dystonia–parkinsonism may be mistaken for a PMD because it follows a static course and is often triggered by a physiological stressor [112]. Other childhood-onset organic movement disorders that may have an abrupt onset include Wilson's disease [113], toxin-induced movement disorders [114], and drug-induced dystonia [115,116]. Acute drug-induced dystonia, which preferentially affects young males, may also be misidentified as a PMD because of its self-limited, remitting course. A relapsing–remitting form of neuroleptic-induced dystonia (occurring despite withdrawal of dopamine receptor-blocking drugs) has recently been described, although its pathophysiological basis remains unknown [117]. Sydenham's chorea, opsoclonus–myoclonus, paroxysmal dyskinesias,

and other pediatric movement disorders may also spontaneously remit [118–120].

Another diagnostic pitfall is to regard any abnormal movement that is incongruent with a conventional organic movement disorder as a PMD. Children occasionally exhibit unusual movements that are neither neurological nor psychogenic, for example pseudo-dystonia from Sandifer syndrome [121], torticollis from atlantoaxial rotatory fixation [122], and stereotypic masturbatory behaviors [123]. Such behaviors and disorders should not be confused with PMDs.

The above examples highlight just a few of the potential difficulties in the diagnosis of PMDs. Consultation with a neurologist who has an expertise in pediatric movement disorders is an essential first step, but a multidisciplinary approach is needed to confirm the diagnosis in some children. Historically, organic movement disorders were misdiagnosed as psychogenic at unacceptably high rates; for example, approximately 40% of (adult) patients with organic dystonia were misdiagnosed as having PMDs [124,125]. Misdiagnosis rates for conversion disorder, however, are now thought to be considerably lower, around 5% [126]. In our experience, children with PMDs are more frequently misdiagnosed as having an organic movement disorder than the converse.

Neurobiology

In 1876, the American neurologist and author S. Weir Mitchell commented that hysteria could "as well be called *mysteria* for all its name teaches us of the host of morbid states which are crowded within its hazy boundaries" [127]. While physicians still do not adequately understand the pathophysiology of somatoform disorders, recent electrophysiological and functional neuroimaging studies have generated a renewed interest in this area and have fueled a shift in our conceptual approach to somatoform disorders from a psychoanalytical to a neurobiological perspective [128].

Two recent case series have used transcranial magnetic stimulation to address the mechanisms underlying paroxysmal and fixed forms of psychogenic dystonia [129,130]. Neither study included children, but two adults with fixed dystonia (not meeting criteria for clinically definite psychogenic dystonia) reported symptom onset during childhood [130]. Both studies found that patients with psychogenic and organic dystonia share similar physiological abnormalities compared with controls, specifically impairments of cortical inhibition (reduced short intracortical inhibition and contralateral silent period). It remains unclear whether these physiological abnormalities are a consequence of the long-standing dystonic posture or a susceptibility trait underlying both psychogenic and organic dystonia; however, one study found that cortical abnormalities were widespread, even in patients with focal symptoms [130]. Accordingly, it seems likely that the observed impairments of cortical inhibition were the cause rather than the result of dystonia. Abnormal motor excitability is also a feature of psychogenic paresis [131–134].

Functional neuroimaging studies of somatoform disorders have been small and have focused predominantly on adults with variable symptom chronicity, different psychiatric comorbidities, and heterogeneous neurological deficits (mostly psychogenic weakness and numbness) [135–149]. Differences in research methodology also encumber comparisons across studies; for example some studies used fMRI, while others utilized positron emission tomography or single photon emission computed tomography (SPECT). Current data, unsurprisingly, do not support a simple consistent pattern of brain activation (or inactivation) underlying psychogenic disorders as a whole. Nonetheless, trends are emerging. For example, psychogenic weakness has been associated with increased activity in the orbitofrontal cortex [137] and diminished activity in the dorsolateral prefrontal cortex [135], right temporoparietal junction [51], thalamus, and striatum [136]. In five patients with astasia–abasia, SPECT imaging showed decreased perfusion in the left temporal and parietal cortices [149]. Also, there is growing literature that functional neuroimaging can distinguish between somatoform disorders and feigned illness, although no imaging technique is currently suitable for diagnostic purposes [138].

There are no studies of the neuroanatomical correlates of PMDs in children. However, functional imaging findings of children with complex regional pain syndrome (CRPS) may be relevant, since CRPS is in some cases associated with movement disorders (often fixed dystonia) that are phenomenologically identical to PMDs [70,150,151]. In one study, fMRI was used to evaluate CNS activation in children during fulminating CRPS and again after their clinical recovery [152]. The authors found distinct patterns of central nervous system activation in response to mechanical and thermal stimuli of body regions both affected and unaffected by CRPS. Some of the observed fMRI abnormalities, including those within the basal ganglia, persisted despite clinical recovery of allodynia, suggesting that CRPS may result in long-standing neuroplastic changes. Whether such changes explain CRPS-related motor symptoms is not known, as none of the children in this study had a movement disorder associated with CRPS. Further research in this area, however, may prove useful in clarifying the neural substrate of fixed dystonia and possibly PMDs in general.

Treatment and prognosis

Role of counseling

The initial and perhaps the most critical element in the treatment of PMDs is to deliver the diagnosis and preliminary counseling optimally [153,154]. This is often difficult and is always time exhaustive. Shortcuts, however, are likely to be unrewarding for the clinician, patient, and family because the outcome is likely to be bleak if the patient does not accept the diagnosis [82]. When discussing PMDs, a few issues should be kept in mind.

A PMD often results in severe disability and suffering [13,155,156]. Clinicians should state this fact explicitly to demonstrate that they recognize the gravity of the patient's situation. One should aim to explain the disorder using non-offensive language that facilitates rapport. This promotes compliance and enhances one's chances of obtaining critical psychosocial information. Terminology that portrays psychiatric diseases as being unreal or feigned should be specifically avoided [157,158]. Unfortunately, many neurologists continue to view patients with psychogenic disorders as being deceptive [159] so it must be expected that some patients will present for a second opinion already disillusioned or with angry parents.

Clinicians should always probe what patients and their loved ones think might be causing their symptoms in order to better understand potential psychodynamic factors and to correct false beliefs and unwarranted fears when possible. Camouflaging the diagnosis with overly complex terminology is counterproductive (e.g., "paroxysmal psychogenic non-kinesiogenic segmental dystonia").

Physicians may acknowledge that, although relatively common, much about PMDs is not understood. It is, however, best to be decisive when communicating the diagnosis. Vacillating between a psychogenic and organic etiology all but guarantees that the family will seek another opinion. In explaining the diagnosis to our patients, we emphasize that PMDs are not caused by a structural lesion, and the movement disorder arises from functional brain changes that may follow stressors. Just as stress may increase blood pressure, it can also cause tremor and other abnormal movements. We always try to convey to the patients and their parents that acceptance of the diagnosis in some cases itself facilitates recovery. We also emphasize that patients should not put their lives on hold while waiting for their movement disorder to remit. We aim to motivate and empower patients to maximize function and quality of life – despite their movement disorder – while treatments are pursued.

Treatment strategies

Prospective treatment trials have not been performed in children with PMDs or other forms of conversion disorder, and the optimal therapeutic strategy is not known. Because PMDs typically do not respond to conventional therapies for organic movement disorders, we generally do not recommend the traditional medications used in the treatment of tremor, dystonia, or other organic movement disorders [160]. In a recent survey of movement disorder neurologists, avoidance of iatrogenic harm was cited as the most important management modality, followed by patient education [82]. We have found this to be particularly germane with regard to children, as the morbidity related to unnecessary medical and surgical therapies may be profound [13]. In our patient cohort, 22% of children had had one or more surgerical procedure for symptoms related to their PMD or for associated symptoms retrospectively determined to have no identifiable organic basis. Surgery, often orthopedic in nature, was particularly common in patients with dystonia and those with prominent pain. Other centers have also reported children with PMDs referred for deep brain stimulation therapy [26].

Pending additional data from controlled trials, we recommend a multidisciplinary approach using a combination of psycho-, physio-, and pharmacotherapy tailored to the individual child's needs. Because effective treatment of conversion symptoms may motivate families to be more committed to therapy, these treatments may be offered concurrently [161].

Two small single-blind trials support the efficacy of psychodynamic psychotherapy and exercise of low–medium intensity in adults with PMDs [162,163].

Cognitive behavioral therapy has proven helpful for adults with other kinds of "medically unexplained symptoms," but has not been adequately studied for PMDs specifically [164,165]. In childhood PMDs, family therapy may be prudent, particularly when specific psychosocial stressors can be identified. One study of children with somatoform disorders linked familial dysfunction with chronicity of disease [59], while another study found that parental psychiatric disorders predicted a poorer outcome [166]. Some centers advocate providing physiotherapy in combination with psychotherapy [167–169]. Hypnosis may be helpful for conversion disorder in children [170], although it is not clear that it provides added benefit when used in conjunction with other psychotherapeutic approaches [167].

In one study, selective serotonin reuptake inhibitors reduced PMD severity in adults with a comorbid mood or anxiety disorder [171]. Additional trials, however, are needed to confirm efficacy and better define which clinical characteristics predict a good response to pharmacotherapy. A prior meta-analysis of antidepressant drugs for medically unexplained symptoms as a whole found that improvements in somatoform symptoms do not necessarily correlate with improvements in mood [172]. In that study, which included medically unexplained symptoms across various body systems, meta-regression found no differential effect among different classes of antidepressant; however, tricyclic antidepressants were associated with a greater likelihood of efficacy than the selective serotonin reuptake inhibitors. How such data apply to children is uncertain, since tricyclic antidepressants are a less established therapy in the treatment of childhood depression, particularly in pre-adolescents [173].

Outcome

Outcome studies of PMDs are difficult to execute for many reasons. Patients often do not return to the clinic owing to a reluctance to accept their diagnosis, the lack of proven therapies, and the sizable distance that many patients must travel to be seen in a subspecialty movement disorders center. Follow-up studies must be relatively long, as the natural history of PMDs may be punctuated by fluctuations and spontaneous remissions. Ideally, studies should also monitor the status of other somatoform symptoms and comorbid psychiatric disease, which is challenging, because motor symptoms may not always mirror patients' overall health status (e.g., tremor might improve coincident with a worsening of pelvic pain or depression). Also, until recently, there was not a validated clinical rating scale for PMDs. A scale, the Psychogenic Movement Disorders Rating Scale (PMDRS), is now available, can be applied to diverse PMD phenomenologies, and includes a measure of PMD-related functional incapacitation [174] (see Chapter 32). The scoring system for the PMDRS, however, requires clarification, and it is not clear how applicable the scale will be for children.

Previous studies of adults suggest that PMD outcomes are better in patients with shorter disease duration [23,27,28,66,175,176], those with a positive perception of their social situation and physician [28], and those with a comorbid DSM axis I disorder [175]. Age of onset may influence PMD outcome, favoring younger patients, but these data are conflicting [3]. Outcomes are poorer in patients who have a personality disorder [66] and secondary gain [175]. In one study of patients with motor conversion symptoms, those with pending litigation faired less well [175], but another study challenged this finding [28]. The association between litigation and outcome may vary regionally or culturally; at least it appears that American physicians find legal information more relevant than their European counterparts [82]. The prognosis for PMDs is less favorable in patients who are suspected to have factitious disorder or malingering rather than a somatoform etiology [3,171]. In a recent survey study, the only variable that movement disorder experts endorsed as extremely important in predicting outcome was whether the patient genuinely accepted the diagnosis. This, of course, may be difficult to gauge and the prognostication of individual patients remains challenging. Overall, the long-term outcome of adults with PMDs is often poor, with remission rates ranging between 5 and 35% [3,23,27,43,75,176]. A larger percentage of patients may report a partial improvement, in one study as high as 57% [28].

The prognosis is more favorable in children with PMDs than in adults. In one cohort of 15 children, nearly 50% recovered completely and 80% showed substantial improvement over time [2]. A recent abstract from the Columbia group (which included adults with childhood-onset PMDs) [26] and a case series of 12 children with acute PMDs [14] also reported a significant improvement in over three-quarters of patients. In an additional 50 previously published cases reviewed by Schwingenschuh and colleagues, 74% of children

recovered fully, 14% improved partially, 8% remained chronically disabled, and in 4% the outcome was not reported [2]. These outcomes are similar to that reported in children with other forms of conversion disorder and psychogenic seizures [20,166,177–179], as well as new data from Rosebush and colleagues in this volume (Chapter 9).

As with adults, the shorter the duration of symptoms prior to diagnosis, the better the outcome. A tremor-dominant PMD phenotype may also predict a more benign course [2], while fixed dystonia follows a more protracted course [70]. Other factors associated with chronicity of childhood somatoform disorders include older age at presentation, depression, parental psychiatric disorders, multiple negative life events, and pain [166,177]. Polysymptomatic presentations of conversion disorder, perhaps a harbinger of somatization disorder, are also associated with a poorer prognosis [59]. Further work is necessary to determine whether children who recover from PMDs have a higher risk of psychiatric or neurological disease in adulthood.

Even though most children with PMDs will improve, many experience severe disability, particularly those with a more protracted course who require referral to a tertiary movement disorder clinic. In one cohort, approximately half of the children became so severely affected that they could not attend school [2]. In our clinic, nearly one-quarter of children with a PMD required home schooling because of their symptoms [13], a rate over 10 times higher than the national average [180]. However, further research hopefully will result in a better understanding of PMD pathogenesis and lead to improved treatment modalities.

References

1. American Psychiatric Association. *Diagnostic and Statistical Manual of Diseases*, 4th edn, text revision. Washington DC: American Psychiatric Press, 2000.

2. Schwingenschuh P, Pont-Sunyer C, Surtees R, *et al.* Psychogenic movement disorders in children: a report of 15 cases and a review of the literature. *Mov Disord* 2008;**23**:1882–1888.

3. Williams DT, Ford B, Fahn S. Phenomenology and psychopathology related to psychogenic movement disorders. *Adv Neurol* 1995;**65**:231–257.

4. Briquet P. *Traité de l'hystérie*. Paris: JB Baillière, 1859.

5. Mai FM, Merskey H. Briquet's treatise on hysteria. A synopsis and commentary. *Arch Gen Psychiatry* 1980;**37**:1401–1405.

6. Nijenhuis ERS, Spinhoven P, van Dyck R, *et al*. Degree of somatoform and psychological dissociation in dissociative disorder is correlated with reported trauma. *J Traum Stress* 1998;**11**:711–730.

7. Roelofs K, Keijsers GPJ, Hoogduin KA, *et al*. Childhood abuse in patients with conversion disorder. *Am J Psychiatry* 2002;**159**:1908–1913.

8. Brown RJ, Schrag A, Trimble MR. Dissociation, childhood interpersonal trauma, and family functioning in patients with somatization disorder. *Am J Psychiatry* 2005;**162**:899–905.

9. Waldinger RJ, Schulz MS, Barsky AJ, *et al*. Mapping the road from childhood trauma to adult somatization: the role of attachment. *Psychosom Med* 2006;**68**:129–135.

10. Spitzer C, Barnow S, Gau K, Freyberger HJ, Grabe HJ. Childhood maltreatment in patients with somatization disorder. *Aust N Z J Psychiatry* 2008;**42**:335–341.

11. Şar V, Akyüz G, Doğan O, *et al*. The prevalence of conversion symptoms in women from a general Turkish population. *Psychosomatics* 2009;**50**:50–58.

12. Fernandez-Alvarez E. Movement disorders of functional origin (psychogenic) in children. *Rev Neurol* 2005;**40**(Suppl 1):S75–S77.

13. Ferrara J, Jankovic J. Psychogenic movement disorders in children. *Mov Disord* 2008;**23**:1875–1881.

14. Dale RC, Singh H, Troedson C, *et al*. A prospective study of acute movement disorders in children. *Dev Med Child Neurol* 2010;**52**:739–748.

15. Tomasson K, Kent D, Coryell W. Somatization and conversion disorders: comorbidity and demographics at presentation. *Acta Psychiatr Scand* 1991;**84**:288–293.

16. Kozlowska K, Nunn KP, Rose D, *et al*. Conversion disorder in Australian pediatric practice. *J Am Acad Child Adolesc Psychiatry* 2007;**46**:68–75.

17. Srinath S, Bharat S, Girimaji S, Seshadri S. Characteristics of a child inpatient population with hysteria in India. *J Am Acad Child Adolesc Psychiatry* 1993;**32**:822–825.

18. Ron MA. Somatisation in neurological practice. *J Neurol Neurosurg Psychiatry* 1994;**57**:1161–1164.

19. Thomas NH. Somatic presentation of psychogenic disease in child neurologic practice. *Neurology* 2002;**58**(Suppl 3):A28.

20. Leary P. M. Conversion disorder in childhood: diagnosed too late, investigated too much? *J R Soc Med* 2003;**96**:436–438.

21. Lieb R, Pfister H, Mastaler M, *et al*. Somatoform syndromes and disorders in a representative population sample of adolescents and young adults: prevalence, comorbidity and impairments. *Acta Psychiatr Scand* 2000;**101**:194–208.

22. Thomas M, Jankovic J. Psychogenic movement disorders: diagnosis and management. *CNS Drugs* 2004;**18**:437–452.

23. Factor SA, Podskalny GD, Molho ES. Psychogenic movement disorders: frequency, clinical profile, and characteristics. *J Neurol Neurosurg Psychiatry* 1995;**59**:406–412.

24. Portera-Cailliau C, Victor D, Frucht S, *et al*. Movement disorders fellowship training program at Columbia University Medical Center in 2001–2002. *Mov Disord* 2006;**21**:479–485.

25. Ahmed MA, Martinez A, Yee A, *et al*. Psychogenic and organic movement disorders in children. *Dev Med Child Neurol* 2008;**50**:300–304.

26. Rotstein M, Pearson T, Williams DT, Frucht S. Psychogenic movement disorders in children and adolescents. *Mov Disord* 2009;**24**(Suppl 1): S130.

27. Feinstein A, Stergiopoulos V, Fine J, *et al*. Psychiatric outcome in patients with a psychogenic movement disorder: a prospective study. *Neuropsychiatry Neuropsychol Behav Neurol* 2001;**14**:169–176.

28. Thomas M, Vuong KD, Jankovic J. Long-term prognosis of patients with psychogenic movement disorders. *Parkinsonism Relat Disord* 2006;**12**:382–387.

29. Shill H, Gerber P. Evaluation of clinical diagnostic criteria for psychogenic movement disorders. *Mov Disord* 2006;**21**:1163–1168.

30. Spierings C, Poels PJ, Sijben N, Gabreëls FJ, Renier WO. Conversion disorders in childhood: a retrospective follow-up study of 84 inpatients. *Dev Med Child Neurol* 1990;**32**:865–871.

31. Ghosh JK, Majumder P, Pant P, *et al*. Clinical profile and outcome of conversion disorder in children in a tertiary hospital of north India. *J Trop Pediatr* 2007;**53**:213–214.

32. Wool CA, Barsky AJ. Do women somatize more than men? Gender differences in somatization. *Psychosomatics* 1994;**35**:445–452.

33. Zadikoff C, Mailis-Gagnon A, Lang AE. A case of a psychogenic "jumpy stump." *J Neurol Neurosurg Psychiatry* 2006;**77**:1101.

34. Skidmore F, Anderson K, Fram D, *et al*. Psychogenic camptocormia. *Mov Disord* 2007;**22**:1974–1975.

35. Valadi N, Morgan JC, Sethi KD. Psychogenic movement disorder masquerading as CJD. *J Neuropsychiatry Clin Neurosci* 2006;**18**:562–563.

36. Williams DR, Cowey M, Tuck K, *et al*. Psychogenic propriospinal myoclonus. *Mov Disord* 2008;**23**:1312–1313.

37. van der Salm SM, Koelman JH, Henneke S, van Rootselaar AF, Tijssen MA. Axial jerks: a clinical

spectrum ranging from propriospinal to psychogenic myoclonus. *J Neurol* 2010 **257**:1349–1355.

38. Pirio Richardson S, Mari Z, Matsuhashi M, *et al*. Psychogenic palatal tremor. *Mov Disord* 2006;**21**:274–276.

39. Cubo E, Hinson VK, Goetz CG, *et al*. Transcultural comparison of psychogenic movement disorders. *Mov Disord* 2005;**20**:1343–1345.

40. Lang AE. General overview of psychogenic movement disorders: epidemiology, diagnosis, and prognosis. In Hallett M, Fahn S, Jankovic J, *et al*., eds. *Psychogenic Movement Disorders Neurology and Neuropsychiatry*. Philadelphia, PA: Lippincott Williams & Wilkins, 2006:35–41.

41. Kirsch DB, Mink JW. Psychogenic movement disorders in children. *Pediatr Neurol* 2004;**30**:1–6.

42. Schrag A, Trimble M, Quinn N, Bhatia K. The syndrome of fixed dystonia: an evaluation of 103 patients. *Brain* 2004;**127**:2360–2372.

43. Ibrahim NM, Martino D, van de Warrenburg BP, *et al*. The prognosis of fixed dystonia: a follow-up study. *Parkinsonism Relat Disord* 2009;**15**:592–597.

44. Munts AG, Koehler PJ. How psychogenic is dystonia? Views from past to present. *Brain* 2010;**133**:1552–1564.

45. Goetz C. Charcot and psychogenic movement disorders. In Hallett M, Fahn S, Jankovic J, *et al*., eds. *Psychogenic Movement Disorders Neurology and Neuropsychiatry*. Philadelphia, PA: Lippincott Williams & Wilkins, 2006:3–13.

46. Marjama J, Troster AL, Koller WC. Psychogenic movement disorders. *Neurol Clin* 1995;**13**:283–297.

47. Reich SG. Psychogenic movement disorders. *Semin Neurol* 2006;**26**:289–296.

48. Chung SS, Gerber P, Kirlin KA. Ictal eye closure is a reliable indicator for psychogenic nonepileptic seizures. *Neurology* 2006;**66**:1730–1731.

49. Stone J, Smyth R, Carson A, *et al*. La belle indifference in conversion symptoms and hysteria: systematic review. *Br J Psychiatry* 2006;**188**:204–209.

50. Stone J, Sharpe M, Carson A, *et al*. Are functional motor and sensory symptoms really more frequent on the left? A systematic review. *J Neurol Neurosurg Psychiatry* 2002;**73**:578–581.

51. Voon V, Gallea C, Hattori N, *et al*. The involuntary nature of conversion disorder. *Neurology* 2010;**74**:223–228.

52. Sheehy MP, Marsden CD. Writers' cramp: a focal dystonia. *Brain* 1982;**105**:461–480.

53. Torres-Russotto D, Perlmutter JS. Task-specific dystonias: a review. *Ann N Y Acad Sci* 2008;**1142**:179–199.

54. Roze E, Soumaré A, Pironneau I, *et al*. Case–control study of writer's cramp. *Brain* 2009 **132**:756–764.

55. Munhoz RP, Lang AE. Gestes antagonistes in psychogenic dystonia. *Mov Disord* 2004;**19**:331–332.

56. Grattan-Smith P, Fairley M, Procopis P. Clinical features of conversion disorder. *Arch Dis Child* 1988;**63**:408–414.

57. Fahn S, Williams DT. Psychogenic dystonia. *Adv Neurol* 1988;**50**:431–455.

58. Lancman ME, Asconape JJ, Graves S. Psychogenic seizures in children. Long term analysis of 43 cases. *J. Child Neurol* 1994;**9**:404–407.

59. Murase S, Sugiyama T, Ishii T, *et al*. Polysymptomatic conversion disorder in childhood and adolescence in Japan. Early manifestation or incomplete form of somatization disorder? *Psychother Psychosom* 2000;**69**:132–136.

60. Balaratnasingam S, Janca A. Mass hysteria revisited. *Curr Opin Psychiatry* 2006;**19**:171–174.

61. Boss LP. Epidemic hysteria: a review of the published literature. *Epidemiol Rev* 1997;**19**:233–243.

62. Cassady JD, Kirschke DL, Jones TF, *et al*. Case series: outbreak of conversion disorder among amish adolescent girls. *J Am Acad Child Adolesc Psychiatry* 2005;**44**:291–297.

63. Powell SA, Nguyen CT, Gaziano J, *et al*. Mass psychogenic illness presenting as acute stridor in an adolescent female cohort. *Ann Otol Rhinol Laryngol* 2007;**116**:525–531.

64. Buttery JP, Madin S, Crawford NW, *et al*. Mass psychogenic response to human papillomavirus vaccination. *Med J Aust* 2008;**189**:261–262.

65. Ranawaya R, Riley D, Lang A. Psychogenic dyskinesias in patients with organic movement disorders. *Mov Disord* 1990;**5**:127–133.

66. Binzer M, Kullgren G. Motor conversion disorder. A prospective 2- to 5-year follow-up study. *Psychosomatics* 1998;**39**:519–527.

67. Pehlivantürk B, Unal F. Conversion disorder in children and adolescents: clinical features and comorbidity with depressive and anxiety disorders. *Turk J Pediatr* 2000;**42**:132–137.

68. Ercan ES, Varan A, VeznedaroGlu B. Associated features of conversion disorder in Turkish adolescents. *Pediatr Int* 2003;**45**:150–155.

69. Zeharia A, Mukamel M, Carel C, *et al*. Conversion reaction: management by the paediatrician. *Eur J Pediatr* 1999;**158**:160–164.

70. Majumdar A, López-Casas J, Poo P, *et al*. Syndrome of fixed dystonia in adolescents: short term outcome in 4 cases. *Eur J Paediatr Neurol* 2009;**13**:466–472.

71. Brown RJ, Cardeña E, Nijenhuis E, *et al.* Should conversion disorder be reclassified as a dissociative disorder in DSM V? *Psychosomatics* 2007;**48**:369–378.

72. Egger HL, Angold A. Common emotional and behavioral disorders in preschool children: presentation, nosology, and epidemiology. *J Child Psychol Psychiatry* 2006;**47**:313–337.

73. Centers for Disease Control and Prevention. Mental health in the United States: prevalence of diagnosis and medication treatment for attention-deficit/hyperactivity disorder – United States, 2003. *MMWR* 2005;**54**:842–847.

74. Ziegler JS, von Stauffenberg M, Vlaho S, *et al.* Dystonia with secondary contractures: a psychogenic movement disorder mimicking its neurological counterpart. *J Child Neurol* 2008;**23**:1316–1318.

75. Deuschl G, Köster B, Lücking CH, *et al.* Diagnostic and pathophysiological aspects of psychogenic tremors. *Mov Disord* 1998;**13**:294–302.

76. Raethjen J, Kopper F, Govindan RB, *et al.* Two different pathogenetic mechanisms in psychogenic tremor. *Neurology* 2004;**63**:812–815.

77. McAuley J, Rothwell J. Identification of psychogenic, dystonic, and other organic tremors by a coherence entrainment test. *Mov Disord* 2004;**19**:253–267.

78. Brown P. Clinical neurophysiology of myoclonus. In Hallett M, Fahn S, Jankovic J, *et al.*, eds. *Psychogenic Movement Disorders Neurology and Neuropsychiatry.* Philadelphia, PA: Lippincott Williams & Wilkins, 2006:131–143.

79. Deuschl G, Raethjen J, Kopper F, *et al.* The diagnosis and physiology of psychogenic tremor. In Hallett M, Fahn S, Jankovic J, *et al.*, eds. *Psychogenic Movement Disorders Neurology and Neuropsychiatry.* Philadelphia, PA: Lippincott Williams & Wilkins, 2006:265–273.

80. Kumru H, Begeman M, Tolosa E, Valls-Sole J. Dual task interference in psychogenic tremor. *Mov Disord* 2007;**22**:2077–2082.

81. Kenney C, Diamond A, Mejia N, *et al.* Distinguishing psychogenic and essential tremor. *J Neurol Sci* 2007;**263**:94–99.

82. Espay AJ, Goldenhar LM, Voon V, *et al.* Opinions and clinical practices related to diagnosing and managing patients with psychogenic movement disorders: an international survey of Movement Disorder Society members. *Mov Disord* 2009 **24**:1366–1374.

83. Canavese C, Ciano C, Zorzi G, *et al.* Polymyography in the diagnosis of childhood onset movement disorders. *Eur J Paediatr Neurol* 2008;**12**:480–483.

84. Bruno MK, Hallett M, Gwinn-Hardy K, *et al.* Clinical evaluation of idiopathic paroxysmal kinesigenic dyskinesia: new diagnostic criteria. *Neurology* 2004;**63**:2280–2287.

85. Sedel F, Saudubray JM, Roze E, *et al.* Movement disorders and inborn errors of metabolism in adults: a diagnostic approach. *J Inherit Metab Dis* 2008;**31**:308–318.

86. Suls A, Dedeken P, Goffin K, *et al.* Paroxysmal exercise-induced dyskinesia and epilepsy is due to mutations in *SLC2A1*, encoding the glucose transporter GLUT1. *Brain* 2008;**131**:1831–1844.

87. Leen WG, Klepper J, Verbeek MM, *et al.* Glucose transporter-1 deficiency syndrome: the expanding clinical and genetic spectrum of a treatable disorder. *Brain* 2010;**133**:655–670.

88. Pons R, Collins A, Rotstein M, Engelstad K, De Vivo DC. The spectrum of movement disorders in Glut-1 deficiency. *Mov Disord* 2010;**25**:275–281.

89. Bandmann O, Marsden CD, Wood NW. Atypical presentations of dopa-responsive dystonia. *Adv Neurol* 1998;**78**:283–290.

90. Wu LJ, Jankovic J. Runner's dystonia. *J Neurol Sci* 2006;**251**:73–76.

91. Ochudło S, Drzyzga K, Drzyzga LR, Opala G. Various patterns of gestes antagonistes in cervical dystonia. *Parkinsonism Relat Disord* 2007;**13**:417–420.

92. Jankovic J, Ashoori A. Movement disorders in musicians. *Mov Disord* 2008;**23**:1957–1965.

93. Jankovic J. Tourette's syndrome. *N Engl J Med* 2001;**345**:1184–1192.

94. Freeman RD, Zinner SH, Müller-Vahl KR, *et al.* Coprophenomena in Tourette syndrome. *Dev Med Child Neurol* 2009;**51**:218–227.

95. Kulisevsky J, Berthier ML, Avila A, Gironell A, Escartin AE. Unrecognized Tourette syndrome in adult patients referred for psychogenic tremor. *Arch Neurol* 1998;**55**:409–414.

96. Kurlan R, Deeley C, Como P. Psychogenic movement disorder (pseudo-tics) in a patient with Tourette's syndrome. *J Neuropsychiatry Clin Neurosci* 1992;**4**:347–348.

97. Dooley JM, Stokes A, Gordon KE. Pseudo-tics in Tourette syndrome. *J Child Neurol* 1994;**9**:50–51.

98. Ojoo JC, Kastelik JA, Morice AH. A boy with a disabling cough. *Lancet* 2003;**361**:674.

99. Bryon M, Jaffe A. Disabling cough: habit cough or tic syndrome? *Lancet* 2003;**361**:1991–1992.

100. Weinberger M. Disabling cough: habit cough or tic syndrome? *Lancet* 2003;**361**:1001.

101. Mejia NI, Jankovic J. Secondary tics and tourettism. *Rev Bras Psiquiatr* 2005;**27**:11–17.

102. Sampaio A, Hounie AG. Organic vs. psychogenic tics. *Rev Bras Psiquiatr* 2005;**27**:163.

103. Irwin RS, Glomb WB, Chang AB. Habit cough, tic cough, and psychogenic cough in adult and pediatric populations: ACCP evidence-based clinical practice guidelines. *Chest* 2006;**129**(Suppl 1):174S–179S.

104. Squintani G, Tinazzi M, Gambarin M, *et al*. Post-streptococcal "complex" movement disorders: unusual concurrence of psychogenic and organic symptoms. *J Neurol Sci* 2010;**288**:68–71.

105. Tan EK. Psychogenic tics: diagnostic value of the placebo test. *J Child Neurol* 2004;**19**:976–977.

106. Shamy MC. The treatment of psychogenic movement disorders with suggestion is ethically justified. *Mov Disord* 2010;**25**:260–264.

107. Deckersbach T, Rauch S, Buhlmann U, *et al*. Habit reversal versus supportive psychotherapy in Tourette's disorder: a randomized controlled trial and predictors of treatment response. *Behav Res Ther* 2006;**44**:1079–1090.

108. Piacentini J, Woods DW, Scahill L, *et al*. Behavior therapy for children with Tourette disorder: randomized controlled trial. *JAMA* 2010;**303**:1929–1937.

109. Walker AR, Tani LY, Thompson JA, *et al*. Rheumatic chorea: relationship to systemic manifestations and response to corticosteroids, *J Pediatr* 2007;**151**:679–683.

110. Ribaï P, Nguyen K, Hahn-Barma V, *et al*. Psychiatric and cognitive difficulties as indicators of juvenile huntington disease onset in 29 patients. *Arch Neurol* 2007;**64**:813–819.

111. Kinugawa K, Vidailhet M, Clot F, *et al*. Myoclonus-dystonia: an update. *Mov Disord* 2009;**24**:479–489.

112. Brashear A, Dobyns WB, de Carvalho Aguiar P, *et al*. The phenotypic spectrum of rapid-onset dystonia-parkinsonism (RDP) and mutations in the *ATP1A3* gene. *Brain* 2007;**130**:828–835.

113. Pendlebury ST, Rothwell PM, Dalton A, *et al*. Strokelike presentation of Wilson disease with homozygosity for a novel T766R mutation. *Neurology* 2004;**63**:1982–1983.

114. Pappert EJ. Toxin-induced movement disorders. *Neurol Clin* 2005;**23**:429–459.

115. Dressler D, Benecke R. Diagnosis and management of acute movement disorders. *J Neurol* 2005;**252**:1299–1306.

116. Gilbert DL. Drug-induced movement disorders in children. *Ann N Y Acad Sci* 2008;**1142**:72–84.

117. Schneider SA, Udani V, Sankhla CS, *et al*. Recurrent acute dystonic reaction and oculogyric crisis despite withdrawal of dopamine receptor blocking drugs. *Mov Disord* 2009;**24**:1226–1229.

118. Bataller L, Graus F, Saiz A, *et al*. Clinical outcome in adult onset idiopathic or paraneoplastic opsoclonus-myoclonus. *Brain* 2001;**124**:437–443.

119. Pranzatelli MR, Tate ED, Kinsbourne M, *et al*. Forty-one year follow-up of childhood-onset opsoclonus-myoclonus-ataxia: cerebellar atrophy, multiphasic relapses, and response to IVIG. *Mov Disord* 2002;**17**:1387–1390.

120. Lotze T, Jankovic J. Paroxysmal kinesigenic dyskinesias. *Semin Pediatr Neurol* 2003;**10**:68–79.

121. Kabakuş N, Kurt A. Sandifer syndrome: a continuing problem of misdiagnosis. *Pediatr Int* 2006;**48**:622–625.

122. Kato Y, Ito S, Kubota M, *et al*. Chronic atraumatic atlantoaxial rotatory fixation with anterolisthesis. *J Orthop Sci* 2007;**12**:97–100.

123. Yang ML, Fullwood E, Goldstein J, *et al*. Masturbation in infancy and early childhood presenting as a movement disorder: 12 cases and a review of the literature. *Pediatrics* 2005;**116**:1427–1432.

124. Marsden CD, Harrison MJ. Idiopathic torsion dystonia (dystonia musculorum deformans). A review of forty-two patients. *Brain* 1974;**97**:793–810.

125. Lesser RP, Fahn S. Dystonia: a disorder often misdiagnosed as a conversion reaction. *Am J Psychiatry* 1978;**135**:349–352.

126. Stone J, Smyth R, Carson A, *et al*. Systematic review of misdiagnosis of conversion symptoms and "hysteria." *BMJ* 2005;**331**:989–991.

127. Mitchell SW. Rest in nervous disease: Its use and abuse. In Seguin EC, ed. *A Series of American Clinical Lectures*, Vol. I, January–December 1875. New York: JP Putnan, 1876.

128. Sharpe M, Carson A. "Unexplained" somatic symptoms, functional syndromes, and somatization: do we need a paradigm shift? *Ann Intern Med* 2001;**134**:926–930.

129. Espay AJ, Morgante F, Purzner J, *et al*. Cortical and spinal abnormalities in psychogenic dystonia. *Ann Neurol* 2006;**59**:825–834.

130. Avanzino L, Martino D, van de Warrenburg BP, *et al*. Cortical excitability is abnormal in patients with the "fixed dystonia" syndrome. *Mov Disord* 2008;**23**:646–652.

131. Yaźići KM, Demirci M, Demir B, *et al*. Abnormal somatosensory evoked potentials in two patients with conversion disorder. *Psychiatry Clin Neurosci* 2004;**58**:222–225.

132. Geraldes R, Coelho M, Rosa MM, *et al*. Abnormal transcranial magnetic stimulation in a patient with presumed psychogenic paralysis. *J Neurol Neurosurg Psychiatry* 2008;**79**:1412–1413.

133. Liepert J, Hassa T, Tüscher O, *et al.* Electrophysiological correlates of motor conversion disorder. *Mov Disord* 2008;**23**:2171–2176.

134. Liepert J, Hassa T, Tüscher O, *et al.* Abnormal motor excitability in patients with psychogenic paresis. A TMS study. *J Neurol* 2009;**256**:121–126.

135. Spence SA, Crimlisk HL, Cope H, *et al.* Discrete neurophysiological correlates in prefrontal cortex during hysterical and feigned disorder of movement. *Lancet* 2000;**355**:1243–1124.

136. Vuilleumier P, Chicherio C, Assal F, *et al.* Functional neuroanatomical correlates of hysterical sensorimotor loss. *Brain* 2001;**124**:1077–1090.

137. Marshall JC, Halligan PW, Fink GR, *et al.* The functional neuroanatomy of a hysterical paralysis. *Cognition* 1997;**64**:B1–B8.

138. Stone J, Zeman A, Simonotto E, *et al.* FMRI in patients with motor conversion symptoms and controls with simulated weakness. *Psychosom Med* 2007;**69**:961–969.

139. Burgmer M, Konrad C, Jansen A, *et al.* Abnormal brain activation during movement observation in patients with conversion paralysis. *Neuroimage* 2006;**29**:1336–1343.

140. Mailis-Gagnon A, Giannoylis I, Downar J, *et al.* Altered central somatosensory processing in chronic pain patients with "hysterical" anesthesia. *Neurology* 2003;**60**:1501–1507.

141. de Lange FP, Roelofs K, Toni I. Increased self-monitoring during imagined movements in conversion paralysis. *Neuropsychologia* 2007;**45**:2051–2058.

142. Ghaffar O, Staines R, Feinstein A. Unexplained neurologic symptoms: a fMRI study of sensory conversion disorder. *Neurology* 2006;**67**:2036–2038.

143. Montoya A, Price BH, Lepage M. Neural correlates of "functional" symptoms in neurology. *Funct Neurol* 2006;**21**:193–197.

144. Vuilleumier P. Hysterical conversion and brain function. *Prog Brain Res* 2005;**150**:309–329.

145. Ballmaier M, Schmidt R. Conversion disorder revisited. *Funct Neurol* 2005;**20**:105–113.

146. Aybek S, Kanaan RA, David AS. The neuropsychiatry of conversion disorder. *Curr Opin Psychiatry* 2008;**21**:275–280.

147. Tiihonen J, Kuikka J, Viinamaki H, *et al.* Altered cerebral blood flow during hysterical paresthesia. *Biol Psychiatry* 1995;**37**:134–135.

148. Spence SA. All in the mind? The neural correlates of unexplained physical symptoms. *Advan Psychiatr Treat* 2006;**12**:349–358.

149. Yaźići KM, Kostakoglu L. Cerebral blood flow changes in patients with conversion disorder. *Psychiatry Res* 1998;**83**:163–168.

150. Birklein F, Riedl B, Sieweke N, *et al.* Neurological findings in complex regional pain syndromes: analysis of 145 cases. *Acta Neurol Scand* 2000;**101**:262–269.

151. Agrawal SK, Rittey CD, Harrower NA, *et al.* Movement disorders associated with complex regional pain syndrome in children. *Dev Med Child Neurol* 2009;**51**:557–562.

152. Lebel A, Becerra L, Wallin D, *et al.* fMRI reveals distinct CNS processing during symptomatic and recovered complex regional pain syndrome in children. *Brain* 2008;**131**:1854–1879.

153. Silver FW. Management of conversion disorder. *Am J Phys Med Rehabil* 1996;**75**:134–140.

154. Stone J, Carson A, Sharpe M. Functional symptoms in neurology: management. *J Neurol Neurosurg Psychiatry* 2005;**76**(Suppl 1):i13–i21.

155. Carson AJ, Ringbauer B, Stone J, *et al.* Do medically unexplained symptoms matter? A prospective cohort study of 300 new referrals to neurology outpatient clinics. *J Neurol Neurosurg Psychiatry* 2000;**68**:207–210.

156. Anderson KE, Gruber-Baldini AL, Vaughan CG, *et al.* Impact of psychogenic movement disorders versus Parkinson's on disability, quality of life, and psychopathology. *Mov Disord* 2007;**22**:2204–2209.

157. Salmon P, Peters S, Stanley I. Patients' perceptions of medical explanations for somatisation disorders: qualitative analysis. *BMJ* 1999;**318**:372–376.

158. Stone J, Wojcik W, Durrance D, *et al.* What should we say to patients with symptoms unexplained by disease? The "number needed to offend." *BMJ* 2002;**325**:1449–1450.

159. Kanaan R, Armstrong D, Barnes P, *et al.* In the psychiatrist's chair: how neurologists understand conversion disorder. *Brain* 2009 **132**:2889–2896.

160. Jankovic J. Treatment of hyperkinetic movement disorders. *Lancet Neurol* 2009;**8**:844–856.

161. Malhi P, Singhi P. Clinical characteristics and outcome of children and adolescents with conversion disorder. *Indian Pediatr* 2002;**39**:747–752.

162. Hinson VK, Weinstein S, Bernard B, *et al.* Single-blind clinical trial of psychotherapy for treatment of psychogenic movement disorders. *Parkinsonism Relat Disord* 2006;**12**:177–180.

163. Dallocchio C, Arbasino C, Klersy C, Marchioni E. The effects of physical activity on psychogenic movement disorders. *Mov Disord* 2010;**25**:421–425.

164. Sumathipala A. What is the evidence for the efficacy of treatments for somatoform disorders? A critical

review of previous intervention studies. *Psychosom Med* 2007;**69**:889–900.

165. Kroenke K. Efficacy of treatment for somatoform disorders: a review of randomized controlled trials. *Psychosom Med* 2007;**69**:881–888.

166. Essau CA. Course and outcome of somatoform disorders in non-referred adolescents. *Psychosomatics* 2007;**48**:502–509.

167. Moene FC, Spinhoven P, Hoogduin KA, *et al.* A randomised controlled clinical trial on the additional effect of hypnosis in a comprehensive treatment programme for in-patients with conversion disorder of the motor type. *Psychother Psychosom* 2002;**71**:66–76.

168. Bragier DK, Venning HE. Conversion disorders in adolescents: a practical approach to rehabilitation. *Br J Rheumatol* 1997;**36**:594–598.

169. Ness D. Physical therapy management for conversion disorder: case series. *J Neurol Phys Ther* 2007;**31**:30–39.

170. Bloom PB. Treating adolescent conversion disorders: are hypnotic techniques reusable? *Int J Clin Exp Hypnosis* 2001;**49**:243–256.

171. Voon V, Lang AE. Antidepressant treatment outcomes of psychogenic movement disorder. *J Clin Psychiatry* 2005;**66**:1529–1534.

172. O' Malley PG, Jackson JL, Santoro J, *et al.* Antidepressant therapy for unexplained symptoms and symptom syndromes. *J Fam Pract* 1999;**48**:980–990.

173. Hazell P, O ' Connell D, Heathcote D, *et al.* Tricyclic drugs for depression in children and adolescents. *Cochrane Database Syst Rev* 2002; (2):CD002317.

174. Hinson VK, Cubo E, Comella CL, *et al.* Rating scale for psychogenic movement disorders: scale development and clinimetric testing. *Mov Disord* 2005;**20**:1592–1597.

175. Crimlisk HL, Bhatia K, Cope H, *et al.* Slater revisited: 6 year follow up study of patients with medically unexplained motor symptoms. *BMJ* 1998;**316**:582–586.

176. McKeon A, Ahlskog JE, Bower JH, *et al.* Psychogenic tremor: long-term prognosis in patients with electrophysiologically confirmed disease. *Mov Disord* 2009;**24**:72–76.

177. Gudmundsson O, Prendergast M, Foreman D, *et al.* Outcome of pseudoseizures in children and adolescents: a 6-year symptom survival analysis. *Develop Med Child Neurol* 2001;**43**:547–551.

178. Pehlivantürk B, Unal F: Conversion disorder in children and adolescents: a four-year follow-up study. *J Psychosom Res* 2002;**52**:187–191.

179. Bhatia MS, Sapra S. Pseudoseizures in children: a profile of 50 cases. *Clin Pediatr* 2005;**44**:617–621.

180. Princiotta D, Bielick S. *Homeschooling in the United States: 2003.* [NCES 2006–042] Washington, DC: US Department of Education. National Center for Education Statistics, 2006, http://nces.ed.gov/pubs2006/2006042.pdf (accessed 12 May 2011).

Chapter

Childhood disorders: another perspective

Kelly M. Isaacs, Matthew D. Johnson, Erica Kao, and Donald L. Gilbert

Introduction

Psychogenic movement disorders (PMDs) cause substantial disability in adults [1] but few studies have characterized pediatric PMDs [2,3]. Challenges to proper diagnosis in children include skill in recognizing complex phenomenology of PMDs and in discerning normal and abnormal movements in children as well as the absence of a gold standard diagnostic test. The study described in this chapter aimed to clarify the characteristics of children and adolescents diagnosed with PMDs to aid clinicians in making an accurate diagnosis.

Methods

Permission for the retrospective study was granted by the Cincinnati Children's Hospital Medical Center Institutional Review Board. Patients evaluated between the years of 2003 and 2007 in the Movement Disorders Clinic at the center were identified from electronic records using the search terms "psychogenic movement disorder" and "conversion disorder." Consistent with recent practice recommendations [4], the diagnostic approach in most cases was based on presence of positive symptoms of PMDs. These included (1) history of sudden onset and offset; (2) observed features of distractibility; (3) entrainability; (4) inconsistent and variable amplitude, frequency, direction of movements; and (5) inconsistent effects of rest, posture, and motion on the movements. Cases were classified as "documented" or "clinically established" [5]. The presence of an identified, temporally related psychosocial stressor was not required for the diagnosis.

Data were abstracted from our New Movement Disorder Consultation Intake questionnaires. Patients were classified as having a "self-model" if their psychogenic movements were superimposed on a pre-existing similar, diagnosed movement disorder or "family model" based on their exposure to a family member with a similar, diagnosed movement disorder. The presence of psychiatric symptoms (e.g., excess worry) and diagnoses was queried directly and systematically. Parents rated current academic performance as failing, below average, average, or above average. Video-taped examinations, when available, were re-reviewed.

The predominant phenomenology was classified as tics, tremor, chorea/athetosis, dystonia, ataxia, or mixed based, as described in Table 8.1.

Results

Out of a total of 1915 patients seen in the clinic from 2003 to 2007, 52 (2.7%) met the diagnostic criteria for PMD, of which 49 had complete data. Age range was 6 to 20 years. The proportion of females was 64.5% in those under 13 years of age and 70% in those over 13 years (not significant). Key characteristics are shown in Table 8.2.

Compliance with recommended follow up with both neurology and with mental health was approximately 60%. Medication was prescribed for 13 (28%) children, mainly selective serotonin reuptake inhibitors to treat anxiety or mood disorders. Twelve children (25%) had been hospitalized for the diagnosis. Predominant stressors were academic, family, and other personal/social [6].

Discussion

The occurrence of aPMD causes significant distress and disruption to a child's life, and such PMDs are usually best understood as abnormal illnesses behaviors

Psychogenic Movement Disorders and Other Conversion Disorders, ed. Mark Hallett, Anthony E. Lang, Joseph Jankovic, Stanley Fahn, Peter W. Halligan, Valerie Voon, and C. Robert Cloninger. Published by Cambridge University Press. © Cambridge University Press 2011.

Table 8.1 Pediatric psychogenic movement disorders: diagnostic features

Predominant phenomenology	Feature of predominant phenomenology	Positive feature of psychogenic movement disorder
Tremor	Oscillation around joint	Direction, amplitude, and/or frequency variable; entrainable
Tic	Paroxysmal, patterned	Urge denied, suppressibility denied, persistence during voluntary action in same body area on examination, rhythmic and entrainable, semi-patterned
Chorea/athetosis	Continuous, random	Entrainable, semi-patterned
Ataxia	Balance difficulty	Astasia abasia, dramatic gait and limb movements, absence of other features of cerebellar disease
Dystonia	Twisting	Posturing inconsistent, position or action effects inconsistent

Table 8.2 Demographics, clinical features, and stressors in the Cincinnati cohort

Characteristics	
Total No.	49
Female/male (No. [% female])	33/16 (68)
Mean age at onset (years [SD])	13 (3.0)
Race (No. [%])	
Caucasian	43 (88)
African-American	2 (4)
Hispanic/other	4 (8)
Neurological disease model (No. [%])	
Self	7 (14)
Family (close relative)	10 (20)
Predominant phenomenology (No. [%])	
Tremor	17 (35)
Tics	17 (35)
Chorea/athetosis	2 (4)
Gait ataxia	2 (4)
Mixed	11 (22)
Psychosocial factors (No. [%])	
Immediate prior stressor	41 (84)
Prior psychiatric diagnoses	20 (41)
Married parents	27 (55)
Above average academically	24 (49)
Medical: hospitalized	12 (25)

in children overwhelmed by some form of stress. Most but not all children with PMDs have experienced identifiable stressors, but many have poor insight into stress as a possible cause. Female gender and high academic achievement appear to be important risk factors [4,7].

The high prevalence of psychogenic tics in our study has not been reported in other samples [2,4,8]. This diagnosis can be challenging [9,10] (of all PMDs, tics are most difficult to differentiate from organic movement disorders). Children usually described these as involuntary, denying premonitory urge or a semi-voluntary component. Onset was often dramatic. Unlike true tics, on examination, these generally did not abate during focused tasks but could be distractable. Videotape review was sometimes helpful for identifying deviations from a pattern (e.g., subtle changes in direction of jerks). Several individuals were also diagnosed with Tourette syndrome or had family members with this diagnosis. Although difficult to validate, the clinicians' impressions were not consistent with malingering (although, like other neurological symptoms such as headaches, some purposeful manipulation may occur with tics). Although the prevalence of psychogenic tics in our sample likely reflects referral bias, we also believe these are underdiagnosed. We suggest psychogenic tics be considered in the differential diagnosis of sudden appearance or worsening of tics.

References

1. Anderson KE, Gruber-Baldini AL, Vaughan CG, *et al.* Impact of psychogenic movement disorders versus Parkinson's on disability, quality of life, and psychopathology. *Mov Disord* 2007;**22**:2204–2209.

2. Schwingenschuh P, Pont-Sunyer C, Surtees R, Edwards MJ, Bhatia KP. Psychogenic movement disorders in children: a report of 15 cases and a review of the literature. *Mov Disord* 2008;**23**:1882–1888.

3. Ferrara J, Jankovic J. Psychogenic movement disorders in children. *Mov Disord* 2008;**23**:1875–1881.

4. Lang AE. General overview of psychogenic movement disorders: epidemiology, diagnosis, and prognosis.

In Hallet M, Fahn S, Jankovic J, *et al.*, eds. *Psychogenic Movement Disorders: Neurology and Neuropsychiatry*. Philadelphia, PA: Lippincott Williams & Wilkins, 2006:35–41.

5. Williams DT, Ford B, Fahn S. Phenomenology and psychopathology related to psychogenic movement disorders. *Adv Neurol* 1995;**65**:231–257.

6. Isaacs KM, Kao E, Johnson MD, Gilbert DL. Precipitating events and significant life stressors of pediatric patients diagnosed with a psychogenic movement disorder. In *37th Annual Meeting of the International Neuropsychological Society*, Atlanta, GA, February, 2009.

7. Grattan-Smith P, Fairley M, Procopis P. Clinical features of conversion disorder. *Arch Dis Child* 1988;**63**:408–414.

8. Ahmed MA, Martinez A, Yee A, Cahill D, Besag FM. Psychogenic and organic movement disorders in children. *Dev Med Child Neurol* 2008;**50**:300–304.

9. Dooley JM, Stokes A, Gordon KE. Pseudo-tics in Tourette syndrome. *J Child Neurol* 1994;**9**:50–51.

10. Kurlan R, Deeley C, Como PG. Psychogenic movement disorder (pseudo-tics) in a patient with Tourette's syndrome. *J Neuropsychiatry Clin Neurosci* 1992;**4**:347–348.

Chapter

9

Clinical features and treatment outcome of conversion disorder in children and adolescents

Teresa Bennett, Patricia I. Rosebush, and Michael F. Mazurek

Introduction

Conversion disorder (CD) in children and adolescents is relatively understudied and, with few exceptions [1,2], reports have focused on those with acute, short-term disturbances of less than a week. The study described here prospectively assessed 23 individuals under 18 years of age who developed CD and whose median duration of illness, at the time of referral, was 12 months.

Methods

Twenty patients were referred by neurologists and three by psychiatrists. All had seen one neurologist and the vast majority had seen more than two, prior to referral. All had been extensively investigated. Patients were assessed psychiatrically (PR, TB) and neurologically (MM) for diagnosis confirmation and to identify concurrent conditions. After assessment, three refused any type of psychiatric intervention. The remaining 20 were treated by the authors. Data were gathered with respect to demographic features, CD type, precipitating and predisposing factors, degree of impairment, medical and psychiatric comorbidity, response to treatment, and long-term outcome.

Results

Clinical features

The patient group included 15 girls and 8 boys, with a mean age of 14.6 years (SE, 2.5; range, 10–18). In those aged 10–13 years, there were essentially equal numbers of boys (4) and girls (3), while girls predominated in the adolescent subgroup (4 boys to 12 girls).

The nature of the primary CD presentation was loss of voluntary movement in one or more limbs in

11, psychogenic non-epileptic seizures (PNES) in 8, ataxia/gait disturbance in 3, and psychogenic blindness in 1. Nine patients displayed more than one type of CD concurrently.

In every child, CD was associated with severe functional impairment and 17 of the 23 (74%) were unable to attend school; 5 of these 17 were completely bedridden and another 5 required a wheelchair for mobilization. Six individuals attended school on a part-time basis only. Ten (43%) had been hospitalized on medical units for investigations, prior to diagnosis.

The more remote psychosocial histories of nine patients (40%) involved sexual, physical or mental abuse, and/or significant neglect. Precipitants, defined as life events that were identified by the patient or a parent/guardian as stressful and that were temporally associated with the onset of CD, were identified in almost every patient (22 of 23) and several had more than one precipitating factor. Psychosocial precipitants were identified in 18 and included parental divorce or loss of a significant other in 8, academic/athletic failure in 4, witnessing extreme violence in 2, being bullied in 2, and the onset of serious medical illness in a family member in 2. Secondary gain, in the form of school avoidance, was identified in four children. In none of the children did we identify sexual abuse as a precipitant to the development of CD, although this may well reflect underreporting, given the difficulties faced by both families and patients in divulging such information.

With respect to comorbid conditions, three children had a known history of seizures. Following referral to our clinic, we diagnosed postconcussive syndrome in three and atypical migraine headaches in one. In total, 19 patients (82%) had either a comorbid

---

Psychogenic Movement Disorders and Other Conversion Disorders, ed. Mark Hallett, Anthony E. Lang, Joseph Jankovic, Stanley Fahn, Peter W. Halligan, Valerie Voon, and C. Robert Cloninger. Published by Cambridge University Press. © Cambridge University Press 2011.

Table 9.1 Comorbid and precipitating medical conditions in 20 youth with conversion disorder

Condition	No. (%)[a]	Type of conversion disorder
Concussion	7 (35)	Mixed
Non-concussive physical injury	7 (35)	Mixed
Seizures	4 (20)	Pseudoseizures in all
Severe influenza/viral illness	3 (15)	Paralysis in all
Atypical migraine headaches	2 (10)	Ataxia

[a] Three individuals had more than one condition.

Table 9.2 Characteristics of children and adolescents with psychogenic non-epileptic seizures versus other conversion disorder type

	Pseudoseizure (*n* = 8)	Other CD (*n* = 15)
Female gender (No. [%])	6 (75)	8 (54)
Mean age (years [SD])	15.13 (2.8)	14.53 (2.4)
Child (< 13 years) (No. [%])	2 (25)	4 (27)
Duration of CD prior to diagnosis (months [SD])	41.25 (41.5)	11.87 (17.3)
GAF score (SD)	46.25 (16.2)	41.43 (14.6)
Full or partial recovery (No. [%])[a]	5 (63)	13 (87)
History of physical trauma (No. [%])	4 (50)	12 (80)
Psychiatric comorbidity (No. [%])	7 (88)	9 (60)
Complete absence from school (No. [%])	5 (63)	12 (80)
History of abuse (No. [%])[b]	2 (25)	7 (47)

CD, conversion disorder; GAF, Global Assessment of Functioning.
[a] Full recovery was defined as remission of all conversion disorder symptoms and return to full functioning. Individuals were classified as "partially recovered" if they had some residual symptoms but significant functional improvement with return to normal activities.
[b] The term "abuse" entailed any history of physical, sexual or emotional abuse or neglect.

or a precipitating medical illness (Table 9.1). Thirteen patients (56%) met DSM-1V [3] diagnostic criteria for one or more additional psychiatric illnesses either prior to, or concurrent with, the development of CD and four others developed another disorder after the resolution of their CD. Anxiety disorder was the most common diagnosis (7), followed by depression (4), personality disorder (4), eating disorder (2), somatization disorder (2), and substance abuse (1).

When the eight patients with PNES were compared with the 15 with other types of CD, with respect to demographic features, duration of illness, psychiatric and neurological comorbidity, psychosocial history, and the presence of identifiable precipitating stresses, there were no significant differences between the two groups (Table 9.2). The phenomenology of the PNES, both convulsive and non-convulsive, in these younger patients was indistinguishable from that described in adults [4]. Important features that pointed to PNES included swooning, thrashing, side-to-side head movements, pelvic thrusting, marked affective expression such as moaning or crying, and memory for the event.

Treatment and outcome

Three patients refused to engage in any type of psychiatric treatment. Of the remaining 20, 14 were treated as outpatients, and 6 were treated on the inpatient psychiatric unit with a mean length of stay of 6.3 weeks (SD, 7.5; range, 1–24). Of the sample of 23 children, 14 (61%) recovered fully and 4 others (17%) responded partially, with significant functional improvement

Table 9.3 Characteristics of children and adolescents with full or partial versus no recovery from conversion disorder

	Full or partial recovery (n = 18)[a]	No recovery (n = 5)[b]
Mean age (years [SD])	14.28 (2.3)	16.40 (2.6)
Child (< 13 years) (No. [%])	5 (28)	1 (20)
CD duration prior to diagnosis (months [SD])	15.89 (26)	44.40 (38)o
GAF score (SD)	41.76 (13)	48.00 (22)
Presence of pseudoseizures (No. [%])	5 (28)	3 (60)
Psychiatric comorbidity (No. [%])	12 (68)	4 (80)
Complete absence from school (No. [%])*	15 (83)	2 (40)
History of abuse (No. [%])[c]	6 (33)	3 (60)

CD, conversion disorder; GAF, Global Assessment of Functioning.
[a] Full recovery was defined as remission of all conversion disorder symptoms and return to full functioning (n = 14); "partially recovered" was defined as continuing to have residual symptoms but significant functional improvement (n = 4).
[b] No recovery was defined as demonstrating minimal or no change in conversion symptoms, with ongoing and significant dysfunction.
[c] The term "abuse" entailed any history of physical, sexual, emotional abuse or neglect, or combination thereof.
* $p < 0.05$.

and return to normal activities, within 6 months. Table 9.3 summarizes the clinical characteristics in those who recovered compared with those who did not. Chi-squared and Fisher's exact tests were performed to determine whether child characteristics or circumstances outlined in Table 9.3 were significantly associated (significance taken as $p < 0.05$) with recovery status. Interestingly, children who were completely absent from school at the time of diagnosis were more likely to recover, either partially or completely (Fisher's exact test, $p = 0.02$). This may reflect the fact that more severe dysfunction triggers more aggressive intervention. Not surprisingly, the mean duration of illness prior to diagnosis and treatment also appeared to differ between the recovery and non-recovery groups (15.89 and 44.40 months, respectively) and approached significance ($p = 0.07$). No other statistically significant associations were found, possibly owing to the small sample size and related power limitations. Treatment included physiotherapy, education about comorbid or underlying conditions, psychoeducation regarding the role of stress in illness and the concept of mind–body interplay, psychotherapy with a focus upon identified precipitants, and medication, when appropriate, for comorbid conditions. The median time of follow-up was 3.3 years (range, 1–12). During the follow-up period, two fully recovered patients relapsed but again enjoyed complete recovery. Four patients subsequently developed depression and anxiety disorder and two others

developed medical problems, the expeditious diagnosis of which was hampered by their prior history of CD. One female patient with a pre-CD history of post-traumatic stress disorder committed suicide at age 22, years after successful treatment of CD at 16 years of age. It is noteworthy that several patients who were treated and recovered fully from CD were subsequently able to cope, without relapse, in the face of new and significant psychosocial stresses, including the murder of a friend, the near fatal illness of a sibling, and a motor vehicle accident. One of the three patients who refused to engage in any type of psychiatric treatment died from the sequelae of prolonged immobility while on a medical unit.

Discussion

A number of conclusions can be drawn from this sample. Female patients with CD outnumbered males in adolescence but not in childhood. In this group of children and adolescents, CD was prolonged prior to treatment and was associated with a considerable burden of suffering and impairment, as previously reported in the literature [1,5].

Despite the severity and duration of illness, CD in these children and adolescents was very responsive to treatment.

In the series described here, there was a very high rate of precipitating or comorbid medical/neurological illness, suggesting that related symptoms may provide a stimulus for the development of a somatoform disorder, in the context of other psychosocial stresses. There are other reports in the literature of a high rate of psychiatric comorbidity, particularly anxiety and depression, in youth with CD [1,6].

Occurrence of CD in children and adolescents merits expeditious diagnosis and treatment because of the severe impairment that can ensue. Investigations and treatment are best carried out in a setting where there is a close working relationship between psychiatry and neurology.

References

1. Ferrara J, Jankovic J. Psychogenic movement disorders in children. *Mov Disord* 2008;**23**:1875–1881.

2. Schwingenschuh P, Pont-Sunyer C., Surtees R., Edwards MJ, Bhatia K. Psychogenic movement disorders in children: a report of 15 cases and a review of the literature. *Mov Disord* 2008;**23**:1882–1888.

3. American Psychiatric Association. *Diagnostic and Statistical Manual of Diseases*, 4th edn. Washington DC: American Psychiatric Press, 1994.

4. Boon P, Williamson P. The diagnosis of pseudoseizures. *Clin Neurol Neurosurg* 1993;**95**:1–8.

5. Kozlowska K, Nunn K., Rose D, Morris A, Ouvrier RA, Varghese J. Conversion disorder in Australian pediatric practice. *J Am Acad Child Adolesc Psychiatry* 2007;**46**:68–75.

6. Wyllie E, Glazer JP, Benbadis S, Kotagal P, Wolgamuth B. Psychiatric features of children and adolescents with pseudoseizures. *Arch Pediatr Adolesc Med* 1999;**153**:224–228.

10
Somatoform disorders and psychogenic movement disorders

Michael Sharpe, Jon Stone, and Alan J. Carson

Introduction

Many of the physical symptoms that patients present to doctors cannot be explained by our current knowledge of bodily disease. A failure to appreciate this has resulted in a large and neglected problem for both medical practitioners and clinical services [1]. Currently there is a lack of consensus on the key questions of what to call these symptoms, how to conceptualize them, and on how to treat them.

This chapter will consider the name and conceptualization of these symptoms and the implications of these for management with special reference to movement disorders judged to be unexplained by organic disease, so-called "psychogenic" movement disorders (PMD).

The prevalence and importance of physical symptoms unexplained by disease in medicine in general and in neurological practice in particular will be considered first. This will be followed by a consideration of the names used to describe the associated conceptualizations as medical or psychiatric conditions. Thirdly, the psychiatric concept of somatoform disorders and the advantages and disadvantages of applying this label to patients with PMD will be described. Our own practical suggestions on the best label and conceptualization of PMD will be offered with, finally, a brief discussion of potential future developments in this area.

Physical symptoms unexplained by disease

The problem in medicine

Medical students may be taught, and even believe, that most of the physical symptoms that patients present with will have a clear basis in identifiable organic disease. It might be expected that if an organic disease was not initially apparent it would always eventually be found if one simply kept on searching. This was surely the best way to serve patients.

But clinical experience and accumulating research evidence tell us that this belief is simply untrue. A very substantial proportion of the physical symptoms that patients present to their doctors are not found, even after extensive and repeated investigation, to be attributable to organic disease, at least within our current state of knowledge [1]. In primary care, such patients make up a substantial number, if not the majority, of presentations [2,3]. In specialist medical care, at least a third of the symptoms patients present with are found to be inadequately explained by organic disease [4,5]. And of the medical specialties, neurology has one of the highest rates of patients presenting with symptoms unexplained by organic disease [5], perhaps in part because of the greater ability of neurologists compared with many other specialists to exclude organic disease.

Do such unexplained symptoms really matter? If one sees one's role as a physician as purely to identify and treat organic disease, perhaps they do not. However, if one sees one's role more broadly as the relief of suffering, they certainly do. Patients with these symptoms are commonly distressed and disabled as well as being symptomatic [6], and consequently they may be judged to be as deserving of medical care as patients with disease are [7].

The problem of symptoms unexplained by organic disease in neurology

In recent years, we have learned much about the symptoms unexplained by organic disease that are seen in neurological practice. We know that approximately

Psychogenic Movement Disorders and Other Conversion Disorders, ed. Mark Hallett, Anthony E. Lang, Joseph Jankovic, Stanley Fahn, Peter W. Halligan, Valerie Voon, and C. Robert Cloninger. Published by Cambridge University Press. © Cambridge University Press 2011.j

10% of patients referred to general neurological clinics have symptoms that are entirely unexplained by organic disease, and about a further 20% have symptoms that, at best, are only partially explained by organic disease [8]. As in other areas of medicine, it has been shown that many of these patients are distressed and disabled and, on average, often more so than patients with organic, neurological disease [9]. These symptoms and the associated disability also often persist despite reassurance [10–12], even in the very long term [13,14].

Consequently, a neurologist who is only interested in disease is likely to be frustrated by a third of the patients who seek his or her help for physical symptoms that are distressing and disabling but which are not explained by organic disease. Indeed, the more unexplained the patient's symptoms are by disease, the more difficulty the neurologists find in helping them [15].

The area of neurological practice that specializes in movement disorders, perhaps unsurprisingly, also sees many patients where a conventional explanation in terms of organic pathology cannot be plausibly applied. These patients are often referred to as having PMDs. The term PMD usually refers to tremor, gait disturbance, and other abnormal movements. However the phenomenon of PMD overlaps with common neurological presentations of weakness and non-epileptic attacks and also with more general symptoms such as pain and fatigue.

How do we describe and understand symptoms unexplained by organic disease?

The practice of medicine requires that we name illnesses by making diagnoses. Diagnoses are essential for communication between doctors, between doctors and patients, and for the generation and application of evidence regarding treatment and prognosis. In areas of medicine where characteristic pathology (e.g., cancer) can be identified, diagnosis is relatively straightforward. However, what do we do when we can find no organic pathology? There are three main strategies, none of which are conspicuously successful in approaching the problem: we say that we do not know what causes them; we say that they are symptoms of organic disease that is not yet manifest, or we say they are physical manifestation of a psychological condition.

We do not know what causes them

One approach is to admit that we have limited understanding of what causes these symptoms. While those adopting this stance may feel scientifically righteous, it is both nihilistic and clinically unhelpful. The patient can only be told that their symptoms are "unexplained" and it remains unclear what is wrong, who will treat the patient, and how.

Symptoms of organic disease that is not yet manifest

Another strategy is to assume that such patients really do have organic, neurological disease (despite this not being demonstrable). It may be assumed that pathology will be found eventually on investigation or will emerge during follow-up. This view has been widely held [16] but has been refuted by modern evidence; not only do long-term follow-up studies show that such patients very rarely develop organic disease that explains their symptoms [8,17,18] but such a suggestion also risks both psychological and physical iatrogenic harm [19].

Physical manifestation of a psychological condition

The third strategy is to assume that if the symptoms are not physical they must be mental or "psychogenic." That is, if no organic pathology can be found there must be mental pathology. The diagnosis of mental pathology may be based on the presence of obvious psychological symptoms such as those of depression or anxiety or, if such symptoms are not prominent, mental pathology may simply be inferred and the symptoms regarded as evidence of a mental condition in somatic form: a somatoform disorder. We will consider the advantages and disadvantages of this in the following section.

Somatoform disorders

Somatoform disorders are a category of diagnoses listed in the *Diagnostic and Statistical Manual* (DSM) of the American Psychiatric Association, the main classification used for psychiatric diagnosis in the USA and much of the world and currently in its fourth edition [20]. The World Health Organization also includes somatoform disorders in its *International Classification of all Diseases* (ICD), currently in its 10th edition [21].

Table 10.1 The somatoform disorders in DSM-IV

Diagnosis	Notes
Somatization disorder	This refers to patients with years of multiple and variable medically unexplained physical symptoms, attributable to a variety of bodily systems. These include pseudoneurological conversion and dissociation symptoms. The threshold for this disorder is high, making it rare. Some regard it as a disorder of personality rather than an illness
Conversion disorder	Despite its psychodynamic origins, the term conversion is retained to describe unexplained symptoms that suggest a neurological condition (including motor symptoms, sensory symptoms and seizures). It is specified that psychological factors are associated
Undifferentiated somatoform disorder	This diagnosis is used for patients who have fewer symptoms than required for somatization disorder and a shorter duration (only 1 year). It is a vaguely specified and rather heterogeneous category
Pain disorder	This diagnosis is used where pain is the predominant symptom and is assumed to be at least partially psychological in origin
Hypochondriasis	An old term which has been retained to describe a preoccupation with the fear or idea of having a serious disease (e.g., motor neuron disease), based on the misinterpretation of bodily symptoms
Body dysmorphic disorder	This is grouped with the others because of the somatic medical presentation. It describes a preoccupation with an imagined or exaggerated defect in physical experience. These patients are commonly seen by plastic surgeons and uncommon in neurology clinics
Somatoform disorder not otherwise specified	This is a catch-all category to allow a diagnosis to be made for patients with unexplained somatic symptoms that do not meet criteria for any of the above disorders

The defining feature of a somatoform disorder in DSM-IV is "the presence of physical symptoms that suggest a general medical condition but are not fully explained by a general medical condition or another mental disorder."

The first psychiatric diagnostic manuals DSM-I and DSM-II did not include a somatoform category. These classifications were strongly influenced by the psychoanalytic theories dominant in American psychiatry at the time and included the concept of a neurosis. Neurosis was quite vaguely defined but encompassed both psychological and physical symptoms (including conversion reaction). Other somatic symptoms such as pain or gastrointestinal symptoms were described under psychophysiological disorders. As part of a move to make psychiatric diagnoses more reliable, DSM-III adopted less theoretical, more operational descriptions of psychiatric disorders with explicit diagnostic criteria for each. It abandoned neurosis as too vague and too associated with psychodynamic theory. However, its removal left no home (and no billing code) for those patients who were referred to psychiatrists with predominantly somatic symptoms considered to be psychological in origin [22]. It was to accommodate these patients that the somatoform category was created.

The creation of a group of conditions under the heading of somatoform disorders was based on the utility of putting somatic presentations of mental illness in one place, rather than on some over-arching theory or evidence of a common etiology. The specific disorders contained within the somatoform disorder group in DSM-IV are shown in Table 10.1.

As can be seen from inspection of these categories, those most relevant to the diagnosis of PMD are somatization disorder, conversion disorder, and perhaps also undifferentiated somatoform disorder.

It should be emphasized that somatoform disorders are only diagnosed when the patient's physical symptoms are not better explained by either a medical disorder or by another psychiatric disorder. Many patients with PMD may have depressive or anxiety disorders. However, determining the extent to which these psychiatric disorders explain the PMD is, of course, not straightforward.

Conceptually important, but in practice hard to operationalize, distinctions are those between somatoform disorders (in which symptoms are deemed to be produced unconsciously), factitious disorder (in which symptoms are consciously stimulated to obtain medical care), and malingering behavior (which is not a psychiatric disorder) [23].

Table 10.2 The potential advantages of a somatoform diagnoses

Advantages	Notes
They transcend medical specialties	Many of the patients with psychogenic movement disorders are likely to have other unexplained symptoms relevant to other medical specialties with different labels, such as non-cardiac chest pain. A somatoform diagnosis can offer one unifying summary as an alternative to multiple medical diagnoses
They indicate that medical care alone may be inadequate	The application of the diagnosis may stop excessive medical investigation and inappropriate medical treatment, and thereby reduce the risk of iatrogenic harm
They indicate a role for psychiatric or psychological treatments	A psychiatric diagnosis points to psychiatric management. The evidence we have suggests that patients with these conditions may benefit from psychological treatments such as cognitive behavioral therapy (see Chapter 39)
They legitimize referral to psychiatry or psychology	Without a psychiatric diagnosis, it may be hard to make a referral, and for the psychiatrist to justify treating the patient (and billing for this treatment)

Advantages of a diagnosing psychogenic movement disorders as somatoform disorder

The question here is if one has a patient with a PMD, are there any advantages in making a psychiatric diagnosis of somatoform disorder? Some potential advantages are listed in Table 10.2.

As we can see these diagnoses can add important additional information. They may allow a change of management. They may also convey additional specific information. This is particularly the case for diagnoses of hypochondriasis (which tells us that as well as symptoms the patient has a severe fear of having disease) and somatization disorder (which puts the current symptoms into a context of a long history of symptoms in many bodily systems).

Disadvantages of diagnosing psychogenic movement disorders as a somatoform disorder

Unfortunately, this solution to the problem of neurological symptoms unexplained by neurological disease also raises a number of difficulties, both theoretical and practical [24]. These are listed in Table 10.3.

Summary

In summary, here we encounter one of the major problems of modern medicine – the parallel worlds of psychiatry and the rest of medicine, including neurology. A neurologist seeing a patient with PMD may confidently state that there is no neurological disease present and the condition is, therefore psychogenic, and outside his or her expertise. The patient may then be referred to a psychiatrist on the presumption that the PMD is a psychiatric illness. The psychiatrist to whom the patient is referred may or may not identify psychological symptoms suggesting a psychiatric diagnosis, such as depression or anxiety, but may also decide that this patient's problems are physical and, therefore, also lie outside his or her expertise [25]. As we have seen, one way of solving this conundrum is to assume that hidden mental pathology is present and that the patient's problems are psychiatric after all. While this approach has some advantages, it is rarely an entirely satisfactory solution, either scientifically [26] or clinically [24]. So how should we proceed?

Practical suggestions for psychogenic movement disorders

The practical question is how should we best describe patients with PMD? The system currently in use by neurologists is based on describing the symptom (e.g., tremor or gait disorder) with an additional descriptor of "psychogenic." This has the advantage of being descriptive but the shortcoming of having few treatment implications. In addition, the description of the symptoms as "psychogenic" is problematic; the term "psychogenic" makes an assumption about the cause that may be both

Table 10.3 The potential disadvantages of a somatoform diagnoses

Problems	Notes
The implication that these conditions are mental illnesses	Although DSM does not say this explicitly, it is the implication of making a diagnosis listed in a book of "mental disorders." However, the absence of a medical explanation is arguably an inadequate reason to give a patient a psychiatric diagnosis
Questionable clinical judgments about psychological etiology are required	For conversion disorder, a judgment of the presence of associated psychological factors is required. Furthermore, any motivation for symptom production (according to the conversion hypothesis) must be judged to be unconscious; consciously produced symptoms are diagnosed as factitious disorder or malingering behavior
There is an unclear boundary with other psychiatric diagnoses	It can be difficult to differentiate a somatoform disorder from somatic symptoms of depression and anxiety, which may be missed. The boundary with dissociative and factitious disorders can be very difficult to define clinically
Pejorative and archaic terms	Despite attempts to purge DSM of archaic and psychodynamic terminology, conversion, somatization and hypochondriasis remain. These are mostly not well accepted by patients and carry substantial theoretical baggage
Lack of a common psychiatric and neurological terminology	These diagnoses are used mainly, and often only, by psychiatrists, whereas the patients are seen mainly by non-psychiatrists
Unclear relationship to the medical "functional" diagnoses	Medicine in general and neurology in particular have a variety of terms used for such patients, such as "functional" and "psychogenic" (as in psychogenic movement disorders) This is a parallel naming system; the precise mapping of somatoform diagnoses onto diagnoses such as psychogenic movement disorders is unclear
Acceptability to patients	Many if not most patients referred to a neurologist for physical symptoms will find a psychiatric diagnosis neither appropriate nor welcome

unjustified and unacceptable to patients. An alternative descriptor such as the term "functional" (reflecting a change in the function of a nervous system, rather than its structure) [27] may be preferable and more acceptable to patients [28]. However, some argue that this term also makes unproven assumptions (see Chapter 37).

The system used by psychiatrists using the DSM-IV psychiatric diagnostic system has the advantage of providing a good description of any associated psychological symptoms such as depression or panic. The patient with PMD may benefit from recognition of these diagnoses. However, for other patients, the psychiatric classification may simply relabel the symptoms with a psychiatric label. Such relabeling may be, perhaps reasonably, resisted by the patient.

Probably the best way forward is to go beyond this "either /or" way of thinking and rather adopt a "both/and" approach. That is, while we have two diagnostic systems we should make best use of both of them: we make a neurological diagnosis that describes the clinical phenomenon and also a psychiatric diagnosis where this is helpful. Simply replacing the term PMD with "somatoform disorder" or "undifferentiated somatoform disorder," or indeed "conversion disorder,"

is of questionable value. However, making a diagnosis of PMD plus panic disorder or somatization disorder adds information and potentially offers the best of both systems.

In summary, our recommendations for practice are as follows.

1. To use a neurological descriptive diagnosis of PMD or similar and describe the symptoms.
2. To consider using a term other than "psychogenic" to qualify the description, ideally one that is less potentially pejorative to the patient and more theoretically neutral. One candidate is "functional" movement disorder. This term is acceptable to patients and can facilitate discussion of both psychological and physiological etiologies [29,30].
3. To add an additional psychiatric diagnosis where this is justified and has useful implications for the management. This is most likely to be the case where the diagnosis of major depressive disorder or anxiety disorder can be made. The diagnosis of somatization disorder, hypochondriasis, or other somatoform disorder may sometimes be useful to make, particularly if it enables the application of a psychological treatment, such as cognitive

behavior therapy [31] as an alternative to further fruitless medical diagnosis and treatment.

The future

What developments can we anticipate in the naming and conceptualization of PMD? Ideally, we might look forward to a unified psychiatric/neurological diagnostic system to describe PMD that does not make strong assumptions about etiology, that is acceptable to patients, and that is useful in clinical practice. Will we get it?

The Task Force charged with defining the diagnoses for the new edition of DSM, DSM-V, which will be published in 2013, includes a group working on the conditions currently referred to as somatoform disorders. The work group aims to achieve a classification of diagnoses that are valid in terms of the limited scientific literature, are useful for psychiatrists, are acceptable to patients, and are also, as far as possible, used by non-psychiatrists, including neurologists. Addressing these requirements will be a major challenge. The view has been expressed that the best solution may be to abolish the somatoform disorders altogether [32,33]. However, the countervailing view is that this would merely lead to even greater neglect of these patients and make it more difficult for psychiatrists to become involved in their management [34]. The new somatoform disorder classification is not yet finalized, but proposals in early 2011 are radically different from that in DSM-V in the following ways.

Overall changes

1. There is an effort to improve the terminology and make it more acceptable: the section is currently called "Somatic Symptom Disorders" rather than Somatoform Disorders and the terms hypochondriasis and somatization disorder will be abolished.

2. There has been a move away from "medically unexplained" as the core criteria for making the diagnosis. This is because the definition of a psychiatric disorder is considered to require more than being unexplained by disease and an unproved assumption that there is underlying mental pathology (i.e., lack of physical does not equal psychological). Consequently, positive psychological criteria such as excessive concern about symptoms have been introduced into the new diagnoses.

3. There has been an attempt to simplify the previous multiple categories into three major disorders: complex somatic symptom disorder, simple somatic symptom disorder, and conversion disorder.

The provisional criteria for the three major new categories proposed are as follows.

Complex somatic symptom disorder. This will describe patients with one or more somatic symptoms (whether judged to be unexplained by organic disease or not) that are distressing or result in significant disruption in daily life and that are accompanied by psychological symptoms such as excessive preoccupation or concern about the symptoms. The symptoms must have lasted at least 6 months. This will incorporate the previous diagnoses of somatization disorder and hypochondriasis.

Simple somatic symptom disorder. This will be used to describe patients with fewer psychological associations or shorter duration.

Conversion disorder. There are a number of specific changes to conversion disorder, which is the diagnosis that may be used most often in relation to PMD. It describes one or more symptoms of altered voluntary motor or sensory function or apparent impaired consciousness that are unexplained by a neurological or other psychiatric condition. It has proved impossible to combine conversion disorder with complex somatic symptom disorder as lack of a disease explanation for the change in function is central to the diagnosis. At present, therefore, conversion disorder remains separate from complex somatic symptom disorder. The criteria for it have been simplified, however, to exclude the requirement for associated psychological factors, which is often unreliable. The differentiation of conversion and other somatic symptom disorders from deliberately and consciously feigned symptoms remains a problematic area. At present, it is likely that the explicit criteria to exclude feigning will be removed from specific conversion disorder criteria but will be retained as a differential diagnosis of all psychiatric disorders. There is debate about retaining the name "conversion disorder" and some support for the term "functional neurological symptoms" [35], although this issue is not resolved. There have also been proposals for the criteria to include the need for positive evidence of internal inconsistency or incongruity with disease in the classification to make explicit the way in which these disorders are diagnosed [35,36]. Finally there has been discussion about whether the category should remain within somatic symptom disorders or move to dissociative disorders [37].

Conclusions

While we do not know what the final version of DSM-V will bring, its shape is starting to become clear. The new version of ICD remains early in development and its form unclear. These new classifications will, hopefully, bring less pejorative terminology, such as somatic symptom disorder, and a simplification of the diagnostic categories. Within conversion disorder, improvements are likely (such as the exclusion of the identification of psychological factors) and the importance of specific neurological assessment should be made clear in the accompanying text, if not in the criteria.

However, there remains a fundamental problem. We still have separate neurological and psychiatric classifications. That means that we still have to make a decision about whether movement disorders are medical or psychiatric. Many, including the authors of this chapter, are of the view that we require a more open mind about the nature of these disorders and that their management requires not a dualistic decision to be made but rather a combined psychiatric/psychological and neurological perspective.

Consequently, trying to solve the problem of naming and understanding PMD simply by changing the psychiatric diagnostic system is arguably doomed to failure. As the old joke goes, the response to the traveler asking "How do I get to Dublin" might be "I wouldn't start from here if I were you." We, therefore, still look forward to a day where we can address this problem not from a purely neurological or psychiatric starting point but rather from a unified position that would facilitate the application of a combination of neurological, psychological, and psychiatric skills to the benefit of these patients.

References

1. Sharpe M. Medically unexplained symptoms and syndromes. *Clin Med* 2002;**2**:501–504.

2. Khan AA, Khan A, Harezlak J, Tu W, Kroenke K. Somatic symptoms in primary care: etiology and outcome. *Psychosom* 2003;**44**:471–478.

3. Fink P, Sorensen L, Engberg M, Holm M, Munk-Jorgensen P. Somatization in primary care: prevalence, health care utilization, and general practitioner recognition. *Psychosom* 1999;**40**:330–338.

4. Hamilton J, Campos R, Creed F. Anxiety, depression and the management of medically unexplained symptoms in medical clinics. *J R Coll Physicians Lond* 1996;**30**:18–20.

5. Nimnuan C, Hotopf M, Wessely S. Medically unexplained symptoms: an epidemiological study in seven specialities. *J Psychosom Res* 2001;**51**:361–367.

6. Lowe B, Spitzer RL, Williams JB, *et al.* Depression, anxiety and somatization in primary care: syndrome overlap and functional impairment. *Gen Hosp Psychiatry* 2008;**30**:191–199.

7. Kroenke K. Somatization in primary care: it's time for parity. *Gen Hosp Psychiatry* 2000;**22**:141–143.

8. Stone J, Carson A, Duncan R, *et al.* Symptoms "unexplained by organic disease" in 1144 new neurology out-patients: how often does the diagnosis change at follow-up? *Brain* 2009;**132**:2878–2888.

9. Carson AJ, Ringbauer B, Stone J, *et al.* Do medically unexplained symptoms matter? A prospective cohort study of 300 new referrals to neurology outpatient clinics. *J Neurol Neurosurg Psychiatry* 2000;**68**:207–210.

10. Carson AJ, Best S, Postma K, Stone J, Warlow C, Sharpe M. The outcome of neurology outpatients with medically unexplained symptoms: a prospective cohort study. *J Neurol Neurosurg Psychiatry* 2003;**74**:897–900.

11. McKenzie P, Oto M, Russell A, Pelosi A, Duncan R. Early outcomes and predictors in 260 patients with psychogenic nonepileptic attacks. *Neurol* 2010;**74**:64–69.

12. Ibrahim NM, Martino D, van de Warrenburg BP, *et al.* The prognosis of fixed dystonia: a follow-up study. *Parkinsonism Relat Disord* 2009;**15**:592–597.

13. Stone J, Sharpe M, Rothwell PM, Warlow CP. The 12 year prognosis of unilateral functional weakness and sensory disturbance. *J Neurol Neurosurg Psychiatry* 2003;**74**:591–596.

14. Reuber M, Pukrop R, Bauer J, *et al.* Outcome in psychogenic nonepileptic seizures: 1 to 10-year follow-up in 164 patients. *Ann Neurol* 2003;**53**:305–311.

15. Carson AJ, Stone J, Warlow C, Sharpe M. Patients whom neurologists find difficult to help. *J Neurol Neurosurg Psychiatry* 2004;**75**:1776–1778.

16. Slater EO. Diagnosis of hysteria. *BMJ* 1965;**i**:1395–1399.

17. Crimlisk HL, Bhatia K, Cope H, *et al.* Slater revisited: 6 year follow up study of patients with medically unexplained motor symptoms. *BMJ* 1998;**316**:582–586.

18. Stone J, Smyth R, Carson A, *et al.* Systematic review of misdiagnosis of conversion symptoms and "hysteria." *BMJ* 2005;**331**:989.

19. Kouyanou K, Pither CE, Wessely S. Iatrogenic factors and chronic pain. *Psychosom Med* 1997;**59**:597–604.

20. American Psychiatric Association. *Diagnostic and Statistical Manual of Diseases*, 4th edn. Washington DC: American Psychiatric Press, 1994.

21. World Health Organization. *The ICD-10 Classification of Mental and Behavioural Disorders,* 10th edn. Geneva: World Health Organization, 1992.

22. Bayer R, Spitzer RL. Neurosis, psychodynamics, and DSM-III. A history of the controversy. *Arch Gen Psychiatry* 1985;**42**:187–196.

23. Sharpe M. Distinguishing malingering from psychiatric disorders. In Halligan PW, Bass C, Oakley DA, eds. *Malingering and Illness Deception*. Oxford: Oxford University Press, 2003:156–170.

24. Sharpe M, Mayou R. Somatoform disorders: a help or hindrance to good patient care? *Br J Psych* 2004;**184**:465–467.

25. Espay AJ, Goldenhar LM, Voon V, *et al*. Opinions and clinical practices related to diagnosing and managing patients with psychogenic movement disorders: an international survey of Movement Disorder Society members. *Mov Disord* 2009;**24**:1366–1374.

26. DeGucht V, Fischler B. Somatization: a critical review of conceptual and methodological issues. *Psychosom* 2002;**43**:1–9.

27. Sharpe M, Carson AJ. "Unexplained" somatic symptoms, functional syndromes, and somatization: do we need a paradigm shift? *Ann Intern Med* 2001;**134**(9 Suppl):926–930.

28. Stone J, Wojcik W, Durrance D, *et al*. What should we say to patients with symptoms unexplained by disease? The "number needed to offend." *BMJ* 2002;**325**:1449–1450.

29. Stone J, Carson A, Sharpe M. Functional symptoms and signs in neurology: assessment and diagnosis. *J Neurol Neurosurg Psychiatry* 2005;**76**(Suppl 1):i2–i12.

30. Stone J, Carson A, Sharpe M. Functional symptoms in neurology: management. *J Neurol Neurosurg Psychiatry* 2005;**76**(Suppl)1:i13–i21.

31. Kroenke K. Efficacy of treatment for somatoform disorders: a review of randomized controlled trials. *Psychosom Med* 2007;**69**:881–888.

32. Mayou R, Levenson J, Sharpe M. Somatoform disorders in DSM-V. *Psychosom Med* 2003;**44**:449–451.

33. Mayou R, Kirmayer LJ, Simon G, Kroenke K, Sharpe M. Somatoform disorders: time for a new approach in DSM-V. *Am J Psychiatry* 2005;**162**:847–855.

34. Rief W, Isaac M. Are somatoform disorders "mental disorders"? A contribution to the current debate. *Curr Opin Psychiatry* 2007;**20**:143–146.

35. Stone J, LaFrance WC, Levenson JL, Sharpe M. Issues for DSM-5: conversion disorder. *Am J Psychiatry* 2010;**167**:626–627.

36. Kanaan RA, Carson A, Wessely SC, *et al*. What's so special about conversion disorder? A problem and a proposal for diagnostic classification. *Br J Psychiatry* 2010;**196**:427–428.

37. Brown RJ, Cardeña E, Nijenhuis E, Şar V, van der Hart O. Should conversion disorder be reclassified as a dissociative disorder in DSM V? *Psychosom Med* 2007;**48**:369–378.

Psychogenic non-epileptic seizures

W. Curt LaFrance, Jr.

Introduction

Psychogenic non-epileptic seizures (PNES) are time-limited, paroxysmal changes in movements, sensations, behaviors, and/or consciousness, presenting like epileptic seizures but not associated with epileptiform activity. Patients with PNES remain one of the most challenging populations to diagnose and treat in medical practice, although clinical findings and laboratory advances are emerging that more clearly establish the diagnosis.

Of the 1% of the US population diagnosed with seizures, presumed epilepsy, 5–20% have PNES [1]. On average, 7 years elapse between a patient's onset of PNES and the correct diagnosis [2]. The misdiagnosis of PNES is costly to patients, the healthcare system, and to society. Repeated workups and treatments for what is mistakenly thought to be epilepsy are estimated to incur $100 to $900 million per year in medical services in the USA [3]. Patients with PNES are prescribed antiepileptic drugs (AEDs) that do not treat, and may exacerbate PNES, have multiple laboratory tests performed, and may not receive the mental healthcare that could benefit them. Delayed diagnosis could lead to adverse effects from unneeded AEDs; iatrogenic complications from invasive procedures in continuous PNES (non-epileptic seizure status); medical costs through unnecessary hospitalization, treatment, and workup; delayed referral for appropriate psychiatric treatment; and employment difficulties and disability [4].

The first step in PNES treatment is proper diagnosis. Video electroencephalography (EEG) remains the gold standard for PNES diagnosis. Certain seizure types, such as frontal lobe epilepsy, may mimic PNES semiology; conversely, ictal characteristics of PNES may resemble epileptic seizures. New diagnostic techniques

may help to distinguish stereotypic semiology seen in frontal lobe seizures that are not seen in PNES. Bedside observations may also be of benefit in augmenting the video–EEG interpretation to establish the PNES diagnosis. In addition to reviewing these issues, this chapter also examines the methodology in PNES treatment trials, describing the challenges in conducting clinical trials with patients with overlapping neurological and psychiatric disorders. Finally, realizing that PNES is one of a spectrum of somatoform disorders, along with psychogenic movement disorders (PMD), the pertinent diagnostic literature in other conversion disorders is reviewed.

Non-epileptic seizures can be physiological or psychogenic in origin and can be difficult to distinguish from epileptic seizures, with both seizure types showing alterations in behavior, consciousness, sensation, and perception [5]. Recent research reveals clinically useful differentiating features at bedside and on video–EEG. Appropriate diagnosis then informs potential treatments.

Diagnosis

Distinguishing non-epileptic from epileptic seizures

The diagnosis and treatment of patients with PNES has long confounded neurologists, psychiatrists, and emergency department physicians. As an adjunct to anamnesis and video–EEG, ictal semiology, neurophysiological tests, patient characteristics, and neuropsychological testing contribute to making the diagnosis of PNES.

Differentiating PNES from epileptic seizures is the first step in appropriate treatment [6] as PNES can

---

Psychogenic Movement Disorders and Other Conversion Disorders, ed. Mark Hallett, Anthony E. Lang, Joseph Jankovic, Stanley Fahn, Peter W. Halligan, Valerie Voon, and C. Robert Cloninger. Published by Cambridge University Press. © Cambridge University Press 2011.

appear similar to epileptic seizures. To distinguish the two types of seizure, monitoring is essential [7]. In a study of raters reviewing one seizure captured on video paired with EEG for 22 individuals, video–EEG has been shown to have substantial interrater reliability for epilepsy and moderate reliability for PNES [8]. The interrater reliability is excellent when incorporating supplemental information, including history, physical, and more ictal segments [9]. Other techniques are used as adjuncts to informing the diagnosis of PNES [10], but admission to a seizure monitoring unit not only provides a definitive diagnosis in almost 90% of patients but also rectifies an incorrect diagnosis of epilepsy and results in treatment change in 79% of patients [11]. Monitoring a patient with seizures in the monitoring unit may also help to identify the 10% of patients who have mixed epilepsy/PNES [12]. Higher numbers of patients with a mixed etiology were listed in the literature in the past, but these appear to have been overestimates based on less stringent criteria for differentiating epilepsy from PNES.

Some physical observations of the ictal semiology used in differentiating PNES from epilepsy are noted in Table 11.1 [13].

Using data from video–EEG monitoring, researchers found that 50 of 52 patients with PNES (96%) closed their eyes during the seizure, compared with 152 of 156 of epileptic patients (97%), who had their eyes open at the beginning of their seizure [14]. This information might help clinicians to differentiate between PNES and epileptic seizures, particularly when the two types of seizures occur in the same patient. Also, other observers, such as family members, could report to physicians if the patient's eyes were open or closed during the ictal event. This observation, however, has been challenged by other authors, who prospectively assessed whether observer or self-report eye closure could predict PNES, prior to video–EEG monitoring [15]. In a seizure monitoring unit, 112 met study criteria and had either PNES (43 [38.4%]) or epilepsy (84 [75%]). The authors recorded eye closure as a percentage of episode duration, rather than the previously studied dichotomous absent versus present. Self-report of eye closure more accurately predicted actual video-recorded eye closure than observer report. The study confirmed that video-recorded eye closure was 92% specific for PNES identification, but not as sensitive (only 64%) as previously reported.

Patients with PNES may also exhibit geotropic eye movements, in which the eyes deviate downward to the side that the head is turned [16]. Eyelids are typically closed for a longer duration (20 s) compared with temporal lobe or frontal lobe seizures (~2 s) [17]. Weeping also is a characteristic with PNES [18,19].

Ictal stuttering and post-ictal whispering voice are seen in PNES [20,21]. Post-ictal nose rubbing and cough, however, have been observed in temporal lobe epilepsy but not in PNES [22]. Similarly, noisy or stertorous breathing can be seen post-ictally in epileptic convulsions but not following PNES convulsions [23]. While helping to differentiate convulsive epilepsy from convulsive PNES, this finding does not apply to partial seizures.

Pelvic thrusting reportedly is as common in frontal lobe seizures as in PNES. Other ictal features associated with PNES are out-of-phase or side-to-side oscillatory movements or chaotic and disorganized thrashing [5]. In contrast, frontal lobe seizures typically arise from sleep, are brief, and often involve vocalization and quick, tonic posturing [24,25]. Occasionally, whole-body trembling may be observed with PNES. These behaviors may wax, wane, and change over many minutes, which is atypical for epileptic seizures.

Physical injury during an ictus was once thought to occur only in patients with epilepsy, but research shows more than 50% of patients with PNES are injured during seizures [26]. The character of the injury is helpful in differentiating epileptic seizures from PNES. Excoriations on long bone surfaces, such as the arm, leg, or cheek, are seen in PNES [27], as opposed to lacerations from epilepsy. Tongue biting, self-injury, and incontinence are commonly associated with epileptic seizures but are also reported by up to two-thirds of patients with PNES, rendering these signs less specific than once thought [28].

Diagnostic measures

A common concern with diagnoses in the *Diagnostic and Statistical Manual of Mental Disorders* IV is that psychiatric diagnoses have no physiological correlates. While aggregate data on depression and anxiety states have revealed alterations in the hypothalamic–pituitary–adrenal axis [29,30], these findings are not applicable to the diagnosis of *individuals* with major depressive disorders or post-traumatic stress disorders. Psychogenic non-epileptic seizures are the neuropsychiatric exception to this rule, with diagnosis validated by a physiological measure and with

Table 11.1 Behaviors to distinguish psychogenic non-epileptic and epileptic seizures

Behavior	Psychogenic non-epileptic seizures	Epileptic seizures
Situational onset	Occasional	Rare
Gradual onset	Common	Rare
Precipitated by stimuli (noise, light)	Occasional	Rare
Purposeful movements	Occasional	Very rare
Opisthotonus "arc de cercle"	Occasional	Very rare
Tongue biting (tip)	Occasional	Rare
Tongue biting (side)	Rare	Common
Prolonged ictal atonia	Occasional	Very rare
Vocalization during tonic–clonic phase	Occasional	Very rare
Reactivity during "unconsciousness"	Occasional	Very rare
Rapid post-ictal reorientation	Common	Unusual
Undulating motor activity	Common	Very rare
Asynchronous limb movements	Common	Rare
Rhythmic pelvic movements	Occasional	Rare
Side-to-side head shaking	Common	Rare
Ictal crying	Occasional	Very rare
Ictal stuttering	Occasional	Rare
Post-ictal whispering	Occasional	Not present
Closed mouth in "tonic phase"	Occasional	Very rare
Closed eyelids during seizure onset	Very common	Rare
Convulsion > 2 min	Common	Very rare
Resisted lid opening	Common	Very rare
Pupillary light reflex	Usually retained	Commonly absent
Lack of cyanosis	Common	Rare
Ictal grasping	Rare	Occurs in frontal lobe and temporal lobe epilepsy
Post-ictal nose rubbing	Not present	Can occur in temporal lobe epilepsy
Stertorous breathing post-ictally	Not present	Common
Self-injury	May be present (particularly excoriations)	May be present (particularly lacerations)
Incontinence	May be present	May be present

Source: from Benbadis and LaFrance, 2010 [13] (assembled from references [14–28]).

adjunctive differentiation from epilepsy using the serum prolactin assay (see below).

Electroencephalography

Diagnosis of PNES is most accurately established by coregistering EEG neurophysiological testing with video. Video–EEG – where the patient's seizure is observed visually with simultaneous EEG – allows data about neurobehavior to be coupled with EEG rhythms. With the history and examination, the absence of expected epileptiform patterns before, during, and after the ictus points to a PNES diagnosis. Rarely, EEG-negative epilepsy on scalp EEG occurs, where a partial simple seizure, a frontal lobe seizure, or a deep temporal lobe seizure does not generate an ictal epileptiform pattern. Without video–EEG, neurologists' ability to differentiate epileptic seizures from PNES by history alone has a specificity of 50% [31].

One study described a method for diagnosing frontal lobe seizures by comparing the video and EEGs in a synchronized, side by side view [32]. Split-screen synchronized display was found to be a simple and valid technique for studying and presenting particular semiological aspects of epileptic seizures. Using this methodology to diagnose PNES may also be of value. Research continues to reveal that magnetoencephalography (MEG) is more useful than EEG for identification and localization of frontal lobe seizures [33], and MEG studies are attempting to develop optimal procedures for localizing interictal epileptiform discharges of patients with localization-related frontal lobe seizures. For those with a negative scalp EEG where the differential diagnosis of frontal lobe seizures and non-epileptic seizures is present, future research could examine the potential to screen for spikes in frontal lobe seizures, which are not seen in PNES.

Neurohumoral techniques

The use of serum prolactin drawn within 30 minutes of the ictus onset is helpful for differentiating generalized tonic–clonic epileptic seizures and partial complex epileptic seizures from PNES, as summarized in a recent report from the Therapeutics and Technology Assessment Subcommittee of the American Academy of Neurology [34]. Trimble first showed that generalized tonic–clonic seizures, but not PNES, raised serum prolactin [35]. Pooling the available data of the 10 studies meeting inclusion criteria, the subcommittee authors found a sensitivity of 60% for generalized tonic–clonic seizures and 46% for complex partial seizures, and a specificity of 96% for both. They found a positive predictive value of 93–99%. Cragar et al. similarly found lack of prolactin elevation has an average 89% sensitivity for PNES [10]. Clinically, this translates into a strong confirmation of a diagnosis of epileptic seizures when elevated serum prolactin is found in patients with generalized tonic–clonic or complex partial seizure-like events suspected of being PNES. The authors concluded that serum prolactin rise is probably a useful adjunct to differentiate generalized tonic–clonic or complex partial epileptic seizures from PNES.

Neuroimaging

Structural neuroimaging abnormalities neither confirm nor exclude epileptic seizures or PNES, as PNES may occur in the presence of focal lesions, as confirmed by case reports of patients with PNES who had central nervous system lesions [36]. One study showed that 10% of patients with PNES alone had structural abnormalities on magnetic resonance imaging (MRI) [37].

A negative ictal single-photon emission computed tomography (SPECT) scan does not imply a diagnosis of PNES nor does an abnormal scan mean epilepsy is present. A small series of ictal and interictal SPECT scans of patients with PNES revealed a few scans with lateralized perfusion abnormalities, but the findings did not change when the ictal and interictal images were compared [38]. Patients with epilepsy, in contrast, have dynamic changes when comparing ictal and interictal changes on functional neuroimaging.

Patient characteristics in psychogenic non-epileptic seizures

Neuropsychological measures

A large number of studies have described the cognitive, emotional, personality, and psychomotor differences between groups with epileptic seizures and with PNES. Cragar et al. reviewed the literature on adjunctive tests for diagnosing PNES and reported sensitivity and specificity of the different measures [10]. A summary of their findings noted that patients with epileptic seizures and PNES perform roughly the same on neuropsychological measures but worse than healthy controls. Patients with PNES performed better than patients with epileptic seizures on certain neuropsychological tests, as described below. Studies examining intelligence, psychomotor function, motivational measures, and personality features in PNES suggest the following.

For cognitive measures, patients with epileptic seizures and PNES show no significant differences on tests of intelligence, learning, and memory, but score lower than healthy control subjects [39]. On psychomotor measures, patients with PNES show reduced motor speed and grip strength compared with healthy controls [40]. Motivational measures reveal patients with PNES score lower than patients with epileptic seizures on some motivational measures, perhaps reflecting a lack of psychological resources necessary to persist with a challenging neuropsychological battery. Some studies show comparable failure rates in PNES and epileptic seizures groups on symptom validity batteries. Frank malingering is thought to occur rarely in non-epileptic seizures [41–43]. The Minnesota Multiphasic Personality Inventory (MMPI) has been used for over 20 years in assessing patients with PNES. Personality testing with instruments such as MMPI-2 show elevations in hypochondria, hysteria, and depression scores in PNES [9,44].

Family and patient traits

Studies comparing family functioning in patients with epileptic seizures and PNES reveal that individuals with PNES view their families as more dysfunctional, particularly in regard to communication, and that family members of patients with PNES reported difficulties defining roles [45]. Individuals with PNES score higher on Symptom Check Lists (a measure of somatic complaints) when compared with other patients with seizures [46]. Pain disorders are also common in patients with PNES. Among patients at an epilepsy clinic, a diagnosis of fibromyalgia or chronic pain has an 85% positive predictive value for PNES [47]. Occurrence of PNES could be thought of as a disorder of communication, where internal distress is conveyed somatically rather than verbally.

Summary of patient characteristics

Compared with healthy controls, patients with epileptic seizures and with PNES perform worse on a number of neuropsychological measures; however, there are few differences between groups with epileptic seizures and those with PNES that would reliably differentiate epileptic seizures from PNES. The impairments in the measures are thought to result from at least three factors: (1) both the patients with epileptic seizures and those with PNES were taking AEDs, which may affect cognition; (2) structural lesions occur in those with epileptic seizures and in some of the patients with PNES; and (3) emotional factors may contribute to cognitive impairment in the PNES group [48]. Psychologically, patients with PNES appear to have personalities with anxiety, cognitive, and somatic distress, with difficulties in expression and communication of that distress to family and others.

Treatment in psychogenic non-epileptic seizures

While many findings continue to be added to the diagnostic literature on PNES, there is limited information on the treatments for PNES with respect to controlled

trials over the past few years. The PNES treatment literature has been systematically summarized in two review articles [49,50] and in a Cochrane database [51], which provided a systematic assessment focused on psychotherapy trials for PNES. The bottom line from the reviews is that to advance the field beyond the numerous case reports, the handful of open label trials, and the few controlled trials involving small numbers of patients, we need controlled treatment trials for PNES. From a prevention perspective, interdisciplinary collaboration to aggressively address the known modifiable risk factor of abuse may have the greatest impact on lowering the incidence of PNES and other chronic psychiatric disorders [50].

Treatment considerations: addressing etiologies

As discussed above, once PNES is definitively diagnosed with video–EEG monitoring, the next step in treatment involves a presentation of the diagnosis of PNES. When done in a clear, non-pejorative, positive manner by the clinician, the presentation can act as a bridge between neurological diagnosis and psychiatric/psychological treatment. The psychiatric treatment that follows the presentation of the diagnosis of PNES begins with an adequate understanding of the individual's developmental history; assessment of comorbid psychiatric diagnoses, personality and coping styles, treatments, and psychosocial environment; and identification of precursors, precipitants, and perpetuating factors in their PNES. Psychogenic non-epileptic seizures are a symptom, not the disease itself. Subgroups of PNES characteristics may respond better to specific interventions directed at the contributing factor to PNES. With an understanding of the etiology of PNES, specific treatments can be directed both at the PNES phenomena and the underlying contributors to PNES. Porter describes a (1) psychopathology, (2) situational, and (3) voluntary basis for PNES [52]. One proposed process is that PNES is a somatic form of communication involving dissociative mechanisms [53]. The seizures are unconscious conversion symptoms which "are nonverbal communications facilitated by nonspecific factors that inhibit a more articulate verbal expression of ideas or emotions" [54].

Despite various references that propose the "heterogeneity" of PNES [55], there are two main "causes" of PNES: post-traumatic and developmental [56]. The heterogeneity that is present can be consolidated or

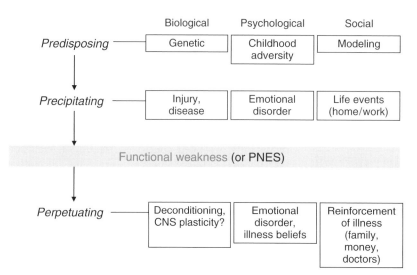

Fig. 11.1. What causes psychogenic non-epileptic seizures (PNES; or "functional weakness")? (From LaFrance and Bjørnæs, 2010 [58]; modified from Stone J. "Paralysis and Sensory Loss," a lecture given at the *Psychogenic Movement Disorders Workshop*, Atlanta GA October, 2003.)

"lumped" into pychiatric comorbidities, personality disorder symptoms, traumatic histories, and neurological symptoms that commonly occur in patients with PNES. Post-traumatic PNES is thought to develop in response to acute or chronic exposure to traumatic experience(s), such as physical or psychological trauma, sexual or physical abuse. Developmental PNES refers to coping difficulties with tasks and milestones along the individual's continuum of psychosocial development. A recent study assessing 288 patients examining potential etiologies confirmed that antecedent trauma and learning disabilities, where an individual may have difficulty with language or expression, were found to be the highest predictors of developing PNES [57].

Some clinicians and family members are suspicious that the individual is "faking it." A very limited number of individuals (< 5%) intentionally produce symptoms, including seizures and movement disorders. Malingering differs from PNES in that malingered seizures are consciously produced. Malingering is not a psychiatric diagnosis; rather, symptoms are feigned and used to get out of service, jail, or to gain benefits or medicine (Fig. 11.1) [58].

Methodological considerations in clinical trials

Regarding clinical trials, one recent methodology article addressed the challenges faced in clinical trials for PNES and other neuropsychiatric populations, such as those with traumatic brain injury and multiple sclerosis [59]. The authors addressed the procedures and limitations of such a trial to inform future PNES

treatment trials, based on their prospective, open label pharmacological feasibility trial. The authors emphasized the importance of monitoring other outcomes and symptoms scales, along with the typical focus of seizure counts. They concluded that an initial comprehensive neuropsychiatric assessment and prospectively assessing cognitive, emotional, behavioral, and psychosocial measures are important for monitoring the outcomes in randomized controlled trials (RCTs) for PNES treatment.

Mood and health-related quality of life (HRQOL) are related in patients with PNES. Along with seizure counts, comorbidities and constitutional symptoms are found to be correlated to quality of life in PNES [60], as they are in epilepsy [61]. The issue of addressing the limited quality of life data seen in the PNES population was underscored in a study by Testa *et al.* [62]. The authors emphasized that treatments designed to improve HRQOL among individuals with intractable seizures should also address chronic psychological symptoms and high levels of somatization.

The utility of antiepileptic drugs

One pharmacological question that has been addressed recently has been the impact of withdrawing AEDs from patients with pure PNES. Given that the majority of patients with PNES are prescribed AEDs, Oto *et al.* studied whether withdrawal of AEDs can be carried out safely in patients with PNES in a prospective evaluation of safety and outcome [63]. Seventy-eight patients with PNES who satisfied a standardized set of criteria for excluding the diagnosis of coexisting or underlying epilepsy had their AEDs withdrawn (64 as outpatients, 14 as inpatients). The frequency of PNES declined in the group as a whole over the period of the study (follow-up 6–12 months) in all individuals except for eight patients in whom there was a transient increase. Fourteen patients reported new physical symptoms after withdrawal; however, no serious adverse events were reported. The authors concluded that with appropriate diagnostic investigation and surveillance during follow-up, withdrawal of AEDs can be achieved safely in patients with PNES.

Potential pharmacological interventions

Reports of pharmacological treatment for PNES [64] using intravenous barbiturates, tricyclic antidepressants, selective serotonin reuptake inhibitors (SSRIs), dopamine receptor antagonists, beta-blockers, analgesics, or benzodiazepines are largely anecdotal in case reports, journal review articles, or book chapters, with only two prospective open label trials [59,65] and one double-blind pilot RCT, discussed below. One proposed approach to managing PNES is to treat the comorbidities accompanying PNES, which may reduce seizure frequency. A feasibility trial of an SSRI to treat comorbid anxiety and depression, which are commonly seen in patients with PNES, provided support for the proposed need to treat the comorbidities [59]. The open label study was followed by a pilot randomized placebo-controlled trial in 38 patients with PNES [66], which revealed a 45% reduction in PNES in the SSRI arm and an 8% increase in the placebo arm, but no difference between the two groups with direct comparison. Fully-powered RCTs are needed to evaluate the potential effect of pharmacological agents for PNES.

Psychotherapy

A number of psychotherapies have been used in case reports and open label trials for PNES, including modalities based on psychodynamic, interpersonal, psychoeducation, family, cognitive, behavioral, and cognitive behavioral approaches, both in individuals and in group formats [51].

Cognitive behavioral therapy

Cognitive behavioral therapy (CBT) has demonstrated preliminary efficacy for PNES. In several trials, medically unexplained symptoms have been shown to be amenable to CBT [67,68]. Behavioral therapy was first

reported in cases of PNES in the late 1960s [69]; however, no class I level of evidence data from RCTs for PNES have been published to date.

Three pilot trials of CBT for PNES have been completed. In Goldstein's open label study, a 12-session CBT intervention for patients with dissociative seizures [PNES] was conducted [70] and was followed by their pilot RCT [71] (described below). Based on data on somatoform and seizure disorders, a cognitive behavioral model was proposed by LaFrance [58] testing the hypothesis that identifying cognitive distortions and environmental triggers for PNES will reduce PNES. The fear-avoidance model first makes connections between triggers, cognitions, and symptoms, and then equips patients to break the cycle. The model was tested in an open label prospective clinical trial of CBT for PNES, involving 21 patients using a CBT for PNES manual, modified with permission from a CBT for epilepsy workbook [72,73]. The 12-session manual-based therapy [74] focuses on gaining control of seizures and includes training in healthy communication, understanding medications, conducting a functional behavioral analysis, and examining internal and external triggers. Treatment involved addressing mood–cognition–environment connections, automatic thoughts, and somatic misinterpretations, targeting issues in PNES.

Intervention feasibility was established in this open label CBT for PNES study [75], where out of 21 subjects enrolled, 17 (81%) completed the CBT weekly intervention over 3 months and 11 of the 17 completers reported no seizures by their final CBT session. Patients with PNES decreased from four seizures per week (median) at enrollment to zero per week upon treatment completion. Mean scores on scales of depression, anxiety, somatic symptoms, quality of life, and psychosocial functioning showed improvement from baseline to the final session ($p < 0.05$). Therefore, CBT for PNES reduced the number of seizures *and* improved psychiatric symptoms, psychosocial functioning, and quality of life [75]. Although a "placebo effect" is possible in any trial, it is unlikely to account for the improvement as this study was conducted in parallel with a pilot pharmacological RCT [66]. In the pilot pharmacological RCT, the placebo group demonstrated no improvements in seizures or other outcome variables. The pilot study revealed that a CBT treatment specifically for the PNES population addressing cognitive distortions and promoting behavioral changes addressed both the comorbidities and the PNES. Independently, a recent pilot RCT by Goldstein *et al.* [71] comparing CBT with standard medical care in a seizure monitoring unit for PNES ($n = 66$) yielded similar results to an earlier trial by Goldstein *et al.* ($n = 20$) [70] and our open pilot trials [75].

Models for treatment of psychogenic movement disorders based on treatment of psychogenic non-epileptic seizures

Like PNES, PMD has limited controlled treatment data. There are fewer data available on the efficacy of CBT in the treatment of PMD, although education of the patient may be important in its treatment [76]. There is a paucity of case reports or clinical trials examining the effect of other non-CBT psychological treatment modalities for PMD and, similar to PNES, open label treatment trials in PMD have incorporated psychodynamic psychotherapy [77] or use of an SSRI [78].

Application of cognitive behavioral therapy

Reviewing the literature revealed one case report using CBT for PMD [79]. The case was a 22-year-old woman who was evaluated for presumed psychogenic dystonia that had been present for 5 years. On consultative examination, she displayed severe dystonic posturing, which consisted of fixed flexion at the abdomen, hips, elbows, and proximal interphalanges, and plantar flexion at both ankles. She displayed lateral- and anterocollis and facial movements consisting of alternating contractions of the risorius, independently. She had full strength without spasticity and normal reflexes. She met Fahn and Williams' diagnostic criteria for probable PMD [80]. She enrolled in treatment and underwent a 12-session weekly CBT for PMD program and had complete resolution of the abdominal and arm dystonia by week 4. Her facial movements persisted on an intermittent basis; however, by week 12, her symptoms had resolved. She has remained symptom free, now 2 years after treatment, and she is off all medications and has returned to work. The CBT used to treat this patient was modified from the CBT manual that has been used in a trial of CBT for patients with PNES, described above. The CBT program used in this case of PMD substituted monitoring the movements for monitoring seizures. During the sessions, the manual-based therapy focused on taking control of movements and followed the outline for the PNES treatment.

Along with complete remission of her chronic symptoms, other significant benefits of the CBT for PMD treatment for her included stopping all medications, returning to work, and avoiding further unnecessary evaluations.

Understanding conversion disorders with neuroimaging and neurophysiological studies

In other conversion disorders, advances in neurophysiology may help to inform further understanding of PNES. For example, Voon *et al.* [81] investigated the relationship between conversion disorder and affect by assessing amygdala activity to affective stimuli in a functional MRI study. The investigators used a block design incidental affective task with fearful, happy, and neutral face stimuli and compared valence contrasts between 16 patients with PMD type conversion disorder and 16 age- and gender-matched healthy volunteers. The findings indicated that greater functional connectivity of limbic regions influencing motor preparatory regions during states of arousal may underlie the pathophysiology of motor conversion symptoms. Further functional neuroimaging examining striato-thalamocortical circuits controlling sensorimotor function and attention may yield insights into the neural connectivity in PNES. Imaging is covered in more detail in other chapters of the book.

Other recent relevant neurophysiological studies include a comparison of serum brain-derived neurotrophic factor (BDNF) in patients with major depressive disorder and patients with a variety of conversion disorders [82]. The mean serum BDNF of the healthy control group was significantly higher than the level in the major depressive disorder group and the conversion group ($p = 0.008$). The conversion group was noted not to have significant levels of depression. Whether BDNF levels may play a similar role in the pathophysiology of depression and conversion disorder remains to be seen. Our laboratory has studied BDNF in patients with epilepsy compared with those with PNES and healthy controls. We found lower BDNF levels in both the group with epilepsy and the group with PNES, compared with the healthy controls, but BDNF did not distinguish epilepsy from PNES [83].

These studies examine the potential neurobiology of conversion disorders. More studies are needed in this area. As in other physiological studies in conversion disorder, and as noted in the hypothalamic–pituitary–adrenal axis study [30], a distinct pattern of hypothalamic–pituitary–adrenal axis dysregulation can be seen in dissociative disorders, emphasizing the importance of further study of stress-response systems in certain forms of psychopathology.

Conclusions

The diagnosis of PNES can be difficult by history alone. Physical signs, patient characteristics, and neuropsychological testing are helpful adjuncts to the video–EEG to confirm the diagnosis. The first phase of treatment begins with the neurologist, as she or he shares the findings of the video–EEG monitoring. Neurologists, psychiatrists, and psychologists must then continue to work together to effectively treat this difficult population. Controlled trials are needed to demonstrate what treatments are effective for patients with PNES. Interdisciplinary research and discussion, along with collaborative sponsorship between neurological and psychiatric institutes, will help to move the field forward to address this difficult-to-treat population. Understanding similarities and differences between patient populations with PMD, with PNES, and with both disorders may help to develop more effective treatments for these patients.

References

1. Gates JR, Luciano D, Devinsky O. The classification and treatment of nonepileptic events. In Devinsky O, Theodore WH, eds. *Epilepsy and Behavior.* New York: Wiley-Liss, 1991:251–263.

2. Reuber M, Fernandez G, Bauer J, Helmstaedter C, Elger CE. Diagnostic delay in psychogenic nonepileptic seizures. *Neurology* 2002;**58**:493–495.

3. Martin RC, Gilliam FG, Kilgore M, Faught E, Kuzniecky R. Improved health care resource utilization following video-EEG-confirmed diagnosis of nonepileptic psychogenic seizures. *Seizure* 1998;7:385–390.

4. LaFrance WC, Jr., Benbadis SR. Avoiding the costs of unrecognized psychological nonepileptic seizures. *Neurology* 2006;**66**:1620–1621.

5. Gates JR, Ramani V, Whalen S, Loewenson R. Ictal characteristics of pseudoseizures. *Arch Neurol* 1985;**42**:1183–1187.

6. LaFrance WC, Jr., Devinsky O. Treatment of nonepileptic seizures. *Epilepsy Behav* 2002;**3**(Suppl 1):S19–S23.

7. Alsaadi TM, Thieman C, Shatzel A, Farias S. Video-EEG telemetry can be a crucial tool for neurologists experienced in epilepsy when diagnosing seizure disorders. *Seizure* 2004;**13**:32–34.

8. Benbadis SR, LaFrance WC, Jr., Papandonatos GD, et al. Interrater reliability of EEG-video monitoring. *Neurology* 2009;**73**:843–846.

9. Syed Tu, LaFrance WC, Jr., Kahriman ES, et al. Can semiology predict psychogenic nonepileptic seizures? A propective study. *Ann Neurol* 2011;**69**:997–1004.

10. Cragar DE, Berry DT, Fakhoury TA, Cibula JE, Schmitt FA. A review of diagnostic techniques in the differential diagnosis of epileptic and nonepileptic seizures. *Neuropsychol Rev* 2002;**12**:31–64.

11. Smolowitz JL, Hopkins SC, Perrine T, et al. Diagnostic utility of an epilepsy monitoring unit. *Am J Med Qual* 2007;**22**:117–122.

12. Benbadis SR, Agrawal V, Tatum IV WO. How many patients with psychogenic nonepileptic seizures also have epilepsy? *Neurology* 2001;**57**:915–917.

13. Benbadis SR, LaFrance Jr WC. Clinical features and the role of video–EEG monitoring. In Schachter SC, LaFrance Jr WC, eds. *Gates and Rowan's Nonepileptic Seizures,* 3rd edn. Cambridge, UK: Cambridge University Press, 2010:38–50.

14. Chung SS, Gerber P, Kirlin KA. Ictal eye closure is a reliable indicator for psychogenic nonepileptic seizures. *Neurology* 2006;**66**:1730–1731.

15. Syed TU, Arozullah AM, Suciu GP, et al. Do observer and self-reports of ictal eye closure predict psychogenic nonepileptic seizures? *Epilepsia* 2008;**49**:898–904.

16. Henry JA, Woodruff GHA. A diagnostic sign in states of apparent unconsciousness. *Lancet* 1978;**ii**:920–921.

17. Donati F, Kollar M, Pihan H, Mathis J. Eyelids position: during epileptic versus psychogenic seizures. *J Neurol Sci* 2005;**238**(Suppl 1):S82–S83.

18. Flügel D, Bauer J, Kaseborn U, Burr W, Elger CE. Closed eyes during a seizure indicate psychogenic etiology: a study with suggestive seizure provocation. *Journal of Epilepsy* 1996;**9**:165–169.

19. Bergen D, Ristanovic R. Weeping as a common element of pseudoseizures. *Arch Neurol* 1993;**50**:1059–1060.

20. Vossler DG, Haltiner AM, Schepp SK, et al. Ictal stuttering: a sign suggestive of psychogenic nonepileptic seizures. *Neurology* 2004;**63**:516–519.

21. Chabolla DR, Shih JJ. Postictal behaviors associated with psychogenic nonepileptic seizures. *Epilepsy Behav* 2006;**9**:307–311.

22. Wennberg R. Postictal coughing and nose rubbing coexist in temporal lobe epilepsy. *Neurology* 2001;**56**:133–134.

23. Sen A, Scott C, Sisodiya SM. Stertorous breathing is a reliably identified sign that helps in the differentiation of epileptic from psychogenic non-epileptic convulsions: an audit. *Epilepsy Res* 2007;**77**:62–64.

24. Kanner AM, Morris HH, Luders H, *et al*. Supplementary motor seizures mimicking pseudoseizures: some clinical differences. *Neurology* 1990;**40**:1404–1407.

25. Jobst BC, Williamson PD. Frontal lobe seizures. *Psychiatr Clin North Am* 2005;**28**:635–651.

26. Reuber M, Pukrop R, Bauer J, *et al*. Outcome in psychogenic nonepileptic seizures: 1 to 10-year follow-up in 164 patients. *Ann Neurol* 2003;**53**:305–311.

27. Trimble MR. Non-epileptic seizures. In Halligan PW, Bass CM, Marshall JC, eds. *Contemporary Approaches to the Study of Hysteria: Clinical and Theoretical Perspectives*. Oxford: Oxford University Press, 2001:143–154.

28. de Timary P, Fouchet P, Sylin M, *et al*. Non-epileptic seizures: delayed diagnosis in patients presenting with electroencephalographic (EEG) or clinical signs of epileptic seizures. *Seizure* 2002;**11**:193–197.

29. Kunugi H, Ida I, Owashi T, Kimura M, *et al*. Assessment of the dexamethasone/CRH test as a state-dependent marker for hypothalamic–pituitary–adrenal (HPA) axis abnormalities in major depressive episode: a multicenter study. *Neuropsychopharmacology* 2006; **31**:212–220.

30. Simeon D, Knutelska M, Yehuda R, *et al*. Hypothalamic–pituitary–adrenal axis function in dissociative disorders, post-traumatic stress disorder, and healthy volunteers. *Biol Psychiatry* 2007;**61**:966–973.

31. Deacon C, Wiebe S, Blume WT, McLachlan RS, Young GB, Matijevic S. Seizure identification by clinical description in temporal lobe epilepsy: How accurate are we? *Neurology* 2003;**61**:1686–1689.

32. Tinuper P, Grassi C, Bisulli F, *et al*. Split-screen synchronized display. A useful video-EEG technique for studying paroxysmal phenomena. *Epileptic Disord* 2004;**6**:27–30.

33. Ossenblok P, de Munck JC, Colon A, Drolsbach W, Boon P. Magnetoencephalography is more successful for screening and localizing frontal lobe epilepsy than electroencephalography. *Epilepsia* 2007;**48**:2139–2149.

34. Chen DK, So YT, Fisher RS. Use of serum prolactin in diagnosing epileptic seizures: report of the Therapeutics and Technology Assessment Subcommittee of the American Academy of Neurology. *Neurology* 2005;**65**:668–675.

35. Trimble MR. Serum prolactin in epilepsy and hysteria. *BMJ* 1978;**ii**:1682.

36. Lowe MR, De Toledo JC, Rabinstein AA, Giulla MF. Correspondence: MRI evidence of mesial temporal sclerosis in patients with psychogenic nonepileptic seizures. *Neurology* 2001;**56**:821–823.

37. Reuber M, Fernandez G, Helmstaedter C, Qurishi A, Elger CE. Evidence of brain abnormality in patients with psychogenic nonepileptic seizures. *Epilepsy Behav* 2002;**3**:249–254.

38. Ettinger AB, Coyle PK, Jandorf L, *et al*. Postictal SPECT in epileptic versus nonepileptic seizures. *J Epilepsy* 1998;**11**:67–73.

39. Binder LM, Kindermann SS, Heaton RK, Salinsky MC. Neuropsychologic impairment in patients with nonepileptic seizures. *Arch Clin Neuropsychol* 1998;**13**:513–522.

40. Kalogjera-Sackellares D, Sackellares JC. Impaired motor function in patients with psychogenic pseudoseizures. *Epilepsia* 2001;**42**:1600–1606.

41. Binder LM, Salinsky MC, Smith SP. Psychological correlates of psychogenic seizures. *J Clin Exp Neuropsychol* 1994;**16**:524–530.

42. Drane DL, Williamson DJ, Stroup ES, *et al*. Cognitive impairment is not equal in patients with epileptic and psychogenic nonepileptic seizures. *Epilepsia* 2006;**47**:1879–1886.

43. Cragar DE, Berry DT, Fakhoury TA, Cibula JE, Schmitt FA. Performance of patients with epilepsy or psychogenic non-epileptic seizures on four measures of effort. *Clin Neuropsychol* 2006;**20**:552–566.

44. Schramke CJ, Valeri A, Valeriano JP, Kelly KM. Using the Minnesota Multiphasic Inventory 2, EEGs, and clinical data to predict nonepileptic events. *Epilepsy Behav* 2007;**11**:343–346.

45. Krawetz P, Fleisher W, Pillay N, *et al*. Family functioning in subjects with pseudoseizures and epilepsy. *J Nerv Ment Dis* 2001;**189**:38–43.

46. van Merode T, Twellaar M, Kotsopoulos IA, *et al*. Psychological characteristics of patients with newly developed psychogenic seizures. *J Neurol Neurosurg Psychiatry* 2004;**75**:1175–1177.

47. Benbadis SR. A spell in the epilepsy clinic and a history of "chronic pain" or "fibromyalgia" independently predict a diagnosis of psychogenic seizures. *Epilepsy Behav* 2005;**6**:264–265.

48. Swanson SJ, Springer JA, Benbadis SR, Morris GL. Cognitive and psychological functioning in patients with non-epileptic seizures. In Gates JR, Rowan AJ, eds. *Non-Epileptic Seizures*, 2nd edn. Boston, MA: Butterworth-Heinemann, 2000:123–137.

49. LaFrance WC, Jr., Devinsky O. The treatment of nonepileptic seizures: historical perspectives and future directions. *Epilepsia* 2004;**45**(Suppl 2):15–21.

50. LaFrance WC, Jr., Barry JJ. Update on treatments of psychological nonepileptic seizures. *Epilepsy Behav* 2005;7:364–374.

51. Baker GA, Brooks JL, Goodfellow L, Bodde N, Aldenkamp A. Treatments for non-epileptic

attack disorder. *Cochrane Database Syst Rev* 2007;(1):CD006370.

52. Porter RJ. Diagnosis of psychogenic and other nonepileptic seizures in adults. In Devinsky O, Theodore WH, eds. *Epilepsy and Behavior*. New York: Wiley-Liss, 1991:237–249.

53. Bowman ES, Coons PM. The differential diagnosis of epilepsy, pseudoseizures, dissociative identity disorder, and dissociative disorder not otherwise specified. *Bull Menninger Clin* 2000;**64**:164–180.

54. Ford CV, Folks DG. Conversion disorders: an overview. *Psychosomatics* 1985;**26**:371–374, 380–383.

55. Baslet G, Roiko A, Prensky E. Heterogeneity in psychogenic nonepileptic seizures: understanding the role of psychiatric and neurological factors. *Epilepsy Behav* 2010;**17**:236–241.

56. Kalogjera-Sackellares D. Psychological disturbances in patients with pseudoseizures. In Sackellares JC, Berent S, eds. *Psychological Disturbances in Epilepsy*. Oxford: Butterworth-Heinemann, 1996:191–217.

57. Duncan R, Oto M. Predictors of antecedent factors in psychogenic nonepileptic attacks: Multivariate analysis. *Neurology* 2008;**71**:1000–1005.

58. LaFrance Jr WC, Bjørnæs H. Designing treatment plans based on etiology of psychogenic nonepileptic seizures. In Schachter SC, LaFrance Jr WC, eds. *Gates and Rowan's Nonepileptic Seizures,* 3rd edn. Cambridge, UK: Cambridge University Press, 2010:266–280.

59. LaFrance WC, Jr., Blum AS, Miller IW, Ryan CE, Keitner GI. Methodological issues in conducting treatment trials for psychological nonepileptic seizures. *J Neuropsychiatry Clin Neurosci* 2007;**19**:391–398.

60. LaFrance WC, Jr., Syc S. Depression and symptoms affect quality of life in psychogenic nonepileptic seizures. *Neurology* 2009;**73**:366–371.

61. Gilliam F. Optimizing health outcomes in active epilepsy. *Neurology* 2002;**58**(Suppl 5):S9–S20.

62. Testa SM, Schefft BK, Szaflarski JP, Yeh HS, Privitera MD. Mood, personality, and health-related quality of life in epileptic and psychogenic seizure disorders. *Epilepsia* 2007;**48**:973–982.

63. Oto M, Espie C, Pelosi A, Selkirk M, Duncan R. The safety of antiepileptic drug withdrawal in patients with non-epileptic seizures. *J Neurol Neurosurg Psychiatry* 2005;**76**:1682–1685.

64. LaFrance Jr WC, Blumer D. Pharmacological treatments for psychogenic nonepileptic seizures. In Schachter SC, LaFrance Jr WC, eds. *Gates and Rowan's Nonepileptic Seizures*, 3rd edn. Cambridge, UK: Cambridge University Press, 2010:307–316.

65. Ataoglu A, Ozcetin A, Icmeli C, Ozbulut O. Paradoxical therapy in conversion reaction. *J Korean Med Sci* 2003;**18**:581–584.

66. LaFrance Jr WC, Keitner GI, Papandonatos GD, *et al.* Pilot pharmacologic randomized trial for psychogenic nonepileptic seizures. *Neurology* 2010;**75**:1166–1173.

67. Kroenke K, Swindle R. Cognitive-behavioral therapy for somatization and symptom syndromes: a critical review of controlled clinical trials. *Psychother Psychosom* 2000;**69**:205–215.

68. Sumathipala A, Hewege S, Hanwella R, Mann AH. Randomized controlled trial of cognitive behaviour therapy for repeated consultations for medically unexplained complaints: a feasibility study in Sri Lanka. *Psychol Med* 2000;**30**:747–757.

69. Gardner JE. Behavior therapy treatment approach to a psychogenic seizure case. *J Consult Psychol* 1967;**31**:209–212.

70. Goldstein LH, Deale AC, Mitchell-O'Malley SJ, Toone BK, Mellers JDC. An evaluation of cognitive behavioral therapy as a treatment for dissociative seizures: a pilot study. *Cogn Behav Neurol* 2004;**17**:41–49.

71. Goldstein LH, Chalder T, Chigwedere C, *et al.* Cognitive-behavioral therapy for psychogenic nonepileptic seizures: a pilot RCT. *Neurology* 2010;**74**:1986–1994.

72. Reiter J, Andrews D, Janis C. *Taking Control of Your Epilepsy. A Workbook for Patients and Professionals.* Santa Rosa, CA: The Basics, 1987.

73. Reiter JM, Andrews DJ. A neurobehavioral approach for treatment of complex partial epilepsy: efficacy. *Seizure* 2000;**9**:198–203.

74. LaFrance Jr WC. *CBT NES Treatment Manual.* Providence, RI: Brown Medical School, 2005.

75. LaFrance WC, Jr., Miller IW, Ryan CE, *et al.* Cognitive behavioral therapy for psychogenic nonepileptic seizures. *Epilepsy Behav* 2009;**14**:591–596.

76. Espay AJ, Goldenhar LM, Voon V, *et al.* Opinions and clinical practices related to diagnosing and managing patients with psychogenic movement disorders: an international survey of Movement Disorder Society members. *Mov Disord* 2009;**24**:1366–1374.

77. Hinson VK, Weinstein S, Bernard B, Leurgans SE, Goetz CG. Single-blind clinical trial of psychotherapy for treatment of psychogenic movement disorders. *Parkinsonism Relat Disord* 2006;**12**:177–180.

78. Voon V, Lang AE. Antidepressant treatment outcomes of psychogenic movement disorder. *J Clin Psychiatry* 2005;**66**:1529–1534.

79. LaFrance WC, Jr., Friedman JH. Cognitive behavioral therapy for psychogenic movement disorder. *Mov Disord* 2009;**24**:1856–1857.

80. Fahn S, Williams PJ. Psychogenic dystonia. *Adv Neurol* 1988;**50**:431–455.

81. Voon V, Brezing C, Gallea C, *et al*. Emotional stimuli and motor conversion disorder. *Brain* 2010;**133**:1526–1536.

82. Deveci A, Aydemir O, Taskin O, Taneli F, Esen-Danaci A. Serum brain-derived neurotrophic factor levels in conversion disorder: Comparative study with depression. *Psychiatry Clin Neurosci* 2007;**61**:571–573.

83. LaFrance Jr WC, Leaver KE, Stopa E, Papandonatos GD, Blum AS. Decreased serum brain-derived neurotrophic factor in patients with epileptic and nonepileptic seizures. *Neurology* 2010:**75**:1285–1291.

Chapter 12

Hypochondriasis and its relationship to somatization

Arthur J. Barsky

The concept of somatization

Somatic symptoms are a prominent, and not uncommonly the exclusive, presenting feature of many psychiatric disorders. Psychiatric patients, particularly those with anxiety and depressive disorders, frequently focus on their somatic discomfort and are less aware of, and less vocal about, their affective and emotional distress. The term somatization originally referred to these patients' selective focus on their bodily distress to the exclusion of their emotional distress. The underlying psychiatric disorder was judged to be the cause of the somatic distress and this judgment was validated when successful treatment of the presumptive psychiatric disorder resulted in somatic relief.

Gradually over time, the construct of somatization was broadened to describe patients with medically unexplained somatic symptoms even when a diagnosable psychiatric disorder could not be established as the cause of the somatic symptoms. Indeed, medically unexplained symptoms were noted to have many sources other than occult psychiatric disorder, such as stressful life events, interpersonal difficulties, learned patterns of behavior, personality traits, and more. Thus the term somatization came to refer more broadly to the presence of a somatic symptom that could not be explained by demonstrable medical disease, that the sufferer believed to have a medical basis, and that prompted medical help-seeking.

As noted above, many medically unexplained symptoms are not caused by a psychiatric disorder. Transient self-limited benign symptoms occur frequently in the course of the daily life of healthy non-patients; back pain, headaches, tinnitus, fasiculations, and dizziness are an endemic part of the human experience. Symptoms without a serious medical cause are a nearly universal human experience, arising and subsiding in perfectly healthy people. Population-based surveys disclose just how frequently bothersome symptoms occur in people who are free of serious medical and psychiatric disorder: 80–90% of the general population experiences at least one symptom every 1–3 weeks [1], and only a very small proportion of people report experiencing no symptoms at all [2,3]. In the USA, 14–15% of adults report being bothered by headache [1,4], 19–39% report fatigue [5,6], 32–50% report back pain [1,7], and 5–23% report dizziness [1]. Most important for our purposes is the finding that the vast majority of such symptoms resolve spontaneously, usually within 1 month [8].

These symptoms constitute an endemic reservoir of distress that generally does not prompt medical help-seeking, but may upon occasion do so. These presentations can be understood from several different perspectives. Some medically unexplained somatic symptoms can be conceptualized as a non-verbal interpersonal communication, in effect a bodily pantomime. These somatizing patients seek recognition and acknowledgement from others that they are in distress and suffering, hoping thereby to secure special attention, support, and consideration. In some cases, a lifetime of medically unexplained complaints can be best conceptualized as a stable personality trait, one that has been associated with other enduring personality characteristics (including alexithymia [9,10] and negative affectivity [11–13], and with several personality disorders [14,15]). Somatization can also be understood as a form of illness and sick role behavior – not something an individual *has*, but rather something he/she *does* [16–19]. From this perspective, the most salient features of somatization are the patients' maladaptive and unproductive utilization of medical care, vigorous

Psychogenic Movement Disorders and Other Conversion Disorders, ed. Mark Hallett, Anthony E. Lang, Joseph Jankovic, Stanley Fahn, Peter W. Halligan, Valerie Voon, and C. Robert Cloninger. Published by Cambridge University Press. © Cambridge University Press 2011.

complaining, activity restrictions, reassurance-seeking, and excessive researching of their condition. The presentation of medically unexplained symptoms is also subject to sociocultural influences. Cultural norms and values encourage the expression of distress in certain forms and discourage it in others; these cultural forces shape the experience and reporting of bodily symptoms by influencing how they are identified, interpreted, described, and reported [20–22]. The search for the neural mechanisms that underlie the somatizer's symptoms is just beginning, and it seems unlikely that a single pathogenic mechanism will explain the wide range of symptoms or disorders. Preliminary investigations have examined the hyperresponsivity of centrally acting proinflammatory cytokines, dysregulation of central and peripheral serotonergic systems, and dysregulation of the hypothalamic–pituitary–adrenal axis [11,23]. Functional brain imaging may eventually elucidate the regulation of afferent somatic and visceral stimuli and the central processing these stimuli undergo at cortical and subcortical levels. Early studies have suggested possible underactivation of the caudate, putamen, and precentral gyrus in somatization disorder [24,25], and hypoactivation of prefrontal cortex [26], thalamus, and basal ganglia [27] in conversion disorder.

In the vast majority of people with medically unexplained somatic symptoms, no specific psychiatric disorder is present. It is only when the symptoms become chronic, excessively distressing, disabling, and impairing (and continue to defy medical diagnosis), that they suggest the presence of psychopathology. Consequently, when the somatic complaints are severe, intense, long lasting, and profoundly disabling, they are more likely to be a manifestation of psychopathology, most often of affective disorder, anxiety disorder, or somatoform disorder. Somatoform disorders are described in the DSM-IV: "The common feature of the somatoform disorders is the presence of physical symptoms that suggest a general medical condition… and are not fully explained by a general medical condition" [28]. In other words, patients with a somatoform disorder appear to have a medical disorder but on closer examination their symptoms seem to be better understood as psychiatric phenomena.

Hypochondriasis

Hypochondriasis is one of the somatoform disorders. It is characterized by the misattribution of benign bodily symptoms to serious disease and the consequent belief that the individual is suffering from an undiagnosed medical illness. Consequently, the hypochondriacal patient has both a bothersome bodily sensation and a cognitive belief about the cause of the sensation, along with anxiety about its putative significance. The cardinal features of the disorder, therefore, are somatic symptoms disproportionate to demonstrable pathology, the firm belief that one has an undiagnosed disease, health-related anxiety or disease fear, and prominent illness and sick role behavior. These behaviors often include repeated self-examination, excessive reassurance seeking, extensive researching of the symptoms (commonly on the Internet), and high levels of medical care utilization that is nonetheless unsatisfactory to both the patients and their doctors.

The DSM-IV defines hypochondriasis as follows:

A. Preoccupation with fears of having, or the idea that one has, a serious disease based on the person's misinterpretation of bodily symptoms.

B. The preoccupation persists despite appropriate medical evaluation and reassurance.

C. The belief in Criterion A is not of delusional intensity… and is not restricted to a circumscribed concern about appearance…

D. The preoccupation causes clinically significant distress or impairment in social, occupational, or other important areas of functioning.

E. The duration of the disturbance is at least 6 months.

F. The preoccupation is not better accounted for by Generalized Anxiety Disorder, Obsessive-Compulsive Disorder, Panic Disorder, a Major Depressive Episode, Separation Anxiety, or another Somatoform Disorder.

This disorder is present in 4–6% of ambulatory patients [29]. In community samples, the prevalence has been reported to be between 0.5% and 4% [30–33]. Little is known about the family histories of hypochondriacal probands. In one study, Noyes et al. [34] found no increase in the prevalence of hypochondriasis in the first-degree relatives of hypochondriacal probands, although they did find a non-significant trend toward an increased prevalence of anxiety disorders. Risk factors for the development of hypochondriasis have been shown to include childhood adversity (including both abuse and neglect) [35], chronic medical illness in the patient him- or herself or in a close relative during childhood [36], and overly solicitous parenting.

The disorder appears to occur as often in men as in women.

The natural history of hypochondriasis is largely unknown, but the onset typically occurs in early or middle adulthood and tends to run a chronic, relapsing and remitting course. The median age of onset appears to be between 20 and 30 years [37–39]. There appears to be both a transient and a more chronic, and persistent form. In one naturalistic, longitudinal study, two-thirds of patients with hypochondriasis as defined by DSM-IV continued to meet diagnostic criteria after 5 years [40]; in another study, two-thirds of such patients continued to meet diagnostic criteria after 1 year [41].

Conceptual models for understanding hypochondriasis

Several pathogenic mechanisms of hypochondriasis have been proposed. They are not mutually exclusive and all may be valid to varying degrees in individual cases. They may also be operative more generally in other forms of somatization as well.

A cognitive-perceptual model suggests that the condition is a self-perpetuating and self-validating disorder of somatic symptom amplification. The clinical condition is precipitated when an individual begins to suspect that a pre-existing, benign but bothersome bodily sensation is not indeed benign but rather is the symptom of a serious disease. This misattribution of benign distress to serious disease may be triggered by a number of factors, including a realistic threat to medical health, the onset of a psychiatric disorder such as panic disorder or major depression, or a stressful life event. Thus a transient, self-limited ailment (e.g., a bruise, tinnitus, or a bout of diarrhea), a normal physiological sensation (e.g., orthostatic dizziness or an ectopic heartbeat), or a somatic symptom of emotional arousal or psychosocial stress is now misunderstood as indicative of serious disease. This mistaken belief that one has a serious disease then amplifies and maintains the initial symptom via several mechanisms. First, it causes more intense scrutiny and more frequent attention to the symptom, which in turn makes it seem increasingly unpleasant, bothersome, and disabling. For example, a headache seems far worse when attributed to a brain tumor rather than to eyestrain. Second, a state of bodily hypervigilance is induced. As a result, other pre-existing, minor bodily discomforts are now re-interpreted as additional evidence of the putative disease. For example, once

a patient suspects he has anemia, then shortness of breath after climbing a flight of stairs seems to confirm his diagnostic impression. In the past, the same breathlessness might not have been noticed at all, or might have been normalized by attributing it to lack of exercise, inadequate sleep, dietary indiscretion, aging, or the "wear and tear" of daily life. Third, through a process of confirmatory bias, information and bodily sensations that disconfirm the suspicion one is sick are ignored and dismissed. The hypochondriacal patient who suspects he or she is working in a "toxic building" notes every time he or she enters the building and has a stuffy nose, but fails to note every time he or she does not have a stuffy nose on entrance. And finally, the growing suspicion that one is sick increases alarm and anxiety, and anxiety produces its own set of somatic symptoms of autonomic arousal. These new symptoms serve only to further convince the hypochondriacal individual that the condition is progressing and the worst fears are well founded. The net result is that the rising somatic distress further substantiates the mistaken belief that an occult disease is present, which then perpetuates the vicious circle of hypochondriacal perception and cognition.

Hypochondriasis can also be understood from an interpersonal perspective, as a non-verbal interpersonal communication. This model, too, may apply more broadly to other forms of somatization. The notion here is that somatic complaints can be viewed as a bodily pantomime, a non-verbal attempt to say something to others. The hypochondriacal individual is asking for special consideration, special care, and support from those around him or her. Hypochondriacal individuals seek others' acknowledgement that they are in distress and are suffering, hoping thereby to secure special attention, nurturance, and assistance they could not otherwise obtain. Illness behaviors can thus be used to negotiate stressful circumstances and secure support and solicit care from others; the hypochondriacal individual is essentially asking others for time-out because he or she finds him or herself facing an insurmountable challenge, obstacle, or responsibility. This is not malingering – the hypochondriacal patient truly experiences the symptom he or she reports and is not lying or feigning illness – but rather a behavioral pattern that has been learned unwittingly over the course of a lifetime, namely that illness exempts one from facing seemingly insoluble obstacles and allows one to avoid obligations and responsibilities that would otherwise have to be met.

Hypochondriasis has also been conceptualized in a very different manner, namely as an intrapsychic process. This is based on the idea that physical distress can hold unconscious meaning and provide unconscious gratification. Three specific formulations have been proposed, revolving around dependency needs, anger, and inadequate self-worth. Childhood experience teaches us all that pain brings love; the sick or ill child is entitled to special nurturance, affection, succor, and privileges. Subsequently, in adulthood, when feeling particularly bereft and uncared for, according to this conceptual model, the hypochondriacal adult develops somatic symptoms in an unconscious attempt to elicit that special care from others. Again, it must be emphasized that this process is entirely unconscious and the hypochondriacal individual is in no way dissembling, lying, or feigning illness. Anger and resentment have also been cited as an unconscious source of hypochondriasis. According to this formulation, the hypochondriacal adult is turning reproach towards someone into complaints to someone. The individual is angry at caretakers in childhood who were felt to have failed him or her; in adulthood he or she then solicits caretaking relationships and expresses anger by thwarting the attempts of others to help. Physicians often experience this indirect but effective expression of hostility as their hypochondriacal patients vividly depict their distress and urgently beseech them for help, but respond to every therapeutic attempt negatively with distressing side effects, an intensification of their presenting symptoms, or new symptoms to replace the old ones. The persistent symptoms and repeated requests for medical attention are combined with a refractoriness, unresponsiveness, and help-rejecting stance that seem to increase in proportion to the physician's attempts to reassure and palliate the distress. The physician consequently feels frustrated, impotent, and defeated. Other psychodynamic observers have conceptualized hypochondriasis as a defense against unbearably low self-esteem and a profound sense of worthlessness. They suggest that it less painful to feel that there is something fundamentally wrong with one's body than to feel there is something wrong with oneself as a human being. The hypochondriacal individual thus believes he or she is friendless because he or she is so ill that they are no fun to be around, and that his or her work is not going well because it is hampered by ill health, not by lack of ability.

Hypochondriasis within the broader context of somatization in general

Hypochondriasis lies mid-way along a continuum. This continuum stretches from patients with somatic distress and minimal concern or worry about the meaning, significance, or cause of their distress at one end, to patients with illness fears and disease convictions that are unaccompanied by any somatic symptoms at the other end. The former is exemplified by patients with somatization disorder and many patients with idiopathic pain. They are primarily concerned with the somatic distress itself – they seek relief of their headache or musculoskeletal pain or fatigue or dizziness – but they do not believe they suffer from a serious, undiagnosed disease and are not morbidly concerned or preoccupied with the etiology of their symptoms. At the other end of the continuum are patients with anxiety disorders such as obsessive-compulsive disorder and disease phobias; they seek relief for disease fears and health-related anxiety rather than for bodily distress or somatic symptoms. Indeed their somatic symptoms may be very mild or even absent entirely. In short, these patients suffer from the *idea* that they are ill, not from somatic distress.

Hypochondriacal patients lie midway along this continuum, since they have *both* distressing somatic symptoms *and* disturbing concerns about the meaning and significance of these symptoms. Indeed, they are preoccupied most with the need for a diagnostic explanation of their physical suffering. This suggests that there may be two subtypes of hypochondriasis. One is characterized by prominent somatic symptoms, a relatively fixed and unassuageable belief that serious occult disease is present, and a primary request for somatic relief. This leads to high levels of medical utilization and great resistance to psychiatric care. The other hypochondriacal subtype is characterized by relatively minor somatic symptoms, high levels of health-related anxiety with prominent illness worry and disease fear, and some degree of insight into the unfounded nature of their fears and the fact that they are not seriously ill. Their profound anxiety leads to an avoidance of medical care while their insight into the groundlessness of their fears leads them to seek psychiatric attention.

This distinction between two subtypes of hypochondriasis may have clinical implications. The somatic subtype may benefit more from cognitive behavior therapy (CBT) to correct their misunderstanding and misattribution of their symptoms and to improve their skills for coping with somatic distress. In contrast, the anxious subtype may be more responsive to the pharmacotherapy used to treat anxiety disorders and obsessive-compulsive disorder.

The goal of CBT is symptom amelioration and palliation of somatic distress, rather than total and outright cure of somatic symptoms. The result of successful therapy is not the absence of all somatic symptoms but rather that the symptoms lose their noxious, intrusive, disturbing, and disabling quality. (As one such patient remarked at the end of therapy, "If I stop to think about it, I still have that lump in my throat; but I just don't think about it anymore.") The CBT approach targets the factors that amplify somatic symptoms: misunderstandings about the causes of symptoms, and mistaken health beliefs; identification and modification of situations, circumstances, and stresses that exacerbate symptoms; alteration of sick role and illness behaviors that lead to symptom amplification; and reductions in bodily hypervigilance and excessive self-scrutiny.

Pharmacotherapy, by comparison, targets the patient's anxiety, emotional arousal, and low threshold for alarm. The selective serotonin reuptake inhibitors and the serotonin norepinephrine reuptake inhibitors appear to be the most effective agents for this condition, but the empirical evidence for their efficacy at the time is relatively scant.

Therefore. careful phenomenological description of hypochondriacal patients may have important implications for therapy – and effective therapies for this condition are sorely needed. Despite its high prevalence in medical populations, and the significant impairment in quality of life that it engenders, hypochondriasis is vastly understudied. Rather, it tends to be disparaged and dismissed as trivial and insignificant. This pejorative and dismissive attitude does a disservice to hypochondriacal patients who are truly distressed and impaired and deserving of treatment.

References

1. Kroenke K, Price RK. Symptoms in the community. *Arch Intern Med* 1993;**153**:2474–2480.

2. White KL, Williams TF, Greenberg BG. The ecology of medical care. *N Engl J Med* 1961;**265**:885–892.

3. Hannay D. Symptom prevalence in the community. *J R Coll Gen Pract* 1978;**28**:492–499.

4. Hammond EC. Some preliminary findings on physical complaints from a prospective study of 1 064 004 men and women. *Am J Pub Health* 1964;**54**:11–23.

5. Buchwald D, Umali J, Kith P, Pearlman T, Komaroff AL. Chronic fatigue and the chronic fatigue syndrome: prevalence in a Pacific Northwest health care system. *Ann Intern Med* 1995;**123**:81–88.

6. Fukuda K, Dobbins JG, Wilson LJ, Dunn RA, Wilcox K, Smallwood D. An epidemiologic study of fatigue with relevance for the chronic fatigue syndrome. *J Psychiatric Res* 1997;**31**:19–29.

7. Loney P, Stratford PW. The prevalence of low back pain in adults: a methodological review of the literature. *Phys Ther* 1999;**79**:384–396.

8. Verbrugge LM, Ascione FJ. Exploring the iceberg: common symptoms and how people care for them. *Med Care* 1987;**25**:539–569.

9. Taylor GJ, Parker JDA, Bagby RM, Acklin MW. Alexithymia and somatic complaints in psychiatric outpatients. *J Psychosom Res* 1992;**36**:417–424.

10. De Gucht V, Heiser W. Alexithymia and somatisation: quantitative review of the literature. *J Psychosom Res* 2003;**54**:425–434.

11. Cohen S, Gwaltney JM, Jr., Doyle WJ, *et al.* State and trait negative affect as predictors of objective and subjective symptoms of respiratory viral infections. *J Pers Soc Psychol* 1995;**68**:159–169.

12. Watson D, Pennebaker JW. Health complaints, stress and distress: exploring the central role of negative affectivity. *Psychol Rev* 1989;**96**:234–254.

13. Vassend O. Dimensions of negative affectivity, self-reported somatic symptoms, and health-related behaviors. *Soc Sci Med* 1989;**28**:29–36.

14. Rost KM, Akins RN, Brown FW, Smith GR. The comorbidity of DSM-III-R personality disorders in somatization disorder. *Gen Hosp Psychiat* 1992;**14**:322–326.

15. Kirmayer LJ, Robbins JM, Paris J. Somatoform disorders: personality and the social matrix of distress. *J Abnorm Psychol* 1994;**103**:125–136.

16. Kirmayer LJ, Looper KJ. Abnormal illness behaviour: physiological, psychological and social dimensions of coping with distress. *Curr Opin Psychiat* 2006;**19**:54–60.

17. Blackwell B. Sick-role susceptibility. *Psychother Psychosom* 1992;**58**:79–90.

18. Stoudemire A. Somatothymia (Part I). *Psychosomatics* 1991;**32**:365–370.

19. Lipowski ZJ. Somatization: the concept and its clinical application. *Am J Psychiat* 1988;**145**:1358–1368.

20. Kleinman A. *Patients and Healers in the Context of Culture.* Berkeley, CA: University of California Press, 1980.

21. Kirmayer LJ. Culture and somatization: clinical, epidemiological, and ethnographic perspectives. *Psychosom Med* 1998;**60**:420–430.

22. Kirmayer LJ. Culture, affect and somatization. Part II. *Transcult Psychiat Res Rev* 1984;**21**:237–262.

23. Rief W, Barsky AJ. Psychobiological perspectives on somatoform disorders. *Psychoneuroendocrinology* 2005;**30**:996–1002.

24. Hakala M, Karlsson H, Ruotsalainen U, *et al.* Severe somatization in women is associated with altered glucose metabolism. *Psychol Med* 2002;**32**:1379–1385.

25. Hakala M, Karlsson H, Kurki T, *et al.* Volumes of the caudate nuclei in women with somatization disorder and healthy women. *Psychiatry Res Neuroimaging* 2004;**131**:71–78.

26. Spence SA, Crimlisk HL, Cope H, Ron MA, Grasby PM. Discrete neurophysiological correlates in prefrontal cortex during hysterical and feigned disorder of movement. *Lancet* 2000;**355**:1243–1244.

27. Vuilleumier P, Chicherio C, Assal F, Schwartz S, Slosman D, Landis T. Functional neuroanatomical correlates of hysterical sensorimotor loss. *Brain* 2001;**124**:1077–1090.

28. American Psychiatric Association. *Diagnostic and Statistical Manual of Mental Disorders*, 4th edn. Washington, DC: American Psychiatric Press, 1994.

29. Barsky AJ, Wyshak G, Klerman GL, Latham KS. The prevalence of hypochondriasis in medical outpatients. *Soc Psychiat Psychiatr Epidemiol* 1990;**25**:89–94.

30. Looper KJ, Kirmayer LJ. Hypochondriacal concerns in a community population. *Psycholog Med* 2001;**31**:577–584.

31. Noyes R, Carney CP, Hillis SL, Jones LE, Langbehn DR. Prevalence and correlates of illness worry in the general population. *Psychosomatics* 2005;**46**:529–539.

32. Bleichardt G, Hiller W. Hypochondriasis and health anxiety in the German population. *BrJ Health Psychol* 2007;**12**:511–523.

33. Martin A, Jacobi F. Features of hypochondriasis and illness worry in the general population in Germany. *Psychosom Med* 2006;**68**:770–777.

34. Noyes R, Jr., Holt CS, Happel RL, Kathol RG, Yagla SJ. A family study of hypochondriasis. *J Nerv Ment Dis* 1997;**185**:223–232.

35. Craig TKJ, Boardman AP, Mills K, Daley-Jones O, Drake H. The South London Somatization Study I: Longitudinal course and the influence of early life experiences. *Br J Psychiat* 1993;**163**:579–588.

36. Noyes R, Stuart S, Langbehn DR, *et al.* Childhood antecedents of hypochondriasis. *Psychosomatics* 2002;**43**:282–289.

37. Barsky AJ, Wyshak G, Klerman GL. Hypochondriasis: an evaluation of the DSM-III criteria in medical outpatients. *Arch Gen Psychiat* 1986;**43**:493–500.

38. Fink P, Ornbol E, Toft T, *et al.* A new, empirically established hypochondriasis diagnosis. *Am J Psychiatry* 2004;**161**:1680–1691.

39. Fallon BA, Petkova E, Skritskaya N, *et al.* A double-masked, placebo-controlled study of fluoxetine for hypochondriasis. *J Clin Pharmacol* 2008;**28**:638–645.

40. Barsky AJ, Fama JM, Bailey ED, Ahern DK. A prospective 4–5 year study of DSM-III-R hypochondriasis. *Arch Gen Psychiat* 1998;**55**:737–744.

41. Noyes R, Kathol RG, Fisher MM, Phillips BM, Suelzer M, Woodman CL. One-year follow-up of medical outpatients with hypochondriasis. *Psychosomatics* 1994;**35**:533–545.

Chapter 13

Movement disorders in complex regional pain syndrome: the pain field perspective

Jacobus J. van Hilten and Johan Marinus

Introduction

Complex regional pain syndrome (CRPS) is characterized by poorly controllable pain, swelling, and changes in skin blood flow and sweating, which usually develop in the distal extremities [1]. The syndrome, which commonly is preceded by a minor to severe trauma or surgical intervention, occurs more frequently in women (~75%) and may occur at all ages. There is compelling evidence that patients with CRPS may develop movement disorders (MDs), including dystonia, myoclonus, and tremor. Studies where selection bias towards MDs was unlikely indicate that 9–49% of the patients with CRPS developed MDs [2–5]. The female predominance in CRPS with MDs is even higher and reaches values of approximately 85% [4]. Additionally, the prevalence of MDs increases as the disease duration lengthens [5]. Here we focus on dystonia because it is the most prevalent MD in CRPS.

Is there a role for psychological factors in movement disorders in complex regional pain syndrome?

Several issues have contributed to a long-lasting controversy concerning the neurological or psychogenic origin of MDs in CRPS. First, studies that applied routine neurophysiological techniques failed to document abnormalities in patients with CRPS type I (CRPS-I) and MDs [6]. However, in view of the complex nature of neural circuits involved in, for example, dystonia, this should not come as a surprise. Second, over the years the concept of particularly dystonia evolved into that of a disorder associated with dysfunction of the basal ganglia–thalamocortical circuitry. Consequently, abnormal postures resulting from sustained muscle contractions that occurred in the absence of basal ganglia pathology were for a long period considered psychogenic. This particularly held for MDs that occurred as a consequence of peripheral trauma or CRPS, where basal ganglia involvement was neither demonstrated nor obvious from a clinical point of view. But how strong is the evidence for psychological factors in patients with CRPS with and without MDs? Research on psychological risk factors requires, at the least, a proper control group, along with reliable information regarding the period before onset. There are only a few studies that followed this approach in CRPS, none of which found differences in psychological characteristics between patients who did and did not develop CRPS after surgery or fractures [7–9]. A case–control study in which patients who developed CRPS were compared with age- and sex-matched patients who did not develop CRPS after a similar trauma showed that there were no psychological factors associated with an increased chance of developing CRPS [10]. A recently performed comprehensive systematic review also showed that there is no evidence of an association between psychological factors and the onset of CRPS-I in adults [11]. There is also no indication that childhood abuse increases the risk of developing CRPS in comparison with other diseases [12], while findings regarding the role of stressful life events are contradictory [12–14]. Cross-sectional studies in patients with CRPS with [15,16] and without [17] dystonia did not find an association with distinct psychological characteristics either; together these studies, therefore, do not support the existence of a unique psychological risk profile for patients with CRPS. Early traumatic experiences were reported in 87% of the patients with CRPS-I, and were found to be moderately related to somatoform dissociative experiences, indicating that

Psychogenic Movement Disorders and Other Conversion Disorders, ed. Mark Hallett, Anthony E. Lang, Joseph Jankovic, Stanley Fahn, Peter W. Halligan, Valerie Voon, and C. Robert Cloninger. Published by Cambridge University Press. © Cambridge University Press 2011.

early traumatic experiences might be a predisposing, although not a necessary, factor for the development of CRPS-I-related dystonia.

Dystonia in complex regional pain syndrome

Clinical characteristics

During clinical examination, it is not unusual to note that the execution of voluntary movement in patients with CRPS is impaired, but generally these disturbances are attributed to the presence of pain. Motor function has been characterized in patients with CRPS without dystonia using kinematic analysis of a standardized reach and grasp paradigm [18]. In this paradigm, specific abnormalities were found during grasping (deceleration and target phase) but not during reaching (acceleration). The target phase, which largely depends on the cortical integration of visual and somatosensory afferent inputs, was prominently prolonged compared with that in controls. These findings were interpreted as a disturbed integration of visual and proprioceptive inputs in the region of the posterior parietal cortex. Another study performed kinematic analysis of a standardized drawing test of the dominant hand of patients who suffered CRPS of the non-dominant arm only [19]. This study showed a poorer execution of movement and an impairment of temporospatial coding (greater variability of segment length and of movement time per segment) compared with controls.

Loss of voluntary control is frequently experienced by patients with CRPS suffering dystonia. Typically these patients report "My mind tells my hand/foot to move, but it won't work" [4]. This so-called loss of voluntary control has been reported in other causes of dystonia [20] and has been ascribed to both dysfunction of attention and abnormal sensorimotor integration [20–22].

Dystonia occurs in approximately 20% of patients with CRPS and is mainly characterized by fixed flexion postures of the fingers, wrist, and feet, which may vary in severity [4,23]. Less severely affected patients may not reveal dystonia at inspection, but this may be provoked by repetitive tasks in some cases. Dystonia of the lower extremity is usually characterized by inversion and/or plantar flexion of the foot, with or without clawing or scissoring of the toes [23]. Dystonia may worsen with exercise of the involved extremity, under circumstances of cold temperatures and humidity, and,

in the more severely affected patients, with tactile and auditory stimuli [23]. A potential pitfall in diagnosing dystonia in CRPS is the possible presence of contractures, which frequently also result in flexion postures. In dystonia in CRPS, however, passive stretching of affected digits provokes a contraction of the stretched muscle, suggesting stretch reflex hyperexcitability [24]. Although patients generally report persistence of their dystonia during sleep, electromyography (EMG) monitoring during sleep revealed no abnormal continuous EMG activity during non-REM or REM sleep [25]. This apparent discrepancy is explained by the fact that abnormal EMG activity immediately recurred at arousal during awakening, as evidenced by EEG.

In most cases, dystonia does not develop simultaneously with CRPS, but appears after a certain interval, which may vary from less than 1 week in 26% of the patients to more than 1 year in 25% of the patients [26]. Patients with CRPS and dystonia have a younger age at onset compared with those without dystonia, and have an increased risk of spread of dystonia to other extremities [26].

Putative mechanisms of disease

Splitting the heterogeneous clinical spectrum of CRPS into clusters of features that are linked to the various biological pathways facilitates understanding of the coherence between the clinical profile and its pathophysiology. Over recent years, knowledge of differentially involved mechanisms underlying inflammatory, vascular, sensory, and motor features of CRPS has gradually been growing. Similarities between the classical symptoms of inflammation and the clinical features of CRPS have led several investigators to suggest an inflammatory origin of the disease [27–29]. Indeed, studies have subsequently demonstrated evidence for aberrant inflammation in CRPS. Tissue injury results in excitation of C- and Aδ-fibres of sensory nerves, which causes release of the inflammatory neuropeptides substance P and calcitonin gene-related peptide from the afferent nerve endings. These neuropeptides induce local vasodilatation and increased capillary permeability, causing edema and an increase of skin blood flow – a process known as neurogenic inflammation [30,31]. In patients with CRPS, several studies have provided evidence implicating involvement of neurogenic inflammation [32,33]. Additionally, there is also involvement of the immune system of the skin, as indicated by elevated levels of tumor necrosis factor-alpha and interleukin-6 in suction blister fluid of affected extremities of patients with CRPS [34]. These cytokines remained elevated at 2–3 years after the onset of CRPS, in spite of an improvement of symptoms and signs [35]. Because neurogenic inflammation is initiated by sensory nerves, which cannot account directly for the development of MDs, it remained unclear how MDs in CRPS evolve. However, nociceptive neurons in the dorsal horns of the spinal cord may become sensitized (central sensitization) by peripheral tissue injury or inflammation, or by nerve lesions [36]. In central sensitization, there is an increased sensitivity of spinal neurons, despite unchanged afferent input. As a result, pain becomes chronic and non-noxious stimuli are painful [36]. On a molecular level, central sensitisation is associated with changes in the release of neuropeptides, neurotransmitters, prostaglandin E_2, and the expression of particularly N-methyl-D-aspartate (NMDA) receptors [36]. It would seem unlikely that central sensitization only involves pathways that deal with perception of pain and not those that mediate a response to pain. Indeed, Ferguson *et al.* [37] found that spinal plasticity associated with central sensitization also impaired motor responses mediated by spinal cord circuitry.

Cutaneous afferents are linked to spinal interneuronal circuits that mediate nociceptive withdrawal reflexes (NWR) [38]. Animal models of neurogenic inflammation have shown that substance P released at the dorsal horn of the spinal cord enhances these withdrawal reflexes [36,39]. Nociceptive withdrawal reflexes have both excitatory and inhibitory components that collectively produce a response appropriate to the specific motor context [40]. There are considerable differences concerning the principles that underlie regulation of the inhibitory and excitatory components. For example, excitatory reflexes are modulated according to the physiological action of each pair of muscles at the respective joint. Inhibitory reflexes are modulated at a more global level by means of a multisegmental spinal network, thus allowing "functional" organization that is linked to the role of proximal and distal muscles in various motor actions [40,41].

In withdrawal reflexes, flexor muscles play a prominent role, and, interestingly, in dystonia of CRPS there is a flexor-dominant pattern in the upper limb, which may hint at involvement of spinal motor programmes that mediate NWRs [23]. However, it is not unusual to note a relative sparing of the thumb and index finger of the hand in dystonia in CRPS. Compared with the flexor

motoneurons of digits III–V, the flexor motoneurons of digits I and II have a larger direct corticomotoneuronal input [42]. It is likely that in the spinal interneuronal circuits that mediates NWRs of the fingers, flexor motoneurons of digits I–V receive a similar interneuronal-motoneuronal input. Under circumstances that impair the interneuronal circuitry of NWRs, the larger proportion of direct corticomotoneuronal connections relative to interneuronal–motoneuronal connections of flexors of digits I and II may contribute to a relative sparing of digits I and II. Patients more affected by CRPS may demonstrate a stereotypical pattern of flexion of the fingers, wrist, and elbow, and adduction of the shoulder. This pattern resembles the bending reflex and Leri sign, which is elicited by forceful and painful passive flexion of the fingers and hand and is accompanied by flexion at the elbow and internal rotation of the shoulder.

The dominant pattern in the leg also seems consistent with NWRs: the withdrawal reflex of the foot is mainly intended to protect the foot when the subject is in an upright position, and the character of the response represents the most appropriate movement for a withdrawal of the stimulated area from an offending stimulus [43]. On excessively strong stimulation of the skin, the differences in reflex responses caused by changes of the stimulus site of the foot become less pronounced, and the reflex movement evoked tends to resemble a stereotyped flexor reflex [44] – plantar flexion/inversion of the foot, knee flexion and hip internal rotation – the dominant leg posture seen in patients with CRPS. A flexor-dominant pattern in the limbs, therefore, may suggest that upregulated or sustained NWRs contribute to the abnormal postures in CPRS.

Central sensitization is generally associated with a decrease of both tonic inhibitory and phasic action of inhibitory interneurons [45]. In patients with CRPS with and without dystonia, neurophysiological studies have found disinhibition along the neuraxis as a key characteristic of central involvement in CRPS [46–49]. Both substance P-sensitized NWRs in animal models and dystonia in CRPS in humans respond to the gamma-aminobutyric acid B ($GABA_B$) agonist baclofen, which enhances spinal GABAergic inhibition [50–52]. Baclofen specifically stimulates the $GABA_B$ receptor, which inhibits sensory input of neurons of the spinal cord.

Together, fundamental and clinical data suggest that peripheral injury or nerve injury may induce central sensitization, which has a prominent impact on sensory transmission and sensorimotor processing in the spinal cord. In view of the new concept of dystonia as a manifestation of aberrant sensorimotor networks involved in the control and execution of voluntary movement [53–55], the consequences of central sensitization on sensorimotor processing may provide a potential explanation for the occurrence of dystonia in CRPS.

To what extent the sudden and rapid onset of symptoms after injury, particularly the dystonic posturing, can be explained by mechanisms underpinning central sensitization remains unclear. However, in animal models it has been shown that within hours following peripheral nerve injury, dramatic chemical and physiological changes occur at the spinal cord level [56,57]. These changes include the upregulation of neuropeptides and neurotransmitters, induction of cyclooxygenase 2, activation of the neurokinin-1 and NMDA receptors, and alterations in gene transcription. Furthermore, in two animal studies of a model of CRPS, nerve injury induced abnormal hind paw postures [58,59]. In the first study, the highest prevalence of postural abnormalities was found after 3 days [58]. However, to date, it is unclear if these postures reflect dystonia and, contrary to the situation in humans, the majority of these "dystonias" in the study of Siegel *et al.* [58] disappeared within 2 weeks.

The hazard of developing dystonia in subsequent extremities in patients with CRPS increases with the number of extremities already affected by dystonia [26]. Apparently, once set into motion, the underlying mechanism of dystonia in CRPS has the capacity to facilitate the occurrence of dystonia in other body parts. This accelerated disease course is a characteristic that may point towards maladaptive neuronal plasticity, as has been documented for pain [60].

A significant association with human leukocyte antigen (HLA)-B62 and HLA-DQ8 was found in 150 patients with CRPS and dystonia [61]. This may be relevant to mechanisms of MDs in CRPS as HLA class I molecules have recently been implicated in mechanisms that mediate neuroplasticity [62,63].

In the context of dystonia as a manifestation of aberrant sensorimotor networks, the question remains whether the pathophysiology of MDs in CRPS is restricted to only spinal involvement. Two studies applied functional magnetic resonance imaging (fMRI) to evaluate cerebral network function during execution of voluntary movement in patients with CRPS with and without MDs [18,64]. One study

that evaluated finger movements in patients without MDs revealed a significant reorganization of central motor circuits, with increased activation of the primary motor cortex and supplementary motor cortices, as well as an increased activation of the ipsilateral motor cortex [18]. Notably, activities of the posterior parietal cortices, supplementary motor cortices, and primary motor cortex correlated with the degree of motor dysfunction as assessed by the maximum finger tapping frequency. Another study evaluated voluntary and imaginary hand movements in patients with CRPS and dystonia [64]. In this study, patients showed altered ipsilateral and contralateral cerebral activation during imaginary movement of the dystonic hand. In this study paradigm, there were no differences between patients and controls when they executed movements, nor when they imagined moving their unaffected hand. Together these fMRI studies have provided important new insights by showing prominent cortical changes of circuitry involved in voluntary and imaginary motor tasks in CRPS. Given the important role of supraspinal sensorimotor processing in the execution of movement, it is seems likely that to some extent these cortical changes indeed contribute to the pathophysiology of MDs in CRPS. Alternatively, the cortical changes could be only adaptive to spinal central sensitization. From the study of Maihöfner *et al.* [18] it is apparent that pain by itself is sufficient to develop such cortical abnormalities.

Acknowledgements

This study is part of TREND (Trauma RElated Neuronal Dysfunction; www.TRENDCONSORTIUM. nl), a knowledge consortium that integrates research on CRPS-I. This project is supported by a Dutch Government grant (BSIK03016).

References

1. Merskey H, Bogduk N. Complex regional pain syndrome, type I (reflex sympathetic dystrophy). *Classification of Chronic Pain: Descriptions of Chronic Pain Syndromes and Definition of Pain Terms*, 2nd edn. Seattle, WA: IASP Press, 1994:41–42.

2. Birklein F, Riedl B, Sieweke N, Weber M, Neundorfer B. Neurological findings in complex regional pain syndromes. *Acta Neurol Scand* 2000;**101**:262–269.

3. Blumberg H, Jänig W. Clinical manifestations of reflex sympathetic dystrophy and sympathetically maintained pain. In Wall P, Melzack R, eds. *Textbook of Pain*, 3rd edn. New York: Churchill Livingstone, 1993:685–698.

4. Schwartzman RJ, Kerrigan J. The movement disorder of reflex sympathetic dystrophy. *Neurology* 1990;**40**:57–61.

5. Veldman PH, Reynen HM, Arntz IE, Goris RJ. Signs and symptoms of reflex sympathetic dystrophy: prospective study of 829 patients. *Lancet* 1993;**342**:1012–1016.

6. Verdugo RJ, Ochoa JL. Abnormal movements in complex regional pain syndrome: assessment of their nature. *Muscle Nerve* 2000;**23**:198–205.

7. Field J, Gardner FV. Psychological distress associated with algodystrophy. *J Hand Surg* 1997;**22**:100–101.

8. Harden RN, Bruehl S, Stanos S, *et al.* Prospective examination of pain-related and psychological predictors of CRPS-like phenomena following total knee arthroplasty: a preliminary study. *Pain* 2003;**106**:393–400.

9. Puchalski P, Zyluk A. Complex regional pain syndrome type 1 after fractures of the distal radius: a prospective study of the role of psychological factors. *J Hand Surg* 2005;**30**:574–580.

10. de Mos M, de Bruijn AGJ, Huygen FJPM, *et al.* The incidence of complex regional pain syndrome: a population-based study. *Pain* 2007;**129**:12–20.

11. Beerthuizen A, van't Spijker A, Huygen FJ, Klein J, de Wit R. Is there an association between psychological factors and the complex regional pain syndrome type 1 (CRPS1) in adults? A systematic review. *Pain* 2009;**145**:52–59.

12. Ciccone DS, Bandilla EB, Wu Wh. Psychological dysfunction in patients with reflex sympathetic dystrophy. *Pain* 1997;**71**:323–333.

13. Geertzen JH, Bruijn-Kofman AT, de Bruijn HP, van de Wiel HB, Dijkstra PU. Stressful life events and psychological dysfunction in complex regional pain syndrome type I. *Clin J Pain* 1998;**14**:143–147.

14. Monti DA, Herring CL, Schwartzman RJ, Marchese M. Personality assessment of patients with complex regional pain syndrome type I. *Clin J Pain* 1998;**14**:295–302.

15. Reedijk WB, van Rijn MA, Roelofs K, *et al.* Psychological features of patients with complex regional pain syndrome type I related dystonia. *Mov Disord* 2008;**23**:1551–1559.

16. van der Laan, van Spaendonck K, Horstink MW, Goris RJ. The Symptom Checklist-90 Revised questionnaire: no psychological profiles in complex regional pain syndrome-dystonia. *J Pain Symptom Manage* 1999;**17**:357–362.

17. DeGood DE, Cundiff GW, Adams LE, Shutty J. A psychosocial and behavioral comparison of reflex sympathetic dystrophy, low back pain and headache patients. *Pain* 1993;**54**:317–322.

18. Maihöfner C, Baron R, DeCol R, *et al.* The motor system shows adaptive changes in complex regional pain syndrome. *Brain* 2007;**130**:2671–2687.

19. Ribbers GM, Mulder T, Geurts AC, den Otter RA. Reflex sympathetic dystrophy of the left hand and motor impairments of the unaffected right hand: impaired central motor processing? *Arch Phys Med Rehabil* 2002;**83**:81–85.

20. Berardelli A, Rothwell JC, Hallett M, *et al.* The pathophysiology of primary dystonia. *Brain* 1998;**121**:1195–1212.

21. Apkarian AV, Thomas PS, Krauss BR, Szeverenyi NM. Prefrontal cortical hyperactivity in patients with sympathetically mediated chronic pain. *Neurosci Lett* 2001;**311**:193–197.

22. Galer BS, Jensen M. Neglect-like symptoms in complex regional pain syndrome: results of a self-administered survey. *J Pain Symptom Manage* 1999;**18**:213–217.

23. van Hilten JJ, van de Beek WJ, Vein AA, van Dijk JG, Middelkoop HA. Clinical aspects of multifocal or generalized tonic dystonia in reflex sympathetic dystrophy. *Neurology* 2001;**56**:1762–1765.

24. van Hilten JJ, Blumberg H, Schwartzman RJ. Movement disorders and dystrophy: pathophysiology and measurement. In Wilson P, Stanton-Hicks M, Harden N, eds. *CRPS: Current Diagnosis and Therapies, Progress in Pain Research and Management*, Vol. 32, Seattle, WA: IASP Press, 2005:119–137.

25. van de Beek WJT, Vein A, Hilgevoord AAJ, van Dijk JG, van Hilten JJ. Neurophysiological aspects of patients with generalized or multifocal dystonia in reflex sympathetic dystrophy. *J Clin Neurophysiology* 2002;**19**:77–83.

26. van Rijn MA, Marinus J, Putter H, van Hilten JJ. Onset and progression of dystonia in complex regional pain syndrome. *Pain* 2007;**130**:287–293.

27. Oyen WJ, Arntz IE, Claessens RM, *et al.* Reflex sympathetic dystrophy of the hand: an excessive inflammatory response? *Pain* 1993;**55**:151–157.

28. Südeck P. Die sogenannte akute Knochenatrophie als Entzündungsvorgang. *Chirurg* 1942;**15**:449–457.

29. van der Laan L, Goris RJ. Reflex sympathetic dystrophy. An exaggerated regional inflammatory response? *Hand Clin* 1997;**13**:373–385.

30. Brain SD, Moore PK (eds). *Pain and Neurogenic Inflammation*. Basel: Birkhauser, 1999.

31. Holzer P, Maggi CA. Dissociation of dorsal root ganglion neurons into afferent and efferent- like functions. *Neuroscience* 1998;**86**:389–398.

32. Birklein F, Schmelz M, Schifter S, Weber M. The important role of neuropeptides in complex regional pain syndrome. *Neurology* 2001;**26**:2179–2184.

33. Leis S, Weber M, Isselmann A, Schmelz M, Birklein F. Substance-P-induced protein extravasation is bilaterally increased in complex regional pain syndrome. *Exp Neurol* 2003;**183**:197–204.

34. Huygen FJ, de Bruijn AG, d e Bruin MT, *et al.* Evidence for local inflammation in complex regional pain syndrome type 1. *Mediators Inflamm* 2002;**11**:47–51.

35. Munnikes RJ, Muis C, Boersma M, *et al.* Intermediate stage complex regional pain syndrome type 1 is unrelated to proinflammatory cytokines. *Mediators Inflamm* 2005;**6**:366–372.

36. Woolf C, Wiesenfeld-Hallin Z. Substance P and calcitonin gene-related peptide synergistically modulate the gain of the nociceptive flexor withdrawal reflex in the rat. *Neurosci Lett* 1986;**66**:226–230.

37. Ferguson AR, Crown ED, Grau JW. Nociceptive plasticity inhibits adaptive learning in the spinal cord. *Neuroscience* 2006;**141**:421–431.

38. Floeter MK, Gerloff C, Kouri J, Hallett M. Cutaneous withdrawal reflexes of the upper extremity. *Muscle Nerve* 1998;**21**:591–598.

39. Parsons AM, Honda CN, Jiay P, *et al.* Spinal NK1 receptors contribute to the increased excitability of the nociceptive flexor reflex during persistent peripheral inflammation. *Brain Res* 1996;**739**:263–275.

40. Don R, Pierelli F, Ranavolo A, *et al.* Modulation of spinal inhibitory reflex responses to cutaneous nociceptive stimuli during upper limb movement. *Eur J Neurosci* 2008;**28**:559–568.

41. Serrao M, Pierelli F, Don R, *et al.* Kinematic and electromyographic study of the nociceptive withdrawal reflex in the upper limbs during rest and movement. *J Neurosci* 2006:**26**;3505–3513.

42. Galea MP, Darian-Smith I. Manual dexterity and corticospinal connectivity following unilateral section of the cervical spinal cord in the macaque monkey. *J Comp Neurol* 1997;**381**:307–319.

43. Pierrot-Deseilligny E, Burke D. *The Circuitry of the Human Spinal Cord: Its Role in Motor Control and Movement Disorders.* New York: Cambridge University Press, 2005.

44. Grimby L. Normal plantar response: integration of flexor and extensor reflex components. *J Neurol Neurosurg Psychiatry* 1963;**26**:39–50.

45. Jones TL, Sorkin LS. Basic chemistry of central sensitisation. *Semin Pain Med* 2003;**1**:184–194.

46. Krause P, Foerderreuther S, Straube A. Bilateral motor cortex disinhibition in complex regional pain syndrome (CRPS) type I of the hand. *Neurology* 2004;**62**:1654.

47. Schwenkreis P, Janssen F, Rommel O, *et al.* Bilateral motor cortex disinhibition in complex regional pain syndrome (CRPS) type I of the hand. *Neurology* 2003;**61**:515–519.

48. Eisenberg E, Chistyakov AV, Yudashkin M, *et al.* Evidence for cortical hyperexcitability of the affected limb representation area in CRPS: a psychophysical and transcranial magnetic stimulation study. *Pain* 2005;**113**:99–105.

49. Avanzino L, Martino D, van de Warrenburg BP, *et al.* Cortical excitability is abnormal in patients with the "fixed dystonia" syndrome. *Mov Disord* 2008;**23**:646–452.

50. Saito K, Konishi S, Otsuka M. Antagonism between Lioresal and substance P in rat spinal cord. *Brain Res* 1975;**97**:177–180.

51. van Hilten JJ, van de Beek WJT, Hoff JI, Voormolen JH, Delhaas EM. Intrathecal baclofen for the treatment of dystonia in patients with reflex sympathetic dystrophy. *N Engl J Med* 2000;**343**:625–630.

52. van Rijn MA, Munts AG, Marinus J, *et al.* Intrathecal baclofen for dystonia of complex regional pain syndrome. *Pain* 2009;**143**:41–47.

53. Huang YZ, Trender-Gerhard I, Edwards MJ, *et al.* Motor system inhibition in dopa-responsive dystonia and its modulation by treatment. *Neurology* 2006;**66**:1088–1090.

54. Mink JW. Abnormal circuit function in dystonia. *Neurology* 2006;**66**:959.

55. Tisch S, Limousin P, Rothwell JC, *et al.* Changes in forearm reciprocal inhibition following pallidal stimulation for dystonia. *Neurology* 2006;**66**:1091–1093.

56. Woolf CJ, Mannion RJ. Neuropathic pain aetiology, symptoms, mechanisms, and management. *Lancet* 1999;**353**:1959–1964.

57. Samad TA, Moore KA, Sapirstein A, *et al.* Interleukin-1b-mediated induction of Cox-2 in the CNS contributes to inflammatory pain hypersensitivity. *Nature* 2001;**410**:471–475.

58. Siegel SM, Lee JW, Oaklander AL. Needlestick distal nerve injury in rats models symptoms of complex regional pain syndrome. *Anesth Analg* 2007;**105**:1820–1829.

59. Tan EC, Bahrami S, Kozlov AV, *et al.* The oxidative response in the chronic constriction injury model of neuropathic pain. *J Surg Res* 2009;**152**:84–88.

60. Woolf CJ, Salter MW. Neuronal plasticity: increasing the gain in pain. *Science* 2000;**288**:1765–1769.

61. de Rooij AM, Gosso FM, Haasnoot GW, *et al.* HLA-B62 and HLA-DQ8 are associated with complex regional pain syndrome with fixed dystonia. *Pain* 2009;**145**:82–85.

62. Corriveau Huh GS, Shatz CJ. Regulation of class I MHC gene expression in the developing and mature CNS by neural activity. *Neuron* 1998;**21**:505–520.

63. Goddard CA, Butts DA, Shatz CJ. Regulation of CNS synapses by neuronal MHC class I. *Proc Natl Acad Sci USA* 2007;**104**:6828–6833.

64. Gieteling EW, van Rijn MA, de Jong BM, *et al.* Cerebral activation during motor imagery in complex regional pain syndrome type 1 with dystonia. *Pain* 2008;**134**:302–309.

Chapter

14

Psychogenic dystonia in psychogenic complex regional pain syndrome

José L. Ochoa

Introduction

Psychogenic movement disorders are established clinical entities, characterized as formally as organically based movement disorders are [1]. These are difficult to differentiate clinically. The same is true for psychogenic versus organic chronic "neuropathic" pain disorders, often labeled descriptively as complex regional pain syndrome types I and II (CRPS-I and CPRS-II). For both movement disorders and "neuropathic" pains, the differential diagnosis between the organic and the psychogenic should not be by exclusion but based on explicit criteria. This requirement is not met for "CRPS-I." From personal knowledge and experience, it is an axiom that when an atypical movement disorder coexists symptomatically with a pseudoneurological CRPS-I, in all likelihood the pathogenesis of *both* conditions is psychogenic and reflects either hysterical conversion/somatization or malingering, or a combination [2].

During an audiovisual presentation to the *Psychogenic Movement Disorders Symposium* in April 2009, I showed evidential videotapes of two patients from the Oregon Nerve Center. One was a certified malingerer displaying a CRPS-I profile following a compensable motor vehicle accident, who embarrassingly failed Collie's yes/no test [3]. The other was also a malingerer communicating chronic pain (CRPS) following a compensable physical injury. She eventually developed grossly atypical, entrainable, and distractible abnormal movements, which were not seen in the video surveillances [4].

Debate around psychogenic complex regional pain syndrome

Although psychogenic movement disorders are unquestionable, there are honest doctors who deny psychogenic CRPS. There are also some who ascribe CRPS to "central neuronal sensitization," a condition that is untestable in humans [5]. Professor Wilfrid Jänig, together with Professor Ralf Baron [6], signed an Editorial for the journal Pain stating: "an extreme view (Ochoa, 1995) is that CRPS I is a pseudoneurological disease, i.e., that many features of CRPS are manifestations of somatoform disorders, malingering and psychiatric pathology. This view is now generally disregarded." This view I rebutted in a letter to the editor [7] and I now take another opportunity to discuss this issue. The pathophysiologies of "neuropathic" pains lie anywhere between sensory nerve endings and the brain; actually, between nerve and psyche. The psyche is neuronal. Many such affected patients are harmed by honest doctors [8]. Supporting evidence for this view now follows.

Taxonomy of pain: causalgia, reflex sympathetic dystrophy, sympathetically maintained pain, and chronic regional pain syndrome types I and II

On behalf of the International Association for the Study of Pain, Merskey and Bogduk [9] classified "neuropathic" CRPS into two types in their current taxonomy of pain. The original causalgia, now known as CRPS-II, is a painful nerve injury. In contrast, in the original reflex sympathetic dystrophy (RSD), now known as CRPS-I, there is no nerve injury. The taxonomy dictum specifies that the clinical course of CRPS-I is variable; the pathology is unknown; the basic pathophysiology is also unknown but is hypothesized to reside somewhere in the nervous system. There is no diagnostic test. The critical diagnostic criterion for CRPS-I is the

Psychogenic Movement Disorders and Other Conversion Disorders, ed. Mark Hallett, Anthony E. Lang, Joseph Jankovic, Stanley Fahn, Peter W. Halligan, Valerie Voon, and C. Robert Cloninger. Published by Cambridge University Press. © Cambridge University Press 2011.

fourth in this taxonomy: "This diagnosis is excluded by the existence of conditions that would otherwise account for the degree of pain and dysfunction." Thus, CRPS-I is a label by default. It is not the explicit diagnosis of a specific biological disease process. Loeser [10] writes:

> The fourth criterion says that CRPS I is a diagnosis that can only be made when another diagnosis cannot be established. This means that if we get better at diagnosing something else, we will reduce the frequency of diagnosing CRPS. Either this entity exists on its own criteria, or it does not and is just a repository for patients who cannot be adequately assessed and labeled.

This could be paraphrased as, "I know what you do not have, but I don't know what is going on; therefore you have CRPS-I."

A retrospective on the concept of RSD and causalgia/CRPS yields useful insights [11]. In the mid 1980s, Roberts [12] proposed that sympathetic maintained pain (SMP) such as RSD and causalgia was subserved by neuronal mechanisms. Natural ongoing sympathetic efferent activity would excite peripheral receptors of low threshold (tactile) mechanoreceptors. Their afferent input would impinge upon pain-signaling dorsal horn neurons, hypothetically already sensitized chronically by a powerful afferent nociceptor barrage during past physical trauma, thus causing sympathetic dependent ongoing pain and tactile allodynia. Although tactile allodynia in neuropathic pain could be partly mediated by low threshold mechanoreceptors, the pain maintenance in patients with SMP was believed to require the interaction between sympathetic efferents and C nociceptors [13]. Campero *et al.* [14] recently used sensitive and specific neurophysiological testing of identified single C nociceptor afferents and neighboring C sympathetic efferents in peripheral nerves serving symptomatic areas in patients with CRPS-I and CRPS-II. During documented activation of sympathetic fibers through reflex maneuvers, no excitation of C nociceptors was ever found. A simplified definition of SMP described it as "all pain syndromes that can be relieved by sympathetic blockade" [15], and the 1994 taxonomy of pain [9] (p. 41), when referring to relief of CRPS, stated: "Sympatholytic interventions may provide temporary or permanent relief." This self-reported subjective "relief" criterion was discredited when it became known that if sympathetic blocks transiently relieve pains, without a cure, they do so through placebo effect [16–19]. The medical world then blushed, but

the pain management industry simply eliminated the term RSD, invented CRPS-I, and carried on, business as usual. In other words, as exposed by Bell [20], "The new-found experts developed therapeutic empires with a vigorous entrepreneurial spirit that was undeterred by the ineffectiveness of their treatment methods." (See below the discussion of Dr. Raja's prediction about who will benefit from intrathecal baclofen in CRPS/dystonia.)

What do patients labeled with complex regional pain syndrome type I have?

Scientific evidence-based differential diagnosis of seemingly neurological conditions tentatively named CRPS-I is generally rewarding, provided a rigorous neurological and neurophysiological evaluation is performed. An illustrated gallery of five archetypical patients with "CRPS-I," who were rigorously differentiated, is given in my chapter in *Surgical Management of Pain* [21]. These cases were summarily presented at the *Psychogenic Movement Disorders Symposium* in April 2009.

Several lessons derived from clinical science can be drawn from consideration of those five patients.

1. All patients were neurological by symptoms, but all had been managed by non-neurologists.
2. All patients had been assumed to carry a sympathetically maintained pain status, but none did.
3. Each patient had a different, specific and diagnosable health disorder, but their medical assessment had bypassed mandatory differential diagnosis.
4. Hysterical conversion/somatization and malingering were both underdiagnosed.
5. Some patients were *curable*.
6. They all had been harmed by invasive treatment addressed at the fantasies of sympathetically maintained pain and/or central sensitization [8].

Again, as defined, CRPS-I is not a discrete disease entity, but rather a non-specific symptom complex, labeled by default. The latest assessment of CRPS-I, generated by the American Medical Association [22] states:

> CRPS is a challenging and controversial concept… Since the hallmark of this diagnosis is a subjective complaint of pain, and since all of the associated physical signs and radiological findings can be the result of disuse, an extensive differential diagnostic process is necessary.

Differential diagnoses that must be ruled out include disuse atrophy, unrecognized general medical problems, somatoform disorders and malingering. The diagnosis of CRPS has not been scientifically validated as representing a specific and discrete health condition. There is no gold standard diagnostic feature that distinguishes CRPS. Scientific findings indicate that whenever this diagnosis is made, it is probably incorrect. The IASP criteria, while sensitive, lack specificity, that is, they would identify patients as having CRPS when they do not.

Therefore, recurrent historical attempts to identify a unique pathophysiological basis for the inhomogeneous clinical category CRPS-I will remain self-defeating, as is the belief that "SMP is first and foremost associated with CRPS" [23,24]. The most recent theory behind CRPS-I envisages an occult small fiber (nociceptor) neuropathy that would explain not just the self-reported pains and allodynias but also the behavioral motor deficits and the movement disorder, plus the remote symptom spread and worsening *contra natura* [25]. This hypothesis, which is incompatible with standard clinical and neurophysiological characteristics of the painful syndrome of hyperexcitable nociceptors [26, 27], has already been countered by movement disorder authorities [28].

Unless patients with CRPS-I are evaluated through expert neurological examination and neurophysiological tests for differential diagnosis of the true source of their sensory, motor, and "autonomic" clinical displays, they are doomed to be adjudicated empirically a culture-bound "*disease process*", on the basis of self-reported subjective symptoms, associated non-specific "autonomic" phenomena, and sensory and motor signs that are unexplainable through neurological pathology. Multiple neurologically differentiable, legitimate primary organic or legitimate psychogenic disorders, plus malingering, may underlie so-called CRPS-I. A chronic pain complaint associated with a false neurological motor and sensory display is one of the favorite clinical presentations of malingerers. They are typically *mis*diagnosed with CRPS and treated inappropriately [29].

It is not uncommon for these psychogenic "CRPS patients" to factitiously self-inflict lesions [30].

Pseudoneurological sensory and motor disorders

The two patients with CRPS-I whose videotapes were presented to the *Psychogenic Movement Disorders Symposium* were both established as psychogenic. Note that in the gallery cited above [21], there are two additional cases of psychogenic CRPS-I: the male malingerer (case 5) and the somatized girl with abnormal movements (case 4). Evidence for a psychogenic diagnosis was obvious in the malingerer, and in the girl it was based on psychiatric assessment. However, from the neurological point of view, all four of these cases were psychogenic because they were pseudoneurological. Shorter [31] commented: "In the present context pseudoneurological illness seems most appropriate for those patients who have the symptoms but not the pathology of an organic lesion of the nervous system."

What are some definite pseudoneurological features:

sensory: false sensory loss or hyperalgesia/allodynia with non-anatomical and variable distribution associated with normal sensorimotor reflexes; normal sensory electrodiagnostics while the patient is displaying deficit; and abolition of the sensory dysfunction with placebo [32,33]

motor: false motor displays with giveway weakness demonstrably (electrodiagnosis) resulting from lack of willful drive from an intact motor cortex, combined with absence of atrophy (except for disuse atrophy); normal sensory-motor reflexes; normal motor electrodiagnostics (except for the electromyographic evidence of interrupted willful drive); and potential abolition of the voluntary weakness with placebo.

Dystonia in complex regional pain syndrome

Movement disorders are fairly common in CRPS. They only occur in patients who today are given the nickname CRPS-I, and who are found after rigorous neurological–neurophysiological differential diagnosis to harbor no organic neuropathology, and to be demonstrably pseudoneurological by semeiology [34]. This movement disorder is atypical. It is distractible, entrainable, and may disappear with placebo. It is highly exceptional for patients with organically based CRPS-II to display atypical movement disorders. Do animal models assist in our understanding of dystonia and CRPS? Importantly, in the experimental model of painful nerve injury, that is CRPS-II, dystonia does not occur and, not unexpectedly from the arguments provided above, legitimate animal models of CRPS-I do not exist.

Theory from the Netherlands

The *Psychogenic Movement Disorders Symposium* programmed a debate on "neuropathic pain." I was asked to present "CRPS and psychogenicity" while Professor J. van Hilten, from the Netherlands, argued for an organic basis for abnormal movements in CRPS. Dr. van Hilten's group had published an article in *Pain* 2 years earlier on dystonia in CRPS [35]. Scientific peer review brings up unassailable concerns about the Netherland's theory. Although the title of the paper mentions CRPS, the Introduction and their Material section specify *CRPS-I* [35]. The authors (p. 288) subscribe to, and quote, the diagnostic criterion 4 for CRPS-I from the Merskey and Bogduk taxonomy [9] (see above). In doing so, the authors ignore better judgment [10]. Moreover, the authors forgot the crucial fact that different kinds of CRPS-I are discerned when patients are examined rigorously, using clinical, neurophysiological, and psychophysical tools while excluding dogma and including the biopsychosocial paradigm. It is, therefore, no surprise that, absent differential delineation of medically meaningful subgroups out of their heterogeneous population of 185 patients with CRPS-I patients, the specific aim of their 2007 study ends in a "hint."

Why did van Rijn and colleagues fail to enlighten the nature of the atypical dystonia often displayed by patients who are descriptively labeled with "CRPS"? First, because the authors chose to construe "CRPS" as one discrete, homogeneous, neuropathophysiological, evidence-based disease entity characterized by self-reported, disproportionate, unexplained, intractable, and paradoxically escalating pains and allodynias, in addition to impaired motor behavior and to non-specific objective changes in the appearance and temperature of skin (assumed to be linked to an "autonomic" pathogenesis of the pains). Such display might be caused by demonstrable structural pathology of the nervous system, or elsewhere, or it may be part of a brain-driven pseudoneurological symptom complex plus disuse signs. And now, dystonia of controversial nature is being promoted as yet another characteristic of "CRPS."

The second reason for concern is that the authors "suggest" that the dystonia necessarily reflects a "maladaptive" neurophysiological aberration of spinal nociceptive withdrawal reflexes secondary to a chain of events that would start with a perturbed function of "C and A delta sensory nerve fibers." In doing so,

the authors turn a blind eye and fail to cite relevant peer-reviewed publications documenting that (1) the dystonia of CRPS-I is atypical compared with neuropathologically demonstrated dystonia; (2) it features explicitly psychogenic attributes; (3) it may be temporally abolished by placebo; (4) it only occurs in patients without demonstrable neuropathology behind their CRPS-I display; and (5) the CRPS-I plus the accompanied dystonia may be malingered or somatized. Van Rijn *et al.* did not examine their patients with CRPS-I for explicit sensory and motor pseudoneurological evidence behind their overall sensory and motor displays, nor for explicit psychogenic "dystonia." It is, therefore, not surprising that the authors trivialized a potential psychogenic etiology for the dystonia of CRPS-I. Van Rijn *et al.* admitted that their study "was not designed to address the question as to what extent psychogenic factors contribute to the onset of trauma related movement disorders… and although a role of psychogenic factors cannot be ruled out in the absence of an established pathophysiological explanation, we consider a major role for psychological factors unlikely for several reasons." The authors' first argument, namely "the phenotype has distinct characteristics which are similar across populations of different cultural background," backfires because those characteristics are uniformly pseudoneurological. The authors' second argument, namely reduced central inhibition in CRPS-related dystonia, starts with an observation and ends with a hypothesis rather than with a thesis validated by experiments and, therefore, is also invalid.

A *third* reason for concern is axiomatic. The method applied in pursuit of the specific clinical/research aim of van Rijn *et al.* is powerless. The expectation that analysis of time intervals between two sequential phenomena might clarify a possible causal link, let alone the medical nature of CRPS–dystonia, is wishful. It is, therefore, surprising that, at the end, the authors propose a causal link based on subsequence rather than consequence: "Our findings suggest that in a proportion of patients, CRPS may trigger a new mechanism which underlies the development of dystonia." They also venture a mechanism for the dystonia in CRPS-I: "The temporal characteristics of dystonia in our patients hint that maladaptive neuroplasticity… may underlie this movement disorder in CRPS." In other words, the authors describe minutely *when* dystonia but they miss the opportunity to clarify *what kind* of dystonia (typically organic versus typically psychogenic), nor do they clarify *in whom* dystonia (neurological versus pseudoneurological CRPS). In sum, the observation of variability in the time interval between onset of CRPS-I in patients not subjected to differential neurological diagnosis, and onset of dystonia, again in patients not subjected to neurological differential diagnosis, amounts, in the eyes of the authors, to sufficient evidence that the dystonia is triggered by CRPS and that it reflects *maladaptive neuroplasticity*. How empirical can it get?

G. Schott [36] from the Institute of Neurology, London, a seasoned scholar of dystonia in neuropathic pains, wrote an invited topical review for *Pain* to analyze CRPS and dystonia in connection with the article by van Rijn *et al.* [35]. As Schott [37] had intuited 20 years earlier, he emphasized the belated recognition of an escalating association of the "twin phenomena" of CRPS and dystonia, to an extreme incidence of 65% of patients with CRPS [35]. After creative speculation regarding hypothetical circuitry subserving CRPS-associated dystonia, and after discussing a potential psychogenic basis (crediting several authors, in particular Schrag *et al.* [38], also from the Institute of Neurology, London), Schott [36] concluded that some of the clinical elements of CRPS–dystonia can only be explained by central nervous system involvement (and he resorts to hypothetical central neuronal sensitization). However, his final point is: "whether peripherally triggered CRPS and dystonia have physiological and psychologically mediated mechanisms in common, remains unclear."

For readers of *Pain* who are not completely informed about CRPS, another recent article from the Netherlands threatens to become uncritically welcome as a breakthrough, particularly since it is endorsed by an Editorial. The article again comes from Professor van Hilten's group and promotes the use of baclofen for dystonia in CRPS [39]. It describes the author's experience with baclofen infusion (intrathecally) in 42 patients with CRPS–dystonia, and the resulting self-reported benefits and complications. The placebo caveat was *not* circumvented, unfortunately. Moreover, again the patient cohort had been named CRPS but not truly differentially diagnosed using scientific medical standards. To the extent that this cohort of patients termed as having CRPS-I must have included unrecognized, unconscious (and conscious) psychogenic cases, the invasive installation of baclofen pumps in those patients is intriguing. Patients with psychogenic CRPS (and dystonia) often welcome invasive procedures when promoted by persuasive physicians. The

Pain editorial supporting van Rijn *et al.* [39], by Raja [40], is remarkable in several ways. The editorialist, an academic physician, is an anesthesiologist. Yet these patients with RSD/CRPS are neurological by nature and require exquisite fund of knowledge and neurological skills on the side of the examiner for their differential diagnosis. Besides, the protocol for intravenous phentolamine block, as applied for attempted diagnosis of "SMP" must be stringently controlled for inert and active placebo effects [18,19], or else it proves misleading [41]. However, nobody could but agree with Dr. Raja's [40] forecast that the present promotion of intrathecal baclofen [39] "is likely to benefit interventional pain practitioners who treat patients with CRPS-associated dystonia."

Acknowledgement

The author was supported by NIH Grant R01NS48932.

References

1. Hallet M, Fahn S, Jankovic J, *et al.* (eds.) *Psychogenic Movement Disorders. Neurology and Neuropsychiatry.* Philadelphia, PA: Lippincott Williams & Wilkins, 2006.

2. Ochoa J. Pseudoneuropathy: conversion versus malingering. In *American Academy of Neurology 61st Annual Meeting, Painful Pain Patients, Education Program Syllabus,* 2009;7A-001-28-38.

3. Collie J. *Malingering and Feigned Sickness.* London: Edward Arnold, 1913.

4. Kurlan R, Brin MF, Fahn S. Movement disorder in reflex sympathetic dystrophy: a case proven to be psychogenic by surveillance video monitoring. *Mov Disord* 1997;**12**:243–245.

5. Ochoa J. The irritable human nociceptor under microneurography: from skin to brain. In Hallett M, Phillips II LH, Schomer DL, Massey JM, eds. *Advances in Clinical Neurophysiology*, Vol 57. New York: Elsevier Science, 2004:15–23.

6. Jänig W, Baron R. Is CRPS I a neuropathic pain syndrome? *Pain* 2006;**120**:227–229.

7. Ochoa J. Letter to the Editor concerning "Is CRPS I a neuropathic pain syndrome?" *Pain* 2006;**123**:332–335.

8. Ochoa J. Neuropathic pain and iatrogenesis. *Am Acad Neurol Cont* 2001;**7**:91–104.

9. Merskey H, Bogduk N. *Classification of Chronic Pain: Descriptions of Chronic Pain Syndromes and Definition of Pain Terms.* Seattle, WA: IASP Press, 1994.

10. Loeser JD. Introduction. In Wilson P, Stanton-Hicks M, Harden N, eds. *CRPS: Current Diagnosis and Therapies, Progress in Pain Research and Management*. Seattle, WA: IASP Press, 2005:3–7.

11. Ochoa J, Verdugo R. Reflex sympathetic dystrophy. Definitions and history of the ideas. A critical review of human studies. In Low PA, ed. *Clinical Autonomic Disorders*. Boston, MA: Little, Brown, 1993:473–492.

12. Roberts WJ. A hypothesis on the physiological basis for causalgia and related pains. *Pain* 1986;**24**:297–311.

13. Torebjörk E, Wahren L, Wallin G, Hallin R, Koltzenburg M. Noradrenaline-evoked pain in neuralgia. *Pain* 1995;**63**:11–20.

14. Campero M, Bostock H, Baumann TK, Ochoa J. A search for activation of C-nociceptors by sympathetic fibers in complex regional pain syndrome. *Clin Neurophysiol* 2010;**121**:1072–1079.

15. Treede RD, Raja SN, Davis KD, Meyer RA, Campbell JN. Evidence that peripheral alpha-adrenergic receptors mediate sympathetically maintained pain. In Bond MR, Charlton JE, Woolf CJ, eds. *Proceedings of the VIth World Congress on Pain*. Amsterdam: Elsevier, 1991:377–382.

16. Jadad AR, Carroll D, Glynn CJ, McQuay HJ. Intravenous regional sympathetic blockade for pain relief in reflex sympathetic dystrophy: a systematic review and a randomized, double-blind crossover study. *J Pain Symptom Manage* 1995;**10**:13–20.

17. Ramamurthy S, Hoffman J. Intravenous regional guanethidine in the treatment of reflex sympathetic dystrophy/causalgia: a randomized, double-blind study. Guanethidine Study Group. *Anesth Analg* 1995;**81**:718–723.

18. Verdugo RJ, Ochoa JL. "Sympathetically maintained pain." I. Phentolamine block questions the concept. *Neurology* 1994;**44**:1003–1010.

19. Verdugo RJ, Campero M, Ochoa JL. Phentolamine sympathetic block in painful polyneuropathies. II. Further questioning of the concept of "sympathetically maintained pain." *Neurology* 1994;**44**:1010–1014.

20. Bell DS. Repetition strain injury: an iatrogenic epidemic of simulated injury. *Med J Aust* 1989;**151**:280–284.

21. Ochoa JL. Pathophysiology of chronic "neuropathic pains." In Burchiel KJ, ed. *Surgical Management of Pain*. New York: Thieme, 2002:25–41.

22. American Medical Association. *Guides to the Evaluation of Permanent Impairment*, 6th edn. Chicago, IL: American Medical Association, 2008:450–454.

23. Jørum E, Ørstavik K, Schmidt R, *et al*. Catecholamine-induced excitation of nociceptors in sympathetically maintained pain. *Pain* 2007;**127**:296–301.

24. Ochoa J. Letter to the Editor concerning "Catecholamine-induced excitation of nociceptors in sympathetically maintained pain." *Pain* 2007;**131**:226–230.

25. Oaklander AL, Fields HL. Is reflex sympathetic dystrophy/complex regional pain syndrome type I a small-fiber neuropathy. *Ann Neurol* 2009;**65**:629–638.

26. Cline MA, Ochoa J, Torebjörk HE. Chronic hyperalgesia and skin warming caused by sensitized C nociceptors. *Brain* 1989;**112**:621–647.

27. Ochoa J L, Campero M, Serra J, Bostock H. Hyperexcitable polymodal and insensitive nociceptors in painful human neuropathy. *Muscle Nerve* 2005;**32**:459–472.

28. Lang AE, Chen R. Dystonia in complex regional pain syndrome type I. *Ann Neurol* 2010;**67**:412–414.

29. Ochoa J, Verdugo R. Neuropathic pain syndrome displayed by malingerers. *J Neuropsychiatry Clin Neurosci* 2010;**22**:278–286.

30. Mailis-Gagnon A, Nicholson K, Blumberger D, Zurowski M. Characteristics and period prevalence of self-induced disorder in patients referred to a pain clinic with the diagnosis of complex regional pain syndrome. *Clin J Pain* 2008;**24**:176–185.

31. Shorter E. The borderland between neurology and history: conversion reactions. In Weintrab MI, ed. *Neurologic Clinics. Malingering and Conversion Reactions*. Philadelphia, PA: W.B. Saunders, 1995:229–239.

32. Mailis-Gagnon A., Nicholson K. Nondermatomal somatosensory deficits (NDSDs): a neuropsychobiological phenomenon? *Clin J Pain* 2009;**145**:12–13.

33. Ochoa JL. Commentary on the nature of nondermatomal somatosensory deficits (NDSDs). *Clin J Pain* 2011;**27**:85–88.

34. Verdugo RJ, Ochoa JL. Abnormal movements in complex regional pain syndrome: assessment of their nature. *Muscle Nerve* 2000;**23**:198–205.

35. van Rijn MA, Marinus J, Putter H, van Hilten JJ. Onset and progression of dystonia in complex regional pain syndrome. *Pain* 2007;**130**:287–293.

36. Schott GD. Peripherally-triggered CRPS and dystonia. *Pain* 2007;**130**:203–207.

37. Schott GD. Induction of involuntary movements by peripheral trauma: an analogy with causalgia. *Lancet* 1986;**27**:712–716.

38. Schrag A, Trimble M, Quinn N, Bhatia K. The syndrome of fixed dystonia: an evaluation of 103 patients. *Brain* 2004;**127**:2360–2372.

39. van Rijn MA, Munts AG, Marinus J, *et al*. Intrathecal baclofen for dystonia of complex regional pain syndrome. *Pain* 2009;**143**:41–47.

40. Raja SN. Editorial. Motor dysfunction in CRPS and its treatment. *Pain* 2009;**143**:3–4.

41. Raja SN. Diagnosis of sympathetically maintained pain. The past, present and future (editorial). *Eur J Pain* 1993;**14**:45–48.

Latah and related syndromes

Philip D. Thompson

The first descriptions of the "culture-related" or "culture-bound" startle syndromes [1–3] included the Jumping Frenchmen of Maine by the North American physician Beard in 1880 [4], Latah in Malays by H. A. O'Brien, an adventurer exploring the Malay Peninsula in 1883 [5], and myriachit in Siberia by W. Hammond [6]. Latah is the most widely recognized and still occurs in Indonesian ethnic groups and Malays, particularly middle-aged married women. Within a community, Latah is often considered a form of social behavior and affected individuals are identified as "a Latah." Many culture-bound syndromes are recognized and similarly embedded in regional folklore or beliefs and accordingly are not necessarily regarded as "illnesses."

The clinical manifestations of the culture-related startle syndromes encompass motor, behavioral, and psychiatric phenomena. The motor phenomenon of an exaggerated startle response is often dramatic. This has often been regarded as a form of hyperekplexia, but, as will be discussed, the culture-related startle syndromes are caused by an exaggeration of the secondary or later component of the startle response, in contrast to hyperekplexia in which the first component of the startle response is enhanced. In addition, the culture-related startle syndromes are associated with a range of complex behavioral and neuropsychiatric manifestations, frequently including anxiety, fear, anger, and rage. Mystical or magical beliefs, somatic delusions, and trance or dissociation are additional accompaniments in some culture-related syndromes [3].

Although many of these syndromes are described in Eastern cultures [1,7], similar behaviors are recorded throughout the world. Examples from Western societies include Jumping Frenchmen [8], Ragin Cajuns [9], Jumpers [7], hyperstartlers [7], and possibly psychogenic myoclonus [10,11]. It is also important to note that comparable exaggerated responses are also observed in daily life from time to time when an unexpected stimulus induces a startle response followed by vocalization, possibly an expletive, and other behavioral phenomena modified by culture, circumstance, and volition. The normal startle response habituates with repeated stimulation, unlike Latah and related syndromes in which successive responses may exhibit increasing complexity.

The startle response

The normal startle response consists of two components [12]. The first component is an abrupt, brief blink, a grimace, then neck and head movement with variable flexion of the upper limbs and trunk. This component occurs at a short latency (50–60 ms) after a startling stimulus and is an involuntary reflex. In normal individuals, this response habituates with repeated stimulation. This component is exaggerated in hereditary hyperekplexia, where there are mutations in the genes for glycine receptors, and in acquired hyperekplexia, which is caused by brainstem diseases affecting the pontine reticular formation [13,14].

The second component of the startle response begins at latencies that overlap with voluntary reaction times (approximately 100–120 ms). The secondary response is longer in duration and subject to voluntary elaboration, incorporating an "orienting" or behavioral reaction toward the startling stimulus [15]. This may include looking in the direction of the stimulus, a voluntary movement away from it, raising the hands (in a defensive or aggressive posture), vocalization (including coprolalia), and dropping or throwing objects. In addition, a transient sensation of fright, anxiety, fear, and autonomic symptoms are normal accompaniments following an unexpected startle. These emotions and the extent of any

Psychogenic Movement Disorders and Other Conversion Disorders, ed. Mark Hallett, Anthony E. Lang, Joseph Jankovic, Stanley Fahn, Peter W. Halligan, Valerie Voon, and C. Robert Cloninger. Published by Cambridge University Press. © Cambridge University Press 2011.

behavioral response will be influenced by the nature of the stimulus, the situation in which it occurs, and the ambient emotional state. The startle response is augmented by states of high emotion and arousal, fear, and anxiety, and it is attenuated by pleasurable relaxation [16]. The level of emotional arousal may further influence the extent of the orienting reaction and voluntary elaboration of the behavioral reaction to the stimulus.

Startle in Latah and the culture-related syndromes appears to be based on augmentation of the second or late component of the startle response. The physical expression of the "jumps" or brisk jerks of the upper body in response to unexpected stimuli in the culture-bound startle syndromes has in the past been the main focus of attention. This led to speculation these conditions might represent a unique form of hyperekplexia. However, video recordings of the stimulus-induced responses in Latah [17] and in descendants of the Jumping Frenchmen [8,9] demonstrate responses beginning much later than the initial component of the startle reflex and the brainstem myoclonus of hyperekplexia. Instead, the observed stimulus-induced responses occur at intervals that overlap the second component of the startle response and fall within voluntary reaction times. In addition, the response in many cases incorporates a prominent behavioral reaction directed towards the triggering stimulus (the "orienting response") that may continue for several seconds.

Behavioral phenomena and the startle response

During the course of the behavioral response, a number of other clinical features appear, including complex motor activities and vocalization with coprolalia or echolalia. Complex motor activities such as forced obedience, imitation behavior, echopraxia, utilization, and other environment-dependent behaviors, including goal-directed and potentially harmful impulsive actions, may be incorporated in the response. Affected individuals may exhibit stimulus-induced vocalizations and complex motor activities at other times. These additional features are common to all culture-bound startle syndromes and were prominently recorded in the original descriptions of Jumping Frenchmen of Maine and of Latah [4,5]. Such behaviors may be prolonged and begin within voluntary reaction times, although they may be experienced as involuntary.

In some reports, the behavioral responses that follow external stimuli are more dramatic than the startle response itself. Similar behavioral accompaniments to startle are recorded in hyperstartlers [7], Tourette syndrome [18], and psychogenic myoclonus [10,11]. An exaggerated startle response has been reported in up to 20% of those with Tourette syndrome and in some cases reflex tics, vocalizations, coprolalia, echolalia, and other complex motor activities are triggered by external stimuli and startle [19]. In one study, stimulus-induced behaviors in Tourette syndrome were recorded at latencies overlapping voluntary reaction times [18]. Accordingly, exaggeration of the second component of the startle responses associated with stimulus-contingent behaviors is expressed in many societies.

Psychiatric conditions with an exaggerated startle response

Modulation of excitability of the auditory startle response also has been demonstrated in post-traumatic stress disorder, "war neurosis," "shell shock," "startle neurosis," schizophrenia, drug withdrawal [16], and psychogenic movement disorders [20]. The experimental paradigms used in these studies captured electromyographic activity from the orbicularis oculi muscle for up to 250 ms after an acoustic stimulus. Depending on when the recording of muscle activity begins, this period will include the blink reflex, the short early component of the startle response, and the longer secondary or late component. The results from studies of affective modulation of the startle response in neuropsychiatric disease, therefore, principally reflect affective modulation of the secondary component of the startle response, which includes the longer orienting and behavioral response to the stimulus.

Linking the startle response and behavior

The startle responses observed in Latah and related syndromes result from augmentation of the second component of the startle response, characteristically triggered by environmental stimuli and accompanied by behaviors that are recognized as neurological signs of frontal lobe dysfunction. In contrast, psychiatric explanations of such phenomena in the past emphasized the role of fright and fear in shaping the response to startle, and construed stimulus contingent behaviors as defense mechanisms against strong emotions, perhaps elaborated by local custom or expectation.

There are strong anatomical links between frontal regions and the startle apparatus in the brainstem.

Reciprocal interconnections between frontal and limbic cortical regions, cortical and ascending brainstem pathways involved in arousal, and the brainstem generators of the startle response provide the anatomical basis for an interaction between the emotional state, the startle response, and behavior [21,22]. The amygdala is particularly important in mediating frontolimbic influence on the excitability of the startle response [23].

A unifying neuropsychiatric postulate based on the anatomy, physiology, and clinical observations is that frontal lobe dysfunction may (1) influence the excitability of the startle response, (2) modify levels of arousal, and (3) augment and elaborate the response to startling stimuli. Enhanced excitability of the startle complex, in turn, may further heighten arousal. The combination of heightened arousal and impulsive (frontal) reactions to environmental (cultural and situational) cues will then determine the subsequent behavioral manifestations.

Conclusions

Startle syndromes resulting from augmentation of the second component of the startle reflex are commonly associated with prominent behavioral phenomena and vocalizations following the startle response or occurring in isolation. It is postulated that frontal lobe dysfunction disinhibits the startle mechanism and releases environmentally triggered startle responses and stimulus-contingent and impulsive behaviors. This hypothesis is amenable to further study in suitable groups. This mechanism, therefore, differs from the internal models of dissociation and conversion in psychogenic movement disorders, although dissociation may also be seen in culture-bound syndromes.

References

1. Yap PM. The Latah reaction: Its pathodynamics and nosological position. *J Mental Sci* 1952;**98**:515–564.

2. Howard R, Ford R. From the jumping Frenchmen of Maine to post-traumatic stress disorder: the startle response in neuropsychiatry. *Psychol Med* 1992;**22**:695–707.

3. Tseng W-S. From peculiar psychiatric disorders through culture bound syndromes to culture related specific syndromes. *Transcult Psychiatry* 2006;**43**:554–576.

4. Beard G. Experiments with the "jumpers" or "jumping Frenchmen" of Maine. *J Nerv Ment Dis* 1880;**7**:487–490.

5. O' Brien HA. Latah. *J Straits Br Asiat Soc* 1883;**11**:143–153.

6. Hammond WA. Miryachit, a newly described disease of the nervous system and its analogues. *NY Med J* 1884;**39**:191–192.

7. Simons RC. The resolution of the Latah paradox. *J Nerv Ment Dis* 1980;**168**:195–206.

8. Saint-Hilaire M-H, Saint-Hilaire J-M. Jumping Frenchmen of Maine. *Mov Disord* 2001;**16**:530.

9. McFarling DA. The "Ragin' Cajuns" of Louisiana. *Mov Disord* 2001;**16**:531–532.

10. Thompson PD, Colebatch JG, Brown P, *et al.* Voluntary stimulus sensitive jerks and jumps mimicking myoclonus or pathological startle syndromes. *Mov Disord* 1992;**7**:257–262.

11. Monday K, Jankovic J. Psychogenic myoclonus. *Neurology* 1993;**43**:349–352.

12. Wilkins D, Hallett M, Wess MM. Audiogenic startle reflex of man and its relationship to startle syndromes. *Brain* 1986;**109**:561–573.

13. Brown P, Rothwell JC, Thompson PD, *et al.* The hyperekplexias and their relationship to the normal startle reflex. *Brain* 1991;**114**:1903–1928.

14. Kimber TE, Thompson PD. Symptomatic hyperekplexia occurring as a result of pontine infarction. *Mov Disord* 1997;**12**:814–816.

15. Gogan P. The startle and orienting reactions in man. A study of their characteristics and habituation. *Brain Res* 1970;**18**:117–135.

16. Grillon C, Baas J. A review of the modulation of the startle reflex by affective states and its application in psychiatry. *Clin Neurophysiol* 2003;**114**:1557–1579.

17. Tanner CM, Chamberland J. Latah in Jakarta, Indonesia. *Mov Disord* 2001;**16**:526–529.

18. Tijssen MAJ, Brown P, Morris HR, Lees A. Late onset startle induced tics. *J Neurol Neurosurg Psychiatry* 1999;**67**:782–784.

19. Seignourel PJ, Miller K, Kellison I, *et al.* Abnormal affective startle modulation in individuals with psychogenic movement disorder. *Mov Disord* 2007, **22**:1265–1271.

20. Eapen V, Moriarty J, Robertson MM. Stimulus induced behaviours in Tourette's syndrome. *J Neurol Neurosurg Psychiatry* 1994;**57**:853–855.

21. Hitchcock JM, Davis M. Efferent pathway of the amygdala involved in conditioned fear as measured with the fear-potentiated startle paradigm. *Behav Neurosci* 2001;**105**:826–842.

22. Swanson LW, Petrovich GD. What is the amygdala? *Trends Neurosci* 1998;**21**:3223–3331.

23. Angrilli A, Mauri A, Palomba D, *et al.* Startle reflex and emotion modulation impairment after a right amygdala lesion. *Brain* 1996;**119**:1991–2000.

Chapter

16

Trauma and dissociation: clinical manifestations, diagnosis, epidemiology, pathogenesis, and treatment

Bethany Brand, Amie Myrick, Vedat Sar, and Ruth A. Lanius

Introduction

The objective of this chapter is to review the clinical manifestations, diagnosis, epidemiology, pathogenesis, and treatment of dissociative symptomatology, often experienced in context with a history of chronic psychological traumatization.

The relationship between stressful/traumatic life events and dissociation

Dissociation is defined in *Diagnostic and Statistical Manual of Mental Disorders*, 4th edition, text revision (DSM-IV-TR) [1] as a disruption of the usually integrated functions of consciousness, memory, awareness of body, and/or self, environment, and identity. The process of dissociation frequently involves psychological protection and detachment from overwhelming experiences, often of a stressful or traumatic nature, and is commonly experienced by adults and children during a traumatic event where fight/flight is impossible [2]. Research has utilized cross-sectional, longitudinal, and meta-analytic designs to extensively validate the relationship between dissociation and stressful or traumatic events in clinical, non-clinical, and large population samples throughout the world (e.g., van Ijzendoorn *et al.*, 1996 [3]).

Dissociation is predicted by trauma, particularly in early childhood, as well as attachment difficulties and parental unavailability [4–7]. Exposure to multiple types of trauma over developmental periods is associated with a range of clinical problems, including post-traumatic stress disorder (PTSD); borderline personality disorder (BPD); dissociative disorders (DD); mood, somatoform, non-PTSD anxiety disorders; and substance abuse [7,8].

The construct of "complex PTSD" has also been used to describe individuals who have been repeatedly traumatized during childhood and includes symptoms of dissociation, emotion dysregulation, somatization, chronic characterological changes, and alterations in systems of meaning [9]. There has also been recent research to suggest a predominantly dissociative subtype of PTSD [10,11]. This subtype is distinguishable from a predominantly hyperaroused subtype and has important treatment and research implications. Research suggests that those who present with the dissociative subtype are likely to have an earlier, more chronic, and repeated trauma history than those with hyperaroused PTSD. Their response to traumatic triggers is more likely to be dissociative in nature, paired with decreased heart rate and skin conductance and delayed cortisol release. This is in direct contrast to hyperemotional PTSD, where patients experience predominantly terror, re-experiencing episodes, and increased autonomic arousal [11] (see pathophysiology below).

Some individuals who fit the complex PTSD construct and/or dissociative PTSD subtype may also be diagnosed with DD. The DSM-IV-TR [1] identifies five DDs: dissociative amnesia, dissociative fugue, depersonalization disorder (DPD), dissociative identity disorder (DID), and dissociative disorder not otherwise specified (DDNOS). Dissociative fugue is thought only to occur in the course of dissociative amnesia or DID [12] and is likely to be removed from the forthcoming DSM-V5 as a separate disorder.

Prevalence of dissociative disorders

Epidemiological studies of DD conducted in North America, Europe, and Asia have found that dissociative

Psychogenic Movement Disorders and Other Conversion Disorders, ed. Mark Hallett, Anthony E. Lang, Joseph Jankovic, Stanley Fahn, Peter W. Halligan, Valerie Voon, and C. Robert Cloninger. Published by Cambridge University Press. © Cambridge University Press 2011.

amnesia is the most prevalent DD in general population studies, with prevalence rates up to 3.0% (reviewed by Dell, 2009 [12]), while DPD is thought to be present in approximately 1–2% [13]. In clinical populations, DDNOS tends to be the most prevalent DD with a prevalence of approximately 9.5% in both inpatient and outpatient samples (reviewed by Dell, 2009 [12]). Dissociative identity disorder, considered the most severe DD, occurs in approximately 1% of the general population [14], 1–20% of psychiatric inpatients [15,16], and 12–38% of outpatients [17,18], depending on the sample.

It is also interesting to note that one-third to one-half of patients with DD have a concurrent conversion disorder [19,20], and several authors have proposed that conversion disorders, therefore, be incorporated into the dissociative disorders section of the upcoming DSM-V [21]. Conversion disorders are known to be common, particularly in non-Western cultures. An epidemiological study conducted in western Turkey found a lifetime prevalence of 5.6% for DSM-IV-defined conversion disorder [21].

Clinical features of dissociative disorders

Depersonalization disorder

Depersonalization is an experience of feeling unreal, detached, or disconnected from one's self and is considered a typical experience, particularly in adolescents. The experience can be an associated feature of other disorders, such as schizophrenia, panic attacks, and substance abuse [1,7,13]. The typical onset of DPD, characterized by persistent or recurrent episodes of depersonalization which cause impairment in one or more areas of functioning, is in adolescence or early adulthood, and it can be acute, although approximately two-thirds of those with DPD have a chronic course [13]. Impairment in attention, memory, and occupational and interpersonal functioning is often reported by these individuals [13,22]. Comorbid mood and anxiety symptoms are also common, although their presence usually follows depersonalization and does not predict severity. Rather, traumatic or severe stress later in life is associated with the onset of DPD in 25% of all cases, and childhood trauma, particularly emotional abuse, uniquely predicts depersonalization severity [23]. This disorder has been hypothesized as

representing the "milder" end of a continuum of dissociative symptoms, with DID representing the more severe end of the continuum [13].

Dissociative amnesia

Dissociative amnesia is characterized as an inability to recall important autobiographical information beyond ordinary forgetfulness [1]. The information is usually of a traumatic or stressful nature, and the memories intrude in disguised forms such as nightmares, flashbacks, or conversion symptoms [7]. Impairment results from reversible psychological inhibition rather than organic factors, as evidenced by the individual's continued ability to learn new information and function cognitively. Dissociative amnesia has been found in documented cases of trauma including combat, the Nazi and Cambodian holocausts, childhood abuse, and adult assault [7,24]. Many patients with dissociative amnesia have a history of depression and suicidality; other predisposing factors may include personal or family history of somatoform or dissociative symptoms, and/or a childhood family setting characterized by rigidly held rules combined with punitive discipline. Dissociative amnesia may be related to avoidance of responsibility (e.g., sexual, legal, financial); fear of combat; avoidance of stressful situations that may evoke feelings of shame, anger, or despair; or urges of a sexual, suicidal, or violent nature.

Dissociative amnesia can present dramatically, as it is frequently portrayed in textbooks or media accounts, with a patient developing sudden, significant amnesia of extensive personal information, appearing disoriented and confused, having altered states of consciousness, and/or wandering [7]. Such patients are often seen in emergency departments and/or inpatient medical or neurology units and resolve within days or months spontaneously, through psychotherapy or through hypnotherapy. The other presentation is more common but receives less attention because it is picked up on with a careful history rather than patient report. In these cases, significant life events are missing from the autobiographical story; the onset and offset are clear, and the patient is aware that there is a gap in his/her memory (e.g., the patient does not recall high school but remembers other school years clearly). This type of dissociative amnesia resolves only through the course of psychotherapy for complex PTSD [7].

Dissociative identity disorder and dissociative disorder not otherwise specified

The diagnosis, phenomenology, etiology, epidemiology, and treatment of DID is covered extensively in the literature. Patients with DID or DDNOS are similar in presenting symptoms, history, clinical course, and treatment response [7], so they are combined here.

Dissociative identity disorder is a post-traumatic developmental disorder beginning in childhood, where the child is unable to formulate a unified sense of self owing to early exposure to repeated trauma. During these traumatic experiences, the child utilizes dissociation as a way to detach from emotional and physical pain. This defense mechanism can result in altered memory encoding and storage, leading to fragmentation of memory and difficulty retrieving information [5,7,25]. In addition, discrete behavioral states develop, persist, and become elaborated over time to develop into DID alternative identities.

The identities in DID have been portrayed in the media such that many clinicians believe that alternative identities are dramatic and that transitions between the identities are obvious. However, these florid presentations only occur in about 5% of patients with DID [26]. More frequently, patients' alternate identities present subtly, with dissociative and PTSD symptoms presented alongside other symptoms including depression, substance abuse, somatoform symptoms, eating disorders, and self-destructive and impulsive behaviors [7,8].

Patients with DID often report a history of multiple treatment providers, hospitalizations, and medication trials that resulted in minimal or no benefit [8]. Experts in treating DD direct treatment so that it focuses less on overt personality states and more on the complex polysymptomatology involved in DID [27]. This focus is based on studies that have demonstrated that overlap and interference between alternative identities into patients' consciousness is more common in DID than obvious "switching." These intrusions into consciousness include both those that are partially excluded (e.g., hearing voices of identities inside the mind) and those that are fully excluded (e.g., time loss) and can be misdiagnosed as psychotic "passive influence" or the schneiderian first-rank symptoms found in schizophrenia [27,28].

Somatoform dissociation and conversion disorder

The essential feature of conversion disorder is the presence of symptoms or deficits affecting voluntary motor or sensory function that suggest a neurological or other general medical condition [1]. Conversion phenomena themselves are conceptualized as types of somatoform dissociation, in contrast to psychological dissociation [29,30]. This notion is in accordance with the BASK model of dissociation, which points out not only the disconnection between *behavior* (B), *affect* (A), and *knowledge* (K), but also between them and *sensation* (S) [31]. While conversion disorder is characterized by objective physical or *pseudoneurological* symptoms (e.g., paralysis, pseudoseizure [1]), the broader concept of somatoform dissociation may include medically unexplained physical complaints beyond the definition of conversion disorder, such as pain, loss of sexual desire, or painful menstruation. Medically unexplained symptoms are associated with high levels of distress and frequent visits to primary care physicians [32], particularly for those with psychiatric disorders [19]. Patients are often dissatisfied with the treatment they receive, particularly when no cause for their symptoms is found [33,34]. The Somatoform Dissociation Questionnaire (SDQ) [30] is a self-rating tool that is able to reliably assess this construct.

Psychogenic non-epileptical seizures (PNES), also called pseudoseizures, is the most prevalent form of conversion disorder in clinical populations. Seizures resembling tonic–clonic convulsions are a hallmark of PNES. Affected patients demonstrate tremors, shaking, and convulsions; most report hearing conversations during the episode without being able to speak. However, seizures resulting in injury or urinary incontinence are uncommon. The duration of the episode is typically 5–10 min to several hours, longer than an epileptic seizure. Screaming and aggressive or self-mutilative behavior may accompany the episode, while crying spells may occur during recovery. In most patients, psychosocial stress factors are observed during the first or last episodes of the conversion disorder.

Comorbidity in dissociative disorders

Patients with DD often meet criteria for multiple comorbid psychiatric and medical problems, including mood disorders, PTSD, anxiety disorders, substance use disorders, and somatoform disorders. Medical problems include headaches, fibromyalgia, chronic fatigue syndrome, gastrointensinal problems (particularly gastroesophageal reflux disease and irritable bowel syndrome), and gynecological problems. The Adverse Childhood Experiences (ACE) study, a longitudinal study that examines the relationship between childhood experiences and biomedical disease, has found that negative childhood experiences are associated with increases in liver disease, chronic pulmonary disease, and heart disease [35]. Researchers have also demonstrated a link between childhood stress and autoimmune disease in adults [35,36]. Patients may also meet criteria for one or more personality disorders. As many as 53–72.5% of patients entering treatment for BPD also have a DD [37,38]. However, this diagnosis is often made when trauma-related symptoms are overwhelming and the patient is severely decompensated. Most no longer meet the criteria after they have been stabilized.

Differential diagnosis

Because patients rarely volunteer information about dissociative symptoms for fear of sounding "crazy" and avoid discussing histories of trauma [39], making the diagnosis of a DD can be difficult. For this reason, a safe, collaborative relationship often must be developed before asking about private and often humiliating experiences. An additional barrier to making a DD diagnosis is lack of training; most clinicians have not been trained in the assessment of dissociation and many fail to ask about trauma history or dissociative symptoms.

For those both trained and untrained in assessing dissociation, a detailed office mental status examination is available for assessing dissociative symptoms [40]. An abridged version of this examination is available in Table 16.1. This examination reviews trauma exposure, as well as post-traumatic, affective, and somatic symptomatology. Additionally, there are several self-report screening instruments available to accurately examine the presence of dissociation. The most widely used is the Dissociative Experiences Scale (DES) [41], which has been used in over 1000 studies to date and translated into more than 40 languages. The DES contains 28 items that assess amnesia, absorption, identity alteration, and depersonalization/derealization. Using a scale ranging from 0 to 100%, patients rate how often they experience each symptom; an average score is then calculated. An average score of 30 or higher is often indicative of more severe DDs such as DID and DDNOS; however, lower scores have also been found in DD. Therefore, screening instruments must be interpreted carefully and within the clinical context; they should never be substituted for clinical judgment. The Multidimensional Inventory of Dissociation (MID) [42] is another self-report measure that assesses partial and full psychological dissociation as well as somatization, and the SDQ, as mentioned above, is used to assess for somatoform dissociation. There are also two DSM-IV-TR structured interviews that can provide formal diagnoses of DD: the Structured Clinical Interview for DSM-IV-TR Dissociative Disorders, revised (SCID-D-R) [22] and the Dissociative Disorders Interview Schedule (DDIS) [43]. Additional information regarding the assessment of dissociation in both children and adults is available [7,44,45].

Often, DID and severe DDNOS are confused with psychotic and affective disorders, as well as BPD. While DD can be comorbid with these disorders, they are not synonymous and differ in many ways. The following list is adapted from Brand and Loewenstein 2010 [46].

- *Psychological trauma histories* tend to be less severe for those with schizophrenia and bipolar disorder than in those with BPD or DD. Patients with DD typically report more severe trauma histories than those with BPD [47].
- *Testing differences* have found that patients with DD and BPD do not differ on the number of traumatic intrusions on the Rorschach. Both patients with DD and those with BPD score higher on traumatic intrusions than those with schizophrenia [47].
- *Presence of dissociative symptoms* is typically highest for those with DD (e.g., DES average score of 44.6), followed by those with BPD (e.g., DES average score of 21.6), then those with schizophrenia (e.g., DES average score of 17.6), and finally those with bipolar disorder [48].
- The *experience of dissociative symptoms* is typically quite different for these groups. Patients with DD often prefer numbness to intense emotions; therefore, they may self-harm to induce dissociation. At times when they are dissociating, they are involved in an elaborate inner world that consists of multiple identities. This experience is very different from that in patients with BPD, who have a low tolerance for numbness and may self-harm to end dissociation rather than initiate

Table 16.1 Office Mental Status Interview for assessing dissociation

Feature	Questions
Blackout/time loss	Do you ever have blackouts, blank spells, memory lapses?
	Do you lose time?
Disremembered behavior	Do you find evidence that you have said and done things that you do not recall?
	Do people tell you of behavior you have engaged in that you do not recall?
Fugues	Do you ever find yourself in a place and not know how you got there?
Unexplained possessions	Do you find objects in your possession (e.g., clothes, groceries, books) that you do not remember acquiring? Out of character items? Items a child might have?
	Do you find that objects disappear from you in ways for which you cannot account?
	Do you find writings, drawings, or artistic productions in your possession that you must have created but do not recall creating?
Changes in relationships	Do you find that your relationships with people frequently change in ways that you cannot explain?
Fluctuations in skill/habits/knowledge	Do you find that sometimes you can do things with amazing ease that seem much more difficult or impossible at other times?
	Does your taste in food, music, or personal habits seem to fluctuate?
	Does your handwriting change frequently? A little? A lot? Childlike?
	Are you right handed or left? Does it fluctuate?
Fragmentary recall of life history	Do you have gaps in your memory of your life? Missing parts of your memory of your life history?
	Do you remember your childhood? When do those memories start? First memory? Next? Next?
Intrusion/overlap/interference (passive influence)	Do you have thoughts or feelings that come from inside or outside you that don't feel like yours? Are outside your control?
	Do you have impulses or engage in behaviors that don't seem to be coming from you?
	Do you hear voices, sounds, or conversations in your mind?
Negative hallucinations	Do you ever *not* see/hear what's going on around you? Can you block out people or things altogether?
Depersonalization/derealization	Do you frequently have the experience of feeling as if you are outside yourself or watching yourself as if you were another person?
	Do you ever feel disconnected from yourself or as if you were unreal?
	Do you experience the world as unreal? As if you are in a fog or daze?
	Do you ever look in the mirror and not recognize yourself?
Psychological trauma	Who made the rules in your family and how were they enforced?
	Did you witness violence between family members?
	Have you ever had unwanted sexual contact with anyone? In childhood? Teenager? Adult?
	As a child what made you feel safe? Was anyone kind or supportive of you?
	Flashbacks – intrusive symptoms – sight, sound, taste, smell, touch: do you ever experience events that happened to you before as if they are happening now?
	Nightmares – how often, since when? Do you awaken disoriented? Find yourself somewhere else?
	Are there specific people, situations, or objects that trigger you? Are these associated with time loss?

Table 16.1 (*Cont.*)

Feature	Questions
	Are you a jumpy person? Easily startled?
	Do you avoid people, situations, or things that remind you of traumatic or overwhelming events? Can you block out feelings?
Somatoform symptoms/ conversion[a]	Are you able to block out physical pain? Wholly? Partly? Always? Sometimes?
	Do you find that your physical responses/capacities (eyesight, blood pressure, response to alcohol, or meds) change in ways you can't explain?
	Did you ever get any of the following physical symptoms that your doctors can't medically explain?
	Seizures and convulsions (fainting fits with or without loss of consciousness)?
	Trouble in walking, paralysis, or muscle weakness?
	Shaking, tremor, or contractures in extremities or entire body?
	Double or blurred vision, or blindness?
	Difficulty in swallowing, vomiting, nausea, or abdominal pain?
	Loss of voice or deafness?
	Pain in extremities, back pain, joint pain?
	Shortness of breath, palpitations, chest pain?
	Have you ever been diagnosed as having migraine headaches?

[a] Includes questions from both Loewenstein [39] as well as from one author (V.S.).
Source: adapted with permission from Loewenstein, 1991 [40].

it. These patients do not experience an inner world of separate identities. When patients with BPD dissociate, they are experiencing a trance-like or depersonalized state.

- *Hypnotizability* is highest in patients with DD, followed by those with BPD, then schizophrenic patients [7].
- *Transformations in identity* also look different amongst these groups. Bipolar patients do not experience such transformations, and patients with BPD do so only with respect to their polarized, intense mood changes in response to situational stress. For example, patients with BPD may feel that they are a worthwhile lovable person when their relationships are going well, but may feel tremendous self-hatred and loathing when a relationship has become conflictual or ended. Neither of these groups experiences amnesia outside of that caused by substance use. However, patients with DD may admit to identity transformations such that they feel as if they act so differently they are like different people, although only patients with DD experience past and present

amnesia. While some schizophrenia patients may indicate they experience transformations in their identity, these perceived changes are related to magical or delusional beliefs.

- *Hallucinatory experiences* are also quite different in these patients. Patients with DD often endorse hearing voices engaged in conversation and may "see" identities or past experiences via flashback, but they understand that these voices are not real. Thus, reality testing remains intact. Bipolar patients experience hallucinations only during episodes of psychotic mania or depression. The voices experienced during psychotic depression are typically persecutory and are not in conflict with one another. Similarly, patients with BPD only experience hallucinations during stress, if at all. These voices represent their polarized values and opinions. Finally, patients with schizophrenia may not be aware of the fact that the voices are not real. These voices typically have less elaborate discussions than the voices experienced in DD, and the voices are not related to abusers or hurt children.

111

- *Affect* also distinguishes these patients, patients with DD experiencing a range of unexplained and rapid mood changes triggered by either internal or external stimuli. This differs from the mood shifts in bipolar disorder, where the changes occur much more slowly (i.e., at least 12 hours), and in BPD, where the changes result from external triggers and can be quite rapid. Patients with BPD also typically demonstrate poor affect modulation [48]. Those with schizophrenia demonstrate flat and/or inappropriate affect. Patients with DD rarely complain of feeling "empty," as opposed to patients with BPD, who regular experience feelings of emptiness and intense anger.
- *Perception* is generally accurate for those with DD. Those with schizophrenia have less logical and organized thinking than those with DD. Those with BPD have significantly less-accurate perception and less logical, organized thinking than those with DD [47]. Those with bipolar disorder only demonstrate poor perception and logical thinking during mood episodes.
- A *working alliance* is achieved more easily by patients with DD, also seen with bipolar patients. Both groups typically demonstrate a capacity to view others as cooperative, to reflect on self, and to develop meaningful relationships. Patients with DD may also choose to avoid relationships and to be alone because being alone may feel safer [47]. Patients with schizophrenia and BPD are less likely to develop a solid working alliance. For schizophrenia patients, this can be because of an expectation of lack of cooperation in relationships, having little interest in others, and/or having less capacity for self-reflection and emotional distancing [47]. While patients with BPD do have an interest in others, they also have difficulty tolerating loneliness and have chaotic relationships because of their devaluation and idealization. Like schizophrenia patients, those with BPD tend to expect a lack of cooperation in relationships and are not as skilled in self-reflection or maintaining emotional distance.

Conversion and somatoform dissociation symptoms also need to be distinguished from neurological disorders by using first-line medical diagnostic procedures. Psychiatric examination alone cannot be a reliable instrument to complete this differential diagnostic task. Epilepsy, cerebrovascular accidents, and multiple sclerosis, as well as several neurological and even general medical disorders, may need to be excluded depending on the predominant symptom. Once the symptom(s) is (are) determined as medically unexplainable, all psychiatric disorders which may lead to conversion (somatoform dissociation) symptoms should be screened in an appropriate order. Patients with any DD may demonstrate conversion symptoms such as pseudoseizures [49]. Whereas conversion and somatoform dissociation symptoms may be superimposed with dissociative or comorbid physical disorders (e.g., neurological disorders including epilepsy), they may also co-occur with other psychiatric disorders such as anxiety, mood, somatization, and even psychotic disorders. They may also stand alone, warranting a diagnosis of conversion disorder.

Neurological etiologies of dissociative symptomatology

Bremner [51] has hypothesized that there may be two subtypes of acute trauma response: failure of cortico-limbic inhibition versus excessive corticolimbic inhibition – emotional under – and overmodulation. These two subtypes comprise one that primarily involves dissociative symptoms and the other predominantly intrusive and hyperaroused; these represent unique pathways to chronic stress-related psychopathology. Data from neuroimaging studies have shown that the two subtypes of response can persist in individuals with chronic PTSD and are associated with distinct patterns of neural activation upon exposure to reminders of traumatic events. Van der Kolk and colleagues define these dissociative subtypes as primary and secondary dissociation [51]. Primary dissociation refers to the re-experiencing/hyperaroused variant of dissociation commonly associated with PTSD symptoms, such as unbidden recollections, flashbacks, and nightmares. In contrast, secondary dissociation is characterized by such symptoms as numbness, amnesia, detachment states, depersonalization, derealization, freezing, analgesia responses, and subjective distance from emotional experience, to which the term dissociation is more commonly applied [51].

Lanius *et al.* [52–56] have researched the neuronal circuitry underlying re-experiencing/hyperarousal (primary dissociation) and depersonalization/derealization dissociative (secondary dissociation) responses in PTSD using the script-driven, symptom-provocation paradigm. In these studies, subjects constructed a narrative of their traumatic experience including as many sensory details as possible. These narratives were later read to the subjects, who were instructed to recall the traumatic memory as vividly as possible during functional magnetic resonance imaging (fMRI). Approximately 70% of subjects relived their traumatic experience, demonstrating predominant primary dissociation (re-experiencing/hyperarousal response) with an increase in heart rate while recalling the traumatic memory [52]. The remaining 30% had a predominant secondary dissociative response with no concomitant increase in heart rate [53,55]. When compared with control subjects, those who had a hyperarousal response and relived their traumatic experience after being exposed to the traumatic script showed significantly less activation of the anterior cingulate gyrus (Brodmann area [BA] 32) and medial frontal gyrus (BA 10 and BA 11) [52]. These brain activation patterns differ markedly from those observed in subjects who exhibited secondary dissociation in response to the traumatic script [53]. These subjects exhibited *higher* levels of brain activation in the following areas: superior and middle temporal gyri (BA 38), the medial prefrontal cortex (BA 9), and anterior cingulate gyrus (BA 24 and BA 32). The neural correlates of re-experiencing/hyperarousal states and depersonalization/ derealization dissociative states, respectively, in patients with PTSD show *opposite* patterns of brain activation in brain regions that are implicated in arousal modulation and emotion regulation. In particular these differential patterns are found in the medial prefrontal cortex, the anterior cingulate cortex, and the limbic system.

Failure of corticolimbic inhibition

Abnormally *low* activation in the medial prefrontal and the anterior cingulate cortex were exhibited in the re-experiencing/hyperaroused PTSD group [56,57]. Consistent with impaired cortical modulation, increased activation of the limbic system, particularly the amygdala, a brain structure that has been shown to play a key role in fear conditioning, has often been observed in patients with PTSD after exposure to traumatic reminders and to masked fearful faces [58]. Studies have also reported direct inhibitory influence of the prefrontal cortex on the emotional limbic system in patients with PTSD. Positron emission tomography studies, for example, have shown a negative correlation between blood flow in the left ventromedial prefrontal cortex and the amygdala during emotional tasks, and negative correlations between medial prefrontal cortex and the amygdala during exposure to fearful faces [58]. Consequently, the *low* activation of medial prefrontal regions described in the re-experiencing/hyperaroused PTSD subgroup is consistent with failed inhibition of limbic reactivity and is associated with re-experiencing/hyperaroused emotional undermodulation. We conceptualize this group of patients as experiencing emotional undermodulation in reaction to traumatic reminders such as a subjective reliving experience of the traumatic events (e.g., flashbacks and reliving nightmares). These symptoms can be viewed as a form of emotion dysregulation that involves emotional undermodulation, mediated by failure of prefrontal inhibition of limbic regions.

Excessive corticolimbic inhibition

In contrast to the re-experiencing/hyperaroused group, abnormally *high* activation in the anterior cingulate cortex and the medial prefrontal cortex was found in the group experiencing secondary dissociative symptoms [53]. Thus, in response to exposure to traumatic memory recall the patients with depersonalization/derealization dissociative PTSD can be conceptualized as having emotional overmodulation. This often involves subjective disengagement from the emotional content of the traumatic memory through depersonalization or derealization or other secondary dissociative responses, which have been hypothesized to be mediated by midline prefrontal inhibition of the limbic regions (Fig. 16.1).

A study by Felmingham *et al.* [59] provides additional evidence for the corticolimbic inhibition model. The impact of dissociation as measured by the Clinician Administered Dissociative State Scale on fear processing was examined using fMRI in two groups of patients with PTSD, one with high and the other with low dissociation scores,. The researchers compared brain activation during the processing of consciously and non-consciously perceived fear stimuli. Compared with patients with low dissociation scores, enhanced activation in the ventral prefrontal cortex during conscious fear processing was found in patients with high dissociation scores. The results of this research led investigators to support the theory that secondary dissociation is a regulatory strategy invoked to cope with extreme arousal in PTSD through hyperinhibition of limbic regions, and that this strategy is most active during conscious processing of threat.

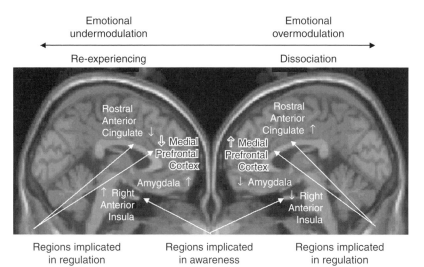

Emotional undermodulation

Emotional overmodulation

Re-experiencing

Dissociation

Regions implicated in regulation of emotion and arousal

Regions implicated in awareness of bodily states

Regions implicated in regulation of emotion and arousal

Fig. 16.1. Re-experiencing/ hyperarousal reactivity to traumatic reminders is viewed as a form of emotion dysregulation that involves emotional *undermodulation*, mediated by failure of prefrontal inhibition of limbic regions. In contrast, the dissociative reactions to traumatic reminders are described as a form of emotion dysregulation that involves emotional *overmodulation*, mediated by midline prefrontal inhibition of the same limbic regions. (From Lanius *et al.*, 2010 [11], with permission from American Psychiatric Press.)

Additional support for the hyperinhibition of the limbic system, including the amygdala during dissociative states, is also provided in the neurobiology literature on pain. For example, decreased amygdala activity in response to painful stimulation during hypnosis-induced states of depersonalization in healthy subjects was reported by Roeder *et al.* [60]. In patients with PTSD and BPD, amygdala deactivation was also observed in response to thermal pain stimuli [61–64]. In addition, trait dissociation as measured by the DES correlated negatively with the right amygdale in a sample of patients with PTSD [65]. We have also used the script-driven imagery paradigm to specifically induce secondary dissociative states in patients with BPD while also assessing pain sensitivity in response to thermal pain stimuli [64]. Higher levels of secondary dissociation, determined by the Dissociation Tension Scale [66], were found during the presentation of these scripts compared with a neutral script. On a neural level, during secondary dissociative states, higher activity in dorsolateral prefrontal cortex was found. A subgroup analysis of 10 patients with both BPD and PTSD was performed, and increased activity was found in right insula and left cingulate cortex, thus providing further evidence for the corticolimbic inhibition model.

Studies of DPD provide additional evidence for the corticolimbic inhibition model. Hollander *et al.* [67] reported a case study of a patient with primary DPD using brain electrical mapping. The results demonstrated left frontal overactivation, which was indicated by increased anteriorized alpha activity. The authors also demonstrated with single-photon emission computed

tomography that this patient showed impaired perfusion in the left caudate and increased activity in posterior frontal areas. A subsequent investigation of a group of patients with DPD examined event-related fMRI to neutral, mild, and intensely happy and sad facial expressions, with simultaneous measurements of skin conductance levels [68]. Compared with healthy controls, patients with DPD showed a decrease in subcortical limbic activity to increasingly intense happy and sad facial expressions. Moreover unlike healthy controls, those with DPD exhibited negative correlations between skin conductance measures and activation in the bilateral dorsal prefrontal cortices for both happy and sad facial expressions. These studies support the hypothesis that subjects with DPD exhibit increased prefrontal activity and/or decreased limbic activity, which results in the hypoemotionality frequently reported in these patients and adds weight to the overmodulation model to explain secondary dissociative states.

The findings described above support the corticolimbic inhibition model of excessive limbic inhibition resulting in secondary dissociation symptoms in PTSD and other trauma spectrum disorders such as BPD, DID, and DD. In addition, these findings are consistent with the phenomenology and clinical presentation of these patients with significant depersonalization/ derealization, amnesias, pain dysregulation, and other secondary dissociation symptomatology. The corticolimbic inhibition model proposes that once a threshold of anxiety and hyperarousal is achieved, the medial prefrontal cortex inhibits emotional processing in limbic structures (including the amygdala). This leads to a significant dampening of sympathetic output and reduced emotional experiencing, resulting in a variety of secondary dissociative symptoms. In contrast, in the subgroup exhibiting secondary dissociative symptoms, increased activation of medial prefrontal structures is consistent with the idea of hyperinhibition of those same limbic regions and pathological emotional overmodulation in response to trauma-related emotions [69].

Treatment of dissociative disorders

Psychological treatment

The current standard of care addresses the complexities of these patients by way of a phasic, multimodel, trauma-focused psychotherapy [7, 70, 71]. However, to date, there are no randomized clinical trials of DD treatment and only one controlled case study. Brand and colleagues [70] reviewed 16 DD treatment outcome studies, as well as four case studies that used standardized measures. Although the data were from non-controlled, observational trials, results demonstrated reductions in symptoms of dissociation, depression, general distress, anxiety, and PTSD when the above-mentioned treatment model was used. Additionally, some studies found that treatment was associated with decreased use of medications and improved occupational and social functioning. A small meta-analysis using eight of the studies found that treatment had a medium to large effect on outcome (e.g., effect size for dissociation, 0.94; 95% confidence interval, −0.27 to 2.18).

Although treatment studies have primarily focused on DID, there has been some limited research published on treatment of the other DD subtypes. For example, placebo-controlled medication trials found that patients with DPD did not respond to fluoxetine or lamotrigine [13]. However, a cognitive behavioral treatment focusing on attention training in addition to traditional psychoeducation and challenging of distortions has shown promise in reducing depersonalization/derealization symptoms and increasing global functioning, with gains maintained at 6 months of follow-up [72]. There has been speculation about the impact that somatoform dissociation may have on treatment effectiveness. For example, Waller and colleagues [73] suggest that somatoform dissociation is likely to impair the effectiveness of exposure-based treatments, which can be successful, unless they are targeted to impact physiological aspects of trauma-related disorders. Further, they suggest that somatoform dissociation may also affect the impact of cognitive treatments where the ability to identify somatic clues and processes is an important part of the therapy.

When considering the treatment outcomes of those with DID, case series studies suggest three treatment trajectories in which some patients can be successfully treated to full "fusion or integration" of all identity states so that they no longer meet criteria for DID; a second group shows reduction in symptoms, and a third group shows mild improvement but continues to be chronically ill [74]. However, full integration of all identities appears to be a relatively infrequent outcome [71].

Non-randomized open DID treatment studies have found reductions in a range of symptoms and number of axis I and II diagnoses when patients receive treatment at specialized trauma/dissociation-focused inpatient units [70,75]. Similarly, promising results have been found for patients with DID and DDNOS treated in the community in an international naturalistic, prospective study of these disorders [76]. Cross-sectional results from this study indicated that treatment was associated with improvements in many areas reported by patients and therapists. The patients in later stages of treatment had fewer dissociative and PTSD symptoms, as well as lower general distress. Patients in the later stages of treatment also had fewer hospitalizations and better general functioning than those early in treatment [77]. Preliminary follow-up data also found that treatment is associated with improvement [70].

There are well-described treatments of DID [e.g., 7,9,44,78–81]. Phase-oriented treatment is the standard of care for the treatment of DD and complex trauma disorders, with three phases typically charting the course of treatment [71]. The first stage emphasizes stabilization and safety, with a focus on symptom, affect and impulse control; education about diagnoses and trauma treatment; and the establishment of a collaborative working relationship. This stage is often considered the most important. The early exposure to trauma and disruptions in attachment for many patients with DD can be re-enacted through self-injurious behaviors, suicide attempts, substance abuse, aggression, or involvement in abusive relationships; consequently, this stage of treatment is often the longest, with some patients remaining in this phase of treatment for years.

Once the patient is stabilized, she or he may choose to move into the next stage of treatment, which involves processing traumatic material. During this stage, therapists assist patients in exploring the meanings and impacts of traumatic experiences, identifying and resolving cognitive distortions, and expressing emotions such as grief, betrayal, terror, anger, helplessness, and shame. Stage three entails "reintegration into life" [9]; the patient integrates previously disowned aspects of his/her self and focuses on his/her present and future life and goals. It is often at this point in treatment that patients fully recognize that their earlier trauma may have altered their development and affected their health in ways that cannot be fully overcome, and yet they can still move forward with their lives.

Pharmacotherapy

Although medication is often used to assist with stabilization and comorbid symptoms, an "anti-dissociative" medication has not yet been found to treat dissociative disorders [13]. No medications have been found to effectively target the symptoms specific to somatoform dissociation or the dissociative subtype of PTSD, although sertraline and paroxetine are approved by the US Food and Drug Administration to stabilize hyperarousal or intrusive symptoms [82]. In this way, a poor medication response may provide a clue that assessment for DD may be warranted. Medications for this population typically result in partial improvement and are considered most useful when targeting hyperarousal and intrusive symptoms of PTSD, as well as comorbid mood disorders and obsessive-compulsive symptoms [7,44,83]. Some success has been reported by those using selective serotonin reuptake inhibitors, tricyclic antidepressants, monoamine oxide inhibitors, beta-blockers, clonidine, prazosin, and anticonvulsants. Benzodiazepines may also be helpful but should be used with caution as there is a high risk for addiction. Neuroleptics are typically ineffective for pseudopsychotic symptoms such as hearing voices in DD; however, low doses of the atypical neuroleptics can be beneficial in cases where severely anxious or intrusive symptoms and/or seriously distorted thinking is present [7]. Experts suggest adjusting medications to attend to the patient's overall needs rather than trying to adjust medications to attend to frequent mood and symptom fluctuations.

Conclusion and implications

Dissociative disorders are disorders characterized by early and often chronic abuse, complex symptom presentations, and comorbidity with other mental health and medical disorders. Corticolimbic pathways have been shown to play an important role in the mediation of dissociative symptomatology. Dissociative patients frequently report unexplained neurological symptoms, which can include movement, making these symptoms one of their most common predecessors to emergency psychiatric admissions [84]. These symptoms can be a source of frustration when no medical cause for their symptoms is found, and this may lead patients to seek out specialists. Therefore, those who treat movement disorders will likely encounter patients with DD. Providers are encouraged to take a careful history, including assessment for trauma and dissociative symptoms and review of past medical treatment. Because childhood trauma has been linked to increased medical problems [e.g., Lin *et al.*, 1991 [34], a complete physical examination and testing should be carried out to exclude medical diseases. Providers should proceed with caution with dissociative patients who have experienced chronic traumatization, meeting patients' questions and concerns with empathy and patience, and referring to mental health professionals who have expertise in assessing and treating dissociation.

References

1. American Psychiatric Association. *Diagnostic and Statistical Manual of Diseases*, 4th edn, text revision. Washington DC: American Psychiatric Press, 2000.

2. Silberg JL, Dallum S. Dissociation in children and adolescents: at the crossroads. In Dell PF, O 'Neill J, eds. *Dissociation and the Dissociative Disorders: DSM-V and Beyond*. New York: Routledge, 2009:67–81.

3. van Ijzendoorn MH, Schuengel C. The measurement of dissociation in normal and clinical populations: meta-analytic validation of the Dissociative Experiences Scale (DES). *Clin Psychol Rev* 1996;**16**:365–382.

4. Gershuny BS, Thayer JF. Relations among psychological trauma, dissociative phenomena, and trauma-related distress: a review and integration. *Clin Psychol Rev* 1999;**19**:631–657.

5. Putnam FW. *Dissociation in Children and Adolescents: A Developmental Perspective*. New York: Guilford Press, 1997.

6. Schore AN. Attachment trauma and the developing right brain: origins of pathological dissociation. In Dell PF, O'Neill J, eds. *Dissociation and the Dissociative Disorders: DSM-V and Beyond*. New York: Routledge, 2009:107–141.

7. Simeon D, Loewenstein RJ. Dissociative disorders. In Sadock BJ, Sadock VA, Ruiz P, eds. *Comprehensive Textbook of Psychiatry*, Vol. 1, 9th edn. Philadelphia, PA: Wolters Kluwer/Lippincott Williams & Wilkins, 2009:1965–2026.

8. Dell PF, O' Neil JA (eds.). *Dissociation and the Dissociative Disorders: DSM-V and Beyond.* New York: Routledge, 2009.

9. Herman JL. *Trauma and Recovery: The Aftermath of Violence from Domestic Abuse to Political Terror.* New York: Basic Books, 1992.

10. Ginzburg K, Koopman C, Butler LD, *et al.* Evidence for a dissociative subtype of post-traumatic stress disorder among help-seeking childhood sexual abuse survivors. *J Trauma Dissoc* 2006;**7**:7–27.

11. Lanius RA, Vermetten E, Loewenstein RL, *et al.* Emotion regulation in PTSD: clinical and neurobiological evidence for a dissociative subtype. *Am J Psychiatry* 2010;**167**:640–647.

12. Dell PF. The long struggle to diagnose multiple personality disorder (MPD): MPD. In Dell PF, O'Neill J, eds. *Dissociation and the Dissociative Disorders: DSM-V and Beyond.* New York: Routledge, 2009:383–402.

13. Simeon D. 2009). Depersonalization disorder. In Dell PF, O 'Neill J, eds. *Dissociation and the Dissociative Disorders: DSM-V and Beyond.* New York: Routledge, 2009:435–444.

14. Ross CA, Joshi S, Currie R. Dissociative experiences in the general population. *Am J Psychiatry* 1990;**147**:1547–1552.

15. Friedl MC, Draijer N. Dissociative disorders in Dutch psychiatric inpatients. *Am J Psychiatry* 2000;**157**:1012–1013.

16. Gast U, Rodewald F, Nickel V, Emrich HM. Prevalence of dissociative disorders among psychiatric inpatients in a German university clinic. *J Nerv Mental Dis* 2001;**189**:249–257.

17. Foote B, Smolin Y, Kaplan M, Legatt ME, Lipschitz D. Prevalence of dissociative disorders in psychiatric outpatients. *Am J Psychiatry* 2006;**163**:623–629.

18. Şar V, Akyüz G, and Doğan O. The prevalence of conversion symptoms in women from a general Turkish population. *Psychosomatics* 2009;**50**:50–58.

19. Şar V, Akyüz G, Kundakçi T, Kiziltan E, Doğan O. Childhood trauma, dissociation, and psychiatric comorbidity in patients with conversion disorder. *Am J Psychiatry* 2004;**161**:2271–2276.

20. Tezcan E, Atmaca M, Kuloglu M, *et al.* Dissociative disorders in Turkish inpatients with conversion disorder. *Compr Psychiatry* 2003;**44**:324–330.

21. Brown RJ, Cardeña E, Nijenhuis ERS, Şar V, van der Hart O. Should conversion disorder be re-classified as a dissociative disorder in DSM-V? *Psychosomatics* 2007;**48**:369–378.

22. Steinberg M. *Interviewer's Guide to the Structured Clinical Interview for DSM-IV Dissociative Disorders – Revised (SCID-D-R),* 2nd edn. Washington, DC: American Psychiatric Press, 1994.

23. Simeon D, Knutelska M, Nelson D, Guralnik O. Feeling unreal: a depersonalization update of 117 cases. *J Clin Psychiatry* 2003;**64**:990–997.

24. Loewenstein RJ. Dissociative amnesia and dissociative fugue. In Micelson LK, Ray WJ, eds. *Handbook of Dissociation: Theoretical, Empirical, and Clinical Perspectives.* New York: Plenum Press, 1996:307–336.

25. Spiegel D, Cardeña E. Disintegrated experience: the dissociative disorders revisited. *J Abnorm Psychol* 1991;**100**:366–378.

26. Kluft RP. The natural history of multiple personality disorder. In Kluft RP, ed. *Childhood Antecedents of Multiple Personality.* Washington DC: American Psychiatric Press, 1985:197–238.

27. Dell PF. The long struggle to diagnose multiple personality disorder (MPD): MPD. In Dell PF, O 'Neill J, eds. *Dissociation and the Dissociative Disorders: DSM-V and Beyond.* New York: Routledge, 2009:383–402.

28. Ross CA, Miller SD, Reagor P, *et al.* Schneiderian symptoms in multiple personality disorder and schizophrenia. *Compr Psychiatry* 1990;**31**:111–118.

29. Nijenhuis ERS, Vanderlinden J, Spinhoven P. Animal defensive reactions as a model for trauma-induced dissociative reactions. *J Traum Stress* 1998;**11**:243–260.

30. Nijenhuis ER, Spinhoven P, van Dyck R, van der Hart O, Vanderlinden J. The development and psychometric characteristics of the Somatoform Dissociation Questionnaire (SDQ-20). *J Nerv Mental Dis* 1996;**184**:688–694.

31. Braun BG. The BASK (behavior, affect, sensation, knowledge) model of dissociation. *Dissociation*, 1988;**1**, 4–23.

32. Gureji O, Simon GE, Ustun TB, Goldberg DP. Somatization in cross-cultural perspective: a World Health Organization study in primary care. *Am J Psychiatry* 1997;**154**:989–995.

33. Hahn SR. Physical symptoms and physician-experienced difficulty in the physician-patient relationship. *Ann Intern Med* 2001;**134**:897–904.

34. Lin EH, Katon W, von Korff M, *et al.* Frusrating patients: physician and patient perspectives among distressed high users of medical services. *J Gen Intern Med* 1991;**6**, 241–246.

35. Felitti VJ, Anda RF, Nordenberg D, *et al.* Relationship of childhood abuse and household dysfunction to many

of the leading causes of death in adults: The Adverse Childhood Experiences (ACES) Study. *Am J Prevent Med* 1998;**14**:245–258.

36. Dube SR, Fairweather D, Pearson WS, *et al.* Cumulative childhood stress and autoimmune diseases in adults. *Psychosom Med* 2009;**71**:243–250.

37. Şar V, Akyüz G, Kugu N, Öztürk E, Ertem-Vehid H. Axis I dissociative disorder comorbidity in borderline personality disorder and reports of childhood trauma. *J Clin Psychiatry* 2006;**67**:1583–1590.

38. Zittel Conklin C, Westen D. Borderline personality disorder in clinical practice. *Am J Psychiatry* 2005;**162**:867–875.

39. Brand BL, Armstrong JG, Loewenstein RJ. Psychological assessment of patients with dissociative identity disorder. *Psychiatr Clin North Am* 2006;**29**:145–168.

40. Loewenstein RJ. An office mental status exam for chronic, complex dissociative symptoms and multiple personality disorder. *Psychiatr Clin North Am* 1991;**14**:567–604.

41. Bernstein EM, Putnam FW. Development, reliability and validity of a dissociation scale. *J Nerv Mental Dis* 1986;**174**:727–735.

42. Dell PF, Multidimensional Inventory of Dissociation (MID): a comprehensive measure of pathological dissociation. *J Trauma Dissoc* 2006;**7**:77–106.

43. Ross CA. *Dissociative Identity Disorder: Diagnosis, Clinical Features, and Treatment of Multiple Personality.* New York: John Wiley, 1997.

44. Chu JA, Loewenstein R, Dell PF, for the International Society for the Study of Dissociation. Guidelines for treating dissociative identity disorder in adults, 2nd revision. *J Trauma Dissoc* 2005;**6**:69–149.

45. Silberg J., Waters F., Nemzer E., *et al.* Guidelines for the assessment and treatment of dissociative symptoms in children and adolescents. *J Trauma Dissoc* 2004;**5**:119–150.

46. Brand BL, Loewenstein RL. Dissociative disorders: an overview of assessment, phenomenology, and treatment. *Psychiatr Times* 2010; October.

47. Brand BL, Armstrong JG, Loewenstein RJ, McNary SW. Personality differences on the Rorschach of dissociative identity disorder, borderline personality disorder, and psychotic inpatients. *Psychol Trauma Theory Re, Pract Policy* 2009;**1**:188–205.

48. Putnam FW, Carlson EB, Ross CA, *et al.* Patterns of dissociation in clinical and nonclinical samples. *J Nerv Mental Dis* 1996;**184**:673–679.

49. Şar V, Koyuncu A, Öztürk E, *et al.* Dissociative disorders in psychiatric emergency ward. *Gen Hosp Psychiatry,* 2007;**29**:45–50.

50. Bremner JD. Acute and chronic responses to psychological trauma: where do we go from here? *Am J Psychiatry* 1999;**156**:349–351.

51. van der Kolk BA, Pelcovitz D, Roth S, *et al.* Dissociation, somatization, and affect dysregulation: the complexity of adaptation of trauma. *Am J Psychiatry* 1996;**153**:83–93.

52. Lanius RA, Williamson PC, Densmore M, *et al.* Neural correlates of traumatic memories in posttraumatic stress disorder: a functional MRI investigation. *Am J Psychiatry* 2001;**158**:1920–1922.

53. Lanius RA, Williamson PC, Boksman K, *et al.* Brain activation during script-driven imagery induced dissociative responses in PTSD: a functional magnetic resonance imaging investigation. *Biol Psychiatry* 2002;**52**:305–311.

54. Lanius RA, Williamson PC, Densmore M, *et al.* The nature of traumatic memories: a 4-T FMRI functional connectivity analysis. *Am J Psychiatry* 2004;**161**:36–44.

55. Lanius RA, Williamson PC, Bluhm RL, *et al.* Functional connectivity of dissociative responses in posttraumatic stress disorder: a functional magnetic resonance imaging investigation. *Biol Psychiatry* 2005;**57**:873–884.

56. Lanius RA, Bluhm R, Lanius U, Pain C. A review of neuroimaging studies in PTSD: heterogeneity of response to symptom provocation. *J Psychiatr Res* 2006;**40**:709–729.

57. Etkin A, Wager TD. Functional neuroimaging of anxiety: a meta-analysis of emotional processing in PTSD, social anxiety disorder, and specific phobia. *Am J Psychiatry* 2007;**164**:1476–1488.

58. Shin LM, Wright CI, Cannistraro PA, *et al.* A functional magnetic resonance imaging study of amygdala and medial prefrontal cortex responses to overtly presented fearful faces in posttraumatic stress disorder. *Arch Gen Psychiatry* 2005;**62**:273–281.

59. Felmingham K, Kemp AH, Williams L, *et al.* Dissociative responses to conscious and non-conscious fear impact underlying brain function in post-traumatic stress disorder. *Psychol Med* 2008;**38**: 1771–1780.

60. Roeder CH, Michal M, Overbeck G, van der Ven VG, Linden DEJ. Pain response in depersonalization: a functional imaging study using hypnosis in healthy subjects. *Psychother Psychosom* 2007;**76**:115–121.

61. Schmahl C, Bohus M, Esposito F, *et al.* Neural correlates of antinociception in borderline personality disorder. *Arch Gen Psychiatry* 2006;**63**:659–667.

62. Geuze E, Westenberg HGM, Jochims A, *et al.* Altered pain processing in veterans with posttraumatic stress disorder. *Arch Gen Psychiatry* 2007;**64**:76–85.

63. Kraus A, Esposito F, Seifritz E, *et al.* Amygdala deactivation as a neural correlate of pain processing in patients with borderline personality disorder and co-occurrent posttraumatic stress disorder. *Biol Psychiatry* 2009;**65**:819–822.

64. Ludaescher P, Valerius G, Stiglmayr C, *et al.* Pain sensitivity and neural processing during dissociative states in patients with borderline personality disorder with and without comorbid PTSD: a pilot study. *J Psychiatry Neurosci* 2010;**35**:177–184.

65. Mickleborough MJ, Daniels J, Coupland NJ, *et al.* Effects of trauma-related cues on pain processing in PTSD: a fMRI investigation. *J Psychiatry Neurosci* 2011;**36**:6–14.

66. Stiglmayr C, Schimke P, Wagner T, *et al.* Development and psychometric characteristics of the Dissociation Tension Scale. *J Personality Assess* 2010;**92**:269–277.

67. Hollander E, Carrasco JL, Mullen LS, *et al.* Left hemispheric activation in depersonalization disorder: a case report. *Biol Psychiatry* 1992;**31**:1157–1162.

68. Lemche E, Surguladze SA, Giampietro VP, *et al.* Limbic and prefrontal responses to facial emotion expressions in depersonalization. *Neuroreport*, 2007;**218**:473–477.

69. Sierra M, Berrios GE. Depersonalization: neurobiological perspectives. *Biol Psychiatry* 1998;**44**:898–908.

70. Brand BL, Classen CC, McNary SW, Zaveri P. A review of treatment outcome studies for dissociative disorders. *J Nerv Mental Dis* 2009;**197**:646–654.

71. Brand BL, Myrick AC, Loewenstein RL, *et al.* submitted). A survey of practices and recommended treatment interventions among expert therapists treating patients with dissociative identity disorder and dissociative identity disorder not otherwise specified. *Psychol Trauma Theory Res Pract Policy* 2011; in press.

72. Hunter ECM, Phillips ML, Chalder T, Sierra M, David AS. Depersonalisation disorder: a cognitive-behavioral conceptualization. *Behav Res Ther* 2003;**41**:1451–1467.

73. Waller G, Hamilton K, Elliott P, *et al.* Somatoform dissociation, psychological dissociation, and specific forms of trauma. *J Trauma Dissoc* 2000;**1**:81–98.

74. Kluft RP, Treatment trajectories in multiple personality disorder. *Dissociation* 1994;**7**:63–76.

75. Ellason JW, Ross CA. Two-year follow-up of inpatients with dissociative identity disorder. *Am J Psychiatry* 1997;**154**:832–839.

76. Brand BL, Classen CC, Lanius R, *et al.* A naturalistic study of dissociative identity disorder and dissociative disorder not otherwise specified patients treated by community clinicians. *Psychol Trauma Theory, Res Pract Policy* 2009;**1**:153–171.

77. Brand BL, Classen CC, Lanius R, *et al.* Treatment outcome of dissociative disorders patients: cross-sectional and longitudinal results of the TOP DD Study. In Proceedings of the Annual Conference of the International Society for the Study of Trauma and Dissociation, Chicago, November, 2008.

78. Chu J. *Rebuilding Shattered Lives: The Responsible Treatment of Complex Post-traumatic and Dissociative Disorders.* New York: John Wiley, 1998.

79. Courtois CA, Ford JD. *Treating Complex Traumatic Stress Disorders: An Evidence-based Guide.* New York: Guilford, 2009.

80. Kluft RP. An overview of the psychotherapy of dissociative identity disorder. *Am J Psychother* 1999;**53**:289–319.

81. Kluft RP, Loewenstein RJ. Dissociative disorders and depersonalization. In Gabbard GO, ed. *Gabbard's Treatment of Psychiatric Disorders,* 4th edn. Washington, DC: American Psychiatric Press, 2007:547–572.

82. Foa EB, Keane TM, Friedman MJ, Cohen JA. *Effective Treatments for PTSD: Practice Guidelines from the International Society of Traumatic Stress Studies.* New York: Guilford, 2009.

83. Loewenstein RJ. Psychopharmacologic treatments for dissociative identity disorder. *Psychiatr Ann* 2005;**35**:666–673.

84. Şar V, Akyüz G, Doğan O. Prevalence of dissociative disorders among women in the general population. *Psychiatry Res* 2007;**149**:169–176.

Chapter

17

Psychogenic movement disorders: illness in search of disease?

Peter W. Halligan

Introduction

Medically unexplained symptoms (MUS) describes a growing number of patient behaviors and symptoms seen by different medical specialties that currently lack an adequate biomedical explanation. Such MUS are among the most common problems in medicine, although current figures probably underestimate the scale, as many doctors remain cautious about excluding physical disease. The search for a biomedical-based diagnosis has resulted in the growth and clinical use of various etiologically agnostic, diagnostically ambivalent descriptors. In most cases, these disorders are described by what they are not, rather than as illnesses in their own right. Central to understanding psychogenic movment disorders (PMD) as a MUS are the social contexts and in particular the beliefs in which the symptoms arise, are given meaning, and are managed.

Many powerful personal, societal and professional beliefs used to explain such illnesses remain strongly linked to primitive forms of intuitive mind–body dualism. Beliefs – many of which are not conscious – are powerful drivers of behavior but also significant shapers of experience and the explanations used to understand and give meaning. Socially credible explanations lie at the heart of reconciling symptom-based syndromes with an adequate understanding of illness and disability that does not necessarily depend on biomedical disease.

In the case of PMD, key issues remain: the contentious historical vacillation between two medical specialty accounts, the potential for deception, and the need to develop a credible framework for understanding and explaining psychogenic movements. Placing PMD in the context of normal (i.e., non-medically related) consciously mediated voluntary actions but as a psychogenic process involving the recruitment of a maladaptive "idea" (e.g., an unconscious belief involving not being able to move the affected limb [paralysis] or the involuntary simulation of dystonic movements) in response to a perceived stressor provides a platform for exploring a "psychological account " that is not far removed from explanations for how we effortlessly generate normal limb movements.

Illness without disease: the big picture

Medically unexplained symptoms describes the common and growing cluster of patient behaviors and symptoms for which biomedical science has yet to find an adequate biomedical cause [1,2]. According to the US National Institutes of Health, MUS present the most common problem for medicine, with most specialties treating at least one MUS [3].

Over the past two decades, many Western countries have experienced what has been described as an "epidemic" of MUS and/or subjective health complaints without verifiable somatic disease [4]. A study of the general population in Nordic countries found prevalence rates of 75% for some subjective health complaints (e.g., musculoskeletal pain; ear, nose, and throat symptoms; abdominal pain and gastrointestinal symptoms; fatigue; and dizziness) with 50% of complaints accounting for long-term sickness compensation and permanent disability [5].

Incapacity benefits have risen significantly in all developed countries since the 1980s, despite improvements in most objective measures of population health [6]. In the UK, the number of people receiving state incapacity benefits through health-related problems rose from 700 000 in 1979 to approximately 2.6 million

Psychogenic Movement Disorders and Other Conversion Disorders, ed. Mark Hallett, Anthony E. Lang, Joseph Jankovic, Stanley Fahn, Peter W. Halligan, Valerie Voon, and C. Robert Cloninger. Published by Cambridge University Press. © Cambridge University Press 2011.

people in 1995 [7]. Many do not demonstrate an underlying recognizable pathological or organic basis that could account for the range and severity of the health complaints reported [8].

In general practice, estimates of MUS indicate that 20–30% lack a demonstrable cause for their symptoms [9–11]. Estimates for those without confirmed disease seen in hospital outpatient clinics range from 30 to 70% [12–14]. These figures are likely to be an underestimate, as doctors understandably remain cautious about excluding physical disease and presenting a patient with a less than definitive diagnosis [13,15,16].

The lack of a confident biomedically based diagnosis, has not (notwithstanding the potential for deception [17]) invalidated the veracity and reality of a patient's experience or precluded the clinical use of various etiologically agnostic, diagnostic descriptors such as PMD, irritable bowel syndrome, tension headache, chronic pelvic pain, multiple chemical sensitivity, and interstitial cystitis. Many of these symptom-based classifications reflect contact with different professional specializations and access to care (i.e., where the patient is first seen) rather than some natural cleavage of MUS [18].

The use of the term MUS describes a social and clinical predicament and not a specific disorder [2]; however, Kendell and Jablensky [19] have commented "once a diagnostic concept… has come into general use, it tends to become reified. That is, people too easily assume that it is an entity of some kind that can be invoked to explain the patient's symptoms and whose validity need not be questioned [in the case of medically unexplained symptoms]… their definitive status in public consciousness and popular discourse contrasts markedly with their uncertain scientific and biomedical status." Unlike their predecessors in the early twentieth century, patients who have these syndromes today are less "relieved by negative findings on medical evaluation and less responsive to explanation, reassurance and palliative treatment" [1]. One reason for this, Barsky and Borus [1] note, is that "the contemporary climate is marked by prominent political, legal, economic and regularity ramifications… functional somatic syndromes form the basis for lawsuits and class actions seeking to attribute liability and fault …" and consequently the area remains a fertile source for disputes over healthcare insurance and the *validity* of current medical diagnosis.

In the absence of a definitive biomedical diagnosis, a presumptive psychological account for the illness becomes the focus of attention and, inevitably, the challenge or barrier for the physician–patient relationship. The clinician's failure to provide a satisfactory explanation in many cases of MUS invariably refocuses attention on the appropriateness of the biomedical model and critical aspects of the doctor–patient interaction [20,21]. Not surprisingly, patient dissatisfaction with the managing physician is "the strongest prognostic risk factor for long-term outcome in PMD" [22].

Problems arising from illnesses without definable biomedical causes are well documented [23–25]. Central to understanding and managing MUS are different powerful societal and professional models used to explain illness. Bracken and Thomas [26] note that considering our mental life as some sort of "enclosed world residing inside the skull does not do justice to the lived reality of human experience [and]… systematically neglects the importance of social context." For example, most biomedical models remain strongly linked to primitive forms of intuitive mind–body dualism. Wade and Halligan [27] have commented that health commissioners, budgetary systems, healthcare professionals, and much of the public "act as if there is some clear, inescapable separation between physical and mental health problems, ignoring evidence that a person's psychological and emotional state always affects their function and presentation of physical symptoms." As a result, separate services typically exist for people with physical problems and those perceived to have mental health problems.

The absence of a unified formulation in the case of MUS, although justified given the potential for multiple interacting causes, results in patients moving between different medical services [28], and substantial differences in expert opinions and practices related to diagnosing and managing patients with PMDs [16]. Irrespective of ultimate explanation(s), the *sine qua non* of *all* illness remains the individual's experience and reporting of a health problem. In attempting to better understand MUS, it is sometimes forgotten that, "as practitioners, we approach our patients and their problems within the framework of a conceptual model that organizes and defines the questions we ask, the information we seek, the diagnostic and therapeutic options, and ultimately the outcome of our interventions" [29].

Locating illness in a social context

The particular model of illness adopted by different specialties and/or society has important consequences for how illness is received and understood, as social acceptance carries implications and responsibilities. Cultural health beliefs and models of illness are particularly important in shaping the perceived importance of presenting symptoms, the nature of the sick role, and the implications for subsequent use of medical resources [27]. In describing their model, derived from the World Health Organization's international classification of functioning framework, Wade and Halligan [27] suggested the need to adopt a more comprehensive, less biologically dependent account of illness.

Traditional biomedical models assume that an organ or bodily function is physically abnormal and that it is this that provides the primary cause of the patient's complaint or presenting symptom(s). The diagnosis of illness, however, does not require the presence of a disease to produce disability, distress, or handicap for the individual. Bass and Mayou [12] reported that fewer than half of the patients referred to emergency departments and cardiac outpatient clinics with chest pain have any evidence of heart disease. Nevertheless, over two-thirds continued to be disabled by their symptoms in the long term, and many remained understandably dissatisfied with their medical care.

When defining disease as an objectively and demonstrable departure from perceived adaptive biological functioning, Albert *et al.* [30] reminded us that "the clinical signs and symptoms do not constitute the disease and that it is not until causal mechanisms are clearly identified that 'we can say we have "really" discovered the disease.'" Consequently, establishing the disease process or pathology thought to be responsible for a patients' illness presentation is a conceptually important, but nevertheless separate, aspect of diagnosis.

Whereas disease is dependent on objective abnormalities of physical structure or function, illness describes the patient's experience, including what they perceive to be involuntary behaviors, and are best considered "a social manifestation, a commentary, a role" [31] that increasingly provides for diagnosis despite relying entirely upon the subjective reports or behaviors of distress, suffering, or disability reported by the subject [4].

One characteristic of the "systems model" proposed by Wade and Halligan [27] is that abnormalities in one system can occur without any of its components

being faulty, and so the model explicitly predicts that illness will occur without discernible pathology. Consequently, the "mystery" of non-organic or functional illness is no longer medically unexplained. This approach does not deny or mitigate the reality of illness as subjectively experienced but rather provides a rationale and support for explanations and treatments that direct their focus to the non-medical reasons why people may feel ill.

Despite lacking evidence of objective disease, there has been growing acceptance of MUS [32] over the past two decades, albeit using different shorthand terms, fuelled by the progressive belief that relevant psychosocial factors play a more significant contributing role in illness presentation that previously thought [33,34]. This "culture shift" in medical practice [35] has been driven in part by the growing numbers of medical specialities confronted with increasing numbers of patients presenting with disabling unexplained somatic and mental symptoms where no relevant pathology or known psychopathology could be established [36,37].

This, in turn, has led to a growing acceptance of illness-based conditions such as "functional somatic symptoms/syndromes," particularly within psychiatry, where many of the mental disorders already described by the DSM–IV [38] remain biomedically unexplained. Therefore, the traditional requirement of an assumed relationship between symptom and demonstrable pathology has changed and become "remedicalized around the notion of a functional disturbance of the nervous system" [39].

A similar shift in social beliefs appears to have occurred with the emergence of, and at times reluctant, acceptance of PMD given the "continuous vacillation between psychogenic and organic explanations" [40]. It is interesting, given the scale of the problem today, that as late as 1975 (and the *First International Dystonia Symposium*) it was not possible to find a proven case of psychogenic dystonia [41], whereas 3 years later, Lesser and Fahn [42] reported the first case of psychogenic dystonia and 10 years later (at the *Second International Dystonia Symposium*) Fahn and Williams [43] presented 21 cases and advocated the degree of certainty scale for PMD diagnosis [44]. Assuming that the prevalence of PMD has not grown significantly over the past 35 years, it seems likely that many patients with movement disorders were misdiagnosed.

In response to the perceived and growing need to consider more complex, interactional, and contextual paradigms, "biopsychosocial models" applied to health sciences emerged in the 1970s [33,45]. These biopsychological models, however, are not ostensibly etiological but rather argue for a process model of illness [7] where the *person*, and *not* the disease is the central focus when defining ill health. Acute and chronic symptoms originating from benign or mild forms of physical or mental impairment are re-experienced as amplified perceptions with accompanying distress, which when filtered through the presenting patient's attitudes, beliefs, coping skills, and occupational or cultural social context can affect patient's perceptions of their impairment and associated disability [34].

The role of beliefs for clinical symptoms and functional outcome

Without evidence of definitive neurobiological or physiological malfunction, acceptance of a set of symptoms as a nominal syndrome (e.g., PMD) and treating it as such ultimately depends on the underlying beliefs of the patient, doctor, and society at large as to the nature of the illness [4]. Despite this, patient and societal beliefs have been little studied in relation to PMD. Although discussion of beliefs can be found in most health psychology [46,47] and biopsychosocial [45] models, the term is often used rather vaguely to describe one of several "psychosocial variables" that impact on health and illness outcome.

Beliefs, however, as basic and relatively stable ideas concerning the nature of reality, provide reasons (conscious) and drivers (unconscious) for behavior and knowing. Inferring a patient's belief can help to predict their subjective experience, capacity to cope, recovery [48], treatment compliance, and behavior [49].

When beliefs are defined as explicit, or more often implicit, mental propositions that help people to understand their lives and experiences, they remain powerful in the light of their use to appraise, explain, and integrate new observations about matters that have to do with the ideas we hold of ourselves [50].

The "power" of beliefs lies in the way they can shape and select evidence for best explanatory fit. Having a belief can change the way evidence is collected and evaluated [51,52]. It is well established that anomalous data (i.e., data that contradict established views) are often ignored or reinterpreted to make them fit established views [53]. It has also been shown in developmental research that students often retain their naive physical [54] and psychological [55] theories, despite receiving appropriate scientific instructions [56].

Although some beliefs are explicit (i.e., consciously endorsed), everyday experience suggests that most beliefs are held implicitly [57]. As Frith [58] points out "Our brains discover what is out there in the world by constructing models and making predictions. Our models are built by combining information from our senses with our prior expectations... [however]... we have no direct contact with the world or even with our bodies... our brain creates this illusion by hiding... all the complex processes that are involved in discovering the world."

Some of the most powerful implicit beliefs (ontological beliefs) become deeply entrenched and hard to change, and these often concern basic properties about the structure of matter [56] and mind–brain relationships [59].

What people believe about the nature of their illness, and its presentation, consequently affects how both they (and their doctors) cope and deal with it [60–62]. Patients' beliefs concerning the causes and prognoses of their illnesses (with and without evidence of organic pathophysiology) remain fundamental for a number of theoretical models of illness behavior [27,63], causation [64], and medication compliance [65].

As explanatory frameworks, beliefs critically provide for future expectancies and shape on-line experiences including the interpretation of symptoms [66,67]. As such, believing is analogous to seeing and, given that not all seeing produces an accurate picture of reality, knowing the role beliefs can play is important since we tend not to look for things that we do not expect (i.e., believe in). The tendency to evaluate incoming evidence in support of current beliefs when new evidence is encountered can provide for serious consequences. Two clinical examples illustrate how patient's pre-existing notions can help to shape experience and expectation.

The first example involves a study by Mittenberg *et al.* [68] designed to see whether symptoms of mild brain damage could be related to what patients believed to be the likely symptoms to follow head injury. In this study, Mittenberg and colleagues asked 223 controls with no personal experience or knowledge of head injury to complete an affective, somatic, and memory checklist as to their expectations of symptoms 6 months after a head injury. A similar checklist was given to 100 patients with head injuries for comparison. Predicted concussion symptoms in the naive controls reliably showed a coherent cluster of symptoms virtually identical to the postconcussion syndrome reported by patients with head trauma, suggesting a possible etiological role for expectations in the experience and expression of symptoms. Patients, by comparison, consistently underestimated the premorbid prevalence of the symptoms compared with controls.

The second example concerns response expectancy – the anticipation of an "automatic subjective response" [66]. When combined with social modeling [69], it has been shown to enhance symptoms by strengthening the expectancy of their occurrence. Although there have been several studies showing how anticipations can elicit expected physical symptoms by manipulating response expectancies [70], the study by Lorber *et al.* [71] was one of the first to target psychogenic symptoms when manipulating psychogenic cues. Using a controlled laboratory design, this study evaluated the effects of expectancy and modeling in generating psychogenic illness. The study induced beliefs by experimental manipulation such that the reported symptoms were those that corresponded to the beliefs about symptoms that a substance could provoke. In their study, students were randomly assigned to inhale or not an inert placebo characterized as a suspected environmental toxin linked to four typical psychogenic symptoms (headache, nausea, itchy skin, and drowsiness). The findings showed that students who inhaled the placebo showed a substantially greater increase in symptoms and that the increase was significantly greater for the specified symptoms than for other symptoms.

Beliefs and the role of healthcare professionals

As indicated above, an adequate understanding of illness and disability cannot ignore the beliefs held by healthcare professionals, academics, and those in wider society regarding what they consider to be the causes of illness, the extent of disability, likely recovery, and the potential for treatment [27]. Not long ago, there was a widespread belief amongst some medical historians that the symptoms of hysteria such as paralysis or blackouts unexplained by disease had become less common over the last century [72].

It is important to recognize that a physician's own behavior can be influenced by patient expectations and other psychosocial factors [73], and that illness beliefs crucially depends on the views of the healthcare professionals and culture involved, all of which collectively contribute to the interpretations of symptoms, patient presentation and treatment outcomes [74]. As pointed out by Barrett [75] (p. 326):

> Psychologists know that people don't contribute to their perceptions of the world in a neutral way. Human brains do not dispassionately look upon the world and carve nature at its joints. We make self-interested observations about the world in all manner of speaking. And what holds true for people in general certainly holds for scientists in particular. Scientists are active perceivers, and like all perceivers, we see the world from a particular point of view (that is not always shared by other scientists). We parse the world into bits and pieces using the conceptual tools that are available at a particular point in time and with a particular goal in mind (often inextricably linked to said conceptual tools). This is not a failing of the scientific method per se – it is a natural consequence of how the human brain sees and hears and feels... and does science.

Two brief clinical examples illustrate how pre-existing notions can shape experience and expectation in medicine. The first concerns "confirmatory bias" and the way in which prior information can bias symptom interpretation. In this study, 20 neurologists were asked to judge a number of plantar responses from film (two of which showed equivocal toe movements presented twice at the same sitting with a fictitious history and examination results (minus the plantar reflex). Van Gijn and Bonke [76] showed that the neurologist's interpretation of the two equivocal toe movements was biased significantly ($p < 0.01$) according to the clinical information provided. Thirty different neurologists who rated the two films without clinical data did not show this bias.

The second example demonstrates the extent to which pre-existing beliefs "can confound treatment outcomes" (e.g., selection bias, observer bias, reporting bias and reviewer bias) in medicine. Schultz *et al.* [77] showed that non-randomized studies tended to overestimate treatment effects by 41% when compared with studies that employed adequately concealed treatment allocations. Cultural aspects were also implicated. Vickers *et al.* [78] showed that acupuncture trials conducted in East Asia were always positive, whereas similar trials in Australia/New Zealand, North America, or Western Europe were positive only half the time.

Psychosocial factors such as beliefs are particularly relevant when managing MUS such as PMD if one considers the prevalent notions (beliefs) within medicine and society regarding the intuitive biomedical causes of illness, expected recovery, and medication efficiency [79,80].

For example "surveys of highly educated samples" suggest that "dualistic" attitudes towards mind–brain relationship are very much alive and "remain very common" in both patients, professionals, and society at large [81]. Two separate but related surveys, one from the University of Edinburgh involving 250 students and the other from the University of Liege involving 1858 healthcare workers and public, showed substantial support for dualistic beliefs highlighting the separateness of mind and brain. In the Liege survey, "more than one-third of medical and paramedical professionals regarded mind and brain as separate entities" [59]. The authors of these surveys suggest that dualism is at work in "clinical practice" and that one of the difficulties patients with somatoform disorders experience in accepting psychological explanations for their symptoms "partly flows from, and reinforces, dualistic attitudes toward the relationship between mind and body."

Similarly, a recent survey of mental-health workers by Miresco and Kirmayer [82] showed how the mind–brain dichotomy was used to reason about patients' responsibility for their condition. Where a clinical problem was categorized as having a psychological etiology, patients were "more often thought to be responsible for their condition, whereas when the problem was thought to have a neurobiological cause, the patients were considered less blameworthy" [59]. In reviewing the Australian epidemic of repetitive strain injury (RSI) in the early 1980s (where New South Wales saw an 11-fold increase in disability claims), Lucire [83] argued that doctors played an important (if unknowing) part in the belief that RSI was the primary result of an occupational injury caused by inhumane working conditions [84]. The role of beliefs is no less relevant in the development of the current psychiatric nosologies, where, as Craddock [85] commented, "many of these categories have found their way into the classifications as a result of impassioned support by eminent and influential psychiatrists during earlier DSM and/or ICD committee meetings, rather than because of robust, relevant and compelling evidence."

Psychogenic movement disorders and the "psychogenesis" of normal movements

Despite being defined and understood as involuntary movements not attributed to known organic causes,

PMD inhabits the contentious hinterland between neurology, psychiatry, and malingering. Accordingly, beliefs of doctors and patients regarding the condition continue to play an important role. Many neurologists consider patient's cultural beliefs about psychological illnesses to play a significant factor in limiting management [16]. Clinicians that engage in the discussion of patients' psychosocial problems are less likely to request investigations, refer patients elsewhere, or offer a drug treatment [16]. Patients with PMD show a "strong belief that whatever causes their symptoms it is definitely not a 'psychological' problem" [22]. In a recent large-scale follow-up of predictors of outcome in patients with symptoms unexplained by disease, the authors suggest that patient beliefs pertaining to poor outcome could play "a causal role in shaping outcome by acting as a self-fulfilling prophecy" [86].

Issues of diagnostic credibility and deception [87] are difficult to avoid when cortical stimulation generates normal movement [15] and such movements are preceded by bereitschaftspotentials suggesting overlap with brain mechanisms responsible for normal voluntary movements [88]. Not surprising, and despite published criteria for PMD diagnoses, opinions and practices relating to diagnosing and managing patients with PMD differ among movement disorders neurologists [16]. Neurologists are often "reluctant to put their thoughts and impressions into clear opinions, let alone share their honest opinion with the patients" [89]. While endorsing psychological accounts, many neurologists do not understand their patients in such terms [87] and accordingly remain reluctant to make the diagnosis for fear of missing an underlying organic and hence a treatable disorder [90].

Having excluded an organic diagnosis, many neurologists turn to psychiatric colleagues or other mental health specialists to establish the responsible underlying psychopathology before discussing the diagnosis with the patient [16]. Currently, the two main international psychiatric classifications consider PMD as a form of "conversion disorder" of the motor subtype (DSM-IV) or a "dissociative disorder" (ICD-10) [91]. Describing such behaviors as a form of conversion has been characterized as accepting "an etiology that is presumptive at best and anachronistic at worst" [92] and holds "the doubtful distinction among psychiatric diagnoses of still invoking 'Freudian' mechanisms as an explanation" [93].

Although the term "psychogenic" provides for a pragmatic and relatively less patient-offensive clinical shorthand than hysteria [94], it remains a "confused, but speciously attractive and convenient concept" [95] and one that provides for a family of different descriptors masquerading as explanation [96]. Moreover, since in some cases "there is no hint of a psychiatric condition" [88] and PMD is not officially recognized and endorsed by all specialties, psychiatrists frequently do not believe the diagnosis [16], lack interest [88], or fail to discover relevant psychopathology [16].

The problem for "psychogenic" accounts, aside from speculative psychodynamic accounts and unwieldy diagnostic criteria (e.g., exclusion of feigning and identification of associated psychological factors) remains how "conversion symptoms could exist in the first place… for if conversion disorder can be purely psychological, why not tension headache?" [92]. This point was well articulated by Ormerod [97], in relation to hysteria, where he indicated that while "it may be necessary, in consequence of our present state of ignorance of the workings of the highest cerebral centers, to speak of these in transcendental terms, yet psychology alone cannot supply an explanation of disease, which, to satisfy the physician, must be physical".

Given the absence of discernible pathology but similarity to neurological-like clinical symptoms, Freud's comment that hysterical phenomena "behave[s] as though anatomy did not exist or though it had no knowledge of it" [98] has sometimes been read in a misleadingly dualist fashion. It is clear that Freud did not mean "without the involvement of central and peripheral nervous systems" [99]. Like Charcot, Freud's explanatory perspective remained firmly rooted in neuroanatomy. Consequently, when Freud [98] suggested that the lesion in hysterical paralyses produced "an alteration of the conception, the idea, of the arm" the implication was not that the (unconscious) ideas and their physical consequences were represented in some form of immaterial mind, but that the way in which such "ideas" could produce effects "lies in the abnormal excitability of the nervous system" [100].

Placing conversion (as a form of "psychogenesis") in the context of normal (i.e., non-medically related) consciously mediated voluntary actions and viewing the psychogenic process as involving a maladaptive "idea" (e.g., a belief of not being able to move the affected limb, albeit unconsciously) in response to a stressor provides a possible "psychological account" not far removed from the intuitive explanations of normal (i.e., non-medical related) limb movements that many of us hold [101].

Engaging in "normal" voluntary actions typically assumes consciousness of the intention to act followed by the voluntary experience of having produced the desired effect [102]. Accordingly, preceding conscious mental states (i.e., psychogenic mechanisms) are attributed "naturally" and often effortlessly to a range of physical movements (actions) or signs, none of which provides an explanatory gap or basis for a dichotomy between somatic and psychological processes. Moreover, these include examples where conscious but unintended signs and actions result (e.g., shame causing blushing; fright causing involuntary immobilization). Moreover, in the exercise of most everyday voluntary movements (actions), the reductionist account of neural engagement (i.e., recruitment of specific brain regions) is meaningfully understood in functional terms (i.e., a volitional cognitive system) without having to assume some form of dualistic gulf between somatic and mental state. Hence, exercising volitional control when performing natural normal limb movements and attributing these experiential observations to a prior mental state, in a functionally intact system, constitutes no less an example of psychogenesis (albeit functionally adaptive) than might be assumed in PMD – save for loss of the subjective sense of volition and the subjective sense of agency, with the associated debilitating consequences. In other words, choosing to make dystonic-like movements or holding a limb still for a period of time (i.e., paralysis-like) by consciously willing it so is not so inexplicable when attributed to conscious (psychogenic) mechanisms.

One problem with this account, however, is that 30 years of evidence from cognitive neuroscience indicates that much of the conscious experience of engaging in a voluntary action such as moving or speaking is relegated to the awareness of the "end product" of complex unconscious processes [103]. As highlighted by Pockett [104] "unconscious and inscrutable mechanisms create both our conscious thought about action and create the action as well, and also produce the sense of will we experience by perceiving the thought as the cause of action… [and therefore] one becomes conscious of what one wants to say only after one has said it."

However, on the assumption that it is "impossible to generate conscious experiences in the absence of neural processing, there is presently no evidence to show that consciousness per se (over and above the neural processing that accompanies it) is essential for any biological function," including initiating movements [104]. In other words, the integration of several prior distinct stages of neural activity (e.g., motor prep-aration, motor command specification, and sensory feedback [102]) remains the product of largely uncon-scious neural processes [105]. Therefore, the impres-sion that actions are freely chosen (i.e., volitional) depends almost entirely upon reports of the subject's awareness of self-agency (i.e., the feelings that one is the cause of one's own actions). Phenomenologically, consciousness simply occurs too late to affect the out-comes of the cognitive processes to which it is appar-ently linked [104,106].

Since Libet's classic experiments in the 1980s which showed that unconscious brain activity in the supplementary motor area preceded the conscious (voluntary) decision to move by several hundred mil-liseconds, claims of "free will" have been regarded as illusionary [104,106,107]. Soon *et al.* [108] have shown that the supplementary motor area is not the only cortical initiation stage in such movements and that an earlier predictive neural information, prior to a subject's conscious awareness of a decision to move, involved regions of the frontopolar and parietal cortex and occurred some 10 seconds before.

The neural indicator for self-generated experience when engaged in body movements is thought to rely on the congruence between the predicted action outcome (feed-forward signal) and relevant sensory feedback located in the inferior parietal cortex [109]. When mov-ing a limb, sensory information appears crucial for pro-ducing the type and extent of proprioceptive awareness associated with the intended movement. This informa-tion arises from a "feed-forward" system that predicts the sensory consequences of a motor command and is monitored directly by comparing the predicted move-ments with those of actual sensory feedback [110]. Accordingly, every time a motor command is issued to a limb, an "efference copy" of that motor command (in other words, a predicted or expected somatosensory experience) is produced in parallel.

According to Frith *et al.* [105], normal awareness and experience of our limb movement (given the latency in translating online information) is largely based on this predicted (expected) state rather than the actual feedback state, unless the system monitoring the actual feedback detects a deviation from that predicted. In patients after limb amputation, such motor com-mands when issued in most cases produce a discernable experience of limb perception, described as a phantom limb [111]. Conversely, when the motor command is not accompanied by confirmatory feedback from the

efference copy, as appears to be the case in some hyp-notically suggested "automatic" limb movements, the self-generated action is experienced (falsely) as a pas-sive movement caused by an external agency [112].

Using a novel within-subject functional neuroim-aging design that compared involuntary movements (PMD tremor) and voluntary mimicked tremor in the same patients, Voon *et al.* [113] suggested that "dys-function" in the normal "sensory prediction signal" comparing predicted versus actual outcomes during involuntary movements provides an explanation for why "conversion movements" may not be perceived as self-generated in such patients.

A role for "maladaptive" beliefs in explaining psychogenic movement disorders

Since one can choose consciously (using normal vol-untary movement systems) to make tremor-like movements at the same frequency and amplitude as psychogenic tremor [114], or hold a limb still for a period of time (i.e., paralysis-like) by willing it so (i.e., engaging the idea), then the recruitment of similar movement systems (albeit outside subject awareness) is no less credible for explaining PMD. Although the range and distinctive pattern of movements in PMD are no doubt multiply determined, the adoption of an unconscious maladaptive "idea" regarding specific movements (e.g., paralysis or dystonia) in response to affective or stress-related factors, by recruiting volun-tary movement systems (but by-passing appropriate feedback confirming self-agency), provides a heuristic account worth considering.

Such an account does not, however, provide a teleo-logical explanation for the range and specific forms of physically behavior observed in different subjects, nor does it explain why disabling the motor system to pre-vent the subject having voluntary control over physio-logically intact limbs provides a way of dealing with a psychological stressor. The consequential societal reaction, however, allows most subjects to enter the sick role and access medical support.

It might be argued that "myoclonic disorders" involving complex and apparently uncoordinated movements are difficult to explain in terms of an "idea" – being less goal directed than say "paralysis" (i.e., removing the ability to voluntarily move). However, assuming that the behavioral expression serves some purpose, albeit one that the subject remains unaware of as a maladaptive response to a psychological stressor, positive "symptom" modeling could potentially provide for mimicking the full range of organic abnormal involuntary movements derived from earlier or learned organic-derived experiences. Therefore, the presentation of what appears to be apparently illogical motor behaviors does not necessarily mean that there is no purpose behind such behaviors.

The involvement of an implicit maladaptive idea for explaining hysteria is hardly new and was central to Charcot's influential explanation of hysteria more than a century ago, whereby psychogenic symptoms were thought to derive from (unconscious) ideas. Charcot's explanation was strongly influenced by the work of the English neurologist John Russell Reynolds [115], who wrote (p. 483):

> that some of the most serious disorders of the nervous system, such as paralysis, spasm, pain, and otherwise altered sensations, may depend upon a morbid condition of emotion, of idea and emotion, or of idea alone… they sometimes associate themselves with distinct and definite diseases of the nervous centres, so that it becomes very important to know how much a given case is due to an organic lesion, and how much to morbid ideation.

Following the concept of "psychical paralysis" introduced by Reynolds [115], Charcot and Marie [116] developed the importance of suggestion, concluding (p. 630) that hysterical (and hypnotic paralysis) could originate when "the idea comes to the patient's mind that he might become paralyzed: in one word through autosuggestion, the rudimentary paralysis becomes real." Recently, and in a similar vein, de Vignemont [117] suggested that patients with conversion paralysis suffer from a delusion (false belief) that they are paralyzed – in the same way that anosognosic patients have the delusion that they are not paralyzed [118]. De Vignemont [117] commented, "Hysterical patients believe that they cannot make any movement due to an organic cause and differs from anosognosia in that part of the hysterical patients' beliefs is true."

A modern take on Charcot's psychogenic account was provided by Hurwitz and Prichard [119], who suggest that hysterical conversion (and presumably PMD) occur when an "idea of illness forms in the mind of a patient and commandeers neuronal machinery to impose a pattern of inhibition or activation which follows that particular persons' idea of illness … reformulated in modern concepts, conversion reactions are fixed beliefs of somatic dysfunction arising from psychological distress that control cortical and subcortical pathways to produce patterns of loss or gain of function that are not organic in the conventional sense."

From a neuropsychological perspective, such an account has been viewed as the activation of nonvolitional stored or learnt behavioral representations, allowing for the direct influence of personal belief on phenomenology [120]. This cognitive account provides for the important role of a subject's belief or idea in shaping the development of symptoms and helps to explain Trimble's comment [121] (p. 203), "the frequent occurrence of symptoms based on earlier physical illness, such as non-epileptic seizures in a patient with prior epilepsy."

According to Brown [120] (p. 231), the chronicity in these conditions is not helped by "deliberately checking to see if a symptom is still present [as this] increases the resting activation level of the underlying symptom's representation… [and can] increase the likelihood of subsequent reselection, setting up a vicious cycle" (see also Page and Weseley, 2003 [25]).

Exploiting the link between suggestion and the role played by "idea" in psychogenic conditions, Charcot was inspired to produce symptoms in patients by the implantation of such ideas using hypnosis [122], and he considered hypnosis an important experimental model for understanding hysteria [123]. Charcot went so far as to propose that similar brain processes were involved in unexplained neurological symptoms and the pseudoneurological behaviors commonly produced by hypnosis. This hypothesis stemmed from Charcot's many years of work using hypnosis where the symptoms of hysteria could be produced, or resolved, and identical symptoms to the post-traumatic symptoms could be reproduced in those with post-traumatic disorders [121].

Although most doctors are aware of (and indeed contribute to) the powerful effects of the placebo response for medical interventions, "few contemplate the significance of suggestion in the development of their own patient's symptomatology" [121] (see also Chapter 41/42). Evidence from the nocebo phenomenon, however, indicates that cultural knowledge regarding medicine (e.g., beliefs) may not only describe conditions of illness but may also foster those same conditions by establishing expectations regarding their occurrence [124]. Recently, several authors have argued for the potential benefits of using "suggestion" as a treatment strategy to change patient beliefs in PMD [125,126] (see also Chapter 42). Interestingly, the last paper published by Charcot dealt with autosuggestion as a means of self-therapy and cure rather than as a precipitant for illness [127].

Since the 1960s, hypnosis has been used as a technique for recreating and studying many neurological and psychiatric symptoms [128,129]. As an experimental tool, targeted hypnotic suggestion has provided for the creation of clinically informed functional analogues or virtual patients delivered through intact cognitive neural systems (see Chapter 21) These include generating subjectively compelling hypnotic analogues for established functional disorders, including blindness, achromatopsia, left leg paralysis, emotional numbing, memory loss, analgesia, auditory hallucinations, hypnotically suggested pain, and, more recently, temporary delusions about the self and the world including clinically relevant hypnotic analogues of delusions of alien and anarchic limb control and mirrored-self misidentification [129].

The use of clinically informed suggestions (ideas) to create virtual patients assumes not only a match between the features of the clinical and the hypnotic conditions but also, more critically, a putative common link to the underlying neurocognitive processes [129]. When studied in conjunction with functional neuroimaging, clinical analogues can provide an important and unique contribution for refining cognitive neuroscience theory [130].

Moreover if a "psychogenesis" account involving the recruitment of maladaptive ideas/beliefs targeting voluntary movement systems provides a tentative "credible explanation" for PMD, then such an account would raise questions for more established neurological symptoms traditionally attributed to organic lesions [15]). Since PMD "symptoms can mimic the full range of organic abnormal involuntary movements" [90,131] and present "like virtually any movement disorder, from myoclonus to bradykinesia" [88], are neurologists capable of ruling out the potential contribution of "psychogenesis" in more established neurological disorders?

Conclusions

Despite the current scale of the problem, neither neurology nor psychiatry has succeeded in advancing the neurobiological understanding or management of PMD disorders [88,132]. There are a "large number of patients" who have been nominally classified with conversion symptoms such as PMDs who do *not* have any established neurological or psychiatric diagnosis

capable of explaining their symptoms [10]. In the case of symptoms unexplained by disease, effective and socially credible explanations lie at the heart of reconciling the reality of symptoms with the absence of disease. Thompson *et al.* [133] commented that the reason is that "for too long, functional diseases have been described by what they are not, rather than as real entities… Not only does this exclusive approach fail to provide the patient with the dignity of a diagnosis, but it also generates needless tests and consultations. The fruitless pursuit of an anatomical cause renders functional disorders diagnoses of exclusion. Their very numbers and cost demand a more positive approach."

The effective engagement with the social context and in particular patient beliefs [86,134,135] and concerns [94,136] regarding illness unexplained by disease provides such an approach. As Kirmayer *et al.* [2] pointed out (p. 669): "the relevant cultural background for explaining unexplained symptoms includes the patient's family and local world, together with global mass media and popular culture. The dynamics of the doctor–patient relationship are played out against a backdrop of social, cultural, and epistemological assumptions that are built into our diagnostic concepts and categories. One of the basic tasks of the clinical encounter is the co-construction of meaning for distress."

References

1. Barsky AD, Borus JF. Functional somatic syndromes. *Ann Intern Med* 1999;**130**:910–921.

2. Kirmayer LJ, Groleau D, Looper KJ, Dao MD. Explaining medically unexplained symptoms. *Can J Psychiatry* 2004;**49**:663–672.

3. Hellhammer DH, Hellhammer J (eds.). *Key Issues in Mental Health*, Vol. 174: *Stress. The Brain–Body Connection*. Basel: Karger, 2008.

4. Halligan PW, Aylward M (eds.). *The Power of Belief: Psychosocial Influence on Illness, Disability and Medicine.* Oxford: Oxford University Press, 2006.

5. Eriksen HR, Svendsrød R, Ursin G, Ursin H. Prevalence of subjective health complaints in the Nordic European countries in 1993. *Eur J Public Health* 1998;**8**:294–298.

6. Waddell G, Aylward M, Sawney P (eds.) *Back Pain, Incapacity for Work and Social Security Benefits: an International Literature Review and Analysis.* London: Royal Society of Medicine Press, 2002.

7. Waddell G, Aylward M. *Models of Sickness and Disability* London: Royal Society of Medicine Press, 2010.

8. Waddell G, Burton AK. *Concepts of Rehabilitation for the Management of Common Health Problems*. London: The Stationery Office, 2004.

9. Carson AJ, Best S, Postma K, *et al*. Outcome of neurology outpatients with medically unexplained symptoms: a prospective cohort study. *J Neurol Neurosurg Psychiatry* 2003;**74**:897–900.

10. Stone J, Vuilleumier P, Friedman JH. Conversion disorder: separating "how" from "why." *Neurology* 2010;**74**:190–191.

11. Spence SA. All in the mind? The neural correlates of unexplained physical symptoms. *Adv Psychiatr Treat* 2006;**12**:349–358.

12. Bass C, Mayou R. ABC of psychological medicine of chest pain. *BMJ* 2002;**325**:588–591.

13. Nimnuan C, Hotopf M, Wessely S. Medically unexplained symptoms syndromes. *J Psychosom Res* 2001;**51**:549–557.

14. Maiden NL, Hurst NP, Lochhead A, Carson AJ, Sharpe M. Medically unexplained symptoms in patients referred to a specialist rheumatology service: prevalence and associations. *Rheumatology* 2003;**42**:108–112.

15. Marsden CD. Hysteria: a neurologist's view. *Psychol Med* 1986;**16**:277–288.

16. Espay AJ, Goldenhar LM, Voon V, *et al*. Opinions and clinical practices related to diagnosing and managing patients with psychogenic movement disorders: an international survey of Movement Disorder Society members. *Mov Disord* 2009;**24**:1366–1374.

17. Halligan, PW, Bass, C, Oakley, DA (eds.). *Malingering and Illness Deception*. Oxford University Press, 2003.

18. Wessely S, White PD. There is only one functional somatic syndrome. *Br J Psychiatry* 2004;**185**:95–96.

19. Kendell R, Jablensky A. Distinguishing between the validity and utility of psychiatric diagnoses. *Am J Psychiatry* 2003;**160**:4–12.

20. Nettleton I, Watt L, O' Malley S, Duffey P. Understanding the narratives of people who live with medically unexplained illness. *Patient Educ Couns* 2005;**56**:205–210.

21. Salmon P. (2006) Explaining unexplained symptoms: the role of beliefs in clinical management. In Halligan PW, Aylward M, eds. *The Power of Belief: Psychosocial Influence on Illness, Disability and Medicine*. Oxford: Oxford University Press, 2006:137–159.

22. Nowak DA, Fink GR. Psychogenic movement disorders: aetiology, phenomenology, neuroanatomical correlates and therapeutic approaches. *Neuroimage* 2009;**47**:1015–1025.

23. Malleson A. *Whiplash and Other Useful Illnesses*. Montreal: McGill-Queens University Press, 2002.

24. Hatcher S, Arroll B. Assessment and management of medically unexplained symptoms. *BMJ* 2008;**336**:1124–1128.

25. Page LA, Wessely S. Medically unexplained symptoms: exacerbating factors in the doctor–patient encounter. *J R Soc Med* 2003;**96**:223–337.

26. Bracken P, Thomas P. Time to move beyond the mind–body split. *BMJ* 2002;**325**:1433–1434.

27. Wade DT, Halligan PW. Do biomedical models of illness make for good healthcare systems? *BMJ*, 2004;**11**;**329**:1398–1401.

28. Wessely S, Nimnuan C, Sharpe M. Functional somatic syndromes: one or many? *Lancet* 1999;**354**:936–939.

29. Dacher E. A systems theory approach to an expanded medical model: a challenge for biomedicine. *J Altern Compl Med* 1995;**1**:187–196.

30. Albert DA, Munson R, Resnik MD. *Reasoning in Medicine*. Baltimore, MD: Johns Hopkins University Press, 1988.

31. Taylor DC. The components of sickness: diseases, illnesses, and predicaments. *Lancet* 1979;**ii**:1008–1010.

32. Ihlebæk C, Eriksen HR. The "myths" of low back pain: status quo in Norwegian general practitioners and physiotherapists. *Spine* 2004;**29**:1818–1822.

33. Engel GL. The need for a new medical model: a challenge for biomedicine. *Science* 1977;**196**:129–136.

34. Waddell G. *The Back Pain Revolution*, 2nd edn. Edinburgh: Churchill Livingstone, 2004.

35. Aylward M, LoCascio J. Problems in the assessment of psychosomatic conditions in social security benefits and related commercial schemes. *J Psychosom Res* 1995;**39**:755–765.

36. Kroenke K, Price RK. Symptoms in the community. Prevalence, classification, and psychiatric comorbidity. *Arch Intern Med* 1993;**153**:2474–2480.

37. Waddell G, Aylward M, Sawney P. *Back Pain, Incapacity for Work and Social Security Benefits: An International Literature Review and Analysis*. London: Royal Society of Medicine Press, 2002.

38. American Psychiatric Association. *Diagnostic and Statistical Manual of Mental Disorders*, 4th edn. Washington DC: American Psychiatric Press, 1994.

39. Sharpe M, Carson A. Unexplained somatic symptoms, functional syndromes, and somatization: do we need a paradigm shift? *Ann Intern Med* 2001;2001;**134**:926–930.

40. Munts AG, Koehler PJ. How psychogenic is dystonia? Views from past to present. *Brain* 2010;**133**:1552–1564.

41. Fahn S, Eldridge R. Definition of dystonia and classification of dystonic states. In Eldridge R, Fahn S,

eds. *Advances in Neurology*, Vol. 14. New York: Raven Press, 1976:1–5.

42. Lesser RP, Fahn S. Dystonia: a disorder often misdiagnosed as a conversion reaction. *Am J Psychiatry* 1978;**153**:349–452.

43. Fahn S, Williams DT. Psychogenic dystonia. *Adv Neurol* 1988;**50**:431–455.

44. Fahn S. The history of psychogenic movement disorders. In Hallett M, Fahn S, Jankovic J, *et al.*, eds. *Psychogenic Movement Disorders: Neurology and Neuropsychiatry*. Philadelphia, PA: Lippincott Williams & Wilkins, 2006:24–32.

45. White P. *Biopsychosocial Medicine: An Integrated Approach to Understanding Illness*. Oxford: Oxford University Press, 2005.

46. Janz NK, Becker MH. The health belief model: a decade later. *Health Educ Q* 1984;**11**:1–47.

47. Ogden J. *Health Psychology,* 3rd edn. Buckingham, UK: Open University Press, 2004.

48. Diefenbach MA, Leventhal H. The common sense model of illness representation: theoretical and practical consideration. *J Soc Distress Homeless* 1996;**5**:11–38.

49. Weinman J, Petrie KJ. Illness perceptions: a new paradigm for psychosomatics? *J Psychosom Res,* 1997;**42**:113–1136.

50. Damasio AR. Thinking about belief: concluding remarks. In Schacter DL, Scarry E, ed. *Memory, Brain and Belief*. Cambridge, MA: Harvard University Press, 2000.

51. Reisberg D, Pearson DG, Kosslyn SM. Institutions and introspections about imagery: the role of imagery experience in shaping an investigator's theoretical views. *Appl Cogn Psychol* 2003;**17**,147–160.

52. Vicente KJ, Brewer WF. Reconstructive remembering of the scientific literature. *Cognition* 1993;**46**:101–128.

53. Lacatos I. Falsification and the methodology of scientific research programmes. In Lakatos I, Musgrave A, eds. *Criticism and the Growth of Knowledge.* Cambridge, UK: Cambridge University Press, 1970:91–196.

54. Levin I, Siegler SR, Druyan S, Gardosh R. Everyday and curriculum-based physics concepts: When does short-term training bring change where years of schooling have failed to do so? *Br J Dev Psychol* 1990;**8**, 269–279.

55. Nemeroff C, Rozin P. The makings of the magical mind: the nature and function of sympathetic magical thinking. In Rosen-Gren KS, Johnson CN, Harris PL, eds. *Imagining the Impossible: Magical, Scientific, and Religious Thinking in Children*. New York: Cambridge University Press, 2000:1–34.

56. Subbotsky E. Magical thinking in judgments of causation: can anomalous phenomena affect ontological causal beliefs in children and adults? *Br J Dev Psychol* 2004;**22**:123–152.

57. Greenwald AG, Banaji MR. Implicit social cognition: attitudes, self-esteem, and stereotypes. *Psychol Rev* 1995;**102**:4–27.

58. Frith C. *Making Up the Mind: How the Brain Creates our Mental World*. Oxford: Blackwell, 2007.

59. Demertzi A, Liew C, Ledoux D, *et al.* Dualism persists in the science of mind. *Ann N Y Acad Sci* 2009;**1157**:1–9.

60. Furze G, Roebuck A, Bull P, Lewin RJP, Thompson D. A comparison of the illness beliefs of people with angina and their peers: a questionnaire study. *BMC Cardiovasc Disord* 2002;**2**(4).

61. Bates MS, Rankin-Hill L, Sanchez-Ayendez M. The effects of cultural context of health care on treatment and response to chronic pain and illness. *Soc Sci Med* 1997;**45**:1433–1447.

62. Stroud MW, Thorn BE, Jensen MP, Boothby JL. The relation between pain beliefs, negative thoughts, and psychosocial functioning in chronic pain patients. *Pain,* 2000;**84**:347–352.

63. Rosenstock IM. Historical origins of the health belief model. *Health Educ Mono* 1974;**2** No. 4.

64. Srinivasan TN, Thara R. Beliefs about causation of schizophrenia: do Indian families believe in supernatural causes? *Soc Psychiatry Psychiatr Epidemiol.* 2001;**36**:134–140.

65. Horne R. Patients' beliefs about treatment: the hidden determinant of treatment outcome? *J Psychosom Res,* 1999;**47**:491–495.

66. Kirsch I (ed.). *How Expectancies Shape Experience.* Washington, DC: American Psychological Association, 1999.

67. Horne R, James D, Petrie K, Weinman J, Vincent R. Patients' interpretation of symptoms as a cause of delay in reaching hospital during acute myocardial infarction. *Heart* 2000;**83**:388–393.

68. Mittenberg W, DiGiulio DV, Perrin S, Bass AE. Symptoms following mild head injury: expectation as aetiology. *J Neurol Neurosurg Psychiatry* 1992;**55**:200–204.

69. Bandura A. *Social Learning Theory*. New York: General Learning Press, 1977.

70. Dalton P. Cognitive influences on health symptoms from acute chemical exposure. *Health Psychol* 1999;**18**:579–590.

71. Lorber W, Mazzoni G, Kirsch I. Illness by suggestion: expectancy, modeling, and gender in the production

of psychosomatic symptoms. *Ann Behav Med* 2007;**33**:112–116.

72. Stone J, Hewett R, Carson A, Warlow C, Sharpe M. The "disappearance" of hysteria: historical mystery or illusion? *J R Soc Med* 2008;**101**:12–18.

73. Buchbinder R, Jolley D, Wyatt M. Population based intervention to change back pain beliefs and disability: three part evaluation. *BMJ* 2001;**322**:1516–1520.

74. Cherkin DC, Deyo RA, Wheeler K, Ciol MA. Physician views about treating low back pain. The results of a national survey. *Spine* 1995;**1**;20:1–9.

75. Barrett LF. The future of psychology: connecting mind to brain. *Perspect Psychol Sci* 2009;**4**, 326–339.

76. van Gijn J, Bonke B. Interpretation of plantar reflexes: biasing effect of other signs and symptoms. *J Neurol Neurosurg Psychiatry* 1977;**40**:787–789.

77. Schultz KF Chalmers I, Hayes, RJ, Altman DG. Empirical evidence of bias: dimensions of methodological quality associated with estimates of treatment effects in controlled trials. *JAMA* 1995;**273**:408–412.

78. Vickers A, Goyal N, Harland R, Rees R. Do certain countries produce only positive results? A systematic review of controlled trials. *Control Clin Trials* 1998;**19**:159–166.

79. Horne R. Beliefs and adherence to treatment: the challenge for research and clinical practice. In Halligan PW, Aylward M, eds. *The Power of Belief: Psychosocial Influence on Illness, Disability and Medicine*. Oxford: Oxford University Press, 2006:115–136.

80. Jorm AF, Griffiths KM. Public and medical beliefs about mental disorders and their treatment. In Halligan PW, Aylward M, eds. *The Power of Belief: Psychosocial Influence on Illness, Disability and Medicine*. Oxford: Oxford University Press, 2006:99–113.

81. Zeman AZJ. What in the world is consciousness? In Laureys S, ed. *Boundaries of Consciousness*. Amsterdam: Elsevier, 2006:1–10.

82. Miresco MJ, Kirmayer LJ. The persistence of mind-brain dualism in psychiatric reasoning about clinical scenarios. *Am J Psychiatry* 2006;**163**:913–918.

83. Lucire Y. *Constructing RSI: Belief and Desire*. Sydney: UNSW Press, 2003.

84. Elliot C. Scrivener's palsy. *London Rev Books* 2004;**26**:21–22.

85. Craddock N. Robust empirical data and clinical utility: the only drivers of change. Commentary on The Classification of Mental Disorders. *Adv Psychiatr Treat* 2010;**16**:20–22.

86. Sharpe M, Stone J, Hibberd C, *et al.* Neurology out-patients with symptoms unexplained by disease: illness beliefs and financial benefits predict 1-year outcome. *Psychol Med* 2010;**40**:689–698.

87. Kanaan R, Armstrong D, Barnes P, Wessely S. In the psychiatrist's chair: how neurologists understand conversion disorder. *Brain* 2009;**132**:2889–2896.

88. Hallett M. Psychogenic movement disorders: a crisis for neurology. *Curr Neurol Neurosci Rep* 2006;**6**:269–271.

89. Friedman JH, LaFrance C. Psychogenic disorders, the need to speak plainly *Arch Neurol* 2010;**67**:753–755.

90. Hinson VK, Haren WB. Psychogenic movement disorders. *Lancet Neurol* 2006;**5**:695–700.

91. World Health Organization. *The ICD-10 Classification of Mental and Behavioural Disorders,* 10th edn. Geneva: World Health Organization, 1992.

92. Kanaan R, Carson A, Wessely S, *et al.* What's so special about conversion disorder? A problem and a proposal for diagnostic classification. *Br J Psychiatry* 2010;**196**:427–428.

93. Ron M. Somatisation in neurological practice. *J Neurol Neurosurg Psychiatry* 1994;**57**:1161–1164.

94. Stone J, Wojcik W, Durrance D, *et al.* What should we say to patients with symptoms unexplained by disease? The "number needed to offend." *BMJ* 2002;**3225**:1449–1450.

95. Lewis A. "Psychogenic": a word and its mutations. *Psychol Med* 1975;**2**:209–215.

96. Ward CD. Better questions, less uneasy answers. *Pract Neurol* 2008;**8**:346–347.

97. Ormerod JA. Hysteria. In Allbutt C, Rolleston HD, eds. *A System of Medicine*, Vol. 8. London; Macmillan, 1911:690–693.

98. Freud S. Quelques considerations pour une étude comparatif des paralysies motrices organiques et hystériques. *Arch Neurol* 1893;**26**:29–43.

99. Halligan PW, David AS. Conversion hysteria: towards a cognitive neuropsychological account. In Halligan PW, David AS, eds. *Conversion Hysteria: Towards a Cognitive Neuropsychological Account*. Hove, UK: Psychology Press, 1999:161–163.

100. Breuer J, Freud S. Über den psychischen Mechanismus hysterischer Phänomene (Vorläufige Mittheilung). In *Neurologische Centralblatt,* Vol. 12. Leipzig: von Veit, 1893:4–10, 43–47.

101. Athwal BS, Halligan PW, Fink GR, *et al.* Imaging hysterical paralysis. In Halligan PW, Bass C, Marshall JC, eds. *Contemporary Approach to the Study of Hysteria: Clinical and Theoretical Perspectives*. Oxford: Oxford University Press, 2001:216–234.

102. Haggard P, Clark S, Kalogeras J. Voluntary action and conscious awareness. *Nat Neurosci* 2002;**5**:382–385.

103. Gazzaniga MS. *The Mind's Past.* Berkley, CA: University of California Press, 1998.

104. Pockett S. Does consciousness cause behaviour? *J Conscious Stud* 2004;**11:** 23–40.

105. Frith CD, Blakemore SJ, Wolpert DM. Abnormalities in the awareness and control of action. *Philos Trans R Soc Lond B Biol Sci*: 2000;**355:**1771–1788.

106. Halligan PW, Oakley D. Greatest myth of all. *New Scientist*, 2000;**2265:**34–39.

107. Wegner D. Self is magic. In Baer J, Kaufman J, Baumeister R, eds. *Are we free? Psychology and Free Will.* New York: Oxford University Press, 2008:226–247.

108. Soon CS, Brass M, Heinze HJ, Haynes JD. Unconscious determinants of free decisions in the human brain. *Nat Neurosci* 2008;**11:**543–545.

109. Blakemore SJ, Goodbody SJ, Wolpert DM. Predicting the consequences of our own actions: the role of sensorimotor context estimation. *J Neurosci* 1998;**18:**7511–7518.

110. Wolpert DM, Ghahramani Z, Jordan MI. An internal model for sensorimotor integration. *Science* 1995;**269:**1880–1882.

111. Halligan PW. Phantom limbs: the body in mind. *Cogn Neuropsychiatry*, 2002;**7:**251–268.

112. Blakemore S-J, Oakley DA, Frith CD. Delusions of alien control in the normal brain. *Neuropsychologia* 2003;**41:**1058–1067.

113. Voon V, Gallea C, Hattori N, *et al*. The involuntary nature of conversion disorder. *Neurology* 2010;**74:**223–228.

114. Voon V, Brezing C, Gallea C, *et al*. Emotional stimuli and motor conversion disorder. *Brain* 2010;**133:**1526–1536.

115. Reynolds JR. Paralysis and other disorders of motion and sensation, dependent on idea. *BMJ* 1869;**2:**483–485.

116. Charcot JM, Marie P. Hysteria. In Hake Tuke D, ed. *Dictionary of Psychololological Medicine.* London: Churchill, 1892.

117. de Vignemont F. Hysterical conversion: the reverse of anosognosia. In Bayne T, Fernandez J, eds. *Delusions and Self-Deception: Affective Influences on Belief- Formation.* Hove, UK: Psychology Press, 2009:241–260.

118. Davies M, Aimola Davies A, Coltheart M. Anosognosia and the two-factor theory of delusions. *Mind Lang* 2005;**20:**241–257.

119. Hurwitz TA, Prichard JW. Conversion disorder and fMRI. *Neurology* 2006;**12;**67:1914–1915.

120. Brown RJ. The cognitive psychology of dissociative states. *Cogn Neuropsychiatry* 2002;**7:**221–235.

121. Trimble R. *Somatoform Disorders: A Medicolegal Guide.* Cambridge, UK: Cambridge University Press, 2004.

122. Merskey H. The importance of hysteria. *Br J Psychiatry* 1986;**149:**23–28.

123. Harris JC. A clinical lesson at the Salpêtrière. *Arch Gen Psychiatry* 2005;**62:**470.

124. Hahn RA. The nocebo phenomenon: concept, evidence and implications for public health. *Prevent Med* 1997;**26:**607–611.

125. Lim E. Ong B, Seet R. Is there a place for placebo in management of psychogenic movement disorders? *Ann Acad Med Singapore* 2007;**36:**208–210.

126. Shamy SC The treatment of psychogenic movement disorders with suggestion is ethically justified. *Mov Disord* 2010;**25:**260–264.

127. Goetz CG. Charcot and psychogenic movement disorders. In Hallet M, Fahn S, Jankovic J, *et al.*, eds. *Psychogenic Movement Disorders: Neurology and Psychiatry*; London: Lippincott Williams & Wilkins, 2006:3–13.

128. Reyher J. A paradigm for determining the clinical relevance of hypnotically induced psychopathology. *Psychol Bull* 1962;**59:**344–352.

129. Oakley DA, Halligan PW. Hypnotic suggestion and cognitive neuroscience. *Trends Cogn Sci* 2009;**13:**264–270.

130. Bell V, Oakley DA, Halligan PW, Deeley Q (2011) Dissociation in hysteria and hypnosis: evidence from cognitive neuroscience. *J Neurol Neurosurg Neuropsychiatry* 2011;**82:**332–339.

131. Reich SG. Psychogenic movement disorders. *Semin Neurol* 2006;**26:**289–296.

132. Rowe JB. Conversion disorder: understanding the pathogenic links between emotion and motor systems in the *brain*. *Brain* 2010;**133:**1295–1129.

133. Thompson WG, Longstreth GF, Drossman DA, *et al*. Functional bowel disorders and functional abdominal pain. *Gut* 1999;**45:**1143–1147.

134. Stone J, Warlow CP, Sharpe M. The symptom of functional weakness: a controlled study of 107 patients *Brain* 2010;**133:**1537–1551.

135. Crimlisk HL, Bhatia KP, Cope H, *et al*. Patterns of referral in patients with medically unexplained motor symptoms. *J Psychosom Res* 2000;**49:**217–219.

136. Stone J, Sharpe M, Rothwell PM, Warlow CP. The 12 year prognosis of unilateral functional weakness and sensory disturbance. *J Neurol Neurosurg Psychiatry* 2003;**74:**591–596.

Chapter 18

Possible genetic approaches to conversion

Torsten Klengel and Elisabeth B. Binder

Introduction

For most psychiatric disorders, both environmental and genetic factors are proposed to contribute to the pathogenesis of the diseases. The genetic risk, often described as heritability (i.e., the proportion of the phenotypic variability in the population explained by genetics), ranges from over 80% for disorders such as schizophrenia, bipolar disorder, and autism, to 30–40% for depression and post-traumatic stress disorder (PTSD), down to around 25% for social phobias and some personality disorders [1]. The degree of genetic and environmental risk load likely varies among affected individuals, with combinations of high environmental risk plus low genetic risk and low environmental risk plus high genetic risk being possible. Once the combined genetic and environmental risk load reaches a certain threshold, individuals would then manifest psychiatric symptoms (Fig. 18.1).

Compared with other psychiatric disorders, very little is known about the genetic contribution to psychogenic movement disorders (PMDs) or conversion disorder, the focus of this book. While these disorders are common, accounting for 1–9% of neurological symptoms observed in the general population, we are not aware of any studies investigating the genetic contribution to PMDs using twin, family, epidemiological, or molecular genetic studies [2].

This is in stark contrast to the majority of other psychiatric disorders. To date, a number of genetic and environmental risk factors and their interaction have been identified in the etiology of psychiatric disorders and behavioral phenotypes [1,3–7].

This chapter begins with a description of the approaches in psychiatric genetics taken in other psychiatric disorders, with results from studies in major

depression and PTSD for illustration. It will then delineate how these could also be applied to PMD. A main focus will be on gene–environment interactions, particularly interactions with early trauma, as trauma experience has been found to have profound impact on the development of PMD [8,9].

Methods in psychiatric genetics

The assumption that genetic variation contributes to the susceptibility for developing psychiatric disorders comes from early genetic epidemiological studies. Large family studies demonstrate the accumulation of a disorder or trait in families but these studies are unable to dissect genetic from environmental influences. This can be done in twin studies, which compare the degree of correlation between an affected individual with the condition and the co-twin with regard to their genetic similarity: monozygotic twins share identical genetic information whereas dizygotic twins have 50% of their genes in common. Comparison of environmental differences in these twins allows estimations of the degree of genetic and environmental influence on a trait or disorder. For most common psychiatric disorders, heritability estimates are between 30% and 80%, with a contribution of multiple different genetic loci as well as a number of environmental influences [1]. Adoption studies can further dissect genetic contributions (i.e., the offspring share genetic similarity to the biological parents but no environmental identity) and environmental factors (i.e., the offspring shares no genetic similarities with the adoptive parents but their environmental influence).

Epidemiological studies can estimate general genetic effects without information on molecular mechanisms, whereas molecular genetics investigate specific

Psychogenic Movement Disorders and Other Conversion Disorders, ed. Mark Hallett, Anthony E. Lang, Joseph Jankovic, Stanley Fahn, Peter W. Halligan, Valerie Voon, and C. Robert Cloninger. Published by Cambridge University Press. © Cambridge University Press 2011.

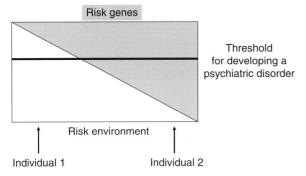

Fig. 18.1. The interplay of environmental exposure and genetic background. Environmental pathogens and, concurrently, genetic predisposition can cause psychiatric phenotypes, with variable combinations of environmental exposure and vulnerability genes leading to the development of the same psychiatric disorder. While both individuals 1 and 2 suffer from the same arbitrary disorder, this results from exposure to a highly traumatic environment and small genetic risk for individual 1 and a high genetic load and little exposure to traumatic environment in individual 2.

variants in the human genome and their implications on symptom presentation [10]. Variations in chromosomal number as seen in Down syndrome are known to be associated with a spectrum of symptoms, including neurobehavioral traits. Smaller chromosomal aberrances such as translocations of chromosomal regions (e.g., *DISC1* and *DISC2* in schizophrenia), deletions (e.g., 22q11 deletion syndrome in schizophrenia), and duplications (e.g., on the long arm of chromosome 15 in autism) have also been shown to contribute to psychiatric phenotypes [11]. These microscopic genetic abnormalities are supplemented by variations at the molecular level: copy number variations can lead to a deletion of genes or multiple copies of genes, resulting in differential gene expression and moderation of psychiatric phenotypes [12]. For example, copy number variations in the cytochrome P450 system have profound influence on the metabolism of psychotropic drugs. Smaller insertion or deletion polymorphisms of the order of a few base pairs can equally contribute to functional differences in risk genes (e.g., the polymorphic region in the serotonin transporter gene [*5-HTTLPR*]). Common polymorphisms are short tandem repeats and variable number of tandem repeats, in which a certain string of bases, such as CG for example, are repeated a variable number of time. The most common genetic polymorphisms are single nucleotide polymorphisms (SNPs), which have become central to current psychiatric genetics [10]. These single base exchanges occur over the whole genome and represent up to 90% of genetic variation in human species. They

are predominantly used as genetic markers in association studies but may have functional consequences when located in regulatory regions, with impact on transcription or translation of different amino acids.

There are different approaches to investigate the genetic basis of psychiatric phenotypes. Initially, linkage analyses were conducted in large families/pedigrees to investigate chromosomal regions that cosegregated with the phenotype. The basic principle underlying the detection of linkage is the recombination of chromosomes during meiosis, with formation of new combinations in the offspring. Linkage analysis is, however, hampered by low genomic resolution and is more successful in highly penetrant and monogenetic disorders than in genetically complex psychiatric diseases [13].

The access to cost-effective high-throughput genotyping techniques for SNPs has spurred an ever-increasing number of genetic association studies, usually in a case–control design. In these, the allele frequency of markers is compared between cases and controls. Their advantage is to provide evidence of disease loci in a much higher resolution than is possible with linkage studies and to identify susceptibility genes with small effects on disease risk [10]. Initially, candidate gene selection was mostly hypothesis driven. Now hypothesis-free genome-wide association studies are possible, currently investigating one million or more SNPs over the genome and requiring careful statistical analysis. While these association approaches are suited to identify common disease alleles with low–moderate effects size, they cannot adequately assess the effects of rare variants contributing to complex phenotypes [14]. In addition, these studies often require very large sample sizes to detect low genetic effect sizes and to be able to correct for a high number of independent statistical tests.

Findings from genome-wide association studies on common variants in neuropsychiatric disorders yielded somewhat sobering results. Using these approaches, new risk genes have been identified in schizophrenia, bipolar disorder, and autism (i.e., disorders with high heritability), but the risk conferred by these variants is usually small, ranging from an increase of 10 to 20%. This would mean that an individual's lifetime risk for schizophrenia would increase from 1% to 1.2%. Nonetheless, these genome-wide approaches have identified interesting candidate systems and have shed new light on the pathophysiology of these disorders. Genome-wide association studies in major depression and anxiety disorders have so far not yielded strong, replicated candidates [15–20].

In the last few years, it has also become apparent that these common genetic variants with small effects are supplemented by other genetic variation in the same genes or pathways. Rare variants or non-SNP variants such as copy number variations have been shown to have strong and reproducible associations [14]. Binder and Cubells [21] give a more in-depth overview of psychiatric genetic methods.

Gene–environment interactions

To date, most studies have focused on a linear genetic approach investigating main effects of variants in the genome on phenotypic presentation, which is certainly not in line with the predicted genetic models of psychiatric disorders in which multiple genetic variants likely interact with the environment to increase risk. In addition to gene–gene interactions, a main focus of psychiatric genetics has now shifted to investigate the interaction of environmental pathogens with the genetic configuration of the patient. Particularly for disorders with less heritability and stronger environmental influence, main genetic effects may only be detected in the presence of a certain environment.

While such gene–environment interactions had been predicted from earlier epidemiological studies, the first molecular proof came from a series of seminal papers by the group led by Avshalom Caspi [22]. In 2003 for example, Caspi and colleagues investigated a polymorphic region in *5-HTTLRP* that has been shown to alter transporter function, with the short allele associated with a decrease in transporter function [23–25]. Because of its putative pathophysiological relevance to depression, a large number of studies have investigated its association with this disorder and related traits, but overall these studies were negative [26–28]. Caspi and colleagues introduced exposure to stressful life events in these analyses. They could show that, while there was no main genetic effect of this polymorphism, carriers of the short allele had a higher risk of developing depressive symptoms and suicidality in response to stressful life events and childhood maltreatment [29]. Together with earlier findings from Lesch *et al.* [23] and Hariri *et al.* [30], this indicated that carriers of the short allele might have an increased stress response and thus susceptibility for depression. The gene–environment interaction of *5-HTTLPR* and stress has been replicated in recent years in different populations with different designs, but is not seen in all studies [19].

A first meta-analysis by Risch *et al.* [27] showing a lack of interaction drew attention to crucial aspects of study design for identifying gene–environment interactions [22]: recording of environmental pathogens by established diagnostic interviews was found to be superior to brief self-reports. In addition, the importance of the type of stressor became apparent – with significant interactions reported for childhood maltreatment and medical illness. In contrast, stressful life events as an environmental variable yielded controversial results, which might reflect the imprecise definition of the included stressors, with a wide range in quantity and quality, duration, and timing.

Besides gene–environment interactions reported for depression, numerous studies have now underlined their impact on other stress-related disorders and phenotypes such as PTSD, post-trauma suicide attempt, alcohol consumption, substance use, sleep disturbances, anxiety sensitivity, and impaired self-regulation of negative affect.

Generally, gene–environment interaction acknowledges that environmental conditions contribute to the development of mental disorders as well as other complex diseases and that genes modulate the influence of environment on an individual basis [22,31–34]. Genetic effects are thus dependent upon variability of the environment [32] and this is reflected by the fact that concordance of monozygotic twins is not 100% even for highly heritable disorders [35].

The pool of environmental risk factors comprises exposures in utero, childhood abuse, toxic exposures, infections, and traumatic life events; a number of other possible factors are also conceivable. Not all individuals exposed to these conditions subsequently develop specific disorders, indicating individual susceptibility or resilience in response to environmental pathogens. In fact, the direction of the genetic moderation can vary with the type of exposure, so that it might be better to use the term plasticity, rather than resilience or vulnerability genes. For example, certain alleles in genes affecting the monoamine neurotransmitters do account for an increased risk in adverse circumstances as well as an enhancement of the positive effects of supportive environments, such as positive life events or sensitive parenting [36]. Finally, gene–environment correlation can affect an individuals' disposition to be exposed to environmental pathogens, which would influence analyses of gene–environment interactions [37].

FKBP5: a common candidate gene for stress-related psychiatric disorders

Because PTSD requires exposure to a traumatic environment for diagnosis, it can serve as prototypical disorder for gene–environment interactions. Although 40–90% of individuals in the general population experience a potentially traumatic event in their lifetime, only 7–12% develop PTSD, a syndrome with a broad range of symptoms and measurable effects on neurobiological pathways [38,39]. Candidate gene studies for main genetic effects have not yielded consistent findings [40,41].

Only a few gene–environment studies have been conducted for PTSD to date [29,42–50] (reviewed by Koenen *et al.*, 2009 [51]). Among them, our group assessed polymorphisms in *FKBP5*, the gene encoding a protein FKBP5, which is involved in immunoregulation and basic cellular processes and interacts with the glucocorticoid receptor. Polymorphisms in this gene have been shown to alter endocrine responses in depression as well as the negative feedback of the stress response in healthy controls [52,53]. While we did not observe main effects of *FKBP5* polymorphisms, they did interact with severity of child abuse to predict adult PTSD symptoms [42], with the effects of child abuse being attenuated in a gene-dose dependent way (Fig. 18.2).

The same genotypes also had an impact on the neuroendocrine signature of PTSD, with an enhanced glucocorticoid receptor sensitivity only reported in carriers of the risk allele with PTSD. These gene–environment interactions were replicated in an independent study, but only in African-American and not in a sample of European descent [54]. This might be linked to population-specific genetic differences but most likely reflects the difference in trauma severity between these cohorts. Moreover, childhood trauma also interacts with *FKBP5* to predict subsequent suicide attempt [55], and a main genetic effect on unipolar depression and bipolar disorder has been reported [56,57]. In an earlier study, *FKBP5* risk alleles were associated with the occurrence of peritraumatic dissociation in medically injured children [58]. Dissociation is thought to be an evolutionary conserved response mechanism to life-threatening stress and has been discussed in the etiology of psychogenic movement disorders.

Two studies indicate that these *FKBP5* polymorphisms moderate stress response in general by decreasing the recovery from a mild psychosocial stressor [53] and by interacting with parent–child attachment in early life to predict stress hormone activity in infants [59]. It is, therefore, possible that these *FKBP5* polymorphisms moderate the effects of environmental stress on the hypothalamic–pituitary–adrenal axis, and that, with repeated or severe exposure, this can result in broad variety of psychiatric phenotypes.

Epigenetic perspective

Besides genetic approaches, epigenetic changes likely play an important role in mediating and moderating the effects of trauma on behavior [60–63]. As mentioned above, even in monozygotic twins with identical genetic and environmental background, discordance

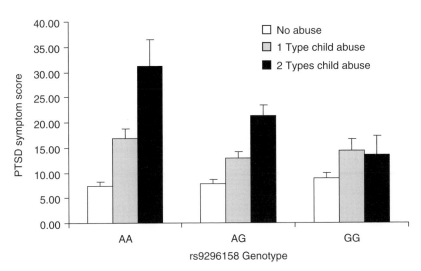

Fig. 18.2. A single nucleotide polymorphism in the gene *FKBP5* moderates the effects of pre-exposure to child abuse on adult symptoms of post-traumatic stress disorder (PTSD). Individuals carrying the A-risk allele of rs9296158 have high PTSD symptoms after exposure to child abuse, while individuals carrying the protective GG genotype show a much smaller increase in symptoms after similar childhood trauma exposure. Note that PTSD symptom scores over 20.0 are considered to reflect clinically relevant symptoms. (The data presented in this figure have been presented in Binder *et al.*, 2008 [42].).

in symptom presentation can be observed [64–66]. Epigenetics refers to the regulation of DNA transcription without alteration of the original sequence and is heritable and controlled by DNA methylation, histone modifications, and non-coding RNAs [67]. The emerging field of epigenetics provides new insight into how environmental factors can influence genetic activity without changing DNA sequence and how this environmental mark can be passed on over generations [68,69]. A number of studies in animals as well as humans have now shown that adverse events early in life can leave persistent marks on the genome without changing DNA sequence but altering gene expression and influencing neurobiological substrates until adulthood [70–74].

This adds a new layer of complexity, as subsequent environmental exposure would not only interact with genetic variation but also with epigenetic marks of previous environmental exposure. It is largely unknown how epigenetic changes interact with genetic variants although first studies are published suggesting a mediation of gene–environment interaction by epigenetic alterations [75].

Genetics and psychogenic movement disorders

To embark on genetic studies in PMD, it would be critical to have some indication on their heritability from twin and family studies, although this might be difficult because of the varying symptom presentation. It will also be important to consider diagnostic issues, such as which inclusion criteria will be applied and which PMDs can be summed together, or not. These should be accepted universally to allow cross-study comparisons and replications, which are critical in genetic association studies, requiring large sample sizes. Even for axis I disorders, it becomes apparent that diagnostic grouping is very important in the success of genetic studies and that it may even be more powerful to look at specific symptom presentations across disorders [16].

The use of biological intermediate or endophenotypes might help to better define diagnostic subgroups, and these are often more powerful in genetic association studies as they are assumed to have higher heritabilities than the psychiatric diagnosis per se.

Environmental factors likely contributing to the phenotype need to be characterized carefully with standardized interviews, which appear superior to self-reports as the latter are prone to selective retention. In addition, gene–environment interactions need to be analyzed separately for different types of stressor.

Animal studies can help in the identification of interesting candidate genes to be tested in humans, and hypothesis-free genome-wide approaches could identify novel candidate systems that can then be further explored using animal models or validated with intermediate phenotypes.

Given the high comorbitiy of PMDs, it might be interesting to investigate known risk genes for these comorbid disorders also in PMD, as similar genetic risk has been shown to be associated with different psychiatric presentations.

Overall, the inclusion of genetic approaches, particularly gene–environment interactions, to research in PMDs could add new insights into the pathophysiology of these disorders.

References

1. Smoller JW, Sheidley BR, Tsuang MT. *Psychiatric Genetics Applications in Clinical Practice*. Washington, DC: American Psychiatric Press, 2008.

2. Nowak DA, Fink GR. Psychogenic movement disorders: aetiology, phenomenology, neuroanatomical correlates and therapeutic approaches. *Neuroimage* 2009;**47**:1015–1025.

3. Lau JY, Eley TC. The genetics of mood disorders. *Annu Rev Clin Psychol* 2010;**6**:313–337.

4. Levinson DF. The genetics of depression: a review. *Biol Psychiatry* 2006;**60**:84–92.

5. Nothen MM, Nieratschker V, Cichon S, Rietschel M. New findings in the genetics of major psychoses. *Dialogues Clin Neurosci* 2010;**12**:85–93.

6. Sullivan PF. The genetics of schizophrenia. *PLoS Med* 2005;**2**:e212.

7. Burmeister M, McInnis MG, Zollner S. Psychiatric genetics: progress amid controversy. *Nat Rev Genet* 2008;**9**:527–540.

8. Brown RJ, Schrag A, Trimble MR. Dissociation, childhood interpersonal trauma, and family functioning in patients with somatization disorder. *Am J Psychiatry* 2005;**162**:899–905.

9. Şar V, Islam S, Öztürk E. Childhood emotional abuse and dissociation in patients with conversion symptoms. *Psychiatr Clin Neurosci* 2009;**63**:670–677.

10. Frazer KA, Murray SS, Schork NJ, Topol EJ. Human genetic variation and its contribution to complex traits. *Nat Rev Genet* 2009;**10**:241–251.

11. MacIntyre DJ, Blackwood DH, Porteous DJ, Pickard BS, Muir WJ. Chromosomal abnormalities and mental illness. *Mol Psychiatry* 2003;**8**:275–287.

12. Stankiewicz P, Lupski JR. Structural variation in the human genome and its role in disease. *Annu Rev Med* 2010;**61**:437–455.

13. Sklar P. Linkage analysis in psychiatric disorders: the emerging picture. *Annu Rev Genom Hum Genet* 2002;**3**:371–413.

14. Cirulli ET, Goldstein DB. Uncovering the roles of rare variants in common disease through whole-genome sequencing. *Nat Rev Genet* 2010;**11**:415–425.

15. Lewis CM, Ng MY, Butler AW, *et al.* Genome-wide association study of major recurrent depression in the UK population. *Am J Psychiatry* 2010;**167**:949–957.

16. McMahon FJ, Akula N, Schulze TG, *et al.* Meta-analysis of genome-wide association data identifies a risk locus for major mood disorders on 3p21.1. *Nat Genet* 2010;**42**:128–131.

17. Muglia P, Tozzi F, Galwey NW, *et al.* Genome-wide association study of recurrent major depressive disorder in two European case–control cohorts. *Mol Psychiatry* 2010;**15**:589–601.

18. Bosker FJ, Hartman CA, Nolte IM, *et al.* Poor replication of candidate genes for major depressive disorder using genome-wide association data. *Mol Psychiatry* 2010;**16**:516–532.

19. Liu Y, Blackwood DH, Caesar S, *et al.* Meta-analysis of genome-wide association data of bipolar disorder and major depressive disorder. *Mol Psychiatry* 2011;**16**:2–4.

20. Sullivan PF, de Geus EJ, Willemsen G, *et al.* Genome-wide association for major depressive disorder: a possible role for the presynaptic protein piccolo. *Mol Psychiatry* 2009;**14**:359–375.

21. Binder EB, Cubells JF. *The American Psychiatric Publishing Textbook of Psychopharmacology,* 4th ed. Arlington, VA: American Psychiatric Association, 2009.

22. Caspi A, Hariri AR, Holmes A, Uher R, Moffitt TE. Genetic sensitivity to the environment: the case of the serotonin transporter gene and its implications for studying complex diseases and traits. *Am J Psychiatry* 2010;**167**:509–527.

23. Lesch KP, Bengel D, Heils A, *et al.* Association of anxiety-related traits with a polymorphism in the serotonin transporter gene regulatory region. *Science* 1996;**274**:1527–1531.

24. Brown GW, Harris TO. Depression and the serotonin transporter *5-HTTLPR* polymorphism: a review and a hypothesis concerning gene–environment interaction. *J Affect Disord* 2008;**111**:1–12.

25. Serretti A, Calati R, Mandelli L, De RD. Serotonin transporter gene variants and behavior: a comprehensive review. *Curr Drug Targets* 2006;**7**:1659–1669.

26. Munafo MR, Durrant C, Lewis G, Flint J. Gene X environment interactions at the serotonin transporter locus. *Biol Psychiatry* 2009;**65**:211–219.

27. Risch N, Herrell R, Lehner T, *et al.* Interaction between the serotonin transporter gene (*5-HTTLPR*), stressful life events, and risk of depression: a meta-analysis. *JAMA* 2009;**301**:2462–2471.

28. Kendler KS, Kuhn JW, Vittum J, Prescott CA, Riley B. The interaction of stressful life events and a serotonin transporter polymorphism in the prediction of episodes of major depression: a replication. *Arch Gen Psychiatry* 2005;**62**:529–535.

29. Caspi A, McClay J, Moffitt TE, *et al.* Role of genotype in the cycle of violence in maltreated children. *Science* 2002;**297**:851–854.

30. Hariri AR, Mattay VS, Tessitore A, *et al.* Serotonin transporter genetic variation and the response of the human amygdala. *Science* 2002;**297**:400–403.

31. Moffitt TE, Caspi A, Rutter M. Strategy for investigating interactions between measured genes and measured environments. *Arch Gen Psychiatry* 2005;**62**:473–481.

32. Caspi A, Moffitt TE. Gene–environment interactions in psychiatry: joining forces with neuroscience. *Nat Rev Neurosci* 2006;**7**:583–590.

33. Uher R, McGuffin P. The moderation by the serotonin transporter gene of environmental adversity in the aetiology of mental illness: review and methodological analysis. *Mol Psychiatry* 2008;**13**:131–146.

34. Amstadter AB, Koenen KC, Ruggiero KJ, *et al.* NPY moderates the relation between hurricane exposure and generalized anxiety disorder in an epidemiologic sample of hurricane-exposed adults. *Depress Anxiety* 2010;**27**:270–275.

35. Dick DM, Riley B, Kendler KS. Nature and nurture in neuropsychiatric genetics: where do we stand? *Dialog Clin Neurosci* 2010;**12**:7–23.

36. Belsky J, Jonassaint C, Pluess M, *et al.* Vulnerability genes or plasticity genes? *Mol Psychiatry* 2009;**14**:746–754.

37. Jaffee SR, Price TS. Gene–environment correlations: a review of the evidence and implications for prevention of mental illness. *Mol Psychiatry* 2007;**12**:432–442.

38. Kessler RC, Sonnega A, Bromet E, Hughes M, Nelson CB. Posttraumatic stress disorder in the National Comorbidity Survey. *Arch Gen Psychiatry* 1995;**52**:1048–1060.

39. Heim C, Nemeroff CB. Neurobiology of posttraumatic stress disorder. *CNS Spectr* 2009;**14**:13–24.

40. Broekman BF, Olff M, Boer F. The genetic background to PTSD. *Neurosci Biobehav Rev* 2007;**31**:348–362.

41. Cornelis MC, Nugent NR, Amstadter AB, Koenen KC. Genetics of post-traumatic stress disorder: review and recommendations for genome-wide association studies. *Curr Psychiatry Rep* 2010;**12**:313–326.

42. Binder EB, Bradley RG, Liu W, *et al*. Association of *FKBP5* polymorphisms and childhood abuse with risk of posttraumatic stress disorder symptoms in adults. *JAMA* 2008;**299**:1291–1305.

43. Amstadter AB, Koenen KC, Ruggiero KJ, *et al*. Variant in RGS2 moderates posttraumatic stress symptoms following potentially traumatic event exposure. *J Anxiety Disord* 2009;**23**:369–373.

44. Kolassa IT, Kolassa S, Ertl V, Papassotiropoulos A, De Quervain DJ. The risk of posttraumatic stress disorder after trauma depends on traumatic load and the catechol-*O*-methyltransferase Val(158)Met polymorphism. *Biol Psychiatry* 2010;**67**:304–308.

45. Grabe HJ, Spitzer C, Schwahn C, *et al*. Serotonin transporter gene (*SLC6A4*) promoter polymorphisms and the susceptibility to posttraumatic stress disorder in the general population. *Am J Psychiatry* 2009;**166**:926–933.

46. Xie P, Kranzler HR, Poling J, *et al*. Interactive effect of stressful life events and the serotonin transporter 5-*HTTLPR* genotype on posttraumatic stress disorder diagnosis in 2 independent populations. *Arch Gen Psychiatry* 2009;**66**:1201–1209.

47. Kolassa IT, Ertl V, Eckart C, *et al*. Association study of trauma load and *SLC6A4* promoter polymorphism in posttraumatic stress disorder: evidence from survivors of the Rwandan genocide. *J Clin Psychiatry* 2010;**71**:543–547.

48. Amstadter AB, Nugent NR, Koenen KC, *et al*. Association between COMT, PTSD, and increased smoking following hurricane exposure in an epidemiologic sample. *Psychiatry* 2009;**72**:360–369.

49. Kilpatrick DG, Koenen KC, Ruggiero KJ, *et al*. The serotonin transporter genotype and social support and moderation of posttraumatic stress disorder and depression in hurricane-exposed adults. *Am J Psychiatry* 2007;**164**:1693–1699.

50. Nelson EC, Agrawal A, Pergadia ML, *et al*. Association of childhood trauma exposure and GABRA2 polymorphisms with risk of posttraumatic stress disorder in adults. *Mol Psychiatry* 2009;**14**:234–235.

51. Koenen KC, Amstadter AB, Nugent NR. Gene–environment interaction in posttraumatic stress disorder: an update. *J Trauma Stress* 2009;**22**:416–426.

52. Binder EB, Salyakina D, Lichtner P, *et al*. Polymorphisms in *FKBP5* are associated with increased recurrence of depressive episodes and rapid response to antidepressant treatment. *Nat Genet* 2004;**36**:1319–1325.

53. Ising M, Depping AM, Siebertz A, *et al*. Polymorphisms in the *FKBP5* gene region modulate recovery from psychosocial stress in healthy controls. *Eur J Neurosci* 2008;**28**:389–398.

54. Xie P, Kranzler HR, Poling J, *et al*. Interaction of *FKBP5* with childhood adversity on risk for post-traumatic stress disorder. *Neuropsychopharmacology* 2010;**35**:1684–1692.

55. Roy A, Gorodetsky E, Yuan Q, Goldman D, Enoch MA. Interaction of *FKBP5*, a stress-related gene, with childhood trauma increases the risk for attempting suicide. *Neuropsychopharmacology* 2010;**35**:1674–1683.

56. Lekman M, Laje G, Charney D, *et al*. The *FKBP5*-gene in depression and treatment response: an association study in the Sequenced Treatment Alternatives to Relieve Depression (STAR*D) cohort. *Biol Psychiatry* 2008;**63**:1103–1110.

57. Willour VL, Chen H, Toolan J, *et al*. Family-based association of *FKBP5* in bipolar disorder. *Mol Psychiatry* 2009;**14**:261–268.

58. Koenen KC, Saxe G, Purcell S, *et al*. Polymorphisms in *FKBP5* are associated with peritraumatic dissociation in medically injured children. *Mol Psychiatry* 2005;**10**:1058–1059.

59. Luijk MP, Velders FP, Tharner A, *et al*. FKBP5 and resistant attachment predict cortisol reactivity in infants: gene–environment interaction. *Psychoneuroendocrinology* 2010;**35**:1454–1461.

60. Tsankova N, Renthal W, Kumar A, Nestler EJ. Epigenetic regulation in psychiatric disorders. *Nat Rev Neurosci* 2007;**8**:355–367.

61. McGowan PO, Szyf M. The epigenetics of social adversity in early life: implications for mental health outcomes. *Neurobiol Dis* 2010;**39**:66–72.

62. Szyf M, McGowan P, Meaney MJ. The social environment and the epigenome. *Environ Mol Mutagen* 2008;**49**:46–60.

63. Petronis A. Epigenetics as a unifying principle in the aetiology of complex traits and diseases. *Nature* 2010;**465**:721–727.

64. Kaminsky ZA, Tang T, Wang SC, *et al*. DNA methylation profiles in monozygotic and dizygotic twins. *Nat Genet* 2009;**41**:240–245.

65. Petronis A, Gottesman II, Kan P, *et al*. Monozygotic twins exhibit numerous epigenetic differences: clues to twin discordance? *Schizophr Bull* 2003;**29**:169–178.

66. Fraga MF, Ballestar E, Paz MF, *et al*. Epigenetic differences arise during the lifetime of monozygotic twins. *Proc Natl Acad Sci USA* 2005;**102**:10604–10609.

67. Jaenisch R, Bird A. Epigenetic regulation of gene expression: how the genome integrates

intrinsic and environmental signals. *Nat Genet* 2003;**33**(Suppl):245–254.

68. Meaney MJ, Szyf M. Environmental programming of stress responses through DNA methylation: life at the interface between a dynamic environment and a fixed genome. *Dialog Clin Neurosci* 2005;**7**:103–123.

69. Weaver IC, Cervoni N, Champagne FA, *et al.* Epigenetic programming by maternal behavior. *Nat Neurosci* 2004;**7**:847–854.

70. Pidsley R, Mill J. Epigenetic studies of psychosis: current findings, methodological approaches, and implications for postmortem research. *Biol Psychiatry* 2011;**69**:146–156.

71. Murgatroyd C, Patchev AV, Wu Y, *et al.* Dynamic DNA methylation programs persistent adverse effects of early-life stress. *Nat Neurosci* 2009;**12**:1559–1566.

72. Tsankova NM, Berton O, Renthal W, *et al.* Sustained hippocampal chromatin regulation in a mouse model of depression and antidepressant action. *Nat Neurosci* 2006;**9**:519–525.

73. Mill J, Tang T, Kaminsky Z, *et al.* Epigenomic profiling reveals DNA-methylation changes associated with major psychosis. *Am J Hum Genet* 2008;**82**:696–711.

74. Petronis A. The origin of schizophrenia: genetic thesis, epigenetic antithesis, and resolving synthesis. *Biol Psychiatry* 2004;**55**:965–970.

75. Hellman A, Chess A. Extensive sequence-influenced DNA methylation polymorphism in the human genome. *Epigenet Chromatin* 2010;**3**:11.

Chapter

19

Functional brain imaging of psychogenic paralysis during conversion and hypnosis

Patrik Vuilleumier and Yann Cojan

Introduction

Conversion disorders have been observed in medical practice for many centuries, but the psychological factors triggering these symptoms and their underlying neurophysiological mechanisms remain poorly understood [1–3]. Formerly called "hysteria" in classic psychiatry terminology, conversion is defined by the presence of neurological symptoms (such as paralysis, anesthesia, blindness, amnesia, neglect, and so forth) that are not explained by organic brain injury but thought to be induced by psychological stress or particular conflicts (DSM-IV-R).

Up to one-third of patients seen in neurology clinics may have symptoms that are only somewhat or not at all explained by an organic disease [4–7], but conversion represents 4% of neurological diagnosis in general practice. A proportion of these patients have weakness or paralysis of a limb that cannot be explained by neurological illness, and in movement disorder practice, the frequency on this diagnosis may range from 6 to 20% [8,9]. A definitive diagnosis usually would require two specialists, both a psychiatrist and a neurologist, and, therefore, needs good collaboration between them. This is sometimes complicated by the fear of misdiagnosis coming from the occasional uncertainties with the neurological diagnosis, but also the limited reliability of psychological features [10,11].

Since the time of Charcot and Freud, a number of speculations have been put forward concerning the possible neural pathways by which emotional states might affect the mind and behavior of patients with conversion [2,3]. Charcot himself considered that the functioning of the nervous system could be altered without any visible pathology under the influence of certain ideas, suggestions, or psychological states [12].

These effects were likened to those induced by hypnosis, whose fascinating power on the mind was also discussed at the same period by authors like William James, who devoted an entire chapter on this phenomenon [13]. Later, his student Babinski added that suggestion factors could produce conversion in specific individuals based on combined influences of the personal significance of emotional triggers and individual predispositions [14]. To underscore this conceptualization, Babinski proposed to replace the term "hysteria" by a newly created word: "pithiatism" (from the Greek *peithô*, persuasion, and *iatos*, curable) – but this term was only rarely taken up in the subsequent literature (unlike his more famous invention of "anosognosia" to describe unawareness of organic neurological deficits, a phenomenon somehow mirroring conversion). Both Charcot and Babinski viewed conversion symptoms as the result of changes in internal representations that normally mediate the subjective experience of movement or sensation – an idea resonating with more modern accounts suggesting that some body maps might be distorted by erroneous information under the effect of emotion or memory [15] or via "as-if" processes normally used to simulate and anticipate future somatic states [16]. In the same period as Charcot, Janet [17] further insisted on the role of a dissociation between conscious and unconscious processes, subserved by distinct (i.e., cortical versus subcortical) neural systems, and with the latter overtaking the former for the control of mental or sensorimotor functions under the influence of strong emotions or during hypnotic induction. This view inspired Freud and Breuer [18], who proposed that physical symptoms might reflect psychological motives or affective motive (often related to sexual issues) that are unconsciously repressed and then

Psychogenic Movement Disorders and Other Conversion Disorders, ed. Mark Hallett, Anthony E. Lang, Joseph Jankovic, Stanley Fahn, Peter W. Halligan, Valerie Voon, and C. Robert Cloninger. Published by Cambridge University Press. © Cambridge University Press 2011.

"converted" into bodily complaints with some symbolic meaning. This interpretation led to the current terminology of conversion to describe psychogenic disorders. However, although this is the only psychiatry condition whose name directly refers to putative mechanisms, the exact processes by which a psychological conflict or stress is transformed or expressed in neurological symptoms are still largely unknown today.

With the advent of more elaborate knowledge about brain functions during the twentieth century, neurologists and theorists proposed more detailed neurophysiological models, but generally based on speculations or analogies with other phenomena rather than empirical findings. Among others, an influential account was put forward according to which conversion deficits (such as paralysis, anesthesia, or blindness) might result from a selective inhibition or "gating" of either sensory inputs or motor outputs, for example at the level the thalamus [19,20], or through the action of attentional mechanisms mediated by anterior cingulate cortex (ACC) or parietal cortex [21–23]. Such inhibition was generally considered to be triggered by unconscious motivational needs or attributed to abnormal responses to stressful events, which might be perceived, recalled, or imagined by the patients in particular situations. Moreover, in line with previous ideas of Charcot and others, similar neuroanatomical models based on inhibition (or sometimes disconnection) were also proposed to account for sensory and motor phenomena induced by hypnosis [24,25]. However, this rich variety of hypotheses has long remained strikingly at odds with the paucity of systematic empirical investigation of conversion disorders using behavioral or neurophysiological measures.

It is only with recent advances in brain imaging methods that clinicians and researchers have begun to more directly probe for distinctive patterns of neural activation in conversion patients. Since the early 1990s, various changes in regional brain activity have been observed with positron emission tomography (PET) or functional magnetic resonance imaging (fMRI), but also with electroencephalography or transcranial magnetic stimulation. However, most imaging studies have concerned small groups of patients with heterogeneous symptoms and very different paradigms, such that the extant findings are still difficult to integrate in a single coherent framework. Nevertheless, some commonalities are progressively emerging. Only a

selective overview of this work will be provided here (for more details, see Vuilleumier, 2005, 2009 [2,3]; Black *et al.*, 2004 [26]; Chapter 20), while neuroimaging and neurophysiology results in psychogenic movement disorders (PMDs) (i.e., positive symptoms such as tremor or dystonia) are discussed elsewhere [9] (see also Chapter 21). The chapter will begin by summarizing the major findings from imaging studies on conversion paralysis conducted by our group and others, then describe new results in a patient with motor conversion, and finally discuss how these data may open the way to new hypotheses and new investigations in this field.

Brain imaging studies

Activation of motor and sensory systems

While the advent of functional neuroimaging techniques has provided tremendous opportunities to investigate the neural bases of cognitive and affective disorders in neurology and psychiatry, it is surprising that only few studies have been conducted in conversion disorders until recently. Furthermore, only a minority of these studies have specifically investigated the theoretical view that inhibition processes and/or emotional processes would be responsible for the generation of symptoms such as motor paralysis. A pioneer study [27] used single photon emission computed tomography (SPECT) in a female patient with left arm anesthesia and showed abnormal hemispheric asymmetries with decreased activity in right parietal areas and increases in right frontal areas, but these results did not suggest any specific causal mechanism for such changes. A subsequent influential study was conducted by Marshall and colleagues [22] using PET in another single patient who had suffered from chronic leg weakness for a few years. When the patient was asked to move one or the other leg on command, no activation was observed in the right motor cortex for attempts with the left/paralyzed limb, in contrast to increases in the left motor cortex for executed movements with the right/unaffected limb. In addition, however, attempts to move the left leg produced a selective activation in orbitofrontal cortex and ACC instead. This finding was taken to suggest that voluntary actions were prevented through an active inhibition of motor pathways by medial prefrontal areas, which are known to be implicated in inhibitory control [28–31] but also in emotional and motivational functions – including pathologies such as depression, aggressive behaviors, and catatonia [31–34].

Other studies using fMRI have also reported decreased activations in motor [35–37] or sensory [38,39] areas in patients with conversion paralysis or anesthesia, respectively, with or without concomitant increases in medial or dorsolateral prefrontal areas (see also Chapter 21). One study [40] found no anomalies in motor areas but reductions in left prefrontal cortex, which was interpreted as a lack of intentional programming or "lack of motor will". Different paradigms have been employed to probe motor functions in these studies, including actual movement attempts, passive movements, motor imagery, motor observation, or somatosensory stimulation. Interestingly, Burgmer et al. [37] examined brain responses during the observation of unilateral hand movement in four patients with psychogenic motor loss and found a lack of "mirror" activation in the motor cortex contralateral to the affected hand, but normal increases on the ipsilateral side, suggesting a lack of covert motor activation even without actual movement execution. However, they did not report changes in other (e.g., prefrontal) brain regions. By contrast, de Lange et al. [41] used an implicit motor imagery task (mental hand rotation) and found normal and symmetric activation of motor cortex for both the affected and unaffected hands (Chapter 20), but performance with the affected hand was associated with an increase (or relative lack of decrease compared with other conditions) in the ventral ACC. Likewise, a recent fMRI study in a patient presenting with left neglect behavior and left sensorimotor disturbances of psychogenic origin revealed a normal activation in parietal areas but increases in ACC during a line bisection task [42]. However, tasks requiring an active participation of the patients are often difficult to interpret since changes in brain activity may reflect either the cause or the consequence of abnormal motor performance. In particular, increases in ACC activity during movement attempts with the affected limb may result from heightened monitoring functions (see Chapter 20) or error detection [43], rather than just inhibition as originally proposed by Marshall and colleagues.

In an early study of seven patients with unilateral motor loss from conversion (with or without additional sensory symptoms), we specifically sought to activate sensorimotor pathways without requiring any voluntary action [44]. Patients were administered a bilateral and symmetric vibratory stimulation (50 Hz) to both hands simultaneously (a procedure known to recruit proprioceptive and motor systems in the brain) while undergoing SPECT imaging. Furthermore, brain scans were obtained in three conditions in each patient: once at rest and once during vibratory stimulation when unilateral motor loss was present, plus once during stimulation again but when motor loss had recovered (after 4–6 months). Comparing brain activation to the stimulation relative to rest in the presence of motor symptoms showed the expected networks of sensory and motor areas in both hemispheres, without any prominent asymmetries. In particular, there was no significant change in the response of the primary motor area contralateral to

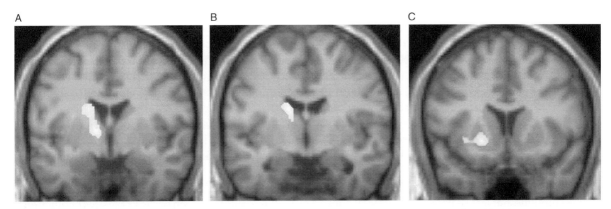

Fig. 19.1. Regional decreases in contralateral hemisphere during unilateral sensorimotor conversion. Data from SPECT scans comparing activity after recovery relative to the presence of symptoms. Scans were obtained in three conditions: at rest (A), during vibratory stimulation when unilateral motor loss was present (B), and during stimulation again but when motor loss had recovered (after 4–6 months) (C). Significant changes were observed in thalamus, caudate, and pallidum/putamen. (Also in color plate section.)

conversion symptoms. More interestingly, comparing brain activation with stimulation in the presence of symptoms relative to recovery revealed highly selective decreases in three brain regions contralateral to the motor loss, including the caudate, putamen, and thalamus (Fig. 19.1, see also color plates). All three regions are interconnected within cortical-basal ganglia circuits that are critically implicated in movement execution, but also receive converging inputs from prefrontal and limbic areas, including orbitofrontal cortex, cingulate, and amygdala. These basal ganglia circuits thus constitute a unique relay within the motor pathways where neural signals related to motor plans can be modulated by concomitant inputs associated with motivational and emotional states [45], which might act to facilitate or suppress specific patterns of behavior [46]. Moreover, changes in basal ganglia activity have been implicated in protective segmental immobility after limb injury [47] and during stereotyped motor arrest elicited by learned stressful situations[47] in animals, but also in motor neglect arising without corticospinal deficits in brain-damaged humans [48]. Taken together, these findings suggest that an "acute" unilateral conversion motor loss may correlate with transient reduction (or inhibition) of motor execution circuits downstream from movement planning in (pre)motor cortex, and that such changes may be driven by modulatory signals from other (e.g., limbic) areas and eventually return to a normal level after symptom recovery.

In this study [44], we also performed a network connectivity analysis using a form of principal component analysis (scaled subprofile modeling), which allows the delineation of functionally distinct networks of regions whose activity tends to covary irrespective of their absolute level of activity. Critically, this analysis identified a network including the thalamus and caudate, together with inferior frontal regions (Brodmann areas [BA] 44/45) and orbitofrontal cortex (BA 11), which was found to exhibit selective increases in coupling during paralysis in the hemisphere contralateral to the motor symptoms (Fig. 19.2, see also color plates). Two other networks were found: one including motor and sensory cortical areas, which showed greater coupling during stimulation irrespective of symptoms, but less so in the contralateral hemisphere during paralysis; and a second of frontoparietal cortical areas, which conversely were more coupled in the ipsilateral hemisphere during paralysis. This network analysis suggests that conversion paralysis does not arise in association with reduced activation of the basal ganglia–thalamic circuits alone, but the latter reduction was accompanied with a distinct pattern of increased functional connectivity with inferior frontal and orbitofrontal cortex. One hypothesis to account for this pattern is that changes in basal ganglia–thalamic circuits might cause a suppression of motor behavior under the influence of affective or stressful signals represented in orbitofrontal or ventral frontal cortex.

Activation of emotion systems

More recent fMRI studies have provided further evidence that emotional brain circuits might be differentially activated in patients with conversion and interact with their motor function. One intriguing single-case study reported transient decreases in motor cortex while the patient was cued to recall traumatic life events associated with the onset of her conversion paralysis [36]. In this patient, a comparison of brain responses to auditory sentences describing traumatic events relative to neutral sentences revealed not only significant reduction in motor areas contralateral to her symptoms but also concomitant increases in the amygdala and hippocampus: These two brain regions are critically associated with memory and emotion, and intimately interconnected with ventromedial prefrontal areas and ventral striatum. This case study is particularly interesting because it suggests that memory retrieval or confrontation with particular stressful events can somehow influence movement representations in cortical motor areas – although no direct evidence or functional connectivity analysis was reported to support this interpretation. Furthermore, similar paradigms involving exposure to traumatic scripts have been used in fMRI studies of post-traumatic stress disorder (PTSD) and showed that the induction of dissociative symptoms by such scripts was associated with modulation of activity in the ventromedial prefrontal cortex (VMPFC). In another recent fMRI study [49], increased amygdala responses to emotional faces was also found in a large group of patients with mixed PMDs (e.g., tremor, dystonia, etc.). However, no systematic anomaly was observed in cortical or subcortical motor regions.

It remains to be seen whether the sites of functional changes (i.e., motor cortex or basal ganglia) may vary with the type of symptoms (psychogenic paralysis versus abnormal movement) and/or their duration, and whether the origin of any inhibition process implicates

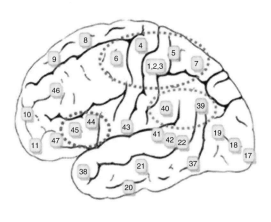
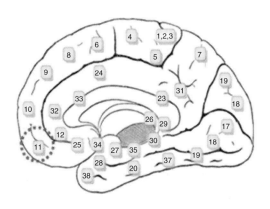

	Network 1 Sensorimotor	Network 2 Attention	Network 3 Limbic-subcortical
Degree of expression:			
Symptom-contra	0.43	-	0.58
Symptom-ipsi	0.59	0.37	-
Recovery-contra	0.77	-	-
Recovery-ipsi	0.80	-	-
Areas included:			
BA 4	0.84		
BA 6	0.90		
BA 8		0.88	
BA 9-44			
BA 44-45			0.66
BA 46			
BA 10			
BA 11			0.66
ACC		0.70	
BA 1-2-3	0.87		
BA 5-7	0.97		
BA 39-40	0.57	0.68	
BA 37		0.76	
BA 17-18			
BA 22			
BA 20-21			
BA 38			
Caudate			0.68
Lenticular			
Thalamus			0.72

Fig. 19.2. Results from a network analysis (subscale profile modeling), comparing brain activation by bilateral stimulation during unilateral sensorimotor conversion and after recovery. Three distinct networks were identified. Network 3 included subcortical nodes in caudate and thalamus that were functionally coupled with areas in inferior and ventral prefrontal cortex (BA 44/45 and BA 11, respectively). (Also in color plate section.)

the amygdala, VMPFC, ACC, or some other brain areas in all types of conversion disorder. Because previous imaging studies were often conducted in single patients or small groups, with symptoms of varying duration (from a few days to several years), and using very different methodologies, all of the above results still remain difficult to generalize.

Activation of inhibition systems

While imaging studies of conversion disorders have proposed that motor loss might result from inhibition of motor pathways (directly or indirectly) by the amygdala [36] or ventromedial prefrontal areas such as ACC [24,42], abundant research on motor inhibition in healthy people and patients with focal brain lesions

has highlighted a key role for more lateral prefrontal regions in inhibitory control, specifically in the right inferior frontal gyrus (IFG) [50]. Moreover, the right IFG has been found to activate not only in conditions requiring voluntary inhibition of prepotent or habitual responses during motor tasks (such as "go–nogo" or "stop" tasks), irrespective of hand side, but also beyond the motor domain, for example in relation to the suppression of verbal responses [51] and memory [52]. In addition, in support of this inhibitory function of the right IFG, neuropsychological studies showed that focal damage to this region can cause selective deficits in response inhibition.

We, therefore, directly tested for the role of the same inhibitory systems in motor conversion by using

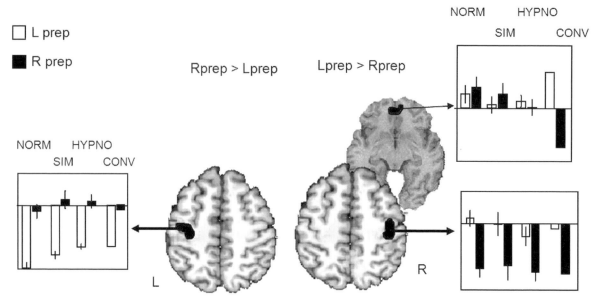

Fig. 19.3. Use of a go–nogo paradigm in a patient with a recent history of psychogenic left arm paresis. Activation during the preparation (prep) phase for the right hand > left paralyzed hand (A) and for the left paralyzed hand > right hand (B). NORM, normal controls; CONV, patient with conversion; SIM, healthy controls simulating paralysis; HYPNO, hypnotically induced paralysis. (A) Contralateral activation of the primary motor cortex was seen in all cases and symmetric across the two hemispheres. (B) In the patients with conversion, additional increases were found in ventromedial prefrontal cortex as well as the left orbitofrontal cortex, for the left/paralyzed hand selectively. (Also in color plate section.)

a go–nogo paradigm in a patient with a recent history of psychogenic left arm paresis [53]. Specifically, our paradigm required motor go–nogo responses with one or the other hand, allowing us to ask whether the failure to execute movements with the affected side (i.e., on a left-go trial) would correspond to an active inhibition associated with recruitment of the right IFG (and other related brain areas), similar to the activation seen during active inhibition for normal participants or for the normal hand. In addition, to investigate the role of "motor will" or intentional programming, we combined our go–nogo task with a motor preparation phase, allowing us to test for any deficit in covert motor activity even without movements [37,40,41].

This experimental design yielded several important findings. First, we found that when required to prepare a unilateral hand movement, our patient showed contralateral increases in motor and premotor regions that were symmetric for the affected and unaffected hands (Fig. 19.3, see also color plates). By contrast, as expected, there was no activation of the contralateral motor cortex during attempted movements with the paralyzed hand. This result is consistent with

preserved activation of motor cortex during mental imagery in other cases [41,54], and accords with the subjective report of patients with conversion, suggesting that their motor intention might be preserved while actual motor execution is experienced as being "blocked". The results for subjects with hypnotically induced paralysis shown in Fig. 19.3 are discussed later in the chapter.

A second important finding was that we found no activation in brain regions usually implicated in motor inhibition (e.g., ACC or right IFG) during attempted movements with the affected limb (i.e., failed go response), although the right IFG as well as the right inferior parietal lobule were significantly activated during the voluntary inhibition of movement with the unaffected hand (i.e., nogo response), as anticipated [50,51]. This result, therefore, suggests that the absence of correct go responses with the paralyzed hand was different from nogo responses, and hence that conversion paralysis does not involve the same inhibitory processes as those recruited by an active conscious suppression of action.

Furthermore, we also tested a group of healthy participants who were required to fake a unilateral left

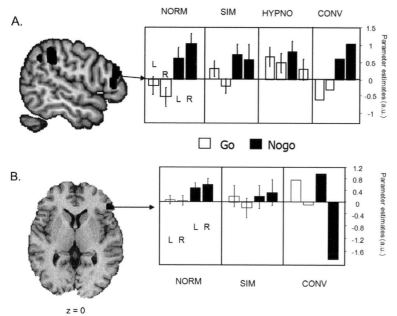

Fig. 19.4. Activation of inhibitory networks. (A) Contrast between nogo > go trials in normal controls (NORM, irrespective of hand side) revealed increased activity in a bilateral but predominantly right hemisphere network including inferior frontal gyrus and inferior parietal lobule. Simulation (SIM) produced similar increases during normal inhibition (nogo trials) and feigned left hand paralysis (left go trials), whereas conversion (CONV) produced a similar pattern to normal condition. (B) Activation of inhibitory processes in conversion. The contrast between left go > right go during conversion revealed a more ventral cluster in anterior lateral prefrontal cortex ($p < 0.001$ uncorrected; k, 10 voxels; xyz coordinates in standard MNI space (Montreal Neurological Institute brain template), 51, 36–3), distinct from the right inferior frontal gyrus activated by nogo trials in normal controls and simulators (see (A), xyz coordinates in standard MNI space, 57, 30, 24). A left hand versus right hand pattern of activation can be observed for the latter region. Plots represent the parameter estimates (betas) in right inferior frontal gyrus for left go and right go (green), plus left nogo and right nogo (red) trials, respectively, in the normal, simulation, hypnosis, and conversion conditions. HYPNO, hypnotically induced paralysis. (Also in color plate section.)

hand paralysis during the same task (they were told that this would allow us to identify mechanisms important for motor effort and recovery in patients with real paralysis). These simulators (SIM in Fig. 19.3) also showed normal activation of right motor cortex during preparation with their "paralyzed" left hand, suggesting an active covert preparation of movement; but unlike the patient with conversion, there was a robust activation of the right IFG during the suppression of left response on go trials, similar to the nogo activation seen in normal conditions (Fig. 19.4A, see also color plates). This result clearly indicates that conversion paralysis differs from feigned paralysis. Notably, in the patient, both preparation and attempts of movement with the right hand activated the contralateral basal ganglia (putamen and thalamus) together with premotor (supplementary motor area) and motor areas, whereas no subcortical activation was found for the left hand.

In addition, the patient also showed a distinctive pattern of activation in the VMPFC during the preparation of movement with the affected left limb (Fig. 19.4), while additional increases were found in the right lateral orbitofrontal cortex during the attempt of left movement on go trials (Fig. 19.4B). None of these effects was seen during motor inhibition on nogo trials in the normal controls or during feigned paralysis on

go trials in simulators. The activation in VMPFC partly overlapped with the regions reported by Marshall *et al.* [22] and de Lange *et al.* [41] but cannot be attributed to active inhibition since it was not recruited during nogo trials in normal conditions or during simulation of left paralysis. By contrast, it is worth noting that similar increases have been found in the right lateral orbitofrontal cortex during motor inhibition in response to negative emotional stimuli (fearful faces) in a study using a stop-signal paradigm in healthy participants [55]. In this study, motor responses had to be withheld on the presentation of an unpredictable color cue paired with either a neutral or fearful face. While the right IFG activated to stop signals on neutral trials but did not predict inhibition success, a more ventral area in the lateral orbitofrontal cortex was activated both to successful stops and to fearful faces irrespective of concomitant stop signals (Fig. 19.5, see also color plates), suggesting that this region might be more specifically involved in integrating emotional inputs with ongoing control of motor actions [55,56].

To further determine whether motor conversion might entail some changes in the functional interaction of motor pathways with other brain areas mediating motor intention or awareness, we performed a connectivity analysis using the time course of activity

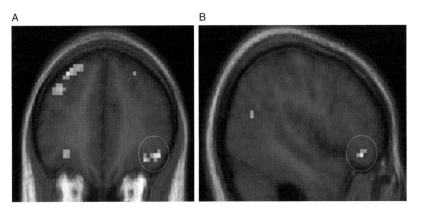

Fig. 19.5. Activation to motor inhibition paired with emotional stimuli in normal subjects. A region in the ventral inferior frontal gyrus/lateral orbitofrontal cortex was selectively engaged during successful inhibition in a speeded stop-signal task (A) and showed a significant interaction between inhibition and emotional significance of the stop stimulus (B, face with fearful versus neutral expression). This region (*xyz* coordinates in standard MNI space (Montreal Neurological Institute brain template), 48, 36–1) overlaps with the cluster activated during motor paralysis (go trials with the affected hand) in our patient with conversion (see Fig. 19.4B). (Also in color plate section.)

in right or left primary motor cortex as a seed, and examined the functional coupling of these with other regions across the whole brain, both in the patient with conversion and in controls. This analysis revealed significant asymmetries in the connectivity of right motor cortex compared with the left motor cortex during conversion, which were not observed in the normal condition and simulation. Whereas the right motor cortex was selectively connected with premotor areas in frontal cortex in normal controls and simulators, there was a reduction of this coupling in the patient with conversion, together with increased connectivity with the VMPFC and precuneus. The two latter areas overlapped with regions found to be differentially activated during left preparation in the patient (see above). This result again suggests that motor pathways might be directly or indirectly modulated by limbic regions involved in emotion regulation (e.g., VMPFC), but perhaps also by medial parietal regions known to be involved in mental imagery and memory (e.g., precuneus). Indeed, similar regions in VMPFC have been found to activate when subjects have to consciously evaluate or regulate their own affective states [57,58], rate their own traits or preferences [59–63], or attribute past or future to the self [64,65], and they are thought to be implicated in long-term memory storage for emotional memories [66]. The precuneus is recruited by mental imagery tasks with egocentric components [67] as well as by self-related episodic memory [68], and its activity is modified during abnormal states of consciousness including coma and minimal consciousness [69,70] and hypnosis [71]. Consequently, the VMPFC and precuneus appear to be associated with distinct aspects of self-related representations.

Taken together, these data indicate that psychogenic paralysis may not only reflect a relative disconnection of motor pathways from premotor systems normally involved in voluntary motor control and voluntary inhibition but also entail greater functional interactions with orbital and medial prefrontal areas as well as posterior midline areas. Remarkably, although partly similar changes have been observed in hypnotically induced paralysis, prefrontal changes might be more specifically observed in conversion (as we further describe below)

Hypnosis and conversion

Since Charcot in the nineteenth century, many authors have speculated on a possible link between hypnosis and hysteria [22,24,25,72]. Charcot considered the ability to be hypnotized as a clinical feature of hysteria, and Janet proposed that both phenomena involved a dissociative state where conscious voluntary control was uncoupled from unconscious automatic processes influencing behavior and cognition. More recently, other authors have also investigated both phenomena with the hypothesis that conversion is a form of autohypnosis [73]. However, there is still little empirical evidence for a true functional relation between hypnotic susceptibility and conversion symptoms. On the one hand, because hypnotic suggestion can also induce striking changes in motor or perceptual behavior unrelated to any organic brain anomalies, it is plausible that conversion may resemble the "dissociation states" induced by hypnosis [72,74]. The subjective feeling of involuntariness that accompanies the motor paralysis under either hypnosis or conversion is one of the main arguments to postulate similar mechanisms [25]. On the other hand, however, it remains unclear whether the degree of hypnotic suggestibility is higher or not in patients with conversion relative to the general population [75].

Recently, a few brain imaging studies have addressed this question by comparing both phenomena in similar task conditions. Following the PET study of Marshall *et al.* [22] in a patient with a left leg paralysis, Halligan *et al.* [72] reproduced the same paradigm with a single subject who received a hypnotic suggestion of unilateral left leg paralysis and was then asked to move either the affected or intact limbs. Activation was found in the ACC during failed movement attempts in both experiments, which was interpreted as reinforcing the idea that conversion and hypnosis involve the same neural mechanisms of motor inhibition. In keeping with this, ACC is also modulated by hypnosis in studies of pain perception [71,76,77]. However, as noted above, ACC activation in the context of induced paralysis may also reflect other processes related to conflict and error monitoring. Furthermore, no activation was found in ACC in a subsequent study of hypnotic paralysis in a larger group of 12 volunteers [77].

More recently, we also investigated both conversion and hypnotic motor loss with the same fMRI paradigm [53], using the go–nogo task described above. Our results pointed to some similarities between the two conditions but also clear differences [53,78]. First, we found that activity in the right IFG, was generally increased across all conditions under hypnosis, for both the go and nogo trials, a pattern that was different from both conversion and simulation (see Fig. 19.4A). More importantly, we found significant increases in activity of the precuneus as well as increases in its connectivity with motor cortex, particularly at the time of motor preparation with the affected hand (see Fig. 19.3) [78]. Therefore, the right motor cortex (contralateral to the left induced paralysis) showed a reduced functional coupling with premotor areas during hypnosis, but greater coupling with the right precuneus. However, there was no differential recruitment of the VMPFC, unlike during conversion. No change was found in ACC.

Our data, therefore suggest only partial similarity between paralysis induced by hypnosis and that in conversion. On the one hand, both phenomena are associated with a greater recruitment of areas mediating self-representations and memory processes, which may be broadly consistent with the hypothesis of Charcot and Janet that motor action becomes governed by internal states and "ideas." On the other hand, the two phenomena appear to differ in terms of the exact nature of the self-representations and executive control processes that are implicated. The VMPFC was not differentially activated during hypnosis, suggesting less involvement of emotion regulation and emotion memories in hypnosis relative to conversion, whereas the more prominent changes in precuneus in hypnosis suggest an important role of egocentric memory and sensory imagery. In addition, hypnosis is accompanied by a distinctive modulation of attentional and executive processes mediated by the right IFG [25,79], which could serve to inhibit responses to the current sensory environment and distracting information, allowing the subject to focus on the experience induced by the hypnotic suggestion. This activity in right IFG appears to be specific to the hypnotic state and, therefore, distinct from the conversion state. These differences were also supported by the distinct patterns of functional connectivity found for the motor cortex, indicating different kinds of influence on motor behavior. Below, we describe additional whole-brain connectivity analyses comparing the effect of hypnosis and conversion on our motor go–nogo task, which further uncover the functional similarities and dissimilarities between these conditions.

Network connectivity in conversion and hypnotic paralysis

Cognitive functions as well as affective states or simple motor acts rely on the coordination of scattered specialized brain regions, and mechanisms of large-scale integration and coordination enable the production of coherent behavior and cognition [80]. Functional connectivity between distributed brain regions can be indirectly assessed by fMRI by measuring the degree and changes in synchronizations (mainly correlations) between regions at different time scales, rather than just comparing changes in the amplitude of regional activity across different conditions [81–83]. Some psychopathological conditions may reflect a modification of dynamic interactions between neural systems involved in specific functions and thus lead to changes in information processing and behavioral responses. In line with the classic view of Charcot, who considered hysteria (conversion) as a "neurosis" where a "dynamic lesion" of the brain was responsible for the paralysis [84], the neuroimaging studies described above have typically assumed that motor deficits in patients with conversion might reflect some change in the functioning of the motor cortex or basal ganglia–thalamic circuits under the influence of affective or stressful signals represented in other regions, such as the VMPFC, ACC, or precuneus. However, the exact pathways and network dynamics underlying these changes remain unknown.

To better determine the pattern of whole-brain connectivity states in motor conversion, we have also performed additional analysis using an independent component analysis (ICA) approach. This technique provides a means of detecting and separating several distinct functional networks at once, based on their independent spatial patterns of fluctuations in activity over time. It does not require any anatomical a priori. While functional networks have first been identified during resting states, they are also present during (and modulated by) the performance of a cognitive task and may vary according to various factors such as pathologies, aging, mood, or affective states [85–88]. We have, therefore, re-analyzed the fMRI data from our previous study, by applying ICA to the same patient (with unilateral hysterical paralysis) as well as our normal control group ($n = 18$) and simulators ($n = 6$). If hysterical conversion involves a functional dissociation or disconnection between discrete brain networks supporting executive and sensorimotor functions [25], then the connectivity patterns of these regions and motor cortical areas should differ between conversion and normal conditions, or between the affected and normal hand side. Importantly, to determine effects specific to conversion, we also investigated a control group of healthy subjects who were instructed to simulate a unilateral hand paralysis.

The ICA was performed using a standard method implemented in the Gift Toolbox as described by Calhoun *et al.* [89] (see also http://icatb.sourceforge. net/groupica.htm). The toolbox supports a group ICA approach, which first concatenates the individual data across time, followed by the computation of the subject-specific components and time courses. The analysis was performed in three stages: (1) data reduction, (2) application of the ICA algorithm, and (3) back-reconstruction for each individual subject. The number of independent components was estimated with the Infomax algorithm, and data were segregated into 21 independent components. After visual inspection, 14 components were considered as artefacts because of their location (e.g., edges of the brain and cerebrospinal fluid), whereas seven represented functionally relevant networks consistent with previous studies (e.g., [89,90]). Individual subject independent component patterns were entered into one-sample random-effects analysis in SPM2 statistical parameter mapping software. A threshold for significance for results of $p < 0.05$ was taken and results were corrected for false discovery rates (FDR) for multiple comparisons. The estimation of each component was specifically compared between the three conditions (conversion, simulation, normal) to determine whether the corresponding network connectivity was modulated as a function of condition. Furthermore, comparisons were made for the different regions found in each component at $p < 0.05$ and FDR corrected, with the assumption that changes in connectivity may selectively affect the participation of some nodes within a given network.

Results showed that the seven independent component patterns (labeled from A to G in Fig. 19.6; see

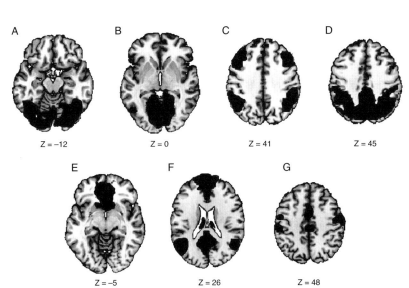

Fig. 19.6. Results from independent component analysis showing seven anatomically plausible networks: A, medial visual component; B, lateral visual component; C, bilateral frontoparietal network; D, superior parietal network; E, posterior ventromedial prefrontal network; F, default-mode network; G, motor network. All components are shown for the normal condition at $p < 0.05$ and false discovery rate corrected. (Also in color plate section.)

also color plates) represented functionally relevant networks [90]. The first two networks (A,B) overlapped with the visual cortex: network A involved lateral and dorsal parts of the occipital lobe, while network B extended in inferior parts of the occipital cortex including the striate area. A third bilateral frontoparietal network C comprised the supramarginal gyrus, middle temporal gyrus, and middle frontal gyrus as well as bilateral frontal areas (Fig. 19.6C), while network D covered the superior parietal lobe and precuneus (BA 7; Fig. 19.6D). Remarkably, network F included anterior medial prefrontal areas, anterior and posterior cingulate cortex, inferior temporal gyrus, and bilateral temporoparietal junction, corresponding to the default-mode network or intrinsic network [91–93]. Another isolated cluster in more posterior medial prefrontal cortex was observed as a distinct component E (see Fig. 19.6E). Finally, network G included several areas relevant for sensorimotor processing in pre- and postcentral gyri, medial frontal cortex in the supplementary motor area and caudal cingulate motor cortex, as well as parts of the superior frontal gyrus [94].

A direct comparison of these components revealed differences between the patient and other groups which selectively affected some regions of the default-mode network (F) and motor network (G). For the cortical part of the default-mode network (including posterior cingulate cortex, VMPFC, and temporoparietal junction), simulators were comparable to normal controls, whereas the patient with conversion showed a dramatic reduction in the connectivity strength of these regions (Fig. 19.7A, see also color plates). Strikingly, for the subcortical part of the default-mode network, namely the caudate nucleus, both the patient and the simulators showed a reduced connectivity compared with normals. Therefore, whereas a general reduction of coherent activity was found within the default-mode network during conversion, only the caudate nucleus demonstrated a selective reduction of coupling with this network during simulation, suggesting that a functional "disconnection" of the caudate from the rest of the default-mode network occurred in both types of paralysis. By contrast, for the motor network (Fig. 19.7B), the patient with conversion showed a specific reduction in connectivity strength in the right motor cortex and the right caudate nucleus, but not the supplementary and motor cingulate areas; the simulators showed a general reduction of connectivity for all clusters of this network (Fig. 19.7B).

No differences were observed in the five other components, in neither the attentional networks (superior parietal and bilateral frontoparietal) nor the isolated VMPFC component (Fig. 19.6E). The lack of effect for the latter region may at first sight appear to contrast with our finding of enhanced coupling with right motor cortex in the patient, as described above, but note that this may be because this independent component was limited to the posterior VMPFC alone and adjacent cortex (distinct from the more anterior region associated with other default-mode network areas). Furthermore, the connectivity measure demonstrated here reflected fluctuations of neural activity in the low-frequency range only (where resting state networks are typically identified by ICA). This may differ from the more phasic, higher-frequency connectivity revealed by our previous seed-based analysis [53].

Taken together, these new connectivity results highlight a dissociation between changes within areas associated with the default-mode network (including posterior cingulate cortex and VMPFC) and the cortical premotor regions, which were differentially modulated by conversion paralysis and simulation. By contrast, both the primary motor cortex and the subcortical motor relays in the caudate nucleus appeared to be commonly affected in both conditions. These data do not only provide further evidence that conversion and simulation involve distinct mechanisms but also indirectly suggest that conversion phenomena are at least partly related to neural processes that are associated with default-mode network activity – which is thought to include interoceptive and memory self-regulation functions and may operate even without conscious awareness [95]. By contrast, simulation of paralysis was found to involve a modulation of a network of premotor areas that are typically related to intentional motor control. Although these findings await replication in additional patients and will need to be compared with results obtained in motor conversion symptoms other than paralysis, such as PMDs [96] (Chapter 21), the current findings may provide new insights into the possible neural mechanisms involved in the conversion of emotional stressors in motor deficits and other "hysterical" behaviors.

Towards a novel neuroanatomical view of conversion

Since the mid 1990s, neuroimaging studies of conversion disorders have begun to pinpoint the neural substrates

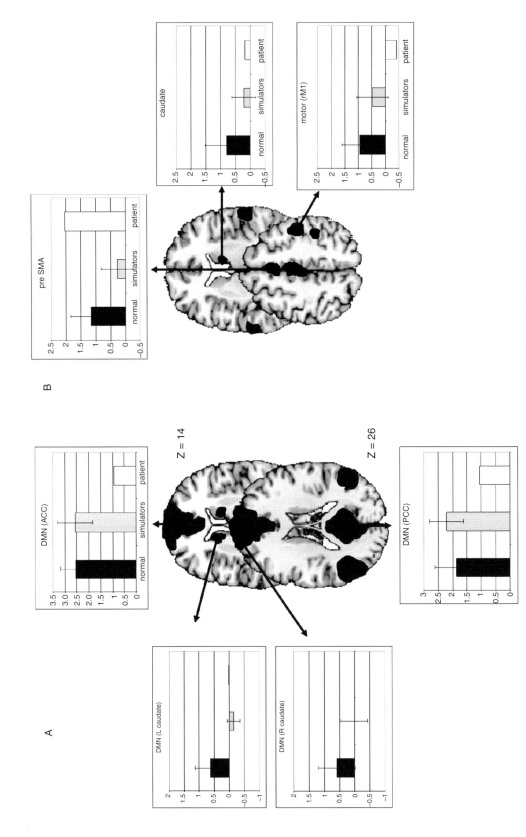

Fig. 19.7. Differences between conversion and other groups in independent component analysis networks. The amplitude of connectivity of individual regions with the network is plotted for different conditions for the default-mode network (DMN; A) and the motor network (B) (mean z-score of the corresponding component expressed in a given area; error bars represent the standard deviation across individuals). Black, normal; gray, simulators; white, patient with conversion. Acc, anterior cingulate cortex; PCC, posterior cingulate cortex; rMI, right motor cortex. (Also in color plate section.).

underlying distortions of sensory, motor, or even cognitive (e.g., memory) functions associated with psychogenic symptoms; however, it remains largely unresolved how such symptoms are actually generated. Although these studies have provided partly divergent results, obtained with different paradigms and methods in different patient groups, some of the available data seem to converge to suggest an important role for a recruitment of midline brain structures including VMPFC (anteriorly) and posterior cingulate cortex or precuneus (posteriorly) across different conditions. In particular, several studies of conversion paralysis [22,41,53,97] as well as the new connectivity analysis described here have demonstrated functional interactions between VMPFC and motor pathways (at cortical and/or subcortical sites) during the presence of motor symptoms. Yet, the exact nature of such interactions remains unresolved.

Remarkably, abundant work in human neuroscience suggests that both the VMPFC and the precuneus play a key role in representations of the self and autobiographical memory [98]. On the one hand, the VMPFC is systematically recruited during tasks that require affective judgments about the self [64,99,100] or the retrieval of personal information from either past or prospective memory [101], including for emotional material [66]. This region also activates when participants introspect about their feelings [59,60,102] or during emotion regulation [103,104], suggesting that it may primarily encode, or mediate the access to, affective representations of self-related information. Importantly, VMPFC responses are evoked even by incidental processing of information related to the self [105], without explicit task demands or conscious will. On the other hand, the precuneus has also been related to autobiographical memory retrieval [101], self-centered strategies during mental imagery [67], attribution of action agency to self versus other [106], as well as preconscious biases determining free motor choices [107]. Taken together, these findings suggest that both the VMPC and the precuneus are pivotal brain regions that hold internal representations about the self, integrating information from personal memory with affective relevance (in VMPFC) and sense of agency (in precuneus). These regions would, therefore, appear well placed to constitute an interface connecting affective and memory self-relevant representations with the ongoing control of behaviors and cognitions.

Nevertheless, the implication of these regions during conversion [22,41,53,97] remains to be confirmed in other studies, and their exact function needs to be more fully elucidated. Based on our own findings and previous results in patients with conversion, we hypothesize that hysterical paralysis might involve a "pathological" activation of affective representations and monitoring functions related to the self (and/or self-initiated behavior), and are mediated by the VMPFC and precuneus under the influence of specific stressors, situations, or memories. These representations might then not only dominate the content of awareness of the patients but also trigger specific patterns of motor behaviors by modulating activity in the motor pathways (through projections to cortical and/or subcortical areas), eventually resulting in an experience of paralysis, abnormal movements, and/or impaired sense of agency. Changes in VMPFC might themselves be triggered by interactions with other brain regions, particularly those implicated in affect and memory, such as the amygdala and hippocampus [36,49]. As already proposed by others [108,109], the conversion symptoms might represent a pathological or exaggerated form of reflexive behavior in response to stressors (somehow analogous to stereotyped motor reactions seen across many animal species, such as feigned death or wrestling flurry, which involve immobility to avoid or paroxystic agitation to escape a threat, respectively), or they could involve the expression of some behaviors learned by prior exposure, experience, or even imagination.

Therefore, after more than a century of conjectures on hysteria or conversion, it is remarkable that neuroimaging findings may now offer a neuroanatomical framework that is surprisingly reminiscent of some of the intuitions of Charcot and his students; while at the same time these data suggest more precise hints to uncover the psychodynamic and neural mechanisms underlying conversion behavior. Importantly, a better understanding of these mechanisms will ultimately be key to improving the clinical management of these patients and hopefully eradicating the current therapeutic despair for so-called "medically unexplained symptoms" [11,110].

Acknowledgements

This work is partly supported by SNF grant 3200B-127560.

References

1. Kozlowska K. Healing the disembodied mind: contemporary models of conversion disorder. *Harv Rev Psychiatry* 2005;**13**:1–13.

2. Vuilleumier P. Hysterical conversion and brain function. *Prog Brain Res* 2005;**150**:309–329.

3. Vuilleumier P. The neurophysiology of self-awareness disorders in conversion hysteria. In Laureys S, Tononi G, eds. *The Neurology of Consciousness*. New York: Academic Press, 2009:282–302.

4. Carson AJ, Ringbauer B, Stone J, *et al.* Do medically unexplained symptoms matter? A prospective cohort study of 300 new referrals to neurology outpatient clinics. *J Neurol Neurosurg Psychiatry* 2000;**68**:207–210.

5. Fink P, Steen Hansen M, Sondergaard L. Somatoform disorders among first-time referrals to a neurology service. *Psychosomatics* 2005;**46**:540–548.

6. Lempert T, Dieterich M, Huppert D, Brandt T. Psychogenic disorders in neurology: frequency and clinical spectrum. *Acta Neurol Scand* 1990;**82**:335–340.

7. Nimnuan C, Hotopf M, Wessely S. Medically unexplained symptoms: an epidemiological study in seven specialities. *J Psychosom Res* 2001;**51**:361–367.

8. Factor SA, Podskalny GD, Molho ES. Psychogenic movement disorders: frequency, clinical profile, and characteristics. *J Neurol Neurosurg Psychiatry* 1995;**59**:406–412.

9. Hallett M. Psychogenic movement disorders: a crisis for neurology. *Curr Neurol Neurosci Rep* 2006;**6**:269–271.

10. Aybek S, Kanaan RA, David AS. The neuropsychiatry of conversion disorder. *Curr Opin Psychiatry* 2008;**21**:275–280.

11. Nicholson TR, Stone J, Kanaan RA. Conversion disorder: a problematic diagnosis. *J Neurol Neurosurg Psychiatry* 2010; E-pub ahead of print.

12. Charcot JM. *Leçons du Mardi à la Salpêtrière (1887–1888)*. Paris: Bureau du progrès médical, 1892.

13. James W. *The Principles of Psychology*. New York: Dover Publications, 1890.

14. Babinsky J, Dagnan-Bouveret J. Emotion et hystérie. *J Psychol* 1912;**9**:146.

15. Brown RJ. Psychological mechanisms of medically unexplained symptoms: an integrative conceptual model. *Psychol Bull* 2004;**130**:793–812.

16. Damasio A. *Looking for Spinoza: Joy, Sorrow and the Feeling Brain*. New York: Harcourt, 2003.

17. Janet P. *L'état Mental des Hystériques*. Paris: Rueff, 1894.

18. Freud S, Breuer J. *Studies on Hysteria*. New York: Hogart Press, 1895.

19. Ludwig AM. Hysteria. A neurobiological theory. *Arch Gen Psychiatry* 1972;**27**:771–777.

20. Sackeim HA, Nordlie JW, Gur RC. A model of hysterical and hypnotic blindness: cognition, motivation, and awareness. *J Abnorm Psychol* 1979;**88**:474–489.

21. Spiegel D. Neurophysiological correlates of hypnosis and dissociation. *J Neuropsychiatry Clin Neurosci* 1991;**3**:440–445.

22. Marshall JC, Halligan PW, Fink GR, Wade DT, Frackowiak RS. The functional anatomy of a hysterical paralysis. *Cognition* 1997;**64**:B1–B8.

23. Sierra M, Berrios GE. Towards a neuropsychiatry of conversive hysteria. In Halligan PW, David AS, eds. *Conversion Hysteria: Towards a Cognitive Neuropsychological Account*. Hove, UK: Psychology Press, 1999:267–287.

24. Halligan PW, Bass C, Wade DT. New approaches to conversion hysteria. *BMJ* 2000;**320**:1488–1489.

25. Oakley DA. Hypnosis and conversion hysteria: a unifying model. *Cogn Neuropsychiatry* 1999;**4**:243–265.

26. Black DN, Seritan AL, Taber KH, Hurley RA. Conversion hysteria: lessons from functional imaging. *J Neuropsychiatry Clin Neurosci* 2004;**16**:245–251.

27. Tiihonen J, Kuikka J, Viinamaki H, Lehtonen J, Partanen J. Altered cerebral blood flow during hysterical paresthesia. *Biol Psychiatry* 1995;**37**:134–135.

28. Bench CJ, Frith CD, Grasby PM, *et al.* Investigations of the functional anatomy of attention using the Stroop test. *Neuropsychologia* 1993;**31**:907–922.

29. Carter CS, Braver TS, Barch DM, *et al.* Anterior cingulate cortex, error detection, and the online monitoring of performance. *Science* 1998;**280**:747–749.

30. Pardo JV, Pardo PJ, Janer KW, Raichle ME. The anterior cingulate cortex mediates processing selection in the Stroop attentional conflict paradigm. *Proc Natl Acad Sci USA* 1990;**87**:256–259.

31. Horn NR, Dolan M, Elliott R, Deakin JF, Woodruff PW. Response inhibition and impulsivity: an fMRI study. *Neuropsychologia* 2003;**41**:1959–1966.

32. Muller JL, Sommer M, Wagner V, *et al.* Abnormalities in emotion processing within cortical and subcortical regions in criminal psychopaths: evidence from a functional magnetic resonance imaging study using pictures with emotional content. *Biol Psychiatry* 2003;**54**:152–162.

33. Northoff G, Kotter R, Baumgart F, *et al.* Orbitofrontal cortical dysfunction in akinetic catatonia: a functional magnetic resonance imaging study during negative emotional stimulation. *Schizophr Bull* 2004;**30**:405–427.

34. Raine A, Yang Y. Neural foundations to moral reasoning and antisocial behavior. *Soc Cogn Affect Neurosci* 2006;**1**:203–213.

35. Stone J, Zeman A, Simonotto E, *et al.* FMRI in patients with motor conversion symptoms and controls with simulated weakness. *Psychosom Med* 2007;**69**:961–969.

36. Kanaan RA, Craig TK, Wessely SC, David AS. Imaging repressed memories in motor conversion disorder. *Psychosom Med* 2007;**69**:202–205.

37. Burgmer M, Konrad C, Jansen A, *et al.* Abnormal brain activation during movement observation in patients with conversion paralysis. *Neuroimage* 2006;**29**:1336–1343.

38. Ghaffar O, Staines WR, Feinstein A. Unexplained neurologic symptoms: an fMRI study of sensory conversion disorder. *Neurology* 2006;**67**:2036–2038.

39. Mailis-Gagnon A, Giannoylis I, Downar J, *et al.* Altered central somatosensory processing in chronic pain patients with "hysterical" anesthesia. *Neurology* 2003;**60**:1501–1507.

40. Spence SA, Crimlisk HL, Cope H, Ron MA, Grasby PM. Discrete neurophysiological correlates in prefrontal cortex during hysterical and feigned disorder of movement. *Lancet* 2000;**355**:1243–1254.

41. de Lange FP, Roelofs K, Toni I. Increased self-monitoring during imagined movements in conversion paralysis. *Neuropsychologia* 2007;**45**:2051–2058.

42. Saj A, Arzy S, Vuilleumier P. Functional brain imaging in a woman with spatial neglect due to conversion disorder. *JAMA* 2009;**302**:2552–2554.

43. Vocat R, Pourtois G, Vuilleumier P. Unavoidable errors: a spatio-temporal analysis of time-course and neural sources of evoked potentials associated with error processing in a speeded task. *Neuropsychologia* 2008;**46**:2545–2555.

44. Vuilleumier P, Chicherio C, Assal F, *et al.* Functional neuroanatomical correlates of hysterical sensorimotor loss. *Brain* 2001;**124**:1077–1090.

45. Haber SN. The primate basal ganglia: parallel and integrative networks. *J Chem Neuroanat* 2003;**26**:317–330.

46. Mogenson GJ, Yang CR. The contribution of basal forebrain to limbic-motor integration and the mediation of motivation to action. *Adv Exp Med Biol* 1991;**295**:267–290.

47. Klemm WR. Drug effects on active immobility responses: what they tell us about neurotransmitter systems and motor functions. *Prog Neurobiol* 1989;**32**:403–422.

48. von Giesen HJ, Schlaug G, Steinmetz H, *et al.* Cerebral network underlying unilateral motor neglect: evidence from positron emission tomography. *J Neurol Sci* 1994;**125**:29–38.

49. Voon V, Brezing C, Gallea C, *et al.* Emotional stimuli and motor conversion disorder. *Brain* 2010;**133**:1526–1536.

50. Aron AR, Robbins TW, Poldrack RA. Inhibition and the right inferior frontal cortex. *Trends Cogn Sci* 2004;**8**:170–177.

51. Xue G, Aron AR, Poldrack RA. Common neural substrates for inhibition of spoken and manual responses. *Cereb Cortex* 2008;**18**:1923–1932.

52. Anderson MC, Ochsner KN, Kuhl B, *et al.* Neural systems underlying the suppression of unwanted memories. *Science* 2004;**303**:232–235.

53. Cojan Y, Waber L, Carruzzo A, Vuilleumier P. Motor inhibition in hysterical conversion paralysis. *Neuroimage* 2009;**47**:1026–1037.

54. de Lange FP, Roelofs K, Toni I. Motor imagery: a window into the mechanisms and alterations of the motor system. *Cortex* 2008;**44**:494–506.

55. Sagaspe P, Schwartz S, Vuilleumier P. Fear and stop: A role for the amygdala in motor inhibition by emotional signals. *Neuroimage* 2011;**55**:1825–1835.

56. Goldstein M, Brendel G, Tuescher O, *et al.* Neural substrates of the interaction of emotional stimulus processing and motor inhibitory control: an emotional linguistic go/no-go fMRI study. *Neuroimage* 2007;**36**:1026–1040.

57. Gusnard DA, Akbudak E, Shulman GL, Raichle ME. Medial prefrontal cortex and self-referential mental activity: relation to a default mode of brain function. *Proc Natl Acad Sci USA* 2001;**98**:4259–4264.

58. Ochsner KN, Knierim K, Ludlow DH, *et al.* Reflecting upon feelings: an fMRI study of neural systems supporting the attribution of emotion to self and other. *J Cogn Neurosci* 2004;**16**:1746–1772.

59. Johnson SC, Baxter LC, Wilder LS, *et al.* Neural correlates of self-reflection. *Brain* 2002;**125**:1808–1814.

60. Kelley WM, Macrae CN, Wyland CL, *et al.* Finding the self? An event-related fMRI study. *J Cogn Neurosci* 2002;**14**:785–794.

61. Mitchell JP, Macrae CN, Banaji MR. Dissociable medial prefrontal contributions to judgments of similar and dissimilar others. *Neuron* 2006;**50**:655–663.

62. Schmitz TW, Kawahara-Baccus TN, Johnson SC. Metacognitive evaluation, self-relevance, and the right prefrontal cortex. *Neuroimage* 2004;**22**:941–947.

63. Zysset S, Huber O, Ferstl E, von Cramon DY. The anterior frontomedian cortex and evaluative judgment: an fMRI study. *Neuroimage* 2002;**15**:983–991.

64. D' Argembeau A, Ruby P, Collette F, *et al.* Distinct regions of the medial prefrontal cortex are associated with self-referential processing and perspective taking. *J Cogn Neurosci* 2007;**19**:935–944.

65. Vogeley K, May M, Ritzl A, *et al.* Neural correlates of first-person perspective as one constituent of human self-consciousness. *J Cogn Neurosci* 2004;**16**:817–827.

66. Sterpenich V, Albouy G, Boly M, *et al.* Sleep-related hippocampo-cortical interplay during emotional memory recollection. *PLoS Biol* 2007;**5**:e282.

67. Cavanna AE, Trimble MR. The precuneus: a review of its functional anatomy and behavioural correlates. *Brain* 2006;**129**:564–583.

68. Lou HC, Luber B, Crupain M, *et al.* Parietal cortex and representation of the mental self. *Proc Natl Acad Sci USA* 2004;**101**:6827–6832.

69. Laureys S, Owen AM, Schiff ND. Brain function in coma, vegetative state, and related disorders. *Lancet Neurol* 2004;**3**:537–546.

70. Voss HU, Uluc AM, Dyke JP, *et al.* Possible axonal regrowth in late recovery from the minimally conscious state. *J Clin Invest* 2006;**116**:2005–2011.

71. Rainville P, Carrier B, Hofbauer RK, Bushnell MC, Duncan GH. Dissociation of sensory and affective dimensions of pain using hypnotic modulation. *Pain* 1999;**82**:159–171.

72. Halligan PW, Athwal BS, Oakley DA, Frackowiak RS. Imaging hypnotic paralysis: implications for conversion hysteria. *Lancet* 2000;**355**:986–987.

73. Bell V, Oakley DA, Halligan PW, Deeley Q. Dissociation in hysteria and hypnosis: evidence from cognitive neuroscience. *J Neurol Neurosurg Neuropsychiatry* 2011;**82**:332–339.

74. Roelofs K, Hoogduin KA, Keijsers GP. Motor imagery during hypnotic arm paralysis in high and low hypnotizable subjects. *Int J Clin Exp Hypn* 2002;**50**:51–66.

75. Roelofs K, Hoogduin KA, Keijsers GP, *et al.* Hypnotic susceptibility in patients with conversion disorder. *J Abnorm Psychol* 2002;**111**:390–395.

76. Derbyshire SW, Whalley MG, Stenger VA, Oakley DA. Cerebral activation during hypnotically induced and imagined pain. *Neuroimage* 2004;**23**:392–401.

77. Faymonville ME, Laureys S, Degueldre C, *et al.* Neural mechanisms of antinociceptive effects of hypnosis. *Anesthesiology* 2000;**92**:1257–1267.

78. Cojan Y, Waber L, Schwartz S, *et al.* The brain under self-control: modulation of inhibitory and monitoring cortical networks during hypnotic paralysis. *Neuron* 2009;**62**:862–875.

79. Egner T, Raz A. Cognitive control processes and hypnosis. In Jamieson G, ed. *Hypnosis and Conscious States*. Oxford, Oxford University Press, 2007:29–50.

80. Varela F, Lachaux JP, Rodriguez E, Martinerie J. The brainweb: phase synchronization and large-scale integration. *Nat Rev Neurosci* 2001;**2**:229–239.

81. Friston KJ, Buechel C, Fink GR, *et al.* Psychophysiological and modulatory interactions in neuroimaging. *Neuroimage* 1997;**6**:218–229.

82. Friston KJ, Harrison L, Penny W. Dynamic causal modelling. *Neuroimage* 2003;**19**:1273–1302.

83. Richiardi J, Eryilmaz H, Schwartz S, Vuilleumier P, van de Ville D. Decoding brain states from fMRI connectivity graphs. *Neuroimage* 2011;**56**:616–626.

84. de la Tourette G. Traité clinique et thérapeuthique de l'hystérie d'après l'enseignement de la Salpêtrière. Paris: Plon, 1891.

85. Damoiseaux JS, Beckmann CF, Arigita EJ, *et al.* Reduced resting-state brain activity in the "default network" in normal aging. *Cereb Cortex* 2008;**18**:1856–1864.

86. Eryilmaz H, van de Ville D, Schwartz S, Vuilleumier P. Impact of transient emotions on functional connectivity during subsequent resting state: a wavelet correlation approach. *Neuroimage* 2011;**54**:2481–2891.

87. Harrison BJ, Pujol J, Ortiz H, *et al.* Modulation of brain resting-state networks by sad mood induction. *PLoS One* 2008;**3**:e1794.

88. Sorg C, Riedl V, Muhlau M, *et al.* Selective changes of resting-state networks in individuals at risk for Alzheimer's disease. *Proc Natl Acad Sci USA* 2007;**104**:18760–18765.

89. Calhoun VD, Adali T, Pearlson GD, Pekar JJ. A method for making group inferences from functional MRI data using independent component analysis. *Hum Brain Mapp* 2001;**14**:140–151.

90. Beckmann CF, DeLuca M, Devlin JT, Smith SM. Investigations into resting-state connectivity using independent component analysis. *Philos Trans R Soc Lond B Biol Sci* 2005;**360**:1001–1013.

91. Damoiseaux JS, Rombouts SA, Barkhof F, *et al.* Consistent resting-state networks across healthy subjects. *Proc Natl Acad Sci USA* 2006;**103**:13848–13853.

92. De Luca M, Beckmann CF, De Stefano N, Matthews PM, Smith SM. fMRI resting state networks define distinct modes of long-distance interactions in the human brain. *Neuroimage* 2006;**29**:1359–1367.

93. Raichle ME, MacLeod AM, Snyder AZ, *et al.* A default mode of brain function. *Proc Natl Acad Sci USA* 2001;**98**:676–682.

94. Grefkes C, Fink GR. The functional organization of the intraparietal sulcus in humans and monkeys. *J Anat* 2005;**207**:3–17.

95. Boly M, Phillips C, Tshibanda L, *et al.* Intrinsic brain activity in altered states of consciousness: how conscious is the default mode of brain function? *Ann N Y Acad Sci* 2008;**1129**:119–129.

96. Voon V, Gallea C, Hattori N, *et al.* The involuntary nature of conversion disorder. *Neurology* 2010;**74**:223–228.

97. Luaute J, Saladinic O, Cojan Y, *et al.* Simulation, conversion or exaggeration. Evolution of the functional investigations. About a case in a

rehabilitation setting. *Ann Medpsychol Rev Psychiatr* 2010;**168**:306–310.

98. Northoff G, Panksepp J. The trans-species concept of self and the subcortical-cortical midline system. *Trends Cogn Sci* 2008;**12**:259–264.

99. Jenkins AC, Macrae CN, Mitchell JP. Repetition suppression of ventromedial prefrontal activity during judgments of self and others. *Proc Natl Acad Sci USA* 2008;**105**:4507–4512.

100. Schneider F, Bermpohl F, Heinzel A, *et al.* The resting brain and our self: self-relatedness modulates resting state neural activity in cortical midline structures. *Neuroscience* 2008;**157**:120–131.

101. Schacter DL, Addis DR, Buckner RL. Remembering the past to imagine the future: the prospective brain. *Nat Rev Neurosci* 2007;**8**:657–661.

102. Macrae CN, Moran JM, Heatherton TF, Banfield JF, Kelley WM. Medial prefrontal activity predicts memory for self. *Cereb Cortex* 2004;**14**:647–654.

103. Lane RD. Neural substrates of implicit and explicit emotional processes: a unifying framework for psychosomatic medicine. *Psychosom Med* 2008;**70**:214–231.

104. Simpson JR, Ongur D, Akbudak E, *et al.* The emotional modulation of cognitive processing: an fMRI study. *J Cogn Neurosci* 2000;**12**(Suppl 2):157–170.

105. Moran JM, Heatherton TF, Kelley WM. Modulation of cortical midline structures by implicit and explicit self-relevance evaluation. *Soc Neurosci* 2009;**4**:197–211.

106. Farrer C, Frith CD. Experiencing oneself vs another person as being the cause of an action: the neural correlates of the experience of agency. *Neuroimage* 2002;**15**:596–603.

107. Soon CS, Brass M, Heinze HJ, Haynes JD. Unconscious determinants of free decisions in the human brain. *Nat Neurosci* 2008;**11**:543–545.

108. Kretschmer E. *Hysteria: Reflex and Instinct*. London: Peter Owen, 1948.

109. Whitlock FA. The aetiology of hysteria. *Acta Psychiatr Scand* 1967;**43**:144–162.

110. Stone J, Smyth R, Carson A, *et al.* Systematic review of misdiagnosis of conversion symptoms and "hysteria." *BMJ* 2005;**331**:989.

Action control in conversion paralysis: evidence from motor imagery

Karin Roelofs, Ivan Toni, and Floris P. de Lange

Introduction

Conversion paralysis (CP) is a frequent and impairing psychiatric disorder characterized by loss of voluntary motor functioning. Although the symptoms may suggest a neuropathological condition, they cannot be adequately explained by known neurological or other organic disorders [1]. Moreover, the onset or exacerbation of symptoms is related to psychological stress, suggesting that psychological mechanisms are implicated. Despite the high prevalence and the long history of speculations about the cause of CP [2], its exact nature remains poorly understood. A few neuroimaging studies have explored objective neural correlates of functional mechanisms that, in the absence of a structural brain lesion, may be able to explain the symptomatology of CP. A straightforward approach used in most of those studies has been to ask patients to try to move their paralyzed limb, which will not distinguish between the cerebral causes of motor alterations and the emotional/motivational consequences of experiencing those alterations [3,4]. In the past few years several attempts have been made to probe motor disturbances in CP in absence of overt movements, either by using "passive" sensorimotor tasks such as action observation [5] or sensory stimulation [3], or by looking at mental movement simulation or "motor imagery" of affected limbs in CP [6,7]. This chapter describe these studies, primarily focusing on motor imagery studies of CP. The results suggest that reduced motor responsivity in CP may be linked to altered action control as well as heightened self-monitoring or self-referential processing and that these two mechanisms are subserved by anatomically distinct parts of the prefrontal cortex. These results will be discussed in relation to the existing literature on emotional and cognitive aspects of conversion disorder and an integrated hypothetical model of factors affecting mental motor representations in CP is presented.

Neural processes in conversion paralysis: from action execution to action observation

A seminal study investigating the functional anatomy of CP by Marshall *et al.* used positron emission tomography to investigate a patient with left-lateralized CP [8]. When she tried to move her unaffected (right) leg, there was a normal pattern of cerebral activity, including activation in the contralateral primary motor cortex. However, when attempting to move the affected (left) leg, there was no activation in the contralateral primary motor cortex, but there was a relative increase in activation of the right anterior cingulate cortex (ACC) and the ventromedial prefrontal cortex (vmPFC). These results were interpreted as suggesting that the loss of voluntary movements observed in CP is caused by increased response inhibition mediated by ACC and vmPFC. Similar results were obtained in a related study, involving a healthy subject with hypnotically induced paralysis of the left leg [9]. When the subject tried to move her "paralyzed" leg, ACC and vmPFC showed increased activity, suggesting that similar mechanisms support hypnotically induced paralysis and CP [9]. In contrast, Spence *et al.* [10] observed that when patients with CP moved their paralyzed limb, there was a de-activation in their dorsolateral prefrontal cortex (dlPFC) compared with healthy control subjects. Burgmer *et al.* [5] did not find any differences in prefrontal or motor cortex activity between patients with CP and healthy controls during

---

Psychogenic Movement Disorders and Other Conversion Disorders, ed. Mark Hallett, Anthony E. Lang, Joseph Jankovic, Stanley Fahn, Peter W. Halligan, Valerie Voon, and C. Robert Cloninger. Published by Cambridge University Press. © Cambridge University Press 2011.

execution of hand movements, and Stone *et al.* [11] observed a more complex and diffuse pattern of activity in motor and frontal regions in CP. These conflicting results may partly reflect the limited sample size (one to four subjects), and the type of comparisons carried out (*within*-subjects versus *between*-subjects). However, on a more fundamental level, it is important to note that the participants in all of these studies were asked to carry out a task ("move/try to move your affected limb") that they could not appropriately perform as part of their condition. Accordingly, these results may reflect brain activity related to the cognitive consequences of a failed movement (such as altered effort, motivation, or error processing), rather than a proximal cause of CP. The increased ACC activity [8,9] may, for instance, reflect enhanced monitoring triggered by movement failure or by conflicting action tendencies [3]. Such interpretation is compatible with our recent findings in an event-related potential study in six patients with unilateral CP, demonstrating increased action monitoring during generation of movements with the affected limb compared with the unaffected limb [4]. To overcome the interpretational limitations imposed by overt motor behavior, Vuilleumier *et al.* [3] assessed brain responsiveness to passive sensory stimulation in patients with CP suffering from unilateral sensorimotor loss in a single photon emission computed tomography study. The results showed decreased activity in the basal ganglia and thalamus contralateral to the affected limb during stimulation of the affected limb compared with stimulation of the unaffected limb. This decrease resolved after recovery of the conversion symptoms, suggesting that differences in sensory processing may play a role in the pathophysiology of CP. Finally, Burgmer *et al.* [5] explored whether CP is associated with abnormal brain activity during observation of hand movements. The authors showed that patients with CP had reduced primary motor cortex activity during observation of hand movements, compared with healthy controls, specifically for the affected hand. However, it remained unclear how these *sensory* and *action observation* deficits relate to the main feature of CP, namely the disturbance of volitional *motor* processes. The next section reviews recent studies examining volitional action simulation by using motor imagery. The rationale of using this approach is to control for processes associated with actual motor execution such as altered sensory feedback or enhanced monitoring of failed movements.

Motor imagery in conversion paralysis

Motor imagery is a widely used paradigm for the study of cognitive aspects of action control, both in the healthy and the pathological brain. Numerous studies have addressed behavioral and cerebral correlates of motor imagery, and its relationship with actual execution and motor planning (reviewed by Jeannerod, 2006 [12]). An influential paradigm that implicitly evokes motor imagery and allows one to quantify performance is the hand-laterality judgment task, in which subjects have to make judgments about the laterality of visually presented rotated images of hands [13,14] (Fig. 20.1 shows an example drawing). Results from many studies have indicated that subjects solve this task by mentally moving their own hand from its current position into the visually presented position, to match the orientation of the stimulus hand [13,15]. Imagined and actually executed hand rotations overlap not only in terms of time course [13,14] and autonomic responses [16] but also with respect to neural architecture [17–19]. Accordingly, previous behavioral studies have used motor imagery tasks to reveal impairments in motoric simulations of the affected limb in patients with CP [20,21]. We have applied the mental hand rotation task to compare motor imagery of affected and unaffected hands in six patients with CP and found

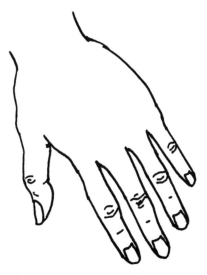

Fig. 20.1. Example of rotated left hand serving as stimulus in the mental hand rotation task. On each trial a back or palm version of a rotated (0–180 degrees leftward or rightward) hand is presented and the participant responds by indicating whether the image displays a left or a right hand.

impaired motor imagery for rotations of the affected hand [21].

In a series of recent studies, we applied this paradigm combined with functional magnetic resonance imaging in eight patients with unilateral CP, allowing for a comparison of cerebral activity evoked by motor imagery of the affected and the unaffected hand [6,7]. In these studies, motor imagery of both the affected and the unaffected hand evoked increased activity in the dorsal parietal and premotor cortex with increasing motor complexity of the imagined movement. This same parietofrontal network has also been isolated in earlier studies using similar motor imagery paradigms [17,22], as well as during the selection and preparation of actual hand movements [23], suggesting that patients with CP can readily imagine actions of both their unaffected and affected hand, using the same cerebral resources as healthy participants. Most importantly, implicit motor imagery of the affected hand led to stronger responses in several regions in dorsomedial prefrontal cortex (dmPFC), dlPFC, and vmPFC [6] compared with the unaffected hand.

Ventromedial prefrontal cortex involvement

At first glance, the involvement of the vmPFC during selection of actions involving a limb affected by CP might seem to replicate findings of previous studies involving this brain region in this pathology [8]). In fact, here the effects reflected a failure to de-activate this region during motor imagery of the affected hand (Fig. 20.2, see color plates). The vmPFC, together with other portions of a so-called "intrinsic" or "default" network [25], has been repeatedly shown to display physiological decreases of metabolic activity during performance of sensorimotor and cognitive tasks [26]. However, our study indicated that when patients with CP simulate actions with the affected hand, their vmPFC activity remains at resting-state levels. This result is not immediately compatible with the theory that vmPFC activity in CP reflects an active and phasic inhibition of the motor system [8,9]. Furthermore, this region has been repeatedly implicated in self-referential processing [27–31], rather than in inhibitory motor control. Accordingly, it appears conceivable that the vmPFC effect is linked to increased self-monitoring during motor processing of the affected hand [3,4,32]. This interpretation points to a crucial link between CP

and heightened self-monitoring during actions with the affected arm [5].

A second study provided further support for this interpretation [7]. We predicted that, if the altered pattern of activity in the vmPFC is related to increased self-monitoring for imagined actions of the affected hand, then *inducing* self-monitoring of actions of the unaffected limb (by means of explicitly cued motor imagery) should boost activity in this region, and potentially abolish the activation differences observed during implicit motor imagery. To test this premise, we induced self-monitoring of actions of both the affected and the unaffected limb by means of explicitly cued motor imagery. Patients were explicitly instructed to mentally rotate their hands from their current position into the position presented on the screen while concentrating on the sensory aspects of the mental actions. In line with our expectations, this explicit motor imagery instruction abolished the activation difference between the affected and the unaffected hand in the vmPFC, suggesting that the differential vmPFC effects found by de Lange *et al.* [6] were indeed related to self-referential processing or increased self-monitoring (Fig. 20.2). Together these findings suggest that, in patients with CP, self-referencing processes persist during the performance of motor simulations involving the affected hand.

Activity in other frontal areas that were specifically involved in implicit mental hand rotations of the affected hands – the dmPFC and the dlPFC – appeared unaffected by the explicit motor imagery instruction.

The next section explores the contribution of each of these three prefrontal subregions by testing frontal–motor connectivity patterns specific for affected hand rotations.

Dorsolateral prefrontal cortex

In order to investigate whether activity in the three prefrontal regions isolated for affected hand rotations (vmPFC, dmPFC, dlPFC) in CP [6] interact with brain areas directly involved in motor control of the affected and unaffected limb, a connectivity analysis (PPI) was conducted with the local maxima of each of the regions as seed regions [33]. Among the three prefrontal regions previously observed to be more activated for imagery of the affected hand, only the dlPFC was functionally connected to the motor system. Moreover, the coupling between this region and various parts of the sensorimotor system was modulated by whether

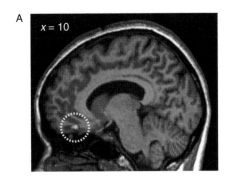

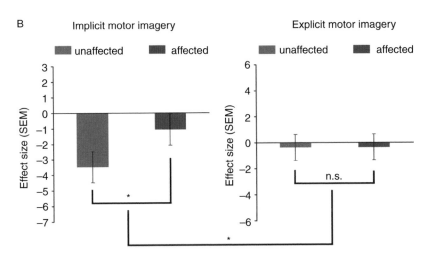

Fig. 20.2. Cerebral differences between motor imagery of the affected and the unaffected hand between implicit and explicit motor imagery. (A) Anatomical localization of a ventromedial prefrontal cluster (10,20,24), showing overall (i.e., not rotation-related) decreased de-activation for the affected hand during implicit motor imagery, but no activation differences between hands during explicit motor imagery. (B) Effect size (±SEM) of activation difference between the affected and unaffected hand during implicit motor imagery (left column) and during explicit motor imagery (right column). As can be seen from the figure, there was a difference between activity for the affected and the unaffected hand in the ventromedial prefrontal cortex during implicit motor imagery, while there was no consistent difference during explicit motor imagery. *Significant interaction; n.s., non-significant. For further details, see de Lange et al. [7]. (Also in color plate section.)

subjects imagined movements of the affected or the unaffected limb. The dlPFC showed a stronger positive coupling with the dorsal premotor cortex, and a stronger negative coupling with the primary somatosensory cortex. Activity in dlPFC was more positively coupled with activity in the premotor cortex during motor imagery of the affected hand. In contrast, it was more *negatively* coupled with activity in the primary somatosensory cortex during motor imagery of the affected hand. The increased coupling between dlPFC and the dorsal premotor cortex during motor imagery of the affected hand may be a cerebral counterpart of the increased attention to action that patients with CP deploy during the generation of action plans of the paralyzed limb [34]. The dorsal premotor cortex is involved in motor imagery and generation of action plan, and the increase in dlPFC–premotor connectivity is likely related to a compensatory mechanism reflecting an increased prefrontal drive towards premotor regions supporting the imagery process. The stronger negative coupling between dlPFC and the

somatosensory cortex may be directly related to the stronger positive coupling between dlPFC and the dorsal premotor cortex. When motor plans are generated (in dorsal premotor cortex), sensory consequences are simultaneously computed, leading to sensory attenuation (in somatosensory cortex). The stronger inhibitory coupling between dlPFC and the somatosensory cortex during motor imagery of the affected hand provides a likely explanation for the decreased excitability of the primary motor cortex that has previously been observed in CP [35]. Activity in the somatosensory cortex can strongly contribute to the excitability of the motor system, as measured by motor evoked potentials [36]. Our results suggest that this reduced excitability may be the result of larger coupling with dlPFC activity during generation of action plans of the affected hand. These results provide a possible link between previous reports of both heightened prefrontal and reduced sensorimotor activity in CP.

A crucial question that emerges next is how these neuropsychological observations may relate to the clinical characteristics of CP. By definition, CP is a psychogenic disorder [1] and it remains unclear how these brain mechanisms may be affected by psychological stress factors. Below we present a hypothetical model integrating neuropsychological findings with clinical observations in CP in order to formulate testable hypotheses for future research.

Towards an integration

It is well known that frontal structures, such as the dlPFC and vmPFC, are sensitive to the effects of emotional stress. For example, vmPFC has close connections not only with motor but also with limbic areas, and it is involved in emotion regulation [24, 37]. We hypothesize that otherwise intact mental motor representations may be modulated or overriden on the basis of emotional or other self-relevant cues in CP [32]. In fact, motor symptoms of CP may be influenced by several environmental (emotional, stress) and individual (cognitive, genetic) factors, as well as by their interactions [38]. Figure 20.3 presents an integrated hypothetical model of these factors and how they may affect neuropsychological mechanisms in CP. At this stage, the model serves to define research questions for future investigations, rather than providing a full-blown theory of this complex disorder.

At present, there is an obvious gap in the literature between what is known about the role of psychological factors in CP (individual and environmental; upper box of Fig. 20.3) and the neuropsychological research findings summarized in the sections above (and displayed in the lower boxes of Fig. 20.3). In our view, it

is a challenge for future studies to bridge this gap and to test the interactions proposed by the model. Below we will highlight one environmental factor that may likely play a role in the causation and/or maintenance of CP – "traumatic stress" – while accepting that contextual learning factors and individual factors such as suggestibility may play a role in the symptom manifestation as well [39–42].

Patients with conversion disorders report relatively high rates of adverse life events such as childhood trauma [43] and show increased threat sensitivity and increased basal levels of the stress hormone cortisol; both are seen particularly in traumatized patients [44–46]. Accordingly, CP may turn out to be one of a range of psychiatric disorders where a transient neurodevelopmental disturbance generates latent neurobiological alterations that can lead to the emergence of a full-blown psychiatric disorder when the individual is later sensitized by an otherwise psychological stressor [47]. For example, Kanaan et al. [48] observed increased limbic activity and reduced motor activity (contralateral to the affected side) in a traumatized patient with unilateral CP during cued recall of a repressed traumatic memory. However, no studies have tested the effects of stress and stress hormones on *frontal* motor regulatory functions in CP, a route that is worth exploring, particularly in light of the enhancing effects of stress/anxiety on frontal action monitoring [49] and self-referential processing [50] – and the fact that enhanced self-monitoring, in turn, is associated with decreased motor performance [51].

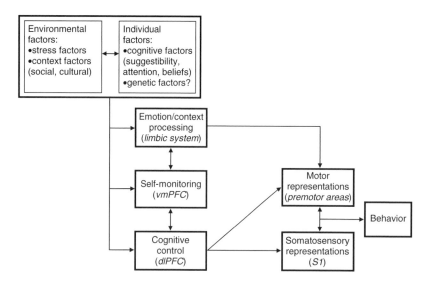

Fig. 20.3. A schematic presentation of predicted effects of individual and environmental factors on volitional motor performance in conversion paralysis. Sensory and motor representations may be modulated by self-monitoring and cognitive control processes (such as self-focused attention and action monitoring), based on these factors and their interactions. These effects might affect sensorimotor processes via dorsolateral prefrontal cortex (dlPFC) involvement. vmPFC, ventromedial prefrontal cortex; S1, primary somatosensory cortex.

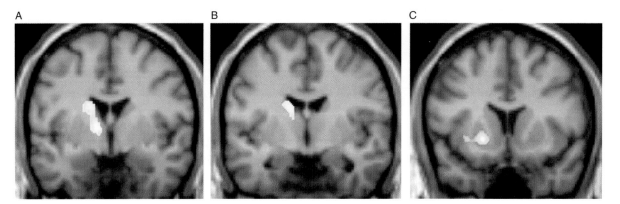

Fig. 19.1. Regional decreases in contralateral hemisphere during unilateral sensorimotor conversion. Data from SPECT scans comparing activity after recovery relative to the presence of symptoms. Scans were obtained in three conditions: at rest (A), during vibratory stimulation when unilateral motor loss was present (B), and during stimulation again but when motor loss had recovered (after 4–6 months) (C). Significant changes were observed in thalamus, caudate, and pallidum/putamen.

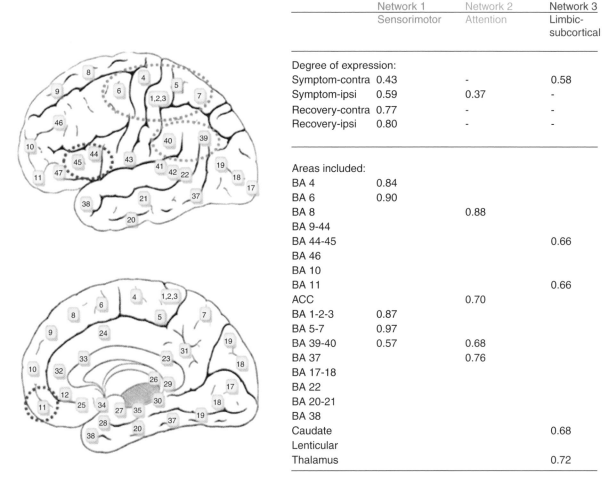

	Network 1 Sensorimotor	Network 2 Attention	Network 3 Limbic-subcortical
Degree of expression:			
Symptom-contra	0.43	-	0.58
Symptom-ipsi	0.59	0.37	-
Recovery-contra	0.77	-	-
Recovery-ipsi	0.80	-	-
Areas included:			
BA 4	0.84		
BA 6	0.90		
BA 8		0.88	
BA 9-44			
BA 44-45			0.66
BA 46			
BA 10			
BA 11			0.66
ACC		0.70	
BA 1-2-3	0.87		
BA 5-7	0.97		
BA 39-40	0.57	0.68	
BA 37		0.76	
BA 17-18			
BA 22			
BA 20-21			
BA 38			
Caudate			0.68
Lenticular			
Thalamus			0.72

Fig. 19.2. Results from a network analysis (subscale profile modeling), comparing brain activation by bilateral stimulation during unilateral sensorimotor conversion and after recovery. Three distinct networks were identified. Network 3 included subcortical nodes in caudate and thalamus that were functionally coupled with areas in inferior and ventral prefrontal cortex (BA 44/45 and BA 11, respectively).

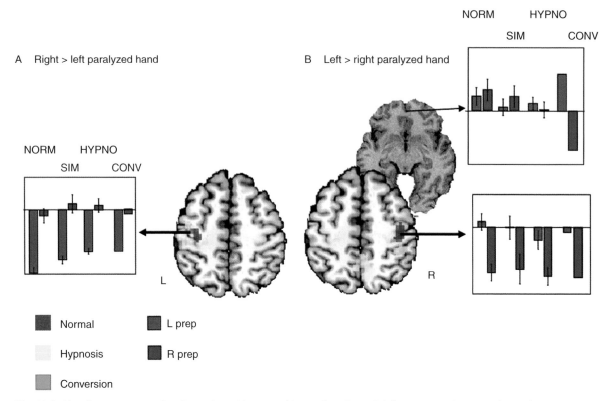

A Right > left paralyzed hand

B Left > right paralyzed hand

NORM HYPNO
SIM CONV

NORM HYPNO
SIM CONV

L

R

Normal

Hypnosis

Conversion

L prep

R prep

Fig. 19.3. Use of a go–nogo paradigm in a patient with a recent history of psychogenic left arm paresis. Activation during the preparation (prep) phase for the right hand > left paralyzed hand (A) and for the left paralyzed hand > right hand (B). NORM, normal controls; CONV, patient with conversion; SIM, healthy controls simulating paralysis; HYPNO, hypnotically induced paralysis. (A) Contralateral activation of the primary motor cortex was seen in all cases and symmetric across the two hemispheres. (B) In the patients with conversion, additional increases were found in ventromedial prefrontal cortex as well as the left orbitofrontal cortex, for the left/paralyzed hand selectively.

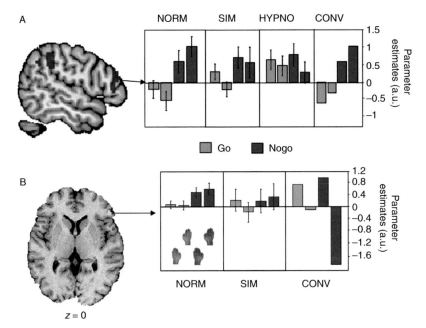

Fig. 19.4. Activation of inhibitory networks. (A) Contrast between nogo > go trials in normal controls (NORM, irrespective of hand side) revealed increased activity in a bilateral but predominantly right hemisphere network including inferior frontal gyrus and inferior parietal lobule. Simulation (SIM) produced similar increases during normal inhibition (nogo trials) and feigned left hand paralysis (left go trials), whereas conversion (CONV) produced a similar pattern to normal condition. (B) Activation of inhibitory processes in conversion. The contrast between left go > right go during conversion revealed a more ventral cluster in anterior lateral prefrontal cortex ($p < 0.001$ uncorrected; k, 10 voxels; *xyz* coordinates in standard MNI space (Montreal Neurological Institute brain template), 51, 36–3), distinct from the right inferior frontal gyrus activated by nogo trials in normal controls and simulators (see (A), *xyz* coordinates in standard MNI space, 57, 30, 24). A left hand versus right hand pattern of activation can be observed for the latter region. Plots represent the parameter estimates (betas) in right inferior frontal gyrus for left go and right go (green), plus left nogo and right nogo (red) trials, respectively, in the normal, simulation, hypnosis, and conversion conditions. HYPNO, hypnotically induced paralysis.

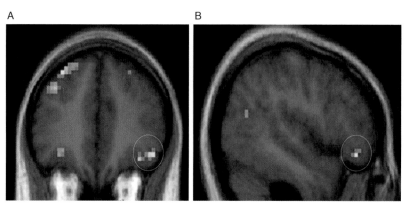

Fig. 19.5. Activation to motor inhibition paired with emotional stimuli in normal subjects. A region in the ventral inferior frontal gyrus/lateral orbitofrontal cortex was selectively engaged during successful inhibition in a speeded stop-signal task (A) and showed a significant interaction between inhibition and emotional significance of the stop stimulus (B, face with fearful versus neutral expression). This region (*xyz* coordinates in standard MNI space (Montreal Neurological Institute brain template), 48, 36–1) overlaps with the cluster activated during motor paralysis (go trials with the affected hand) in our patient with conversion (see Fig. 19.4B).

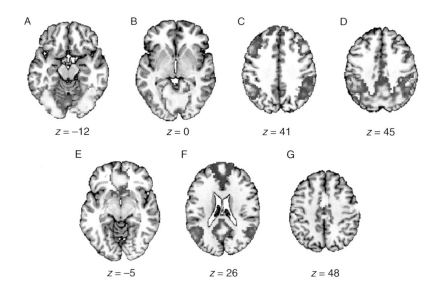

Fig. 19.6. Results from independent component analysis showing seven anatomically plausible networks: A, medial visual component; B, lateral visual component; C, bilateral frontoparietal network; D, superior parietal network; E, posterior ventromedial prefrontal network; F, default-mode network; G, motor network. All components are shown for the normal condition at $p < 0.05$ and false discovery rate corrected.

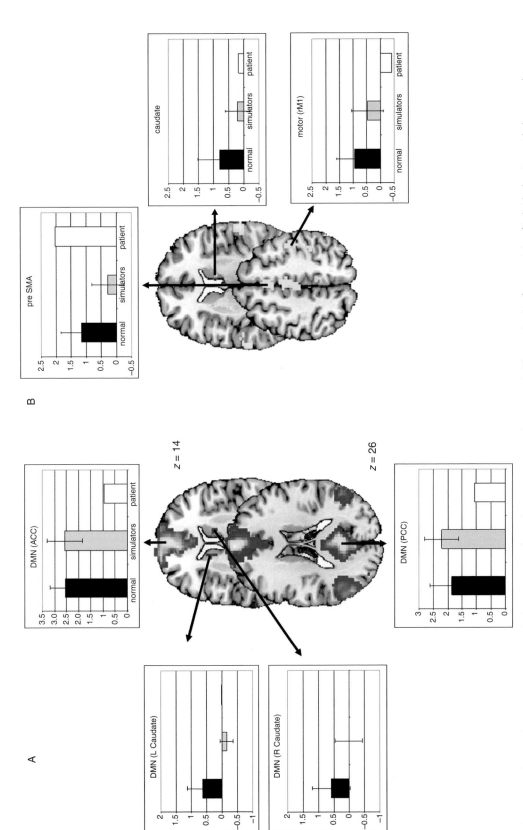

Fig. 19.7. Differences between conversion and other groups in independent component analysis networks. The amplitude of connectivity of individual regions with the network is plotted for different conditions for the default-mode network (DMN; A) and the motor network (B) (mean z-score of the corresponding component expressed in a given area; error bars represent the standard deviation across individuals). Black, normal; gray, simulators; white, patient with conversion. ACC, anterior cingulate cortex; PCC, posterior cingulate cortex; rMI, right motor cortex.

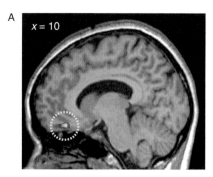

B

| Implicit motor imagery | Explicit motor imagery |

Implicit motor imagery

☐ unaffected   ■ affected

Explicit motor imagery

☐ unaffected   ■ affected

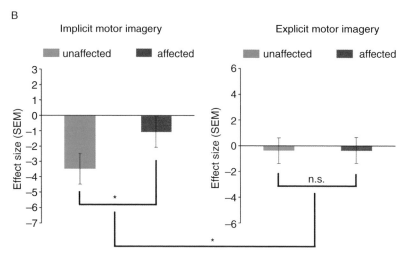

Fig. 20.2. Cerebral differences between motor imagery of the affected and the unaffected hand between implicit and explicit motor imagery. (A) Anatomical localization of a ventromedial prefrontal cluster (10,20,24), showing overall (i.e., not rotation-related) decreased de-activation for the affected hand during implicit motor imagery, but no activation differences between hands during explicit motor imagery. (B) Effect size (±SEM) of activation difference between the affected and unaffected hand during implicit motor imagery (left column) and during explicit motor imagery (right column). As can be seen from the figure, there was a difference between activity for the affected and the unaffected hand in the ventromedial prefrontal cortex during implicit motor imagery, while there was no consistent difference during explicit motor imagery. *Significant interaction; n.s., non-significant. For further details, see de Lange *et al.* [7].

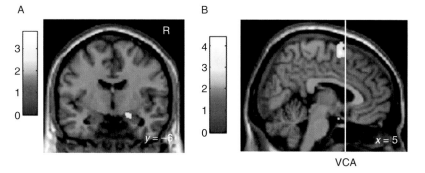

VCA

Fig. 21.1. Functional magnetic resonance imaging in motor conversion disorder. (A) Loss of the normal greater amygdala activity to negative affective stimuli relative to positive affective stimuli. (B) Greater limbic–motor functional connectivity between the right amygdala and supplementary motor area to affective stimuli relative to neutral stimuli.

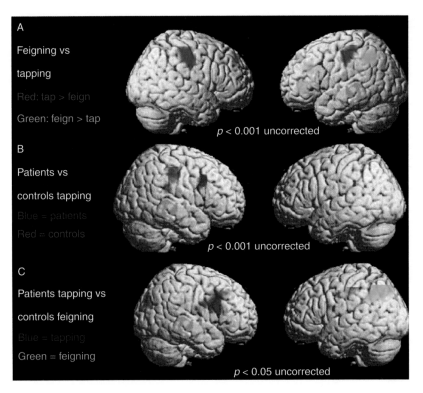

A

Feigning vs

tapping

Red: tap > feign

Green: feign > tap

$p < 0.001$ uncorrected

B

Patients vs

controls tapping

Blue = patients

Red = controls

$p < 0.001$ uncorrected

C

Patients tapping vs

controls feigning

Blue = tapping

Green = feigning

$p < 0.05$ uncorrected

Fig. 23.1. Group analyses comparing combined left, right, and bilateral conditions in patients with conversion disorder and controls. Activations have been rendered on a canonical brain. (A) Feigned weakness versus normal tapping in controls; (B) patients tapping versus controls tapping; (C) patients tapping versus controls feigning. The thresholds used for each comparison are indicated in the figure. Functional imaging was carried out on a GE Signa 1.5 T scanner, using single-shot gradient-echo echo planar sequences (echo time, 40 ms; repetition time, 2000 ms; flip angle, 90 degrees; eight slices thickness, 5 mm (10 mm gap); field of view, 240 mm; resolution 64 × 64). Each series contained 128 volumes and consisted of six alternating 20 s blocks of rest and activity.

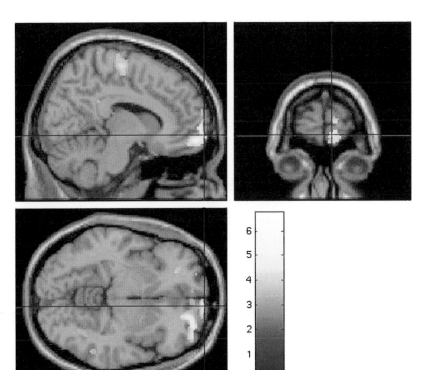

Fig. 24.1. Pattern of orbitofrontal activation identified by functional neuroimaging of a patient with motor conversion disorder comparing recall of their "conversion" event with recall of a "control" event of equivalent severity from the same time period.

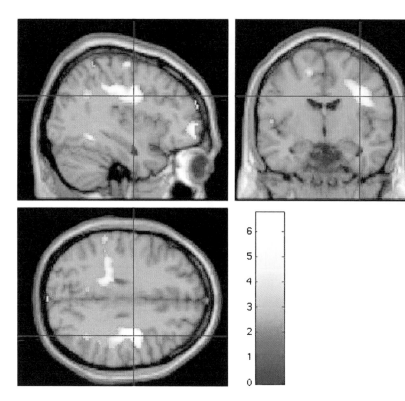

Fig. 24.2. Pattern of parietal activation identified by functional neuroimaging of a patient with motor conversion disorder comparing recall of their "conversion" event with recall of a "control" event of equivalent severity from the same time period.

Discussion and suggestions for future studies

Motor imagery provides a reliable and fruitful method to test neural correlates of motor planning and preparation in CP. On the basis of a first series of studies, a hypothetical integrated model of CP has been developed and is outlined here. Follow-up studies are needed to further test the interactions proposed by the model. Ideally, such studies would involve pre- as well as post-treatment assessments in CP, in order to test the validity of the currently proposed mechanisms. Future studies should also test whether the proposed mechanisms are specific for CP or whether they may apply also to patients with conversion disorder with positive motor symptoms or sensory symptoms. Finally it would be interesting to test possible implications of the model. For, example, if heightened self-monitoring and self-focused attention interfere with motor processes, by altering or overriding otherwise intact sensorimotor representations, one implication could be the choice of interventions that bypass the explicit attempt to move or train the affected body-part.

Conclusions

Patients with CP are able to perform mental movements with affected limbs. This finding offers a starting point for interventions, such as mental movement training.

Increased vmPFC activity is one of the most robust findings in CP and likely reflects enhanced self-monitoring or increased self-referential processing in CP. Future research should clarify the nature of the interactions between vmPFC and the sensorimotor system in CP, testing whether vmPFC mediates the disproportionate effects that self-relevant emotional and context-related cues have on otherwise intact motor representations. The dlPFC shows extensive functional connectivity with the sensorimotor system and altered its connectivity as a function of whether patients with CP engaged in motor imagery of the affected or the unaffected hand. The dlPFC may be more directly involved in mediating the altered sensory and motor symptoms observed in CP, and it might offer a target for intervention (using transcranial magnetic stimulation, for instance).

Future studies are needed to systematically test effects of emotion and stress-related factors as well as cognitive factors on volitional motor processes in CP, preferably before and after successful treatment.

Acknowledgements

KR, IT and FdL are supported by the Netherlands Science Foundation (NWO: grant number 451-02-115 awarded to KR, 452-03-339 awarded to IT, and 446-07-003 awarded to FdL) and the Dutch Brain Foundation (Hersenstichting Nederland: grant number 12F04(2).19 awarded to KR and FdL).

References

1. American Psychiatric Association. *Diagnostic and Statistical Manual of Mental Disorders*, 4th edn. Washington DC: American Psychiatric Press, 1994.

2. Halligan PW, Bass C, Marshall JC (eds.). *Contemporary Approaches to the Study of Hysteria: Clinical and Theoretical Perspectives*. Oxford: Oxford University Press, 2001.

3. Vuilleumier P, Chicherio C, Assal F, *et al.* Functional neuroanatomical correlates of hysterical sensorimotor loss. *Brain* 2001;**124**:1077–1090.

4. Roelofs K, de Bruijn ER, van Galen GP. Hyperactive action monitoring during motor-initiation in conversion paralysis: an event-related potential study. *Biol Psychol* 2006;**71**:316–325.

5. Burgmer M, Konrad C, Jansen A, *et al.* Abnormal brain activation during movement observation in patients with conversion paralysis. *Neuroimage* 2006;**29**:1336–1343.

6. de Lange FP, Roelofs K, Toni I. Increased self-monitoring during imagined movements in conversion paralysis. *Neuropsychologia* 2007;**45**:2051–2058.

7. de Lange FP, Roelofs K, Toni I. Motor imagery: a window into the mechanisms and alterations of the motor system. *Cortex* 2008;**44**:494–506.

8. Marshall JC, Halligan PW, Fink GR, Wade DT, Frackowiak RS. The functional anatomy of a hysterical paralysis. *Cognition* 1997;**64**:B1–B8.

9. Halligan PW, Athwal BS, Oakley DA, Frackowiak RSJ. Imaging hypnotic paralysis: implications for conversion hysteria. *Lancet* 2000;**355**:986–987.

10. Spence SA, Crimlisk HL, Cope H, Ron MA, Grasby PM. Discrete neurophysiological correlates in prefrontal cortex during hysterical and feigned disorder of movement. *Lancet* 2000;**355**:1243–1244.

11. Stone J, Zeman A, Simonotto E, *et al.* fMRI in Patients With motor conversion symptoms and controls with simulated weakness. *Psychosom Med* 2007;**69**:961–969.

12. Jeannerod M. *Motor Cognition: What Actions Tell to the Self.* Oxford: Oxford University Press, 2006.

13. Parsons LM. Imagined spatial transformations of one's hands and feet. *Cogn Psychol* 1987;**19**:178–241.

14. Sekiyama K. Kinesthetic aspects of mental representations in the identification of left and right hands. *Percept Psychophys* 1982;**32**:89–95.

15. Parsons LM. Temporal and kinematic properties of motorbehavior reflected in mentally simulated action. *J Exp Psych Hum Perc Perf* 1994;**20**:709–730.

16. Decety J, Jeannerod M, Germain M, Pastene J. Vegetative response during imagined movement is proportional tomental effort. *Behav Brain Res* 1991;**42**:1–5.

17. de Lange FP, Hagoort P, Toni I. Neural topography and content of movement representations. *J Cogn Neurosci* 2005;**17**:97–112.

18. de Lange FP, Helmich RC, Toni I. Posture influences motor imagery: an fMRI study. *Neuroimage* 2006;**33**:609–617.

19. Jeannerod M. The representing brain: neural correlates of motor intention and imagery. *Behav Brain Sci* 1994;**17**:187–245.

20. Maruff P, Velakoulis D. The voluntary control of motor imagery. Imagined movements in individuals with feigned motor impairment and conversion disorder. *Neuropsychologia* 2000;**38**:1251–1260.

21. Roelofs K, Näring GWB, Keijsers GPJ, *et al.* Motor imagery in conversion paralysis. *Cogn Neuropsychiatry* 2001;**6**:21–40.

22. Johnson SH, Rotte M, Grafton ST, *et al.* Selective activation of a parietofrontal circuit during implicitly imagined prehension. *Neuroimage* 2001;**17**:1693–1704.

23. Thoenissen D, Zilles K, Toni I. Movement preparation and motor intention: an event-related fMRI study. *J Neurosci* 2001;**22**:9248–9260.

24. Ochsner KN, Gross JJ. The cognitive control of emotion. *Trends Cogn Sci* 2005;**9**:242–249.

25. Raichle ME, Mintun MA. Brain work and brain imaging. *Annu Rev Neurosci* 2006;**29**:449–476.

26. Gusnard DA, Raichle ME, Raichle ME. Searching for a baseline: functional imaging and the resting human brain. *Nat Rev Neurosci* 2001;**2**:685–694.

27. Goldberg II, Harel M, Malach R. When the brain loses its self: prefrontal inactivation during sensorimotor processing. *Neuron* 2006;**50**:329–339.

28. Amodio DM, Frith CD. Meeting of minds: the medial frontal cortex and social cognition. *Nat Rev Neurosci* 2006;**7**:268–277.

29. Gilbert SJ, Spengler S, Simons JS, *et al.* Functional specialization within rostral prefrontal cortex (area 10): a meta-analysis *J Cogn Neurosci* 2006;**18**:932–948.

30. Lombardo MV, Chakrabarti B, Bullmore ET, *et al.* Atypical neural self-representation in autism. *Brain* 2010;**133**:611–624.

31. Northoff G, Heinzel A, de Greck M, *et al.* Self-referential processing in our brain: a meta-analysis of imaging studies on the self. *Neuroimage* 2006;**15**:440–457.

32. Cojan Y, Waber L, Carruzzo A, Vuilleumier P. Motor inhibition in hysterical conversion paralysis. *Neuroimage* 2009;**47**:1026–1037.

33. De Lange F, Toni I, Roelofs K. Altered connectivity between prefrontal and sensorimotor cortex in conversion paralysis. *Neuropsychologia* 2010;**48**:1782–1788.

34. Rowe JB, Toni I, Josephs O, Frackowiak RS, Passingham RE. The prefrontal cortex: response selection or maintenance within working memory? *Science* 2000;**288**:1656–1660.

35. Liepert J, Hassa T, Tüscher O, Schmidt R. Abnormal motor excitability in patients with psychogenic paresis: a TMS study. *J Neurol* 2009;**256**:121–126.

36. Avenanti A, Bolognini N, Maravita A, Aglioti SM. Somatic and motor components of action simulation. *Curr Biol* 2007;**17**:2129–2135.

37. Urry HL, van Reekum CM, Johnstone T, *et al.* Amygdala and ventromedial prefrontal cortex are inversely coupled during regulation of negative affect and predict the diurnal pattern of cortisol secretion among older adults. *J Neurosci* 2006;**26**:4415–4425.

38. Roelofs K, Spinhoven Ph. Trauma and medically unexplained symptoms: towards an integration of cognitive and neuro-biological accounts. *Clin Psych Rev* 2007;**27**:798–820.

39. Cojan Y, Waber L, Schwartz S, *et al.* The brain under self-control: modulation of inhibitory and monitoring cortical networks during hypnotic paralysis. *Neuron* 2009;**62**:862–875.

40. Oakley DA. Hypnosis and conversion hysteria: a unifying model. *Cogn Neuropsychiatry* 1999;**4**:243–265.

41. Roelofs K, Hoogduin CAL, Keijsers GPJ. Motor imagery in hypnotic paralysis. *Int J Clin Exp Hypnosis* 2001;**50**:51–66.

42. Roelofs K, Hoogduin CAL, Keijsers GPJ, *et al.* Hypnotic susceptibility in patients with conversion disorder. *J Abn Psychol*;2002;**3**:390–395.

43. Roelofs K, Keijsers GPJ, Hoogduin CAL, Näring GWB, Moene FC. Childhood abuse in patients with conversion disorder. *Am J Psychiatry* 2002;**159**:1908–1913.

44. Bakvis P, Roelofs K, Kuyk J, *et al.* Trauma, stress and preconscious threat processing in patients with psychogenic non-epileptic seizures. *Epilepsia* 2009;**50**:1001–1011.

45. Bakvis P, Spinhoven Ph, Giltay EJ, *et al.* Basal hypercortisolism and trauma in patients with psychogenic non epileptic seizures. *Epilepsia* 2010;**51**:752–759.

46. Voon V, Brezing C, Gallea C, *et al*. Emotional stimuli and motor conversion disorder. *Brain* 2010;**133**:1526–1536.

47. Niwa M, Kamiya A, Murai R, *et al*. Knockdown of DISC1 by in utero gene transfer disturbs postnatal dopaminergic maturation in the frontal cortex and leads to adult behavioral deficits. *Neuron* 2010;**65**:480–489.

48. Kanaan RA, Craig TK, Wessely SC, David AS. Imaging repressed memories in motor conversion disorder. *Psychosom Med* 2007;**69**:202–205.

49. Gehring WJ, Himle J, Nisenson LG. Action-monitoring dysfunction in obsessive–compulsive disorder. *Psych Sci* 2000;**11**:1–6.

50. Liao W, Chen H, Feng Y, *et al*. Selective aberrant Functional connectivity of resting state networks in social anxiety disorder. *Neuroimage* 2010;**52**:1549–1558.

51. Jordet G, Hartman E, Visscher C, Lemmink KA. Kicks from the penalty mark in soccer: the roles of stress, skill, and fatigue for kick outcomes. *J Sports Sci* 2007;**25**:121–129.

Chapter

21

Imaging in psychogenic movement disorders

Valerie Voon and Mark Hallett

Introduction

Psychogenic movement disorders (PMD) are a fascinating condition characterized by unexplained movement symptoms without a neurological or medical cause. This chapter focuses on insights from neuroimaging that may shed light on underlying mechanisms. There are several questions that arise in addressing the pathophysiology of PMD using neuroimaging. How and why are the symptoms generated? Why are specific symptoms expressed and not others? Why is the symptom experienced as involuntary? The how and why can be divided into several broad questions. Is motor control impaired, and, if so, how and what regions are implicated? Specifically, is planning, execution, or inhibition impaired? Is there a similar mechanistic impairment for different motor presentations (e.g., tremor, dystonia, myoclonus, gait disorder, tic)? How is this similar or different from that of organic movement disorders? How is this similar or different from conversion paralysis, or the absence of movement or other conversion symptoms such as sensory deficits? Is there an abnormal upstream process such as an affective or arousal mechanism or internal thought processes that may facilitate or interfere with normal motor function? If so, how does the limbic–motor interaction occur (i.e., functional connectivity, limbic–motor nodal points, structural differences in white matter integrity)? Are there abnormalities in neurotransmitter function that can be measured using ligand-based imaging modalities?

Neurophysiology has provided insights suggesting that symptoms such as psychogenic myoclonus and tremor, although experienced as involuntary, utilize the same voluntary motor pathways for execution. For instance, psychogenic myoclonus is associated with

a normal bereitschaftspotential, a slowly rising negativity occurring 1 to 2 s before the electromyography-detected motor onset, indicating normal involvement of the premotor cortex and supplementary area in preparation of movement [1]. Psychogenic tremor has the same frequency in different body parts [2] and entrainment, or the observation that a psychogenic tremor matches the frequency of voluntary tapping of another body part, suggests that psychogenic tremor uses the same central oscillatory mechanism and hence the same neural network as that of voluntary movement. Overall, these observations suggest that PMD utilizes voluntary motor pathways, leading to the intriguing question of why the symptom is experienced as involuntary. Neuroimaging has provided insight into some of these mechanisms.

Insights from conversion paralysis

Most functional imaging studies in conversion motor disorders have focused on conversion paralysis characterized by the absence of movement, the mechanisms of which may differ from that of aberrant or excessive movement. Studies have used different paradigms, different imaging modalities and had small sample sizes (one to eight). Nevertheless, imaging studies support several intriguing hypotheses to explain conversion paralysis. The main hypotheses put forward include (1) impairments in the generation of motor intention [3] or conceptualization [4], (2) disruption of motor execution [5,6], (3) impairments in self-monitoring [6,7] or limbic processing [5,8], or (4) top-down regulation from higher-order frontal regions [9,10] may interfere with motor execution. These studies are extensively discussed in Chapters 19 and 20 and are only briefly reviewed here.

Competing hypotheses postulate that neither motor intention nor motor conceptualization is impaired, or that motor intention is intact but execution impaired. For example, a study employing a paced self-selected joystick paradigm demonstrated left dorsolateral prefrontal hypoactivity, which was interpreted as impaired motor intention [3]. Similarly, movement observation (hand movements) was associated with contralateral motor cortex hypoactivity for the affected hand whereas there were no differences during movement execution (observation and copying of movements), leading the authors to suggest an impairment in movement representation [11]. However, in contrast, in a case report, preparation to move an affected leg activated premotor, cerebellar, and dorsolateral prefrontal cortical regions, whereas attempted movement failed to activate premotor or primary motor cortices; this suggested intact motor preparation but impaired motor execution [8]. Supporting this hypothesis, a recent study comparing one patient with conversion with 24 healthy volunteers demonstrated normal contralateral primary motor cortex activity during the preparatory go phase of a go–nogo task despite lack of movement, which the authors suggest represented intact motor intention and motor imagery [6]. Put together, the studies are not clear on whether motor planning, conceptualization, or execution is impaired in conversion paralysis.

Neuroimaging studies have also focused on possible upstream impairments in self-monitoring [6,7,12], limbic processing, or higher-order regulation [8,9], which have been proposed to inhibit motor execution. For instance, during motor imagery, conversion paralysis is associated with greater activity of regions associated with the resting state network, the ventromedial prefrontal cortex and superior temporal cortex, which authors have suggested may represent hyperactive action monitoring [7,12]. Along similar lines, during motor preparation, greater functional connectivity between the right motor cortex and posterior cingulate during preparation was suggested to represent internal monitoring of memories or internal states that may interfere with motor execution [6]. In another study, abnormal activation of the right ventromedial prefrontal cortex was suggested to play a role in a top-down higher-order inhibition of motor execution from regions involved with higher-order motor control [8]. A more recent study demonstrated that conversion paralysis during motor imagery is characterized by lower functional connectivity between the

ventromedial prefrontal cortex and the sensorimotor cortex, and increased connectivity between the dorsal prefrontal cortex and sensorimotor cortex; this led the authors to speculate that different prefrontal cortical regions may play a top-down regulatory role in higher-order motor control [10]. Data from neuroimaging studies have implicated possible networks engaging limbic and motor regions that may be involved in conversion paralysis. Studies demonstrate the engagement of regions in the limbic–motor interface with attempted or imagined movement (ventromedial prefrontal cortex) and non-noxious brush stimuli (caudate/putamen) in conversion paralysis. These regions have been suggested as potential nodal points for emotional stimuli to influence motor mechanisms [5,7,8,12]. Furthermore, a patient with conversion paralysis was demonstrated to have greater amygdala activity and lower motor cortex activity to recall of a personal emotionally distressing event [13]. As a result, distinct mechanisms have been postulated. How these interact remains to be established.

Studies in psychogenic movement disorders

Patients with PMDs have greater eye blink startle response to arousing stimuli relative to healthy volunteers, linking arousal to a reflexive motor response [14]. These findings are consistent with the observation that patients with conversion disorder with mixed symptoms have greater arousal during the illness state, as measured using galvanic skin response [15,16], baseline cortisol [17,18], reduced heart rate variability [18] and greater threat vigilance [18]. In a functional magnetic resonance imaging (fMRI) study with a large sample size (16), patients with motor conversion disorder (which only included those with PMD and aberrant or excessive motor symptoms such as tremor or gait disorders, not patients with conversion paralysis) had loss of the normal greater amygdala activity to negative relative to positive affective stimuli (Fig. 21.1A, see the color plates). The authors suggested these findings represent greater amygdala activity to arousing stimuli [19]. The impairment in amygdala habituation dovetails with reports of a failure of habituation of galvanic skin response to acoustic stimuli in patients with both active and remitted conversion disorder [15,16]. Furthermore, greater limbic–motor functional connectivity was observed between the right amygdala and supplementary motor area to affective stimuli

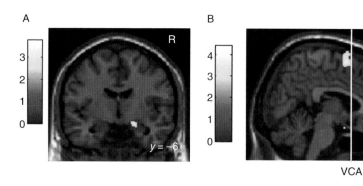

Fig. 21.1. Functional magnetic resonance imaging in motor conversion disorder. (A) Loss of the normal greater amygdala activity to negative affective stimuli relative to positive affective stimuli. (B) Greater limbic–motor functional connectivity between the right amygdala and supplementary motor area to affective stimuli relative to neutral stimuli. (Also in color plate section.)

relative to neutral stimuli (Fig. 21.1B). The supplementary motor area is implicated in motor initiation, particularly self-initiation, and in non-conscious motor response inhibition. This study addresses aspects of why and how PMD symptoms develop: greater amygdala activity to arousal and potential impairments in amygdala habituation may have a downstream influence on a motor region involved in motor initiation and non-conscious response inhibition. Consequently, a model of the contributors to PMD may include either positive or negative emotional events, major personally relevant crises or minor repeated daily stressors, exposure to physiologically arousing events such as lack of sleep or a neurobiological recurrence of depression symptoms; all of these may lead to greater arousal and the onset or exacerbation of conversion motor symptoms. Whether this represents a premorbid (i.e., endophenotypic state), and hence a risk factor, or is primary (i.e., causative) or secondary (i.e., secondary to the disorder itself) is not possible to conclude from the study. Although patients with conversion disorder were included in this study (i.e., patients whose psychological issues were believed to play a role in initiation or exacerbation of symptoms), the study also suggests that potentially highly idiosyncratic and subjective events or stressors can lead to this state of arousal, and that these events or stressors may not necessarily be recognizable or diagnosable by clinicians or patients. This is in line with the diagnostic criteria of PMD, in which the identification of psychological factors is a supportive but not a necessary diagnostic criterion. It also provides evidence supporting the removal from conversion disorder of the diagnostic criterion of requiring the judgment that psychological factors are associated with the conversion symptoms.

In a separate study, the question of the involuntary nature of the symptom was indirectly addressed. Using a within-subject fMRI design, non-intentional tremor versus intentional mimicked tremor in eight patients with psychogenic tremor was associated with lower right temporoparietal junction activity [20]. While there is a range of potential explanations, a crucial role of the temporoparietal junction is to act as a comparator of predicted versus actual outcomes. The sense of agency, or the sense that one is in control of one's movements, is believed to be predicated on a match between the predicted outcome and the actual sensory outcome of a movement. The authors speculated that the temporoparietal junction hypoactivity may result from lack of an appropriate prediction outcome signal for the conversion tremor. Without the predicted outcome signal, there would be no comparison between the predicted and actual sensory outcome of the conversion movement. This lack of comparison would lead to temporoparietal junction hypoactivity and the perception that the movement is not under one's control. Further studies using carefully designed paradigms investigating agency will shed more light on the nature of involuntariness in PMD.

Limitations in neuroimaging studies of psychogenic movement disorders

There are several difficulties that arise in the study of PMD using fMRI. The presence of hyperkinetic movements can result in movement artefacts in fMRI studies, which may be less of an issue with positron emission tomography (PET) imaging but at the expense of poorer temporal resolution. Assessing patients with chronic PMD may also be an issue as the chronicity itself may result in neuroplastic changes and as such may represent downstream changes rather than reflect causal factors. This has been an issue in the electrophysiological studies in dystonia [21,22] but equally is an issue for the study of all chronic psychiatric disorders. Whether studies should focus only on specific movement symptoms, hence affecting recruitment, or study a more general range of symptoms depends on the hypotheses. For instance, in one study we focused on the influence of affective or arousing stimuli; the inclusion of a range of psychogenic movement symptoms was felt to be justified as we were investigating common mechanisms. Highly specific inclusion criteria may limit recruitment and generalization. For example, recruitment for the above tremor study took place over 7 years despite the availability of over 150 subjects in the database of the Human Motor Control Section Clinic, a tertiary center which subspecializes in PMD and recruits from across North America. Another issue is determining appropriate controls for the movement symptoms, which again depends on the hypothesized question. In the tremor study, we used a within-subject design with the patient performing the same mimicked voluntary movement as their own control. Other options include the use of patients with organic movement disorders as a control for movement symptoms; however, this poses its own issues as patients with PMD have variable presentation of movements. Subjects can be studied at rest assuming there are no movements at rest; however, this also means the study no longer focuses on active symptoms. As depressive symptoms are common in PMD, and depression itself has specific neural markers commonly overlapping with regions identified in conversion disorders, ideally patients without comorbid major depression diagnosis should be recruited – or depression scores can be used as covariates of no interest. However, an argument can also be made that major depression itself may also contribute to psychogenic symptoms and may be worthy of study.

Conclusions

Studies of PMD using functional imaging are in a nascent stage. Neurophysiological studies have suggested that psychogenic tremor and myoclonus may utilize the same motor pathways as voluntary movement. Further studies in psychogenic dystonia have suggested that either chronic dystonic symptoms may result in similar neuroplastic changes as organic dystonia or that these neuroplastic differences represent an endophenotypic risk marker for development of dystonic symptoms. Based on fMRI studies, we can tentatively suggest that patients with PMD may have

greater limbic activity to arousing stimuli along with greater limbic–motor connectivity (amygdala–supplementary motor area), suggesting a potential mechanism whereby arousing internal or external stimuli may lead to PMD symptoms. We also speculate that impairments in a prediction outcome signal accompanying the psychogenic movement, despite the use of the same voluntary motor network, may lead to the feeling that the movement is involuntary or not under one's control. These studies in pathophysiology can hopefully lead towards formulating specific treatments targeting this debilitating disorder.

References

1. Terada K, Ikeda A, Van Ness PC, *et al*. Presence of Bereitschaftspotential preceding psychogenic myoclonus: clinical application of jerk-locked back averaging. *J Neurol Neurosurg Psychiatry* 1995;**58**:745–747.

2. O'Suilleabhain PE, Matsumoto JY. Time-frequency analysis of tremors. *Brain* 1998;**121**:2127–2134.

3. Spence SA, Crimlisk HL, Cope H, Ron MA, Grasby PM. Discrete neurophysiological correlates in prefrontal cortex during hysterical and feigned disorder of movement. *Lancet* 2000;**355**:1243–1244.

4. Roelofs K, de Bruijn ER, van Galen GP. Hyperactive action monitoring during motor-initiation in conversion paralysis: an event-related potential study. *Biol Psychol* 2006;**71**:316–325.

5. Vuilleumier P, Chicherio C, Assal F, *et al*. Functional neuroanatomical correlates of hysterical sensorimotor loss. *Brain* 2001;**124**:1077–1090.

6. Cojan Y, Waber L, Carruzzo A, Vuilleumier P. Motor inhibition in hysterical conversion paralysis. *Neuroimage* 2009; **47**:1026–1937.

7. de Lange FP, Roelofs K, Toni I. Increased self-monitoring during imagined movements in conversion paralysis. *Neuropsychologia* 2007;**45**:2051–2058.

8. Marshall JC, Halligan PW, Fink GR, Wade DT, Frackowiak RS. The functional anatomy of a hysterical paralysis. *Cognition* 1997;**64**:B1–B8.

9. Tiihonen J, Kuikka J, Viinamaki H, Lehtonen J, Partanen J. Altered cerebral blood flow during hysterical paresthesia. *Biol Psychiatry* 1995;**37**:134–135.

10. de Lange FP, Toni I, Roelofs K. Altered connectivity between prefrontal and sensorimotor cortex in conversion paralysis. *Neuropsychologia*;**48**:1782–1788.

11. Roelofs K, van Galen GP, Keijsers GP, Hoogduin CA. Motor initiation and execution in patients with conversion paralysis. *Acta Psychol* 2002;**110**:21–34.

12. de Lange FP, Roelofs K, Toni I. Motor imagery: a window into the mechanisms and alterations of the motor system. *Cortex* 2008;**44**:494–506.

13. Kanaan RA, Craig TK, Wessely SC, David AS. Imaging repressed memories in motor conversion disorder. *Psychosom Med* 2007;**69**:202–205.

14. Seignourel PJ, Miller K, Kellison I, *et al.* Abnormal affective startle modulation in individuals with psychogenic [corrected] movement disorder. *Mov Disord* 2007;**22**:1265–1271.

15. Horvath T, Friedman J, Meares R. Attention in hysteria: a study of Janet's hypothesis by means of habituation and arousal measures. *Am J Psychiatry* 1980;**137**:217–220.

16. Lader M, Sartorius N. Anxiety in patients with hysterical conversion symptoms. *J Neurol Neurosurg Psychiatry* 1968;**31**:490–495.

17. Bakvis P, Spinhoven P, Giltay EJ, *et al.* Basal hypercortisolism and trauma in patients with psychogenic nonepileptic seizures. *Epilepsia* 2010;**51**:752–759.

18. Bakvis P, Roelofs K, Kuyk J, *et al.* Trauma, stress, and preconscious threat processing in patients with psychogenic nonepileptic seizures. *Epilepsia* 2009;**50**:1001–1011.

19. Voon V, Brezing C, Gallea C, *et al.* Emotional stimuli and motor conversion disorder. *Brain* 2010;**133**:1526–1536.

20. Voon V, Gallea C, Hattori N, *et al.* The involuntary nature of conversion disorder. *Neurology* 2010;**74**:223–228.

21. Espay AJ, Morgante F, Purzner J, *et al.* Cortical and spinal abnormalities in psychogenic dystonia. *Ann Neurol* 2006;**59**:825–834.

22. Hallett M. Physiology of psychogenic movement disorders. *J Clin Neurosci* 2010;**17**:959–965.

Imaging in hysterical, hypnotically suggested, and malingered limb paralysis

David A. Oakley, Quinton Deeley, Vaughan Bell, and Peter W. Halligan

Introduction

One of the most distinctive patterns of behavior displayed by patients attending Franz Anton Mesmer's clinics in the late 1700s was the "crisis," typically involving a series of motor convulsions resembling those of epilepsy [1,2]. The Royal Commissions established to examine Mesmer's practices concluded there was no evidence in them for the involvement of "animal magnetism," as he claimed, and dismissed the phenomena produced, including apparent "cures," as a product of expectation, compliance, and most importantly of "imagination." The seizures, along with other physical and psychological effects, could in other words be seen as psychogenic. It is also clear from contemporary accounts that suggestion, both explicit and implicit, was a central feature of the mesmeric performances (see also Chapter 41). A century later the eminent neurologist Jean Martin Charcot saw similar patterns of convulsive behavior in hysterical patients under his care, particularly when they were in contact with individuals diagnosed with neurologically based epilepsy. Charcot also noted that his hysterical patients were highly susceptible to suggestion and that many of their symptoms, particularly limb paralyses, contractures, and anesthesias, were psychogenic and could be reproduced using suggestion in hypnosis (as mesmerism had become known). His explanation for the similarity of hypnotic phenomena and hysterical symptoms was that hypnotism was a form of hysteria and that both were characterized by suggestibility based on an underlying neurological predisposition. His observations had a profound effect on an influential group of neurologists working at the Salpêtrière Hospital in Paris, including Georges Gilles de la Tourette, Joseph Babinski, Alfred Binet, and Pierre Janet. Among a series of eminent visitors to the Salpêtrière was Sigmund Freud, who, with Joseph Breuer, adapted Charcot's views on both hypnosis and hysteria to develop their own influential theory that gave us the term "conversion hysteria" and laid the foundations for psychoanalysis [3].

An important aspect of Charcot's approach was his belief that hypnosis and hysteria shared common mechanisms and his use of hypnosis to create specific analogues of conversion disorder symptoms. This latter instrumental use of hypnosis as a tool to explore clinical conditions and psychological processes generally has been advocated by a number of researchers since. Reyher [4], for example, argued the case for "hypnotically induced psychopathology" and provided a paradigm to ensure its clinical relevance, and Kihlstrom [5] contributed an optimistic review of the past and future uses of hypnosis as a clinical research tool. More recently, hypnosis has been used, often in combination with neuroimaging, to create and explore functional pain and disorders of volition/motor control [6–9]; as a tool for exploring more general processes of interest to cognitive neuroscientists, such as delusions, synesthesia, color processing, attentional conflict, and memory [10–12]; and to create effective experimental analogues of clinical and neuropsychological conditions [11] (see also Chapter 17).

The use of hypnosis to produce experimental analogues for psychogenic/conversion disorders is particularly promising in that hypnotically suggested phenomena have a number of features in common with conversion disorder symptoms [13,14]. Notably, both produce neurological-like changes (paralyses, tremor, blindness, etc.) in the absence of demonstrable anatomical or physiological pathology. In addition they both show preservation of implicit processing and are experienced as involuntary (or "real") while

Psychogenic Movement Disorders and Other Conversion Disorders, ed. Mark Hallett, Anthony E. Lang, Joseph Jankovic, Stanley Fahn, Peter W. Halligan, Valerie Voon, and C. Robert Cloninger. Published by Cambridge University Press. © Cambridge University Press 2011.

remaining demonstrably "pseudoneurological" on the basis of objective tests [13]. Also, one form of dissociation ("compartmentalization") has been implicated in both sets of phenomena [15,16].

Neuropsychological evidence on the relationship between dissociation, conversion disorder, and hypnosis is reviewed by Bell *et al.* [16]. Their review included studies derived from the conversion disorder literature on functional motor disorders (limb paralysis, motor weakness, tremor, dystonia, and gait problems), functional sensory symptoms (anesthesia and vision loss), and amnesia, as well as studies in which some of these have been modeled using hypnosis. The present review follows the path outlined by Charcot and takes a closer look at motor conversion disorder in relation to hypnotizability and studies in which groups of researchers have explored both conversion disorder and the use of hypnotic suggestion to create a direct analogue of this clinical condition.

Hypnosis, hysteria and movement disorders

A clear prediction from Charcot's work is that patients diagnosed with a range of hysteria (conversion disorder) symptoms should be higher in hypnotizability and many studies have provided support for that prediction [17–19]. The more specific prediction that individuals who present clinically with psychogenic (non-epileptic or pseudoepileptic) seizures should also score highly on tests of hypnotic suggestibility is less consistently supported. Kuyk *et al.* [20] reported that patients with non-epileptic seizures had higher hypnotizability than those with epilepsy, but two subsequent studies [21,22] failed to confirm this relationship.

There has also been interest in testing Charcot's proposal for commonality in brain processes in hypnotic and hysterical phenomena. In 1997, Marshall *et al.* [23] used positron emission tomography (PET) in a study of a right-handed female patient who met all the clinical criteria for conversion disorder and who presented with paralysis of her left leg in which no movement had been observed for the previous 2.5 years. Tendon reflexes were intact in the affected limb but there was no somatosensory loss. Both legs were restrained to control for actual movement of the right leg during scanning. Preparation to move the right leg as expected activated sensorimotor brain areas with the exception of left primary sensorimotor cortex. Preparation to move the left leg activated a subset

of the same areas, notably left lateral premotor cortex and the cerebellar hemispheres bilaterally, which the authors took as evidence of the patient's readiness to move her paralyzed limb and an indication against feigning. When she moved her right leg (against the restraint), brain activations included dorsolateral prefrontal cortex (DLPFC) and cerebellar areas bilaterally, left lateral premotor areas, left primary sensorimotor cortex (S1 and M1), and bilateral secondary somatosensory areas. Electromyography (EMG) recordings confirmed the absence of muscle activity in the affected limb when the patient attempted to move it, and there was no activation of right premotor areas or of primary sensorimotor cortex. Activation was seen in left DLPFC and cerebellum bilaterally, and this was taken as further evidence against faking. Interestingly, there was also distinct right-sided activation of anterior cingulate and orbitofrontal cortices compared with the preparation to move the same leg. These two prefrontal cortical areas were the only differentially activated areas when the attempted movement condition for the left (paralyzed) leg was compared with attempted movement condition for the right leg. The authors noted that these two areas had been previously implicated in action, emotion, and motor control and concluded that, in their patient, they serve to "actively inhibit movement of the left leg despite DLPFC activation and downstream activation of the cerebellum." The possibility that the anterior cingulate activation, in particular, was associated with distress experienced by the patient at being asked to attempt to move her paralyzed leg was discounted on the grounds that she displayed no evidence of anxiety at any stage of scanning and that there were no other activations of limbic structures that might have been expected to accompany increased emotional response.

In a follow-up to the Marshall *et al.* study [23], Halligan *et al.* [24] used hypnotic suggestion in another single case study to create a comparable complete paralysis of the left leg in a right-handed male participant. The participant had experienced hypnotically suggested motor paralysis previously and was familiarized with the scanning environment to minimize the possibility of anxiety or distress during the procedure. Initial neurological assessment confirmed normal function of both limbs. The hypnotic induction and deepening, carried out before scanning commenced, involved a standardized eye closure and counting (1–10) procedure and included suggestions of muscle relaxation. Suggestions were then given to create an equivalent flaccid paralysis to that presented by the patient with conversion disorder with no somatosensory loss in the affected limb. Neurological assessment was repeated following these suggestions and confirmed that the participant could not move his left leg when requested to do so, although he could still move his right leg normally. As in the previous study both legs were restrained, and the same statistical analyses, PET technology, and experimental protocol as used by Marshall *et al.* [23] were adopted.

Activations in motor and premotor areas were found as expected, with right leg movements against the restraint in the "attempt to move" condition. When attempting to move the paralyzed left leg, lack of muscle activity was confirmed by EMG recordings and motor cortex activations did not occur. However, in confirmation of the Marshall *et al.* [23] finding, selective activations were found in right orbitofrontal and right anterior cingulate cortices, which were not seen with attempted movement in the right leg. A recent study using single and paired-pulse transcranial magnetic stimulation to examine corticospinal motor excitability in patients with conversion disorder paralysis and controls [25] also provides evidence of motor inhibition. In the patients, imagining body movements was associated with a reduction of corticospinal motor excitability, whereas it was associated with an increased excitability in healthy controls.

Taken together these results provide clear support for Charcot's assertion that there are commonalities in mechanisms underlying both hypnotic and conversion disorder phenomena, at least in the case of limb paralysis, and that these involve contralateral prefrontal regions. Halligan *et al.* [24] also concurred with Marshall *et al.* [23] in proposing that the most likely interpretation of the result was that the anterior cingulate and orbitofrontal activations "represent neural activity responsible for inhibiting the participant's voluntary attempt to move his left leg." They also raised the possibility that there are other commonalities between the hypnotic and hysterical conditions, such as mental dissonance or internal conflict, that might in this case be generated in both by a presumably subjectively generated experience of being unable to move but making an active attempt to do so when requested. Such an interpretation could account for the congruence of brain activity observed and might apply to hypnotic phenomena and conversion disorder generally rather than being specific to limb paralysis.

More recently Cojan *et al.* [26] reported a single case of a female patient with medically unexplained (conversion) weakness in her left hand and wrist, with some preservation of finger movements but without sensory deficit. Using functional magnetic resonance imaging (fMRI) they found preparatory activations in right-sided motor cortex when she attempted movement of her "weak" left hand, along with increases in ventromedial prefrontal cortical areas associated with motivational and affective processing. In a go–nogo task, failure to move the left hand on go trials was accompanied by activations in precuneus and ventral lateral prefrontal gyrus but not by activation in right frontal areas normally associated with inhibition. These latter areas were, however, activated as expected on nogo trials with her normally functioning right hand. Connectivity analysis revealed enhanced linkages in their patient between right motor cortex and posterior cingulate cortex, precuneus, and ventromedial prefrontal cortex. The authors concluded, in contrast to the interpretation of Marshall *et al.* [23], that the conversion symptom in their patient was not mediated via the usual cognitive inhibitory circuits but involved activations in brain areas associated with "self-related representations" and "the regulation of emotion."

The same group reported a parallel study involving 12 participants in an fMRI go–nogo design experiencing either hypnotically suggested left hand paralysis (motor weakness) or normal motor function in both hands in a no-hypnosis condition [27]. As in the previous studies of conversion disorder paralysis [23,26], a preparatory activation of right motor cortex consistent with an intention to move was seen when participants attempted to move their "paralyzed" left limb. Also, in common with their patient with conversion disorder [27], they found in the hypnotic group increases in precuneus activity usually associated with imagery and self-awareness, as well as evidence of enhanced functional connectivity between precuneus and right motor cortex. Similarly, and again as in their patient with conversion disorder, on go trials for the "paralyzed" left hand, no evidence was found of contralateral motor cortex activation or of increased activation of brain areas associated with cognitive or motor inhibition,. Inhibitory activations were seen, however, on nogo trials with the left hand in the same subjects in the no-hypnosis condition.

Malingering

Aside from suggestion, there is a further possibility that might explain similar brain activity in both conversion disorder and hypnotically suggested analogues irrespective of the specific presenting symptom or suggested effect. Terao and Collinson [28] proposed that the reason for the finding of apparently common brain mechanisms in the clinical case of conversion hysteria reported by Marshall *et al.* [23], and the parallel experimental case of hypnotically suggested leg paralysis [24], was that in both cases the individuals were feigning their condition. They supported their argument using the findings of a PET study by Spence *et al.* [29], published just after the paper by Halligan *et al.* [24]. Spence *et al.* [29] reported that when two male patients with a conversion disorder diagnosis, showing unexplained weakness in their left arms, attempted to carry out a joystick movement task (which they could do but with difficulty), their attempts were consistently accompanied by left-sided hypoactivity in DLPFC compared with two individuals feigning the same condition and with six volunteer participants carrying out the task normally. Using the same comparisons, the feigners showed hypofunction of right anterior prefrontal cortex. A single male with a hysterical weakness of the right arm and two participants feigning the same right-sided weakness were added to their sample and the combined data analysis showed that left prefrontal hypofunction was common to all three hysteria patients during task performance irrespective of the laterality of their symptoms. In contrast, conscious feigning of the same symptoms in normal volunteers was associated with right frontal hypofunction, irrespective of the laterality of the simulated disability. While acknowledging the difference in task demands between the two sets of studies, Terao and Collinson [28] argued that, in terms of laterality alone, the finding of an "abnormality in right cortex" in both the hysterical patient of Marshall *et al.* [23] and the hypnotized participant of Halligan *et al.* [24] were more consistent with the feigning condition in the study by Spence *et al.* [29]. In their response, Halligan *et al.* pointed out [30] that, laterality aside, different cortical areas were involved in the two sets of studies. Moreover, they noted that Terao and Collinson's criticism [28] seemed to imply not only that their own hypnotic subject had been faking his paralysis but that, despite similar clinical diagnostic criteria being applied in the two studies, the patient in the study by Marshall *et al.* [23] had been incorrectly identified as displaying conversion disorder whereas the three patients studied by Spence *et al.* [29] had been correctly diagnosed.

The possibility of malingering or faking, however, remains an important issue and one that needs to be addressed directly. The evidence from the Spence *et al.* [29] PET study clearly supports the conclusion that brain activations in patients diagnosed as having conversion disorder limb weakness are different when performing a motor task from those of normal volunteers feigning the same condition. Arguably, the need for a similar demonstration is even more urgent in the case of hypnosis, where the validity of the suggested response is based primarily on the informal testimony of the subject alone; by comparison, the categorization of symptoms as a product of conversion disorder is founded on well-established diagnostic criteria commonly supported by neurophysiological and neuroanatomical investigation. It is also particularly important to eliminate the possibility of feigning or malingering in the case of hypnosis, particularly if it is to be advanced as an effective means of creating credible analogues of conversion disorder symptoms.

The question of malingering was tackled directly in a PET study by Ward *et al.* [31] in a group of 12 hypnotized participants tested in a single session under two conditions: (1) with a suggested left leg paralysis and (2) when feigning the same disability. In order to approximate to the reality of malingering, participants were offered a financial reward if an independent neurological examination failed to distinguish their simulated performance from the hypnotically suggested paralysis. Although the neurological examination failed to reliably distinguish the two conditions, increased brain activation was seen in right orbitofrontal cortex, right cerebellum, left thalamus, and left putamen in the hypnotically suggested paralysis compared with the simulation condition. In contrast, the simulation condition showed increased relative activation in left ventrolateral prefrontal cortex and some right posterior cortical areas. In common with earlier studies, participants in the suggested paralysis condition showed preparatory activations in motor control areas, indicating that failures to move in both cases were the products of a failure of movement initiation rather than of movement preparation. This outcome clearly supports the view that subjectively experienced hypnotic paralysis is generated by different mechanisms to its intentionally simulated counterpart. It is also worth noting that right orbitofrontal cortex, one of the activations previously reported for attempted movement during both hysterical (Marshall *et al.* [23]) and hypnotically suggested [Halligan *et al.* [30]) paralysis, was also found in the larger group, although previously reported activation in right anterior cingulate cortex was not.

In their single case study, Cojan *et al.* [26] also included normal control subjects who were asked to feign weakness of the left hand. Unlike the patient, the controls showed the same inhibitory activations of inferior frontal gyrus on go trials with their "weak" left hand as on nogo trials with either hand. This indicated that the feigned weakness was mediated via different mechanisms than the conversion symptom.

In their hypnotic paralysis study, Cojan *et al.* [27] found that, although no activation of contralateral inhibitory areas was seen on go trials for the "paralyzed" left hand in the experimental group, a control group of six non-hypnotized participants who were asked to feign a similar left-sided motor weakness (to act "as if" they were suffering from motor weakness and unable to move their fingers) did show activation of right-sided inhibitory regions (such as the inferior frontal gyrus and inferior parietal lobe) during the left go condition. Again, this indicated that the mechanism underlying the hypnotic paralysis differed from that underlying the voluntary simulation of the same condition.

Discussion

There are three major outcomes from the five main studies reviewed in this chapter [23,24,26,27,31]. First, although there are some reported differences within each research group [26,27,31], there is overall a striking level of congruence in terms of brain activity between the conversion disorder condition and the comparable paralysis condition produced by hypnotic suggestion. Second, and equally striking perhaps, are the different patterns of brain activity reported between the two groups in association with the failure to move the paralyzed limb in both conversion and hypnosis when this movement was required by the experimental design – and the interpretations that followed from this. Third, is the consistent conclusion that intentionally simulated limb paralysis or weakness is accompanied by different brain activity to that in the corresponding conditions seen in conversion disorder or produced by suggestion in hypnosis.

The first of these outcomes serves as a clear endorsement of Charcot's original position. Irrespective of differences between the five studies, they all support the use of suggestion in hypnosis as a convincing and potentially useful analogue for dissecting

and understanding conversion disorder [11], as well as suggesting therapeutic approaches [14]. A major strength of hypnotic suggestion used in this way is that it provides the possibility of tuning the analogue condition to the target symptom presented by a patient with a conversion disorder. The suggestions given in hypnosis by Halligan *et al.* [24] to create, for example, a complete flaccid paralysis of the left leg were different from those used by Cojan *et al.* [27] to produce a paralysis characterized by heaviness and stiffness in the left hand. The studies we have reviewed have been concerned primarily with the "product" of conversion disorder or hypnotic suggestion: the conversion symptom or its hypnotically suggested counterpart. Hypnotic suggestion may also provide a model for the process of developing functional disorders. In which case, their development would be predicted to require a receptive state of focused absorption similar to the state of mind produced by the hypnotic induction procedure. Also, some form of internally or externally generated suggestion is required that carries with it a circumscribed suspension of reality testing.

As well as the broad similarities between conversion disorder symptoms and hypnotically suggested phenomena, there are of course some important [16]. The most notable of these is the chronicity that is typical of the conversion disorder symptoms and easy reversibility over much shorter time course in the hypnotically suggested phenomena. Also, whereas hypnotic phenomena typically arise from an interaction with another individual, conversion disorder symptoms may be seen as "autosuggested," with their roots in psychodynamic conflict or distress [13].

With reference to the second of the listed outcomes, failure to move was attributed by both Marshall *et al.* [23] and Halligan *et al.* [24] to inhibition associated with activity in right anterior cingulate and orbitofrontal cortices, activations that were not seen by Cojan *et al.* [26,27] in association with attempts to move the paralyzed limb. This last group instead found activation of precuneus and other brain areas associated with enhancement of self-monitoring processes, which they proposed might allow internal representations generated by suggestion to guide behavior and they attributed the failure to move to these. Although both sets of studies involved the left limb as the affected body part, there are a number of differences such as the limb itself (leg versus arm), the presenting condition for that limb ("paralysis" in conversion versus "weakness" in hypnosis), and the duration of the condition (chronic in conversion versus acute in hypnosis). None of these, on the face of it perhaps, would be expected to produce such a marked difference in the location of brain activations reported. Also, there were possibly more significant differences in the experimental procedures used (attempted movement on verbal instruction against restraint versus button pressing in a go–nogo design). It is also worth returning briefly at this point to the speculation by Halligan et al. [24] that the activations they reported in anterior cingulate and orbitofrontal cortex might reflect "mental dissonance or internal conflict" associated with hypnotically suggested effects and conversion disorder symptoms rather than more specific forms of cognitive or motor inhibition. One further implication of this is that these activations might be common to all suggested and autosuggested phenomena (hypnotic and conversion). It is also a possibility on this basis that the activations reported by Cojan et al. [26,27] related more generally to mechanisms of suggestion rather than those concerned specifically with inhibition of motor movement. Clearly, again, more research is needed with a wider range of conversion disorder symptoms and their hypnotically suggested counterparts to resolve questions of this sort. It is interesting, however, that Cojan et al. [27] did find increased activation in right anterior cingulate cortex and bilaterally in orbitofrontal cortex when comparing the hypnosis-plus-paralysis suggestion condition with a no-hypnosis no-suggestion condition, indicating perhaps that these areas may be related to hypnosis, suggestion, or a combination of the two – and by extension to conversion disorder irrespective of the presenting symptom.

Finally, there is the reassuring evidence that the clinically and hypnotically suggested phenomena we are interested in are not the product of either malingering, where "symptoms" are fabricated for material gain [31], or the simple request to simulate the target condition [26,27]. It is also worth noting that in the case of hypnotically produced "functional" pain, brain activations are similar to those seen with a physically induced pain stimulus [8,32] but are clearly different from those seen when the same hypnotized individuals are simply instructed to "imagine clearly" the same pain experience [8]. It would be interesting to make the same comparison between both conversion disorder and hypnotically suggested paralysis and their imagined counterparts. In the case of intentional simulation, although the evidence to date seems

clear-cut for motor paralysis/weakness, researchers should consider including simulation or malingering controls in future studies of the sort reviewed above. A further consideration is whether the simulation in the case of hypnotically suggested phenomena should be conducted outside hypnosis, as Cojan et al. [27] did to control for the fact that hypnosis could be feigned and the paralysis, therefore, voluntarily simulated, or should be in hypnosis, as Ward et al. [31] did with their "malingering" condition, to control for intentional simulation with hypnosis kept as a constant. Similarly, there is the choice of whether to use a separate group of simulators [27] or to adopt a within-subjects approach [31]. Although hypnotic suggestion offers greater flexibility and control (as the suggestion producing the "symptom" can be readily removed), in principle the same design choices also apply to conversion disorder, although in this case the simulation would have to be applied to another body part for the within-subject option.

References

1. Gauld A. *A History of Hypnotism*, Cambridge, UK: Cambridge University Press, 1992.

2. Pintar J, Lynn SJ. *Hypnosis: A Brief History*, Chichester, UK: Wiley-Blackwell, 2008.

3. Ellenberger HF. *The Discovery of the Unconscious: The History and Evolution of Dynamic Psychiatry*. London: Fontana, 1994.

4. Reyher J. A paradigm for determining the clinical relevance of hypnotically induced psychopathology. *Psychol Bull* 1962;**59**:344–352.

5. Kihlstrom JF. Hypnosis and psychopathology: retrospect and prospect. *J Abnorm Psychol* 1979;**88**:459–473.

6. Blakemore S-J, Oakley DA, Frith CD. Delusions of alien control in the normal brain. *Neuropsychologia* 2003;**41**:1058–1067.

7. Derbyshire SWG, Whalley MG, Stenger VA, Oakley DA. Cerebral activation during hypnotically induced and imagined pain. *Neuroimage*, 2004;**23**:392–401.

8. Derbyshire SWG, Whalley MG, Oakley DA. Fibromyalgia pain and its modulation by hypnotic and non-hypnotic suggestion: an fMRI analysis. *Eur J Pain* 2009;**13**:542–550.

9. Haggard P, Cartledge P, Dafydd M, Oakley DA. Anomalous control: when 'free-will' is not conscious. *Conscious Cogn* 2004;**1**:646–654.

10. Oakley DA. Hypnosis as a tool in research: experimental psychopathology. *Contemp Hypnosis*, 2006;**23**:3–14.

11. Oakley DA, Halligan PW. Hypnotic suggestion and cognitive neuroscience. *Trends Cogn Sci* 2009;**13**:264–270.

12. Terhune DB, Cardeña E, Lindgren, M. Disruption of synaesthesia by posthypnotic suggestion: an ERP study. *Neuropsychologia* 2010;**48**:3360–3364.

13. Oakley DA. Hypnosis and conversion hysteria: a unifying model. *Cogn Neuropsychiatry* 1999;**4**, 243–265.

14. Oakley DA. Hypnosis and suggestion in the treatment of hysteria. In Halligan PW, Bass C, Marshall JW, eds. *Contemporary Approaches to the Study of Hysteria: Clinical and Theoretical Perspectives.* Oxford: Oxford University Press, 2001:312–329.

15. Holmes EA, Brown RJ, Mansell W, *et al.* Are there two qualitatively distinct forms of dissociation? A review and some clinical implications. *Clin Psychol Rev* 2005;**25**:1–23.

16. Bell V, Oakley DA, Halligan PW, Deeley Q. Dissociation in hysteria and hypnosis: evidence from cognitive neuroscience. *J Neurol Neurosurg Psychiatry* 2011;**82**:332–339.

17. Bliss EL. Hysteria and hypnosis. *J Nerv Mental Dis* 1984;**172**:203–206.

18. Roelofs K, Hoogduin KA, Keijsers GP, *et al.* Hypnotic susceptibility in patients with conversion disorder. *J Abnorm Psychol* 2002;**111**:390–395.

19. Roelofs K, Keijsers GP, Hoogduin KA, Näring GW, Moene FC. Childhood abuse in patients with conversion disorder. *Am J Psychiatry* 2002;**159**:1908–1913.

20. Kuyk J, Spinhoven P, van Dyck R. Hypnotic recall: a positive criterion in the differential diagnosis between epileptic and pseudoepileptic seizures. *Epilepsia,* 1999;**40**:485–491.

21. Goldstein LH, Drew C, Mellers J, Mitchell-O' Malley S, Oakley DA. Dissociation, hypnotizability, coping styles and health locus of control: characteristics of pseudoseizure patients. *Seizure* 2000;**9**:314–322.

22. Litwin R, Cardeña E. Demographic and seizure variables, but not hypnotizability or dissociation, differentiated psychogenic from organic seizures. *J Trauma Dissoc* 2001;**1**:99–122.

23. Marshall JC, Halligan PW, Fink GR, Wade DT, Frackowiak RSJ. The functional anatomy of a hysterical paralysis. *Cognition* 1997;**64**:B1–B8.

24. Halligan PW, Athwal BS, Oakley DA, Frackowiak RSJ. Imaging hypnotic paralysis: Implications for conversion hysteria. *Lancet* 2000;**355**:986–987.

25. Liepert J, Hassa T, Tüscher O, Schmidt R. Motor excitability during movement imagination and movement observation in psychogenic lower limb paresis. *J Psychosom Res* 2011;**70**:59–65.

26. Cojan Y, Waber L, Carruzzo A, Vuilleumier P. Motor inhibition in hysterical conversion paralysis. *Neuroimage* 2009;**47**:1026–1037.

27. Cojan Y, Waber L, Schwartz S, *et al.* The brain under self-control: modulation of inhibitory monitoring cortical networks during hypnotic paralysis. *Neuron* 2009;**62**:862–875.

28. Terao T, Collinson S. Imaging hypnotic paralysis. *Lancet* 2000;**356**:162–163.

29. Spence SA, Crimlisk HL, Cope H, Ron MA, Grasby PM. Discrete neurophysiological correlates in prefrontal cortex during hysterical and feigned disorder of movement. *Lancet* 2000;**355**:1243–1244.

30. Halligan, PW, Oakley DA, Athwal BS, Frackowiak RSJ. Imaging hypnotic paralysis: authors' reply. *Lancet* 2000;**356**:163.

31. Ward NS, Oakley DA, Frackowiak RSJ, Halligan PW. Differential brain activations during intentionally simulated and subjectively experienced paralysis. *Cogn Neuropsychiatry,* 2003;**8**, 295–312.

32. Raij TT, Numminen J, Narvanen S, Hiltunen J, Hari R. Brain correlates of subjective reality of physically and psychologically induced pain. *Proc Natl Acad Sci USA* 2005;**102**:2147–2151.

Chapter 23

Functional imaging of psychogenic and feigned weakness

Graeme D. Hammond-Tooke, Alexandra Sebastian, Jill Oliver, James Fulton, Richard Watts, and Elizabeth E. Franz

Introduction

Psychological factors are crucial in the pathogenesis of conversion syndrome, but the neural mechanisms by which they are converted into physical symptoms are poorly understood. Functional imaging studies with positron emission tomography and magnetic resonance imaging have yielded variable and inconclusive results [1–6]. This chapter reports preliminary findings from five people with conversion weakness by DSM IV criteria and 10 healthy volunteers using unimanual and bimanual tapping tasks with and without feigned weakness.

Methods

Three patients with conversion weakness on the left (two female) and two with conversion weakness on the right (both female) were compared with 10 healthy control subjects (six female) using functional magnetic resonance imaging. The mean age of the patients was 41 years (±14) and the mean age of the controls was 38 years (±14). Participants carried out right, left, and bilateral thumb tapping or thumb tapping with feigned weakness, at a rate of 1 Hz, paced by an auditory tone, with blocks of rest and activity. Analysis was carried out using SPM5 software (Wellcome Trust Centre for Neuroimaging, London) [7], and preprocessing included stereotactic normalization to the brain template created by the Montreal Neurological Institute (MNI) and spatial smoothing using a Gaussian kernel (full width half maximum, 8 mm). Movement parameters were included as regressors. Group analysis was carried out using a random effects second-level analysis of the individual results of the control group in order to compare normal tapping and feigned tapping, and the results of patients and controls were combined in a second-level analysis in order to compare conversion weakness with normal and feigned weakness in controls.

Results

Control subjects produced the required number of taps, but patients with conversion missed occasional taps, particularly on the affected side. Here, we report preliminary findings from combined unilateral and bilateral tapping conditions.

Combined left, right, and bilateral tapping in controls was associated with activation of motor areas including the pre-and postcentral gyri, left medial frontal gyrus, and anterior cerebellum (z-scores 3.43–7.28; significance $p < 0.001$; false discovery rate) (data not shown). When tapping with feigned weakness was contrasted with normal tapping in controls, there was reduced activation of sensorimotor cortices and cerebellum and enhanced activation of the left middle frontal gyrus and inferior parietal lobule (Figure 23.1A (see color plates) and Table 23.1).

The contrast of tapping (combined left, right, and bilateral) in patients versus controls suggests that the postcentral gyri and right insula were activated more in controls and the right middle frontal gyrus was activated more in patients (Fig. 23.1B and Table 23.1). Compared with controls feigning weakness, patients showed less activation of left inferior parietal lobule, left cingulate gyrus, right insula, left precentral gyrus, and right medial frontal gyrus. Patient tapping was associated with more activation of the right inferior frontal gyrus (Fig. 23.1C and Table 23.1).

Discussion

The sample was small but comparable to previous studies, reflecting the difficulties in recruiting patients with

---

Psychogenic Movement Disorders and Other Conversion Disorders, ed. Mark Hallett, Anthony E. Lang, Joseph Jankovic, Stanley Fahn, Peter W. Halligan, Valerie Voon, and C. Robert Cloninger. Published by Cambridge University Press. © Cambridge University Press 2011.

Table 23.1 The most significant activations for comparisons from group analyses comparing combined left, right, and bilateral conditions in patients and controls[a]

Area	BA	Action	MNI coordinates			Voxels	z-score	p value
			x	y	z			
Controls tapping versus feigning								
Right precentral gyrus	4	Tap > feign	40	−20	55	68	5.08	< 0.005
Left postcentral gyrus	2	Tap > feign	−52	−20	45	37	4.83	< 0.005
Left inferior parietal lobule	40	Feign > tap	−48	−56	45	26	4.13	< 0.01
Left middle frontal gyrus	10	Feign > tap	−40	44	5	6	3.57	< 0.05
Left middle frontal gyrus	9	Feign > tap	−40	32	30	3	3.53	< 0.05
Right postcerebellum								
Patients tapping versus controls tapping		Tap > feign	12	−52	-40	3	3.52	< 0.05
Right postcentral gyrus	40	Controls > patients	−42	−24	48	52	4.94	< 0.02
Right insula	13	Controls > patients	−48	−36	21	15	3.63	< 0.001[b]
Right middle frontal gyrus	9	Patients > controls	−51	15	33	20	3.47	< 0.001[b]
Left postcentral gyrus	2	Controls > patients	−60	−24	42	16	3.40	< 0.001[b]
Patients tapping versus controls pretending								
Left inferior parietal lobule	40	Control feign > patient tap	−48	−57	51	357	4.44	< 0.05
Left cingulate	24	Control feign > patient tap	−27	−12	42	19	3.76	< 0.05
Right insula	13	Control feign > patient tap	51	−33	21	19	3.62	< 0.05
Left precentral gyrus	44	Control feign > patient tap	−54	3	0	12	3.62	< 0.05
Right medial frontal gyrus	6	Control feign > patient tap	6	9	51	11	3.28	< 0.001[b]
Right inferior frontal gyrus	44	Patient tap > control feign	−57	12	21	2	3.16	< 0.001[b]

MNI, Montreal Neurological Institute brain template; BA, Brodmann area.
[a] Details of functioning imaging are given in Fig. 23.1.
[b] Uncorrected.

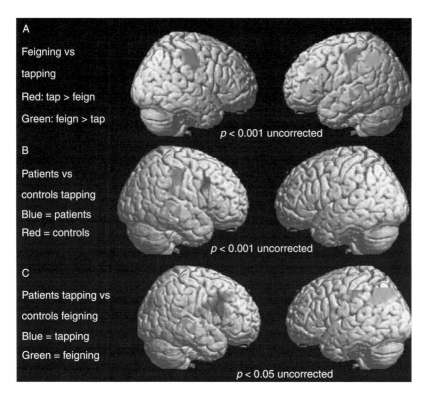

Fig. 23.1. Group analyses comparing combined left, right, and bilateral conditions in patients with conversion disorder and controls. Activations have been rendered on a canonical brain. (A) Feigned weakness versus normal tapping in controls; (B) patients tapping versus controls tapping; (C) patients tapping versus controls feigning. The thresholds used for each comparison are indicated in the figure. Functional imaging was carried out on a GE Signa 1.5 T scanner, using single-shot gradient-echo echo planar sequences (echo time, 40 ms; repetition time, 2000 ms; flip angle, 90 degrees; eight slices thickness, 5 mm (10 mm gap); field of view, 240 mm; resolution 64 × 64). Each series contained 128 volumes and consisted of six alternating 20 s blocks of rest and activity. (Also in color plate section.)

this disorder [1–6]. The patients had unilateral weakness, this varying side, but the images were not flipped; this means that activations independent of the side of the weakness have been emphasized at the expense of side-dependent differences.

Psychogenic and feigned weaknesses were both associated with decreased activation of the sensorimotor cortex and cerebellum, a finding consistent with most previous studies [5–6]. In contrast, Burgmer and colleagues [1] found normal activation of the motor cortex during movement execution in patients with conversion, which they attributed to simultaneous contraction of antagonists and agonists.

Conversion and feigned weakness were both associated with activation of dorsolateral prefrontal cortices. Together with areas such as the pre-supplementary motor area, anterior cingulate cortex, inferior parietal lobule, insula, and temporoparietal junction, these may represent an inhibitory system activated in go–nogo tasks [8,9]. Activation of this system may be associated with movement inhibition in general and may not be specific for conversion syndrome.

Comparison of feigned weakness in controls and functional weakness in patients with conversion

suggests that activation of the left cingulate gyrus is more strongly associated with feigned weakness, while the right inferior frontal gyrus is more strongly activated in psychogenic weakness. Although activation of the inhibitory system appears to be a feature of both psychogenic and deliberately feigned weakness, there may be differences pertinent to the pathogenesis of conversion disorder, and further analysis of these data should yield further insights into this.

References

1. Burgmer M, Konrad C, Jansen A, *et al.* Abnormal brain activation during movement observation in patients with conversion paralysis. *Neuroimage* 2006;**29**:1336–1343.

2. Marshall JC, Halligan PW, Fink GR, Wade DT, Frackowiak RS. The functional anatomy of a hysterical paralysis. *Cognition* 1997;**64**:B1–B8.

3. Spence SA, Crimlisk HL, Cope H, Ron MA, Grasby PM. Discrete neurophysiological correlates in prefrontal cortex during hysterical and feigned disorder of movement. *Lancet* 2000;**355**:1243–1244.

4. Halligan PW, Athwal BS, Oakley DA, Frackowiak RS. Imaging hypnotic paralysis: implications for conversion hysteria. *Lancet* 2000;**355**:986–987.

5. Ward NS, Oakley DA, Frackowiak RS, Halligan PW. Differential brain activations during intentionally simulated and subjectively experienced paralysis. *Cognit Neuropsychiatry* 2003;**8**:295–312.

6. Stone J, Zeman A, Simonotto E, *et al*. fMRI in patients with motor conversion symptoms and controls with simulated weakness. *Psychosom Med* 2007;**69**:961–969.

7. Members and Collaborators of the Wellcome Trust Centre for Neuroimaging. *SPM5*. London: Wellcome Trust Centre for Neuroimaging, University College London, 2010 http://www.fil.ion.ucl.ac.uk/spm/software/spm5/ (accessed 12 May 2011).

8. Nakata H, Sakamoto K, Ferretti A, *et al*. Somato-motor inhibitory processing in humans: an event-related functional MRI study. *Neuroimage* 2008;**39**:1858–1866.

9. Coxon JP, Stinear CM, Byblow WD. Stop and go: the neural basis of selective movement prevention. *J Cogn Neurosci* 2009;**21**:1193–1203.

Chapter

24

An fMRI study of recall of causal life events in conversion disorder: preliminary evidence of increased orbitofrontal and parietal activation

Timothy R. J. Nicholson, Selma Aybek, Fernando Zelaya, Tom K. Craig, Anthony S. David, and Richard A. Kanaan

Introduction

Conversion disorder has been hypothesized to be caused by overwhelming psychological stress resulting from significant life events, but the neural mechanism of "conversion" from psychological trauma to neurological symptoms is not understood. There are emerging data supporting the role of the frontal cortex in this mechanism, potentially, in the case of motor symptoms, by disruption of motivation or motor planning/execution [1]. There is also evidence for the role of other brain areas particularly elsewhere in the motor pathway and in areas involved in attentional awareness such as the parietal cortex [2]. However, there is as yet no proven connection between psychological stress or significant life events and such potential mechanisms. Recall of a traumatic event has been shown to be linked to emotional arousal with activation of the right inferior lobe in a single case pilot study [3]. This chapter describes an investigation of recall of life events to examine this postulated etiological link between functional anatomy and motor conversion disorder.

Method

Patients with an onset of motor conversion disorder within 2 years were assessed for the presence of preceding psychological stressors using the Life Events and Difficulties Schedule (LEDS) semi-structured interview [4] and invited to participate in a functional neuroimaging study. The 2-year period preceding symptom onset was studied and life events were rated blindly by a consensus panel for potential etiological significance, taking into account (1) the temporal relationship of the event to symptom onset; (2) the potential for avoiding unwanted circumstances ("escape" or "secondary gain"); and (3) the relative underreporting of the severity of the event by the patient ("repression"). Such events, if identified, were assigned "conversion event" status. "Control events" from the same time period, of low potential etiological significance, were selected for similar contextual (as opposed to reported) severity to the patient's conversion event. Contextual ratings were based on research into the severity of specific life events and their association with depression [4] and other psychological disorders and reflect how a specific event would affect the average person. A comprehensive dictionary of all known stressors was used to rate each event.

Two to four weeks prior to scanning, details of conversion and control events were obtained to generate 24 length-matched statements of each event, six (25%) of which were rendered incorrect by changing key facts in the narrative (e.g., "It was a cold rainy day" was changed to "It was a warm sunny day") that required immersive recall of the event [5]. Subjects underwent functional magnetic resonance imaging at 3 T while they were visually presented with the statements, having been instructed to decide if the events were true or false and respond with a button-press device. Activations during recall of conversion events were compared with control events using a block design in SPM5 software (Wellcome Trust Centre for Neuroimaging, London). Healthy age- and sex-matched controls were recruited from local primary care services and underwent the

---

Psychogenic Movement Disorders and Other Conversion Disorders, ed. Mark Hallett, Anthony E. Lang, Joseph Jankovic, Stanley Fahn, Peter W. Halligan, Valerie Voon, and C. Robert Cloninger. Published by Cambridge University Press. © Cambridge University Press 2011.

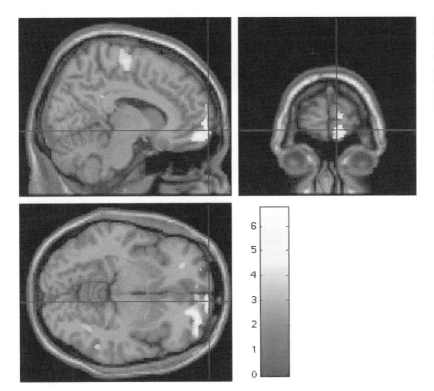

Fig. 24.1. Pattern of orbitofrontal activation identified by functional neuroimaging in a patient with motor conversion disorder comparing recall of their "conversion" event with recall of a "control'"event of equivalent severity from the same time period. (Also in color plate section.)

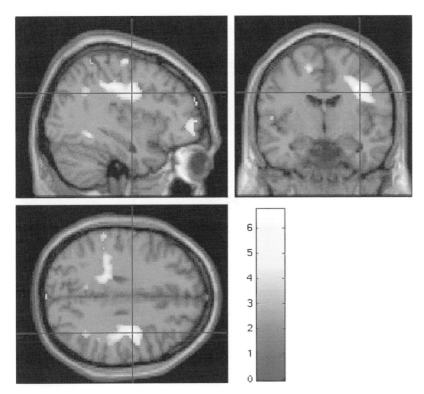

Fig. 24.2. Pattern of parietal activation identified by functional neuroimaging in a patient with motor conversion disorder comparing recall of their "conversion" event with recall of a "control'" event of equivalent severity from the same time period. (Also in color plate section.)

same procedures before being selected for scanning if they had a severe event of escape potential (but with no resultant conversion disorder) and/or a severe event with no escape potential.

Results

Three patients with motor conversion disorder, two with right-sided hemiplegia and one with paraplegia, were recruited with an identifiable conversion and control event. The two patients with hemiplegia were still significantly symptomatic at the time of scanning. Two age- and sex-matched controls were recruited, each with two identifiable control events. In the two symptomatic patients a fixed-effects model revealed significant ($p < 0.001$, corrected) increases in cerebral activation bilaterally in orbitofrontal and parietal cortex when comparing recall of the conversion event with recall of the control event. This pattern of activation was significant for the three patients as a group but was not seen in the recovered patient. The pattern of activation for one of the symptomatic patients can be seen in Figs. 24.1 and 24.2 (see color plate), showing orbitofrontal activation and parietal activation, respectively. This pattern was not seen in the two control subjects when comparing their two severe (control) events.

Conclusions

This study provides further evidence for the role of the frontal and parietal lobes in the mechanism of motor conversion disorder. The frontal activation may indicate inhibition of motor or emotional processing and the parietal activation differences in attentional awareness. The presence of these differential activations only in symptomatic patients may indicate that these areas are involved in the etiology and/or maintenance of conversion symptoms. Alternatively, this may reflect differential emotion processing of conversion events that normalizes with recovery. Further work is required to establish if these preliminary findings are consistent across other patients with conversion.

References

1. Veuillemier P. Hysterical conversion and brain function. *Prog Brain Res* 2005;**150**:309–329.

2. Sierra M, Berrios GE. Conversion hysteria: the relevance of attentional awareness. In Halligan PW, Bass C, Marshall J, eds. *Contemporary Approaches to the Study of Hysteria: Clinical and Theoretical Perspectives*. Oxford: Oxford University Press, 2001:192–202.

3. Kanaan RA, Craig TK, Wessley SC, David AS. Imaging repressed memories in motor conversion disorder. *Psychosom Med* 2007;**69**:202–205.

4. Brown G, Harris T. *The Social Origins of Depression: A Study of Psychiatric Disorder in Women*. London: Tavistock, 1978.

5. Maguire EA, Mummery CJ, Buchel C. Patterns of hippocampal–cortical interaction dissociate temporal lobe memory subsystems. *Hippocampus* 2000;**10**:475–482.

Chapter

25

Cortisol, trauma, and threat vigilance in patients with psychogenic non-epileptic seizures

Patricia Bakvis and Karin Roelofs

Introduction

Psychogenic non-epileptic seizures (PNES) have been considered as paroxysmal dissociative symptoms characterized by an alteration of cognitive functions. Although PNES is by definition associated with psychological stress factors (reviewed by Roelofs and Spinhoven, 2007 [1]), little is known about the effects of stress on cognitive processing in PNES. In a series of studies, we recently investigated whether patients with PNES showed indications of increased cognitive and neurobiological stress sensitivity. This chapter provides a brief summary of findings from four recent experimental studies on cognitive and neurobiological stress sensitivity in PNES, followed by some directions for future research.

Cognitive stress sensitivity

The first study examined cognitive stress sensitivity in patients with PNES by testing their attentional processing of social threat cues. A masked emotional Stroop test, comparing color-naming latencies for pictures of backwardly masked angry, happy, and neutral faces, was administered to 19 unmedicated patients with PNES and 20 matched healthy controls. In contrast to healthy controls, patients displayed a positive attentional bias specific for angry faces. The magnitude of the attentional bias was positively correlated with sexual trauma rates in the patients [2]. These results suggest a state of hypervigilance to threat in patients with PNES and offer a first indication that increased cognitive stress sensitivity in PNES may be linked to psychological trauma. A second study showed that working memory performance was disturbed by distracting face stimuli in those with PNES but not in healthy controls [3].

Neurobiological stress sensitivity

Only a few studies have examined the associations between PNES and neurobiological stress systems, such as the hypothalamus–pituitary–adrenal (HPA) axis and its end product cortisol. The majority of these studies focused on the effects of seizure activity on cortisol levels and found mostly increased cortisol levels in patients with PNES related to seizures [4,5]. So far, only two studies have investigated *basal* activity of the HPA axis in patients with PNES [5,6], and the results are conflicting. We, therefore, further tested basal diurnal cortisol levels (at seven time points) using saliva sampling in 18 patients with PNES and 19 matched health controls and found indications for increased basal cortisol levels in patients with PNES. The effects remained significant when relevant factors, such as depressive symptoms, use of medication, and acute stress (including seizures), were controlled. Moreover, this effect was most pronounced in patients reporting sexual trauma, who displayed slightly increased cortisol levels compared with patients without a sexual trauma report [7]. These findings point to basal HPA axis activity as a significant neurobiological marker for PNES.

Relationship of cognitive and neurobiological stress sensitivity

Because elevated cortisol levels have been shown to enhance the processing of angry faces [8], we further tested whether the previously observed attentional bias for angry faces was positively related to basal (pretask) cortisol levels in patients with PNES [2]. We reanalyzed previous data on attentional threat vigilance in patients with PNES [2] and related the attentional bias for angry faces to newly analyzed baseline cortisol levels [9]. We

Psychogenic Movement Disorders and Other Conversion Disorders, ed. Mark Hallett, Anthony E. Lang, Joseph Jankovic, Stanley Fahn, Peter W. Halligan, Valerie Voon, and C. Robert Cloninger. Published by Cambridge University Press. © Cambridge University Press 2011.

also added a new control group of 17 patients with epileptic seizures. The results showed a positive correlation between baseline cortisol levels and the attentional bias for threat stimuli in patients with PNES. Such effects were not present for the healthy controls or the epilepsy control group [9]. A second study showed that mild stres induction enhanced working memory performance in healthy subjects but not in patients with PNES [3]. Stress-induced cortisol was related to worsening performance.

Discussion and future directions

The findings of increased cognitive and neurobiological stress sensitivity in patients with PNES provide a first empirical basis for integrated psychoneurobiological theories for this complex disorder [1]. Such theories will provide a starting point to fine-tune pharmacological and psychological interventions for PNES. To further specify the association between cortisol and increased cognitive stress sensitivity in patients with PNES, it is relevant to investigate the effects of exogenous cortisol administration [8] in addition to stress-induced cortisol on threat processing in patients with PNES. It is also relevant to examine how threat cues interfere with actual behavior and complex cognitive functions in patients with PNES. Additionally, to gain more insight into the neural correlates of increased threat processing in patients with PNES, neuroimaging could examine whether increased threat processing in patients with PNES is associated with increased amygdala activity [10,11] or with decreased frontal regulatory functions, or both. Finally, in order to test the clinical relevance of the findings described in this chapter, the association between patients' increased cognitive and neurobiological stress sensitivity and their symptomatology should be studied by assessing patients before and after (successful) treatment and to examine the link with seizure frequency.

Acknowledgements

These studies were supported by the "Teding van Berkhout Fellowship/Christelijke Vereniging voor de Verpleging van Lijders aan Epilepsie" (PB) and a VIDI grant (452-07-008) from the Netherlands Organization for Scientific Research (KR).

References

1. Roelofs K, Spinhoven P. Trauma and medically unexplained symptoms towards an integration of cognitive and neuro-biological accounts. *Clin Psychol Rev* 2007;**27**:798–820.

2. Bakvis P, Roelofs K, Kuyk J, *et al.* Trauma, stress, and preconscious threat processing in patients with psychogenic nonepileptic seizures. *Epilepsia* 2009;**50**:1001–1011.

3. Bakvis P, Spinhoven P, Putman P, *et al.* The effect of stress induction on working memory in patients with psychogenic nonepileptic seizures. *Epilepsy Behav* 2010;**19**;448–454.

4. Mehta SR, Dham SK, Lazar AI, *et al.* Prolactin and cortisol levels in seizure disorders. *J Assoc Physicians India* 1994;**42**:709–712.

5. Tunca Z, Ergene U, Fidaner H, *et al.* Reevaluation of serum cortisol in conversion disorder with seizure (pseudoseizure). *Psychosomatics* 2000;**41**:152–153.

6. Tunca Z, Fidaner H, Cimilli C, *et al.* Is conversion disorder biologically related with depression?: A. DST study. *Soc Biol Psychiatry* 1996;**39**:216–219.

7. Bakvis P, Spinhoven P, Giltay EJ. *et al.* Basal hypercortisolism and trauma in patients with psychogenic non epileptic seizures. *Epilepsia* 2010;**51**:752–759.

8. Van Peer JM, Roelofs K, Rotteveel M, *et al.* The effects of cortisol administration on approach-avoidance behavior: an event-related potential study. *Biol Psychol* 2007;**76**:135–146.

9. Bakvis P, Spinhoven P, Roelofs K. Basal cortisol is positively correlated to threat vigilance in patients with psychogenic nonepileptic seizures. *Epilepsy Behav* 2009;**16**:558–560.

10. Kanaan RA, Craig TK, Wessely SC, David AS. Imaging repressed memories in motor conversion disorder. *Psychosom Med* 2007;**69**:202–205.

11. Voon V, Brezing C, Gallea C, *et al.* Emotional stimuli and motor conversion disorder. *Brain* 2010;**133**:1526–1536.

Chapter

26

Components of voluntary action

Elisa Filevich and Patrick Haggard

Introduction

Psychogenic movement disorders (PMDs) are, almost by definition, pathologies of the relation between conscious thought and action. The experiences of intention, movement, and agency that accompany normal voluntary action appear to become dissociated from the circuits that generate movement. This chapter starts by briefly reviewing the relation between conscious thought and action. The nature of this relation in normal action is unclear – and a topic of dispute in both neuroscience and philosophy. However, the existing data point toward an experience of conscious intention being a consequence of activity in medial frontal and parietal brain circuits. Then a simple model of voluntary action with three components is proposed: intention, action control, and agency attribution. The model is used to examine many pathologies of volition, including some PMDs, considering them either as deficits in a single component within the model or communication failures between components.

Motor physiology

Actions can be classified as being either *stimulus driven* or *voluntary*. Stimulus-driven actions are those that are more or less direct responses to an external stimulus. This external stimulus, through an association, however arbitrary, specifies a movement to be done. Voluntary actions, by comparison, do not appear to be elicited by any obvious external stimulus. Instead, they can be seen as resulting from the integration of many different sources of information, without any single obvious cause being sufficient. Folk psychology often explains, or fails to explain, the origins of voluntary actions by comments such as " 'I' did it." Therefore,

voluntary actions are less predictable than stimulus-driven actions, and less easy to explain.

Distinct neural circuits have been implicated in stimulus-driven and voluntary actions. In stimulus-driven actions, stimuli activate early sensory cortices. This activation then drives the flow of information from the sensory cortices to "intermediate areas," notably the parietal and premotor cortices, which link stimuli to responses. Another, rather different, system underlies voluntary action. It is based on the basal ganglia and the presupplementary motor area (pre-SMA). These structures show higher levels of activation when voluntary or self-paced actions are compared with instructed movements that are physically similar [1]. Neural firing in these and other premotor areas is thought to underlie the well-known readiness potential of the electroencephalography (EEG) signals recorded from the scalp prior to voluntary action [2].

Voluntary action and conscious experience

Conscious experience is an important aspect of motor control. We are normally aware of our voluntary actions. The neural mechanisms that contribute to conscious awareness of voluntary actions have been reviewed extensively elsewhere [3]. Two findings are particularly relevant here. First, an experience that one is about to perform a voluntary action, which we can call conscious intention, can occur after the onset of the readiness potential but prior to the moment of action itself.

In Benjamin Libet's now famous experiment, subjects were asked to press a button whenever they "felt the urge" to do so, while they were looking at a clock hand rotating on a screen [4]. They were then asked to

Psychogenic Movement Disorders and Other Conversion Disorders, ed. Mark Hallett, Anthony E. Lang, Joseph Jankovic, Stanley Fahn, Peter W. Halligan, Valerie Voon, and C. Robert Cloninger. Published by Cambridge University Press. © Cambridge University Press 2011.

report the time at which they became aware of their intention to act. The basic findings of this experiment show that an unconscious preparatory brain activity (a negativity that has been called readiness potential) begins well before (> 500 ms) the report of awareness of intention. These results seem to deny a causal function of intentions, contradicting the everyday concept of "conscious free will," by which our intentions are the triggering factors of actions.

The second finding is that direct stimulation of the cortex can produce a conscious urge to make a specific bodily movement. If the stimulating current is increased, actual movement occurs. While this fascinating effect has been obtained using epicortical grids covering the pre-SMA [5], it has also been reported intraoperatively following more lateral premotor stimulation [6], and recently during parietal stimulation [7]. The stimulation results suggest that conscious intention is a result of the frontal motor activity that normally leads to voluntary movement. Thus, the mechanisms of voluntary action could, in principle, be recruited without conscious intention. The person's "voluntary" action might then seem to them to be involuntary, as has been claimed for some forms of PMD [8].

Role for inhibition

Inhibitory mechanisms of both intentions and actions are important components of voluntary action. Inhibition of action can be studied with external stop signals [9] or with paradigms that require more "internally generated" inhibition [10].

Interestingly, in addition, cortical stimulation in humans can also produce movement arrest. This has been shown chiefly by exploratory stimulation in epileptic patients who have an implanted subdural grid [11]. Two main areas (namely, the inferior frontal gyrus and the SMA) have been reported to generate arrest or significant slowing of an ongoing voluntary movement when they are stimulated directly. These areas have been called the "negative motor areas" and appear to have some degree of somatotopic organization.

A functional model of volition for psychogenic movement disorders

We identify three orthogonal but interacting components within the voluntary action system, and relevant to the experience of voluntary action. The three components can be named and distinguished according to their different functions: *intention, action,* and *attribution.*

The intention component comprises the mechanisms for intention generation (i.e., action planning and initiation). In a classical view of voluntary action, intentions should appear before actions. The definition of intention has been the subject of long-standing discussion, but for the purposes of this chapter, by "intentions" we mean the conscious mental state associated with initiating voluntary actions. Intentions are thus clearly linked to advance planning for action. For example, recent accounts [12] describe a cascade of intentions containing increasing levels of detail, recalling the advance specification of motor parameters in an action plan.

The action component is associated with motor execution. This is the acknowledged centerpoint of voluntary movement.

The third component of volition is attribution of agency (which we here call attribution, but is also sometimes referred to as "authorship of action" [13]). Attribution refers to explicit judgment or knowledge about whether one is oneself the cause of an action or not.

These three components have been linked by recent computational theories of motor control [14]. These theories suggest that sensory consequences of self-initiated actions are predicted by an internal model on the basis of *efference copy* of motor commands. The efference copy corresponds to the readout of intentions. A comparator then compares sensory feedback during the action itself to the feedback predicted from the efference copy. If these cancel out exactly, it follows that the sensory feedback was caused by the efferent command, and the action can be attributed to the self.

The model outlined in Fig. 26.1 shows the interaction of the three components, intention, action, and attribution, and where certain disorders, discussed below, might fall within this breakdown of the voluntary action system.

Neural substrates

If this tripartite model of volition is of value, we might expect each component to have distinct neural correlates. Further, these should interact to produce a coherent experience of voluntary action.

The readiness potential has classically been considered the neural correlate of intention and preparation.

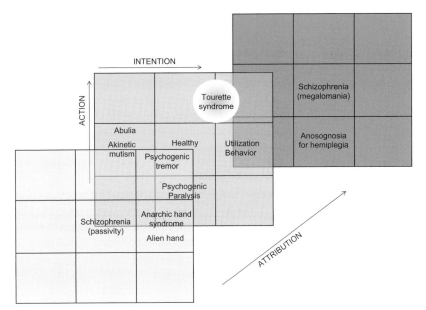

Fig. 26.1. A proposed model of volitional movement disorders. The three components of voluntary action (intention, action execution, and action attribution) represent three orthogonal axes. Components can be independently altered, producing a range of different disorders (and suggesting other potential disorders not known in the literature) (see text for more details).

This event-related potential was the focus of the studies by Libet and colleagues mentioned above. It can be identified (and appears to arise from the pre-SMA, SMA, and other premotor areas [15]) when human participants are asked to do simple movements (such as finger tapping) at their own pace, but not when they do the same movements in response to external stimuli.

The physiological mechanisms mediating monitoring and attribution of self-initiated actions have also been studied. The predictions of the efference copy theory fit nicely with data from schizophrenia patients [16]. Identifying the location of efference copies in the brain has proved difficult, and indeed the general principle of an efference copy may apply at several levels. However, Haggard and Whitford [17] reported that a transcranial magnetic stimulation pulse on the SMA reduced sensory suppression of a proprioceptive stimulus. This strongly suggests a role of the SMA in mediating the generation of the efference copy.

Pathologies of volition: a three-way classification

If the three components of this model (intentions, actions, and attribution) are truly independent, a distinct pathology of volition should arise from damage to each.

Not all combinations of the three factors have been identified with specific movement disorder symptoms.

However, the set of possibilities within the model can nevertheless be informative about the possible functional organization of brain systems for voluntary action.

Therefore, the discussion below provides an analysis of some of the known disorders of volition in this context and argues for the necessity and sufficiency of three functional modules and the connections between them to account for a brain system for voluntary action.

Abulia

Abulia is defined as a lack of will or motivation [18]: typically decreased spontaneity in activity and speech; prolonged latency in responding to queries, directions and other stimuli; and reduced ability to persist with a task.

Abulia is, therefore, a condition in which the intention-generating system is impaired. Actions are not willed and are, therefore, not done. In principle, there is no dysfunction of either of the remaining two modules. This is, however, sometimes difficult to establish, as a lack of motivation for action means that actions and attribution cannot easily be analyzed.

Akinetic mutism

In extreme cases, akinetic mutism can be taken for coma [19]. Patients can respond to queries accurately but they only do so with monosyllables and with a long delay. Movements tend to be few and slow. Patients with akinetic mutism can withdraw a limb if a noxious stimulus is delivered to it, but no sign of emotions (face expression, tears, or vocalization) is apparent. This situation is very similar to abulia, with a strong decrease in the intention-generating functions but no apparent deficit in the remaining functional components.

Psychogenic paralysis

Psychogenic paralysis is one of the syndromes within the grouping of conversion disorders: conditions for which there appears to be no underlying structural pathology. When asked to perform a movement with the "paralyzed" limb, patients typically report to be "trying hard" but are unable to move. There is, however, no traceable physiological deficit in the motor circuitry. In one case of hysterical paralysis, Marshall *et al.* [20] presented neuroimaging evidence that motor plans and movement preparation were present when the patient was asked to try to move her paralyzed leg. However, there was also an increased activation of inhibition-related areas (orbitofrontal cortex and anterior cingulate). Marshall *et al.* proposed that these areas effectively inhibit a prepared action plan. In our proposed model for intentional action, hysterical paralysis would represent a situation in which intentions and attribution functions are preserved, but action modules are impaired, because of an abnormal level of frontal inhibition.

Schizophrenia

For the purpose of the present analysis, two different forms of schizophrenia should be discriminated. Delusions of control, on the one hand, can lead schizophrenia patients to feel that thoughts, intentions, or actions have been "implanted" into them. They experience passivity as they do not feel themselves to be responsible for movements or actions that seem to an external observer to be completely voluntary. On the other hand, schizophrenia patients can sometimes claim authorship for events that lie absolutely out of their reach, a condition referred to as megalomania [21].

In both cases, there is a misattribution of agency. In the first case (delusions of control) the individual fails to recognize their actions as being generated from the self. In the second case (megalomania), the individual overattributes events to the self. The core of this deficit lies in the attribution component: the action and intention modules are, in principle, preserved.

A disorder of communication between the intention and agency modules would explain this disorder. Intentional actions are being generated, but the action monitoring system would fail to detect the corresponding intentions. This would lead to the patient denying the authorship of actions that would otherwise appear to be voluntary. Indeed, precisely this explanation has been given to account for the abnormal sense of agency in schizophrenia [22].

Utilization behavior

Utilization behavior is characterized by behaviors that are automatically elicited by external cues [23]. For example, a patient with utilization behavior presented with a nail and hammer would proceed to nail the nail to the wall and hang a panting that was lying on the floor [24], even though they were not asked to do so. These stimulus-elicited actions are not simply an artefact of the strange experimental setting, or a misunderstanding on the patients' part of what they are asked to do, because they are also found incidentally [25].

Importantly, the actions are not voluntary or internally generated, in the stronger sense proposed at the start of this chapter, but they always involve an interaction triggered by an object in the environment.

Interestingly, patients suffering from utilization behavior do not complain of lack of control. To the extent that there is a problem with volition, we suggest that there is lack of intentional inhibition and hence intentions are generated "in excess." However, patients do not seem to experience an external agent to be controlling their actions. The attribution system appears unaffected.

Anarchic hand syndrome

A different situation is presented in patients with anarchic hand syndrome. This is diagnosed when a patient performs reflexive grasping or compulsive tool manipulation with their hand, which they report being unable to prevent [26].

In anarchic hand syndrome, the hand performs actions "by itself." These "anarchic" actions are, as in the case of patients with utilization behavior, driven by clear cues in the external environment. However, in clear contrast to patients with utilization behavior, patients with anarchic hand syndrome clearly recognize that their hand moves contrary to their intentions. Indeed, the patient often uses their unaffected hand to restrain their anarchic hand. So in anarchic hand syndrome, stimulus-driven intentions are generated in excess, but the patient does not attribute these intentions to him- or herself. Consequently, in anarchic hand syndrome, both intention and attribution systems fail to function normally.

Alien hand syndrome

A syndrome related to the previous two has been called alien hand. Alien and anarchic hand are not always distinguished in the literature so some confusion might emerge. The alien hand resembles the anarchic hand with the additional sense of disownership of their "alien" limb. They may, in fact, fail to recognize it as their own when obvious visual cues are removed, suggesting a disorder of body ownership, as well as a disorder of action [27].

Perhaps the key distinction between the alien hand and the anarchic hand syndromes involves two different kinds of attribution. In anarchic hand syndrome, patients fail to attribute *intentions*, and might say that the hand has "a mind of its own." However, they correctly attribute the *action* to themselves and recognize that the hand that is moving is theirs, rather than another's. In alien hand syndrome, both intention attribution and action attribution are impaired.

Psychogenic tremor

Psychogenic tremor may resemble organic tremor, but the two are distinguishable mainly on the basis of the higher distractibility and suggestibility of psychogenic tremor [28]. The distractibility of psychogenic tremor and the lack of an obvious organic explanation have led to the suggestion that the movements are, from a neurophysiological point of view, voluntary. One interesting possibility consistent with the clinical presentation would be that the tremor movements of PMD arise from the neurophysiological pathways for voluntary action but are nevertheless *experienced* by the participants as involuntary. This would place psychogenic tremor within our model as a pathology of attribution of intention, as in the case for anarchic hand syndrome. Previous experimental results with other groups confirm the plausibility of voluntary movements not being perceived as voluntary in the normal way. First, Haggard *et al.* [29] showed that hypnotic suggestion might be able to dissociate the processes that initiated voluntary action from conscious experience. Second, Sirigu *et al.* [30] studied the perceived time of conscious intention to perform voluntary actions in patients with focal parietal lesions. Their results suggest that the patients lacked any normal anticipatory experience of their own intention to do a clearly voluntary movement.

On this evidence, we conjecture that psychogenic tremor could be caused by the voluntary motor system. Unknown abnormalities might keep voluntary motor system activity from triggering the normal subjective experience of voluntary action.

Gilles de la Tourette syndrome

Gilles de la Tourette syndrome is a movement disorder characterized by tics, which can range from relatively simple movements to more elaborated movement sequences [31]. Tics are of an explosive nature and are usually reported to be done to satisfy a strong urge. Some controversy has arisen over whether tics are voluntary [32,33]. Because of this controversy, it is unclear where to locate Tourette syndrome within the model. Since patients have no difficulty in recognizing themselves as the agents of the tics, it follows that the attribution module is unaffected. Also, there is no doubt that actions are excessive. What remains unclear is whether the intention module is affected. As patients' introspective reports can vary, it is likely that patients with Tourette syndrome present a graded situation where intention generation is affected to varying degrees.

Anosognosia for hemiplegia

Anosognosia for hemiplegia represents an interesting challenge for the model. Patients are typically unaware of their paralyzed limbs. They might claim they have moved when in fact they have not, or they may attribute the lack of movement to other causes (minor aches etc.) [34].

There is a controversy related to what mechanisms can account for anosognosia for hemiplegia. On one view, there is an important role of the feedforward component. If there are no intentions to move in the first place, there is no way to recognize a failure [35]. Another view favors the role of attribution mechanisms to account for the emergence of the condition [36]. Aiming at resolving this discrepancy, a recent experiment [37] evaluated whether patients would be more accurate in detecting movement of a (prosthetic) limb depending on whether they had planned to move their limb or not. The findings indicate that patients were more likely to ignore the visual feedback information (of a motionless rubber hand) and instead base their judgment on their intentions to move it. These results provide support for the idea that patients with anosognosia for hemiplegia indeed generate intentions. The problem seems to be that the intention is "misinterpreted" as a completed movement [38].

Anosognosia for hemiplegia would, therefore, be understood as an overattribution of actions, as opposed to a lack of intention generation.

Conclusions

An evidence-based account of psychogenicity requires a scientific approach to volition. Although problematic, some recent progress has been made in quantifying experiences of voluntary action, and in identifying their neural substrates. Implicit measures are desirable to avoid such measures being dominated by the ubiquitous influence of people's narratives and beliefs about volition. We have presented a three-component model of volition that provides a useful conceptual framework for comparing different disorders of voluntary action, both neurological and psychogenic.

Acknowledgements

We are grateful to Mark Edwards for useful comments on a previous version of this article. Writing of this article was supported by a PhD studentship from the Wellcome Trust and an ORS award from the British Council (E.F.), and by an Economic and Social Research Council project grant and a Leverhulme Trust Research Fellowship (P.H.).

References

1. Jahanshahi M, Jenkins IH, Brown RG, *et al.* Self-initiated versus externally triggered movements: I. An investigation using measurement of regional cerebral blood flow with PET and movement-related potentials in normal and Parkinson's disease subjects. *Brain* 1995;**118**:913–933.

2. Shibasaki H, Hallett M. What is the Bereitschaftspotential? *Clin Neurophysiol* 2006;**117**:2341–2356.

3. Haggard P. Human volition: towards a neuroscience of will. *Nat Rev Neurosci* 2008;**9**:934–946.

4. Libet B, Gleason CA, Wright EW, Pearl DK. Time of conscious intention to act in relation to onset of cerebral activity (readiness-potential): the unconscious initiation of a freely voluntary act. *Brain* 1983;**106**:623.

5. Fried I, Katz A, McCarthy G, *et al.* Functional organization of human supplementary motor cortex studied by electrical stimulation. *J Neurosci* 1991;**11**:3656–3666.

6. Penfield W, Rasmussen T. *The Cerebral Cortex of Man.* New York: Macmillan, 1950:149.

7. Desmurget M, Reilly KT, Richard N, *et al.* Movement intention after parietal cortex stimulation in humans. *Science* 2009;**324**:811.

8. Peckham EL, Hallett M. Psychogenic movement disorders. *Neurol Clin* 2009; **27**:801–819.

9. Logan GD, Cowan WB. On the ability to inhibit thought and action: a theory of an act of control. *Psychol Rev* 1984;**91**:295–327.

10. Brass M, Haggard P. To do or not to do: the neural signature of self-control. *J. Neurosci* 2007;**27**:9141–9145.

11. Lüders HO, Dinner DS, Morris HH, Wyllie E, Comair YG. Cortical electrical stimulation in humans. The negative motor areas. *Adv Neurol* 1995;**67**:115.

12. Pacherie E. The phenomenology of action: a conceptual framework. *Cognition* 2008;**107**:179–217.

13. Wegner DM. *The Illusion of Conscious Will.* Cambridge, MI: MIT Press, 2003.

14. Blakemore SJ, Wolpert D, Frith C. Why can't you tickle yourself? *Neuroreport* 2000;**11**:R11.

15. Yazawa S, Ikeda A, Kunieda T, *et al.* Human supplementary motor area is active before voluntary movement: subdural recording of bereitschaftspotential from medial frontal cortex. *Exp Brain Res* 2000;**131**:165–177.

16. Frith C. The self in action: lessons from delusions of control. *Conscious Cogn* 2005;**14**:752–770.

17. Haggard P, Whitford B. Supplementary motor area provides an efferent signal for sensory suppression. *Cogn Brain Res* 2004;**19**:52–58.

18. Al-Adawi S, Dawe GS, Al-Hussaini AA. Aboulia: neurobehavioural dysfunction of dopaminergic system? *Med Hypotheses* 2000; **54**:523–530.

19. Shetty AC, Morris J, O' Mahony P. Akinetic mutism: not coma. *Age Ageing* 2009;**38**:350–351.

20. Marshall JC, Halligan PW, Fink GR, Wade DT, Frackowiak RSJ. The functional anatomy of a hysterical paralysis. *Cognition* 1997;**64**:B1–B8.

21. Koehler K, Jacoby C. Acute confabulatory psychosis: a rare form of unipolar mania? *Acta Psychiatr Scand* 1978;**57**:415–425.

22. Farrer C, Franck N, Frith CD, *et al.* Neural correlates of action attribution in schizophrenia. *Psychiatry Res Neuroimaging* 2004;**131**:31–44.

23. Lhermitte F. "Utilization behaviour" and its relation to lesions of the frontal lobes. *Brain* 1983;**106**:237.

24. Lhermitte F. Human autonomy and the frontal lobes. Part II: Patient behavior in complex and social situations: the "environmental dependency syndrome." *Ann Neurol* 1986;**19**:335–343.

25. Shallice T, Burgess PW, Schon F, Baxter DM. The origins of utilization behaviour. *Brain* 1989;**112**:1587.

26. Della Sala S, Marchetti C. The anarchic hand syndrome. In Freund H-J, Jeannerod M, Hallett M, Leiguarda R, eds. *Higher-Order Motor Disorders: From Neuroanatomy and Neurobiology to Clinical Neurology*. New York: Oxford University Press, 2005:293–301.

27. Marchetti C, Della Sala S. Disentangling the alien and anarchic hand. *Cogn Neuropsychiatry* 1998;**3**:191–207.

28. Kenney C, Diamond A, Mejia N, *et al.* Distinguishing psychogenic and essential tremor. *J Neurol Sci* 2007;**263**:94–99.

29. Haggard P, Cartledge P, Dafydd M, Oakley DA. Anomalous control: when "free-will" is not conscious. *Conscious Cogn* 2004;**13**:646–654.

30. Sirigu A, Daprati E, Ciancia S, *et al.* Altered awareness of voluntary action after damage to the parietal cortex. *Nat Neurosci* 2004; **7**:80–84.

31. Robertson MM. The Gilles de la Tourette syndrome: an update. *Psychiatry* 2004;**3**:3–7.

32. Obeso JA, Rothwell JC, Marsden CD. Simple tics in Gilles de la Tourette's syndrome are not prefaced by a normal premovement EEG potential. *BMJ* 1981;**44**:735–738.

33. Fattapposta F, Restuccia R, Colonnese C, *et al.* Gilles de la Tourette syndrome and voluntary movement: a functional MRI study. *Psychiatry Res Neuroimaging* 2005;**138**:269–272.

34. Marcel AJ, Tegnér R, Nimmo-Smith I. Anosognosia for plegia: specificity, extension, partiality and disunity of bodily unawareness. *Cortex* 2004;**40**:19–40.

35. Heilman KM, Barrett AM, Adair JC. Possible mechanisms of anosognosia: a defect in self-awareness. *Philos Trans R Soc Lond B Biol Sci* 1998;**353**:1903–1909.

36. Frith CD, Blakemore SJ, Wolpert DM. Abnormalities in the awareness and control of action. *Philos Trans R Soc Lond B Biol Sci* 2000;**355**:1771–1788.

37. Fotopoulou A, Tsakiris M, Haggard P, *et al.* The role of motor intention in motor awareness: an experimental study on anosognosia for hemiplegia. *Brain* 2008;**131**:3432–3442.

38. Jenkinson P, Fotopoulou A. Motor awareness in anosognosia for hemiplegia: experiments at last! *Exp Brain Res* 2010;**204**:295–304.

Action selection in psychogenic movement disorders

Christina A. Brezing, Valerie Voon, and Mark Hallett

Conversion disorder, or unexplained neurological symptoms related to a psychological cause, dates to the beginning of psychiatry and neurology with archetypal descriptions by Freud and Janet. Despite its long history of recognition, high morbidity, and financial burden, conversion disorder is still very poorly understood [1,2]

Previous functional imaging studies in conversion disorders have focused on conversion paralysis characterized by the absence of movement. The main hypotheses to explain conversion paralysis include either impairments in the generation of motor intention [3–5] or that motor intention is intact but execution is disrupted [6,7]. Conversion paralysis has also been associated with lower cortical excitability relative to rest during motor imagery to move an affected finger compared with an unaffected finger. It is suggested that the findings are reminiscent of greater intracortical inhibition in response to volitional inhibition of a prepared action ("nogo" signals relative to "go" signals using imagined movements) in healthy volunteers, thus supporting a potential role for a cortical inhibitory function [8,9].

Impairments in self-monitoring [7,10,11] limbic processing [6,12] or higher order regulation [6,13] have been proposed to inhibit motor execution (reviewed by Nowak and Fink, 2009 [14]). Greater ventromedial prefrontal activity has been demonstrated with motor preparation [7], attempted movement [6], and motor imagery [10,11], although not in all studies [15]. This activity has been interpreted in different ways. Aberrant ventromedial prefrontal cortex activity along with orbitofrontal cortex and anterior cingulate activity during attempted movement has been interpreted to play a role in inhibition of motor execution from higher-order regions [6]. Alternatively,

it has been suggested that these regions lie in a motor–limbic interface as a path for limbic modulation of motor networks [6]. Patients with conversion paralysis showed additional recruitment of the ventromedial prefrontal cortex and superior temporal cortex when performing an implicit mental imagery task with the affected compared with the unaffected hand; this activity was abolished using an explicit imagery task, thus suggesting the activity represented greater self-monitoring [10]. Those with conversion paralysis also had additional recruitment of the ventromedial prefrontal cortex, orbitofrontal cortex, and posterior cingulate cortex during motor preparation, along with greater functional connectivity between the posterior cingulate and motor cortex [7]. This ventromedial prefrontal cortex and posterior cingulate activity have been proposed to represent aberrant self-monitoring of internal representations or memories related to self, which may interfere with motor execution [7,10,11]. Notably whether these findings represent the maintenance of conversion symptoms as opposed to causal effect is not clear.

Whereas most imaging studies have focused on conversion symptoms of paralysis or sensory symptoms and why an intended action fails, more recent studies have focused on symptoms of aberrant or excessive movements, including tremor, dystonia, chorea, tics, and gait disorders, and how these motor symptoms are generated. The generation of positive conversion motor symptoms may be characterized by abnormalities in the conversion motor representation, possibly through implicit learning processes, or may implicate abnormal action selection processes. Similar to the hypotheses in conversion paralysis, upstream inputs such as emotion, arousal, or hyperactive self-monitoring may play a role in interfering with these processes. Regarding these upstream inputs, it was recently demonstrated that patients with positive conversion motor symptoms without concurrent depression may have greater right amygdala activity and impaired habituation to arousing positive and negative stimuli compared with that seen in healthy volunteers [16]. This greater right amygdala activity has greater functional connectivity towards the right supplementary motor area during arousing stimuli than with neutral stimuli compared with the response seen in healthy volunteers. This finding is consistent with a previous study demonstrating that repressed memories in motor conversion disorder were associated with greater amygdala activity along with connectivity between the amygdala and sensorimotor cortex [17].

Additionally, the clinical sign of entrainment, which describes the observation that the frequency of conversion tremor entrains to the same frequency as any voluntary rhythmic movement made by patient, is a cardinal and diagnostic feature of conversion tremor [18]. Entrainment is not a feature of involuntary tremor from neurological disorders such as Parkinson's disease or essential tremor. This observation suggests that conversion tremor utilizes the same central oscillatory mechanism and pathways as that of voluntary movement. A recent study examined the mechanisms underlying the generation of voluntary movement in patients with conversion motor disorders presuming that abnormalities in this process may shed light on the generation of involuntary movement [18]. This study found that, relative to healthy subjects, during voluntary action selection of internally and externally generated movements, patients with conversion motor disorder had lower activity in a region associated with motor preparation and inhibition, the left supplementary motor area, and greater activity in regions associated with emotional processing, including the right amygdala, left anterior insula, and bilateral posterior cingulate. These findings suggest that the representation of conversion motor symptoms, which may be aberrantly learned or encoded, may be triggered by abnormally salient internal states (e.g., worrying about a previous event) or externally arousing stimuli (e.g., observing a stressful event) and be either aberrantly facilitated or improperly inhibited during action selection. The abnormally salient states may either play a role in facilitating the specific conversion motor representation or in influencing the general activity of the limbic-motor regions engaged in action selection.

References

1. Bass C, Peveler R, House A. Somatoform disorders: severe psychiatric illnesses neglected by psychiatrists. *Br J Psychiatry* 2001;**179**:11–14.

2. Carson AJ, Ringbauer B, Stone J, *et al.* Do medically unexplained symptoms matter? A prospective cohort study of 300 new referrals to neurology outpatient clinics. *J Neurol Neurosurg Psychiatry* 2000;**68**:207–210.

3. Burgmer M, Konrad C, Jansen A, *et al.* Abnormal brain activation during movement observation in patients with conversion paralysis. *Neuroimage* 2006;**29**:1336–1343.

4. Spence SA, Crimlisk HL, Cope H, Ron MA, Grasby PM. Discrete neurophysiological correlates in prefrontal cortex during hysterical and feigned disorder of movement. *Lancet* 2000;**355**:1243–1244.

5. Roelofs K, van Galen GP, Keijsers GP, Hoogduin CA. Motor initiation and execution in patients with conversion paralysis. *Acta Psychol* 2002;**110**:21–34.

6. Marshall JC, Halligan PW, Fink GR, Wade DT, Frackowiak RS. The functional anatomy of a hysterical paralysis. *Cognition* 1997;**64**:B1–B8.

7. Cojan Y, Waber L, Carruzzo A, Vuilleumier P. Motor inhibition in hysterical conversion paralysis. *Neuroimage* 2009;**47**:1026–1027.

8. Liepert J, Hassa T, Tüscher O, Schmidt R. Electrophysiological correlates of motor conversion disorder. *Mov Disord* 2008;**23**:2171–2176.

9. Liepert J, Hassa T, Tüscher O, Schmidt R. Abnormal motor excitability in patients with psychogenic paresis. A TMS study. *J Neurol* 2009;**256**:121–126.

10. de Lange FP, Roelofs K, Toni I. Increased self-monitoring during imagined movements in conversion paralysis. *Neuropsychologia* 2007;**45**:2051–2058.

11. de Lange FP, Roelofs K, Toni I. Motor imagery: a window into the mechanisms and alterations of the motor system. *Cortex* 2008;**44**:494–506.

12. Vuilleumier P, Chicherio C, Assal F, *et al.* Functional neuroanatomical correlates of hysterical sensorimotor loss. *Brain* 2001;**124**:1077–1090.

13. Tiihonen J, Kuikka J, Viinamaki H, Lehtonen J, Partanen J. Altered cerebral blood flow during hysterical paresthesia. *Biol Psychiatry* 1995;**37**:134–1345.

14. Nowak D, Fink G. Psychogenic movement disorders: aetiology, phenomenology, neuroanatomical correlates and therapeutic approaches. *Neuroimage* 2009;**47**:1015–1025.

15. Stone J, Zeman A, Simonotto E, *et al*. FMRI in patients with motor conversion symptoms and controls with simulated weakness. *Psychosom Med* 2007;**69**:961–969.

16. Voon V, Brezing C, Gallea C, *et al*. Emotional stimuli and motor conversion disorder. *Brain* 2010; **133**:1526–1536.

17. Kanaan RA, Craig TK, Wessely SC, David AS. Imaging repressed memories in conversion disorder. *Psychosom Med* 2007;**69**:202–205.

18. Hallett M. Physiology of psychogenic movement disorders. *J Clin Neurosci* 2010;**17**:959–965.

Insights from physiology: tremor and myoclonus

John C. Rothwell

Introduction

Psychogenic tremors and myoclonus are examples of excess movements that occur without any perception of volitional effort and which cannot be influenced by conscious control. By definition, they can be distinguished from malingering in that the latter is accompanied by an awareness of control [1]. Crucially, like other psychogenic movement disorders, psychogenic tremors and myoclonus differ from pathological forms in that they can disappear quickly after appropriate psychological intervention.

Electrophysiological approaches to psychogenic movement disorders usually view the healthy motor system as a set of circuits that transform volitional commands into specific patterns of muscle contraction. For the purposes of this chapter, we can imagine these consist of the premotor, supplementary motor, and motor cortices, together with their associated basal ganglia and cerebellar loops, plus brainstem and spinal circuits. Pathological tremors and myoclonus are caused by abnormalities within these intrinsic motor circuits. This leads to a range of problems such as inappropriate muscle activity in response to a given volitional input (e.g., action myoclonus) or continuous output in the absence of any input (such as resting tremor) (Fig. 28.1).

Psychogenic movements, in contrast, are not associated with any deficits in the movement circuits themselves. Instead, it is supposed that they result from abnormal inputs to those circuits. These psychogenic motor commands differ from volitional motor commands because they are not accompanied by any awareness of conscious effort and cannot be changed by effort of will. Note that the model shown in Fig. 28.1 does not specify whether the inputs that initiate psychogenic movements are a type of volitional input of which the individual is unaware or whether they are produced by another system entirely. Exactly how a movement is perceived as being voluntary is a question that has been dealt with by others [1].

As discussed below, although this model has worked well as a basis for identifying certain forms of psychogenic movement, it appears to fail to explain some of the observations that have been made in some recent studies. However, it is useful to begin by summarizing the field as it currently stands conventionally.

Electrophysiological methodologies to identify psychogenic tremors and myoclonus

The scheme in Fig. 28.1 offers two approaches to the identification of psychogenic tremors and myoclonus. The first employs the logic that pathological processes can change the operation of motor circuits such that involuntary movements have a *unique pathophysiological signature*, such as hypersynchronous electromyography (EMG) bursts or high-frequency electroencephalography (EEG) activity. Psychogenic movements by definition are produced by circuits that operate normally and, therefore, cannot have such signatures. Conversely, it may be that movements initiated by the normally operating circuits have a unique signature that would be absent for pathophysiological movements. A potential candidate for this is the bereitschaftspotential (BP), the slowly rising EEG negativity that precedes self-initiated voluntary movement (but see below) [2].

The second approach to identifying psychogenic tremors or myoclonus makes use of the assumption

Psychogenic Movement Disorders and Other Conversion Disorders, ed. Mark Hallett, Anthony E. Lang, Joseph Jankovic, Stanley Fahn, Peter W. Halligan, Valerie Voon, and C. Robert Cloninger. Published by Cambridge University Press. © Cambridge University Press 2011.

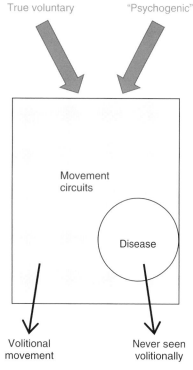

True voluntary   "Psychogenic"

Movement
circuits

Disease

Volitional
movement

Never seen
volitionally

Fig. 28.1. Standard model used by physiologists to identify psychogenic tremors and myoclonus. Motor circuitry is represented by the gray box and can be accessed by voluntary commands. Volitional commands give rise to the bereitschaftspotential (BP), an electromyographic "signature" of a voluntary movement. Organic disease causes parts of the circuit to behave abnormally; the movements produced by these mechanisms can, therefore, be distinguished by their abnormal physiology. They do not have a BP. Psychogenic movement commands can access the same motor circuits as volition; this leads to interference between attempted voluntary movement and psychogenic tremor or myoclonus. Psychogenic movements should have a BP.

that they employ the same circuits as are accessed by volitional movement. If this is the case, then there should be *interference between a volitional movement and a psychogenic movement* when both occur at the same time.

Unique physiology of organic tremors and myoclonus

Tremors

Unfortunately, many organic tremors, except for those associated with peripheral neuropathy and impaired nerve conduction, do not have a unique pathophysiological signature. Consequently, volitional tremors have much the same frequency and EMG burst patterns as the organic tremors of patients with Parkinson's

disease or essential tremor. In fact there is only one clear exception: orthostatic tremor, which is typically a 16 Hz tremor in leg muscles that is so rapid that it cannot be induced voluntarily [3,4].

In the particular case of bilateral organic tremors, there is one other characteristic that can sometimes be used to distinguish psychogenic tremors: in almost all pathological tremors (apart from orthostatic and some cases of palatal tremor that have minor additional tremors in the limbs [5]), oscillations occur independently in each limb with no coherence between limbs [1]. Additionally, the frequency of tremor is often subtly different in different limbs, being, for example, 4.5 Hz in the left arm and 5 Hz in the right arm. In contrast, most volitional bilateral tremors are the same frequency in each limb and are coherent with each other.

A final characteristic of some forms of tremor is insensitivity to inertial loading [6,7]. Many experiments have shown that tremors that are driven primarily by reflex inputs slow in frequency when the limb is loaded with additional inertia. In contrast, the frequency of centrally generated tremors, such as those in Parkinson's disease or the central component of essential tremor, is unaffected by inertial loads, although the amplitude usually declines. However, these distinctions cannot reliably separate organic and volitional tremors since the latter may respond in either way to loading.

All other forms of tremor, particularly dystonic tremor, have no distinguishing physiology. They may vary in amplitude and frequency within the same individual, particularly in response to changing levels of stress [8,9]. They are conventionally identified using the interference approach below.

Myoclonus

A number of forms of myoclonus have unique features in either EMG or EEG that distinguish them from volitional muscle jerking. For example, cortical myoclonus typically is produced by hypersynchronous EMG bursts, particularly in hand muscles, that are as short as 50 ms in duration [10–12]. In contrast, the shortest volitional EMG bursts such as are seen in rapid ballistic movements are usually 80 ms or more [13,14]. Cortical myoclonus is also accompanied by EEG spikes in the contralateral sensorimotor cortex that precede the jerks by approximately 25 ms in the hand or 40 ms in the leg.

A second feature of organic myoclonus is the reproducibility and latency of EMG onset in different muscles. For example, stimulus-induced jerks (reflex myoclonus) in cortical myoclonus have a latency of 50 ms or so in hand muscles, with little variation from trial to trial, whereas voluntary reaction times to sensory stimuli are invariably in excess of 100 ms and vary by 10–20% from trial to trial. This reasoning has been used successfully to distinguish organic and psychogenic hyperekplexia [15]. In hyperekplexia, the latency of the reflex jerks to startle stimuli is relatively long and within the range of rapid voluntary reaction times. However, the pattern of muscle recruitment from trial to trial as well as the intermuscular delays between muscles activated in each jerk is relatively constant [16–18]. Patients with psychogenic jerks have more variable recruitment patterns and onset latencies. The same argument has been made to distinguish organic propriospinal myoclonus, which classically begins in midabdominal muscles and then spreads caudal and rostral at a relatively slow spinal conduction velocity [19,20].

Myoclonus in association with dystonia, like dystonic tremor, has little physiology that distinguishes it from volitional jerking. In most cases, the EMG bursts are long and variable in timing and recruitment; in addition there is no sign of cortical involvement in the EEG [21,22]. At the present time there is no reliable way of separating organic and psychogenic myoclonus-dystonia with neurophysiological methods.

The bereitschaftspotential

The BP is a slowly rising negative potential in the EEG that starts 1–1.5 s prior to the onset of self-initiated voluntary movements. It consists of an early slowly rising phase (BP1), which is thought to reflect activity primarily in the supplementary and presupplementary motor area, and a second more rapidly rising phase (BP2) that probably reflects activity in the premotor and motor areas [2]. Many authors in the past have argued that absence of a BP is a hallmark of a pathophysiological movement whereas presence of a BP (particularly if the BP1 can be identified) usually indicates involvement of the voluntary motor system. The corollary was that if a suspected psychogenic movement had a BP then it was definitely psychogenic whereas if there was no BP then it was likely to be organic. For example, simple motor tics of patients with Tourette syndrome were reported not to have a BP, hence their tics were thought to be produced by a mechanism that differed from that of volitional movement [23,24]. In contrast, abdominal jerks in some patients with apparent propriospinal

myoclonus of the trunk were preceded by a BP. In this case, the jerks were suspected to be psychogenic [25].

Interference between volitional movements and psychogenic tremors or myoclonus

An interference approach is often used to provide evidence that an unusual tremor may have a psychogenic origin [1]. Several groups have pointed out that the frequency of a unilateral organic tremor is unaffected by rhythmic volitional movements of unaffected limbs. In contrast, most unilateral voluntary tremors become entrained by a second volitional rhythm started in another limb. Consequently, the frequency of a psychogenic tremor should change if patients are asked to produce a rhythmic volitional movement of another limb. This argument is similar to that put forwards to differentiate bilateral psychogenic tremors. Consistent with this, McAuley and Rothwell [26] reported that the "coherence entrainment test," in which volitional rhythmic movements such as tapping or waving entrained unilateral psychogenic tremors, occurred in all clinically definite and clinically probable cases of psychogenic dystonic tremors that they studied.

A second method to detect psychogenic tremor (unilateral or bilateral) is to ask subjects to react to a stimulus as fast as possible with an unaffected part of the body. In patients with psychogenic tremor, reaction times are longer than normal and there is a transient interruption of tremor in affected limbs [27,28]. Again it seems likely that such dual task interference is a consequence of the shared motor circuitry in psychogenic and volitional movement.

A final example of the interaction between volitional movement and tremor comes in the special case of voluntarily initiated clonus. An example of this is the tremor at the ankle that it is possible to produce by holding the posture of the leg in a particular position, usually when seated. Although the tremor itself is involuntary, it can be distinguished from true clonus by inspecting its onset: in volitionally initiated clonus, the tremor is preceded by a short period of co-contraction, which is sometimes referred to as the "co-contraction sign" [6].

There are no clear examples of interaction between voluntary movement and myoclonus. Myoclonic jerks are usually sporadic and of short duration, making it impossible to guarantee that a voluntary movement is initiated to coincide with a myoclonic jerk.

Problems with the notion of physiological signatures for pathological or volitional movements

Myoclonus

Pathological jerks are said to have less variability in their timing, duration, and order of muscle jerks than those of a volitional movement. However, physiologists in practice will admit that the dividing line is remarkably murky. In fact, there are few data available to characterize the normal variation in these parameters in either healthy subjects or in people who have organic muscle jerks. The jerks of hyperekplexia and propriospinal myoclonus are frequently variable in onset latency and even in the pattern of muscle recruitment; hence, in practice, it is difficult to distinguish these from volitional jerks.

Tremor

Bilateral organic tremors are usually non-coherent between limbs; however, Raethjen *et al.* [29] reported that that 50% of the individuals they identified with psychogenic tremor had different frequencies in each arm. Based on the model shown in Fig. 28.1, it is possible to argue that highly trained healthy subjects (such as pianists) can maintain different volitional tremor frequencies in each arm, and in this case psychogenic tremors can still be seen to behave as normal voluntary movement. The problem is that it is unlikely that many of the patients with different frequencies of tremor in each arm were trained pianists who could volitionally produce such tremors. It is possible that for some reason they trained themselves to generate such non-coherent tremors before they were diagnosed, or that the "training" occurred subconsciously during the course of tremor. Alternatively, it may be that psychogenic inputs to the voluntary motor system can address different patterns of output to those in volitional effort, as shown in the revised model below (e.g., by employing mechanisms of clonus or physiological tremor).

The bereitschaftspotential

It is probably true to say that identification of a BP, particularly the early BP1, is a good indicator that a movement has some volitional component. However, the converse is not true: absence of a BP is not a guarantee

that a movement is pathological. There are two reasons for this. The first is that the BP is not easy to record, particularly in patients with movement disorders, and, therefore, the possibility of false negatives is high. The second reason is that many volitional movements, such as those made in response to a reaction signal, do not have a clear BP. As an example of the problem, Esposito *et al.* [25] recently examined 20 patients with spinal and/or propriospinal myoclonus and found little correspondence between presence or absence of a BP and suspected psychogenic versus organic jerks. The only positive conclusion that they could make was that the jerks in a number of patients who were thought to have organic jerks were preceded by a BP and hence were likely to be psychogenic. They also used this argument to conclude that a number of patients who were clinically thought to have organic axial muscle jerks may instead have had psychogenic jerks.

Problems with the concept of interference

As with the BP, the concept of interference works well if interference is observed. In this case it is likely that the two movements share some volitional component. However, absence of interference is no guarantee that a tremor or jerk is organic. This is clear from the example of bilateral psychogenic tremors above, which in some cases may be of different frequency in each arm, and from the example of trained musicians, who can play different rhythms in each hand.

Is the model correct?

An important question that is left unanswered by the model outlined in Fig. 28.1, and which is highly relevant to the practical problems discussed above, is whether volitional inputs have access to all parts of the motor circuits, or are there parts that are not usually available to voluntary command and which, therefore, could potentially be addressed only by psychogenic inputs? If we were to assume (as in Fig. 28.1) that volitional inputs can address all motor circuits, then it would be correct that any psychogenic movement could be imitated by a voluntary movement and that psychogenic and volitional movements should interfere with each other if they attempt to address the same circuitry at the same time. However, is it possible for psychogenic inputs to access motor circuits that are either not accessible to volition or are accessible only after intense training (Fig. 28.2)? In this case, psychogenic movements can

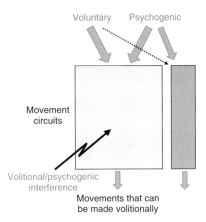

Fig. 28.2. Proposed model to explain why some presumed psychogenic tremors and myoclonus may not interfere with voluntary movement or give rise to a bereitschaftspotential (BP). In this scheme, the movement circuits consist of those that can be accessed easily by volition (light gray) and a subsection that is normally inaccessible to volition (dark gray, dotted line), or which requires intense training before voluntary control is achieved. If a psychogenic movement is produced via activity in the circuits that can be accessed easily by volition, then the movements will behave as in Fig. 28.1 and show a BP, interference, and so on. If psychogenic commands can access the subsection that is normally inaccessible to volition, then they may have no BP and show no interference with voluntary movement.

exist that cannot be mimicked voluntarily and that do not interfere with volitional movement.

The scheme outlined in Fig. 28.2 does not identify the location and nature of the motor circuits that are accessible by psychogenic commands but which cannot be addressed voluntarily. In fact, we might ask why such circuits would exist if they are not normally used in voluntary movement. One possibility is that they are circuits that are usually used in automatic movements such as the anticipatory contractions of postural muscles in the trunk that precede volitional movement of the arm [30,31]. Another is that they are subcircuits of those normally addressed at a higher level by volitional commands. The latter would be equivalent to a radio in which volitional movement accesses circuits by turning a switch on or off, while psychogenic movements, or volitional movements of a highly trained individual, can access subcircuits by removing the back cover to reveal the electronics inside.

The scheme in Fig. 28.2 is also relevant for the problem of the relationship of the BP to psychogenic movement. The logic that a BP should be present in psychogenic movements is correct only if we imagine that the BP is produced by activity within the motor circuits addressed by volitional and psychogenic motor commands. If, however, the BP is produced by activity responsible for the volitional command (i.e., the input arrow), then there may be no BP in a psychogenic movement. Similarly in Fig. 28.2, if the BP is produced by activity in volitional motor circuits then movements produced by the circuits that are not normally accessible by volitional commands will not be accompanied by a BP. The conclusion is that absence of a BP does not mean that an involuntary movement is necessarily organic.

Conclusions

There are presently three main ways in which neurophysiological methods have been used to differentiate psychogenic from organic tremors and myoclonus: unique physiology, the BP, and presence/absence of interference between voluntary and involuntary movement. All of them are based on the scheme outlined in Fig. 28.1, and in all cases, a positive finding is useful. Thus, a tremor or muscle jerk with a unique physiology can be identified as organic whereas presence of a BP or interference with volitional movement can be used to detect a psychogenic movement. Unfortunately, the inverse is not very informative. This is partly because measurements of the BP or of interference effects are difficult and subject to error. However it is also possible that our model (Fig. 28.1) of volitional, psychogenic, and organic varieties of tremor or myoclonus is too simple. Figure 28.2 represents an alternative formulation in which parts of the motor system are not normally accessible to volitional input, or perhaps require long periods of training before coming under voluntary control. It may be that these circuits can be accessed by psychogenic commands, in which case they will fail the usual physiological tests that we use to identify psychogenic movements. They movements may also be perceived as being different to volitional movements and "uncontrollable."

References

1. Hallett M. Physiology of psychogenic movement disorders. *J Clin Neurosci* 2010;**17**:959–965.

2. Shibasaki H, Hallett M. What is the bereitschaftspotential? *Clin Neurophysiol* 2006;**117**:2341–2356.

3. Gerschlager W, Munchau A, Katzenschlager R, *et al.* Natural history and syndromic associations of orthostatic tremor: a review of 41 patients. *Mov Disord* 2004;**19**:788–795.

4. Thompson PD, Rothwell JC, Day BL, *et al.* The physiology of orthostatic tremor. *Arch Neurol* 1986;**43**:584–587.

5. Deuschl G, Toro C, Valls-Sole J, *et al.* Symptomatic and essential palatal tremor. 1. Clinical, physiological and MRI analysis. *Brain* 1994;**117**:775–788.

6. Deuschl G, Koster B, Lucking CH, *et al.* Diagnostic and pathophysiological aspects of psychogenic tremors. *Mov Disord* 1998;**13**:294–302.

7. Deuschl G, Raethjen J, Lindemann M, *et al.* The pathophysiology of tremor. *Muscle Nerve* 2001;**24**:716–735.

8. Munchau A, Schrag A, Chuang C, *et al.* Arm tremor in cervical dystonia differs from essential tremor and can be classified by onset age and spread of symptoms. *Brain* 2001;**124**:1765–1776.

9. Deuschl G. Dystonic tremor. *Rev Neurol* 2003;**159**:900–905.

10. Cassim F, Houdayer E. Neurophysiology of myoclonus. *Neurophysiol Clin* 2006;**36**:281–291.

11. Hallett M, Chadwick D, Marsden CD. Cortical reflex myoclonus. *Neurology* 1979;**29**:1107–1125.

12. Shibasaki H, Hallett M. Electrophysiological studies of myoclonus. *Muscle Nerve* 2005;**31**:157–174.

13. Hallett M, Marsden CD. Ballistic flexion movements of the human thumb. *J Physiol (Lond)* 1979;**294**:33–50.

14. Berardelli A, Rothwell JC, Day BL, *et al.* Duration of the first agonist EMG burst in ballistic arm movements. *Brain Res* 1984;**304**:183–187.

15. Thompson PD, Colebatch JG, Brown P, *et al.* Voluntary stimulus-sensitive jerks and jumps mimicking myoclonus or pathological startle syndromes. *Mov Disord* 1992;**7**:257–262.

16. Brown P, Rothwell JC, Thompson PD, *et al.* The hyperekplexias and their relationship to the normal startle reflex. *Brain* 1991;**114**:1903–1928.

17. Matsumoto J, Fuhr P, Nigro M, *et al.* Physiological abnormalities in hereditary hyperekplexia. *Ann Neurol* 1992;**32**:41–50.

18. Tijssen MA, Voorkamp LM, Padberg GW, *et al.* Startle responses in hereditary hyperekplexia. *Arch Neurol* 1997;**54**:388–393.

19. Brown P, Thompson PD, Rothwell JC, *et al.* Axial myoclonus of propriospinal origin. *Brain* 1991;**114**:197–214.

20. Chokroverty S. Propriospinal myoclonus. *Clin Neurosci* 1995;**3**:219–222.

21. Kinugawa K, Vidailhet M, Clot F, *et al.* Myoclonus-dystonia: an update. *Mov Disord* 2009;**24**:479–489.

22. Roze E, Apartis E, Clot F, *et al.* Myoclonus-dystonia: clinical and electrophysiologic pattern related to SGCE mutations. *Neurology* 2008;**70**:1010–1016.

23. Hallett M. Neurophysiology of tics. *Adv Neurol* 2001;**85**:237–244.

24. Obeso JA, Rothwell JC, Marsden CD. Simple tics in Gilles de la Tourette's syndrome are not prefaced by a normal premovement EEG potential. *J Neurol Neurosurg Psychiatry* 1981;**44**:735–738.

25. Esposito M, Edwards MJ, Bhatia KP, *et al.* Idiopathic spinal myoclonus: a clinical and neurophysiological assessment of a movement disorder of uncertain origin. *Mov Disord* 2009;**24**:2344–2349.

26. McAuley J, Rothwell J. Identification of psychogenic, dystonic, and other organic tremors by a coherence entrainment test. *Mov Disord* 2004;**19**:253–267.

27. Kumru H, Begeman M, Tolosa E, *et al.* Dual task interference in psychogenic tremor. *Mov Disord* 2007;**22**:2077–2082.

28. Kumru H, Valls-Sole J, Valldeoriola F, *et al.* Transient arrest of psychogenic tremor induced by contralateral ballistic movements. *Neurosci Lett* 2004;**370**:135–139.

29. Raethjen J, Kopper F, Govindan RB, *et al.* Two different pathogenetic mechanisms in psychogenic tremor. *Neurology* 2004;**63**:812–815.

30. Forget R, Lamarre Y. Anticipatory postural adjustment in the absence of normal peripheral feedback. *Brain Res* 1990;**508**:176–179.

31. MacKinnon CD, Bissig D, Chiusano J, *et al.* Preparation of anticipatory postural adjustments prior to stepping. *J Neurophysiol* 2007;**97**:4368–4379.

Physiology of psychogenic dystonia

Robert Chen and Alfredo Berardelli

Introduction

Dystonia is a syndrome characterized by sustained muscle contraction, frequently causing twisted postures and repetitive movements. Dystonia has multiple causes. Many genes have been identified as causes of primary dystonia [1]. Dystonia may also be secondary to focal brain lesions, metabolic diseases, or neurodegenerative diseases such as Parkinson's disease. Dystonia may also be classified according to the distribution of symptoms, as focal, segmental, or generalized dystonia. The majority adult-onset focal dystonia has no identifiable cause and is considered idiopathic. It is thought that dystonia in these adults may be caused by a combination of factors such as genetic predisposition and environmental factors such as repeated practice.

Psychogenic dystonia is a common disorder in subspeciality movement disorders clinics. Rapid onset of symptoms and presence of fixed dystonia with painful posturing are common features of psychogenic dystonia, and it is frequently associated with other psychiatric disorders. It often causes considerable disability and is difficult to treat. This chapter will review the pathophysiology of organic dystonia and the recent studies on the pathophysiology of psychogenic dystonia.

Pathophysiology of organic dystonia

Dystonia is associated with physiological changes at multiple levels in the nervous system [2]. At the level of the muscles, electromyographic (EMG) studies have demonstrated co-contraction of agonist and antagonist muscles, and overflow of muscle activities to muscles not required for the performance of the motor task [3]. Moreover, EMG bursts are often prolonged and patients with dystonia may take a longer time to switch

from one complex task to another. These features likely contribute to the slowness and variability of movements seen in dystonia.

Several studies have tested spinal inhibition in dystonia. Reciprocal inhibition measures the normal reciprocal innervation of agonist and antagonist muscles. In the upper limbs, it is often tested by examining how a stimulus to the radial nerve, which innervates the wrist extensor muscles, changes the H-reflex elicited by median nerve stimulation recorded in the flexor carpi radialis muscle. Depending on the time between the conditioning radial nerve stimulus and the median nerve stimulus, three phases of reciprocal inhibition can be identified. The first phase involves glycine-mediated disynaptic inhibition; the second phase results from presynaptic inhibition, but the physiology of the third phase is not known. Previous studies found that spinal reciprocal inhibition is reduced in dystonia and the abnormality is present on both the affected and unaffected sides of patients with focal, task-specific dystonia [4,5]. Another measure of spinal inhibition is the cutaneous EMG silent period (CuSP), which refers to the period of interruption of EMG activity following cutaneous stimulation. One study has shown that the cutaneous silent period is prolonged on both the affected and unaffected sides in patients with brachial dystonia [6].

Inhibition at the brainstem level is also impaired in dystonia. For example, patients with dystonia showed faster blink reflex recovery, consistent with reduced inhibition [7].

Many studies reported cortical abnormalities in dystonia. Paired pulse transcranial magnetic stimulation studies have found reduced short-interval intracortical inhibition, likely mediated by gamma-aminobutyric acid (GABA) $GABA_A$ receptors [8].

Psychogenic Movement Disorders and Other Conversion Disorders, ed. Mark Hallett, Anthony E. Lang, Joseph Jankovic, Stanley Fahn, Peter W. Halligan, Valerie Voon, and C. Robert Cloninger. Published by Cambridge University Press. © Cambridge University Press 2011.

Long-interval intracortical inhibition and the cortical silent period, likely mediated by $GABA_B$ receptors, are also impaired in dystonia [9,10]. Recently, surround inhibition was found to be impaired during movement initiation in patients with focal dystonia [11].

There is also evidence that brain plasticity is abnormal in dystonia. Long-term potentiation, like plasticity induced by a protocol known as paired associative stimulation, was found to be increased in focal dystonia [12,13]. In addition, long-term depression, like plasticity, is also enhanced [13].

In summary, physiological studies in dystonia have found deficient inhibition at multiple levels in the nervous system. This likely correlates with the overactivity of muscles seen in dystonia and may be secondary to abnormalities in the basal ganglia [2]. Excessive plasticity may contribute to the development of dystonia.

Pathophysiology of psychogenic dystonia

The pathophysiology of psychogenic dystonia was first investigated by Espay *et al.* [14]. Ten patients with clinically definite psychogenic dystonia were studied and the findings were compared with eight patients with organic dystonia and 12 age-matched healthy controls. In both patients with organic dystonia and patients with psychogenic dystonia, the short-interval intracortical inhibition was reduced compared with controls both at rest and during muscle contraction. Similarly, there was a trend for reduction of the long-interval intracortical inhibition for both organic and psychogenic dystonia. The cortical silent period was reduced in both organic and psychogenic dystonia. For spinal inhibition, the EMG cutaneous silent period was increased whereas reciprocal inhibition was decreased in both organic and psychogenic dystonia. Therefore, this study largely confirmed the abnormal cortical and spinal inhibitions reported in previous studies in organic dystonia, but showed that patients with psychogenic dystonia also have similar abnormalities.

While the study of Espay *et al.* [14] only examined the affected side of patients with psychogenic or organic dystonia, the study by Avanzino *et al.* [15] examined 12 patients with fixed dystonia on both the affected and unaffected sides and compared the findings in these patients with those in 10 patients with typical dystonia and age-matched controls. Eight of the patients with fixed dystonia fulfilled the diagnostic criteria for probable or clinically definite psychogenic dystonia [16]. It was found that patients with fixed dystonia had reduced short-interval intracortical inhibition and cortical silent period, similar to the findings in patients with typical dystonia. Interestingly, the abnormalities were present on both the clinically affected and unaffected side. Spinal inhibition was not examined in this study.

Quartarone *et al.* [17] used paired associated stimulation to study long-term potentiation-like plasticity in 10 patients with psychogenic dystonia, 10 patients with organic dystonia, and 10 healthy controls. The authors confirmed that short-interval intracortical inhibition was reduced in both groups of patients with dystonia. The interesting finding was that while long-term potentiation-like plasticity was abnormally increased in organic dystonia, as previously reported [12,13], it was normal in psychogenic dystonia.

Interpretations of the studies

The physiological studies in psychogenic or fixed dystonia demonstrated that abnormal cortical and spinal inhibition previously found in patients with organic dystonia are also present in psychogenic dystonia [14,15]. There are several possible interpretations of these findings and they are not mutually exclusive. One possibility is that these physiological changes may be a consequence of maintaining dystonic postures for prolonged periods. Brain plasticity is known to occur in adults in response to manipulations such as transient ischemic nerve block [18,19], amputation [20], and muscle transfer [21]. The finding that subjects with fixed dystonia had reduced cortical inhibition on the unaffected side does not exclude this possibility because physiological changes may occur on the side contralateral to the dystonic posturing.

Another interpretation is that the abnormal inhibition and excitability may represent an endophenotypic trait and these features may predispose the subjects to both organic and psychogenic dystonia. Consistent with this hypothesis is the finding of reduced cortical inhibition in non-manifesting carriers of the gene *DYT1* [22] and subjects with fixed dystonia had reduced cortical inhibition on the unaffected side [15]. However, spinal inhibition was found to be normal in non-manifesting carriers of *DTY1* [22] and it is not known if spinal inhibition is abnormal on the unaffected side of patients with psychogenic dystonia.

The physiological abnormalities in psychogenic dystonia may also represent underlying psychiatric disorders. For example, reduced cortical inhibition has been reported in schizophrenia [23] and Tourette syndrome [24]. However, it is unlikely that abnormal spinal inhibition can be explained by psychiatric disturbance.

The finding of abnormally increased long-term potentiation-like plasticity in organic dystonia but normal plasticity in organic dystonia [17] suggests that excessive long-term potentiation plasticity may be a hallmark of organic dystonia. It is possible that the symptoms of organic dystonia are related to a combination of increased plasticity and reduced inhibition, while in psychogenic dystonia it is related to deficient cortical and spinal inhibition together with other features such as psychological factors.

Conclusions

Patients with psychogenic dystonia have demonstrable physiological abnormalities and the findings in cortical and spinal inhibitory circuits are similar to patients with organic dystonia, but cortical plasticity is increased in organic but not in psychogenic dystonia. Future studies are needed to address the physiological differences between organic and psychogenic dystonia. The findings also raise the question whether therapies aimed at correction of the physiological abnormalities in psychogenic dystonia can be effective in this treatment-resistant condition.

References

1. Muller U. The monogenic primary dystonias. *Brain* 2009;**132**:2005–2025.

2. Berardelli A, Rothwell JC, Hallett M, *et al.* The pathophysiology of primary dystonia. *Brain* 1998;**121**:1195–1212.

3. van der Kamp W, Berardelli A, Rothwell JC, *et al.* Rapid elbow movements in patients with torsion dystonia. *J Neurol Neurosurg Psychiatry* 1989;**52**:1043–1049.

4. Nakashima K, Rothwell JC, Day BL, *et al.* Reciprocal inhibition between forearm muscles in patients with writer's cramp and other occupational cramps, symptomatic hemidystonia and hemiparesis due to stroke. *Brain* 1989;**112**:681–697.

5. Panizza ME, Hallett M, Nilsson J. Reciprocal inhibition in patients with hand cramps. *Neurology* 1989;**39**:85–89.

6. Pullman SL, Ford B, Elibol B, *et al.* Cutaneous electromyographic silent period findings in brachial dystonia. *Neurology* 1996;**46**:503–508.

7. Berardelli A, Rothwell JC, Day BL, Marsden CD. Pathophysiology of blepharospasm and oromandibular dystonia. *Brain* 1985;**108**:593–608.

8. Ridding MC, Sheean G, Rothwell JC, Inzelberg R, Kujirai T. Changes in the balance between motor cortical excitation and inhibition in focal, task specific dystonia. *J Neurol Neurosurg Psychiatry* 1995;**39**:493–498.

9. Chen R, Wassermann EM, Caños M, Hallett M. Impaired inhibition in writer's cramp during voluntary muscle activation. *Neurology* 1997;**49**:1054–1059.

10. Curra A, Romaniello A, Berardelli A, Cruccu G, Manfredi M. Shortened cortical silent period in facial muscles of patients with cranial dystonia. *Neurology* 2000;**54**:130–135.

11. Beck S, Richardson SP, Shamim EA, *et al.* Short intracortical and surround inhibition are selectively reduced during movement initiation in focal hand dystonia. *J Neurosci* 2008;**28**:10363–10369.

12. Quartarone A, Bagnato S, Rizzo V, *et al.* Abnormal associative plasticity of the human motor cortex in writer's cramp. *Brain* 2003;**126**:2586–2596.

13. Weise D, Schramm A, Stefan K, *et al.* The two sides of associative plasticity in writer's cramp. *Brain* 2006;**129**:2709–2721.

14. Espay AJ, Morgante F, Purzner J, *et al.* Cortical and spinal abnormalities in psychogenic dystonia. *Ann Neurol* 2006;**59**:825–834.

15. Avanzino L, Martino D, van de Warrenburg BP, *et al.* Cortical excitability is abnormal in patients with the "fixed dystonia" syndrome. *Mov Disord* 2008;**23**:646–652.

16. Fahn S, Williams DT. Psychogenic dystonia. *Adv Neurol* 1988;**50**:431–455.

17. Quartarone A, Rizzo V, Terranova C, *et al.* Abnormal sensorimotor plasticity in organic but not in psychogenic dystonia. *Brain* 2009;**132**:2871–2877.

18. Ziemann U, Corwell B, Cohen LG. Modulation of plasticity in human motor cortex after forearm ischemic nerve block. *J Neurosci* 1998;**18**:1115–1123.

19. Levy LM, Ziemann U, Chen R, Cohen LG. Rapid modulation of GABA in sensorimotor cortex induced by acute deafferentation. *Ann Neurol* 2002;**52**:755–761.

20. Chen R, Corwell B, Yaseen Z, Hallett M, Cohen LG. Mechanisms of cortical reorganization in lower-limb amputees. *J Neurosci* 1998;**18**:3443–3450.

21. Chen R, Anastakis DJ, Haywood CT, Mikulis DJ, Manktelow RT. Plasticity of the human motor system following muscle reconstruction: a magnetic

stimulation and functional magnetic resonance imaging study. *Clin Neurophysiol* 2003;**114**:2434–2446.

22. Edwards MJ, Huang YZ, Wood NW, Rothwell JC, Bhatia KP. Different patterns of electrophysiological deficits in manifesting and non-manifesting carriers of the *DYT1* gene mutation. *Brain* 2003;**126**:2074–2080.

23. Daskalakis ZJ, Christensen BK, Chen R, *et al.* Evidence for impaired cortical inhibition in schizophrenia using

transcranial magnetic stimulation. *Arch Gen Psychiatry* 2002;**59**:347–354.

24. Ziemann U, Paulus W, Rothenberger A. Decreased motor inhibition in Tourette's disorder: evidence from transcranial magnetic stimulation. *Am J Psychiatry* 1997;**154**:1277–1284.

Chapter

30

Evoked potentials in the assessment of patients with suspected psychogenic sensory symptoms

Alan D. Legatt

Introduction

Sensory evoked potentials (EPs) are the electrical signals produced by the nervous system in response to a sensory input. Evoked potentials to stimulation that is visual (VEP), auditory (AEP), or somatosensory (SEP) are most often employed clinically. They are used to assess the function of the eyes, the ears, and the sensory pathways within the nervous system.

When using EPs for the evaluation of patients with suspected psychogenic sensory symptoms, several questions must be considered: Will EPs always be abnormal in patients with pathology affecting the anatomical substrate for that sensory modality, or can pathology cause abnormal sensory perception without causing EP abnormalities? If the latter is true, normal EPs may not prove that the subjective deficits are psychogenic. If a patient has sensory symptoms that are caused by organic disease but is reporting deficits that are more severe, can EPs detect the psychogenic exaggeration of the symptoms? And, particularly important in a patient who may be malingering, is there anything that a neurologically normal person can do to make the EP results appear to be abnormal? As will be shown, the answers to these questions vary for the different EP modalities.

In order to answer these questions, it is important to understand several aspects of the manner in which EPs are recorded and evaluated. Evoked potential latencies are highly consistent from one subject to another as long as the same recording paradigm is used, whereas EP amplitudes vary considerably among subjects. The latter reflects the fact that many EP components are recorded as near-field potentials, and intersubject differences in brain anatomy and electrode placement can cause substantial variability in the recorded amplitudes.

Also, stimuli for EP recordings are not supramaximal, and a different percentage of the afferent fibers may be activated in different subjects. Therefore, interpretation of EPs is based on component latencies and not on absolute component amplitudes [1]. If pathology blocks the function of a subset of the sensory fibers but the remaining fibers are conducting at normal velocity, the EP may be smaller in amplitude but normal in latency, and therefore it will be interpreted as normal, even though the partial loss of function can cause symptoms.

Evoked potentials are typically recorded by electrodes placed on the scalp and, for SEPs, over peripheral nerves and over the spine. These electrodes also pick up other electrical signals from a variety of sources, such as (1) the electroencephalogram (EEG), representing ongoing electrical activity from the brain that is not related to the response to the sensory input; (2) the electrocardiogram from the heart; (3) electrical signals from muscles near the recording electrodes, the electromyogram (EMG); (4) line frequency artifact (predominantly 60 Hz in the Western hemisphere and 50 Hz elsewhere, or a harmonic thereof) from power lines, fluorescent lights, and leakage currents in equipment; and (5) noise from other sources. Large VEPs elicited by strobe flash stimulation are sometimes visible in the raw EEG as a photic driving response, but VEPs cannot be adequately evaluated in the raw data, and brainstem AEPs (BAEPs) and SEPs are not visible in the raw data from scalp recordings. Signal averaging (Fig. 30.1) is used to extract the EPs from the other electrical signals produced by the recording electrodes. Multiple stimuli are administered and data epochs recorded after each stimulus are averaged together (after artefact rejection to discard those epochs which are contaminated by an unacceptable level of noise).

Psychogenic Movement Disorders and Other Conversion Disorders, ed. Mark Hallett, Anthony E. Lang, Joseph Jankovic, Stanley Fahn, Peter W. Halligan, Valerie Voon, and C. Robert Cloninger. Published by Cambridge University Press. © Cambridge University Press 2011.

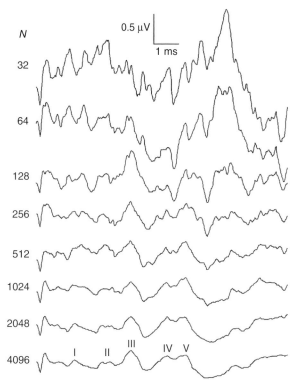

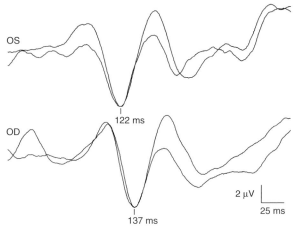

Fig. 30.1. Averaged brainstem auditory evoked potentials (BAEPs) with a progressively increasing number of stimuli in the averages, showing the effect of signal averaging in improving the signal-to-noise ratio. *N* indicates the number of sweeps in the average; the improvement in the signal-to-noise ratio is proportional to the square root of *N*. Right ear stimulation, vertex-to-right mastoid recording. In this and subsequent BAEP figures, positivity at the vertex is plotted as an upward deflection and the roman numerals indicate the component peaks labeled according to the convention of Jewett and Williston [2]. (Modified from Legatt [3].)

Fig. 30.2. Pattern-reversal visual evoked potentials recorded in a 27-year-old woman with multiple sclerosis. She had previously had an attack of optic neuritis in the right eye but her vision had subsequently recovered; at the time of testing her visual acuity was 20/20 in each eye. In this and subsequent figures showing visual evoked potentials, positivity at the occipital electrode, relative to the mastoid reference electrode, is plotted as a downward deflection, and the P100 components are marked with their peak latencies. The latency of the P100 to left eye stimulation is within normal limits, but the P100 to right eye stimulation is abnormally delayed, despite the improvement of the visual acuity in that eye to normal. (Reprinted from Legatt 2003 [3] with permission.)

The EPs, which are consistent from epoch to epoch, are preserved during the averaging process. The noise, which is random with respect to stimulus delivery, is progressively reduced by averaging – the magnitude of the noise in the average is the amount of noise in the raw data divided by the square root of the number of epochs included in the average [3,4]. Thus, the residual noise decreases with continued averaging but never equals zero. Since residual noise could resemble an EP component, averaged EP waveforms should be replicated to confirm that the peaks truly represent an EP [1].

Increasing the number of epochs to further reduce noise becomes impractical after a point. (For example, to cut the residual noise in half, one has to record four times as many epochs. If the average already includes 250 epochs, that would require an additional 750 epochs, giving a total of 1000. Another halving of the residual noise would require 3000 additional epochs, and a further halving would require another 12 000 epochs.) If the raw data are very noisy (e.g., because the patient's muscles are tensed), then the residual noise in the average may be sufficient to block evaluation of the EP, even if the EP itself is normal.

In patients with nervous system pathology, the relationship between that pathology, the sensory EP findings, and the patient's symptoms are complex, depending on the anatomical location of the pathology in relation to the sensory pathways and the manner in which the pathology is affecting neural function. Pathology can cause slowing of conduction in afferent fibers without conduction block, or it can cause loss of afferent signals through conduction block or through actual destruction of neural tissue. Conduction slowing without conduction block, such as might be caused by demyelinating disease, would in general be asymptomatic, since the afferent signals are still reaching the sensory cortex and the patient, therefore, still has sensory perception. This includes imperfect remyelination following an episode of demyelination that did cause symptoms (Fig. 30.2) (i.e., a prior exacerbation that was followed by a remission), as well as subclinical demyelination (demyelination that never reached the degree that caused conduction block and symptoms). The effects of such conduction slowing would also be undetected on routine neurological examination. It is precisely because EPs can detect subclinical demyelination that they have been so useful in the diagnosis of demyelinating disease.

Loss of afferent signals through conduction block or destruction of neural tissue would be correlated with negative sensory symptoms such as numbness. Pathology that caused spontaneous firing of sensory neurons would cause positive symptoms such as paresthesias. If pathology causing spontaneous firing did not at the same time block normal conduction of afferent sensory signals, then it would not alter the EPs.

The activity of a single neuron is too small to be identified at the scalp; the EPs that we record are the summated activity of hundreds or thousands of neurons firing in synchrony. Uniform conduction slowing would lead to prolongation of the EP peak latencies. Non-uniform conduction slowing would cause temporal dispersion, which could make the EPs undetectable despite the persistence of conduction within the sensory pathway. Therefore, the complete absence of an EP peak does not mean that there is no afferent neural activity at the level of its generator, but it does indicate that there is pathology within the afferent sensory pathway.

Brainstem auditory evoked potentials

A transient acoustic stimulus will produce a complex series of AEPs with latencies of up to hundreds of milliseconds. The short-latency AEPs, with latencies of under 10 ms in normal adults, have the greatest clinical utility because they are easy to record and are highly consistent across normal subjects. Although they are not entirely generated within the brainstem, they are commonly called brainstem AEPs. The BAEPs are recorded between the vertex and the earlobes or mastoids, and the positive peaks in the vertex-to-ipsilateral ear waveform are typically shown as upward deflections and are labeled with roman numerals according to the convention of Jewett and Williston [2] (Fig. 30.3). The most clinically useful peaks are waves I, III, and V. Wave I is generated in the distal eighth nerve. Wave III predominantly reflects activity in the lower pons, at the level of the superior olivary complex. Wave V predominantly reflects activity in the mesencephalon, at the

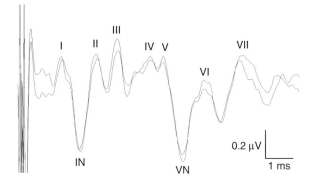

Fig. 30.3. Normal brainstem auditory evoked potentials recorded between the vertex and the right earlobe following right ear stimulation in a 23-year-old woman. Downward traces after waves I and V are labeled IN and VN, respectively. An electrical stimulus artefact appears at the beginning of the tracings. See Fig. 30.1 for plotting method. (Reprinted from Legatt [5])

level of the inferior colliculus [6]. Waves VI and VII have been ascribed to the medial geniculate nucleus and the auditory radiations, respectively. While they may receive contributions from these structures, they also receive contributions from activity at the level of the mesencephalon, which may persist in the presence of more rostral damage [6]. Conversely, waves VI and VII may be absent in normal subjects. Therefore, waves VI and VII do not reliably assess auditory structures rostral to the mesencephalon, and BAEPs can only be used to assess the auditory pathways up through the level of the mesencephalon. A patient with auditory symptoms caused by pathology that is only affecting the auditory pathways rostral to the mesencephalon would have normal BAEPs. Normal BAEPs have been reported in a patient who was completely deaf as the result of bilateral auditory cortex lesions [7].

Ascending auditory projections become bilateral at and above the level of the superior olivary complex, in the lower pons. In a patient with pathology affecting the ear, the eighth nerve, or the cochlear nucleus, BAEP abnormalities will be found with stimulation of the ear ipsilateral to the lesion. With more rostral unilateral lesions within the brainstem, unilateral BAEP abnormalities are most often, although not invariably, present to stimulation of the ear ipsilateral to the lesion [5]. However, the presence of bilateral ascending auditory pathways within the brainstem permits generation of apparently normal BAEPs to stimulation of each ear in the presence of a unilateral brainstem lesion. In addition, there is a functional subset of the brainstem auditory pathways in which the neurons

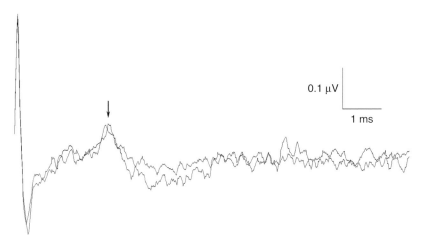

Fig 30.4. Brainstem auditory evoked potentials to left ear stimulation recorded during surgery for a left vestibular schwannoma, showing persistence of wave I (arrow) but absence of waves III and V after transection of the intracranial eighth nerve. The nerve was intentionally sacrificed to permit total resection of the tumor. Vertex to left earlobe recording. See Fig. 30.1 for plotting method. (Modified from Legatt [11])

have morphological and physiological features that minimize temporal dispersion, which is necessary for sound localization, and these are the neurons that generate the BAEPs [8–10]. Pathology affecting the other, more temporally dispersed neuronal subsystem, may not be reflected in the BAEPs. Because of these aspects of auditory system anatomy and physiology, recording of normal BAEPs in a patient with subjective hearing loss in most cases does not rule out the possibility of brainstem pathology. There is one exception to this, however.

Since the ascending brainstem auditory pathways above the lower pons and the projections to auditory cortex are bilateral, unilateral deafness can only result from pathology at the level of the ear, the eighth nerve, or the cochlear nucleus. Complete unilateral deafness implies that no afferent signal reaches the level of cerebral cortex, and, therefore, that there is no outflow from the cochlear nucleus. Wave I may be present if the distal eighth nerve is intact (Fig. 30.4), but waves III and V would be absent. The presence of hearing in the other ear would argue that there are functioning projections from the lower pons to auditory cortex. Therefore, the presence of normal BAEPs (including wave V) to stimulation of one ear would be incompatible with deafness in that ear and would indicate that a reported unilateral deafness in that ear was psychogenic.

Since BAEPs are small (typically less than 1 μV in amplitude), if subjects maintain a degree of tension in their cranial and neck muscles, the EMG activity may be sufficient to obscure the BAEPs. However, patients cannot volitionally make their BAEPs abnormal (i.e., with some components delayed or absent).

Somatosensory evoked potentials

Following electrical stimulation of a mixed peripheral nerve, such as the median nerve in the arm or the posterior tibial nerve in the leg, SEP components generated in peripheral nerve, spinal cord, brainstem (dorsal column nucleus), and cerebral cortex can be recorded [12]. The earliest cortical SEP components, which arise from the earliest activation of primary somatosensory cortex, are named according to their scalp polarity and typical peak latency in normal adult subjects: N20 for median nerve stimulation at the wrist and P37 for posterior tibial nerve stimulation at the ankle. The opposite polarities of these primary cortical SEPs are related to the three-dimensional orientations of their anatomical generators. Longer-latency cortical components show more intrasubject variability and are less useful for routine neurological diagnosis. The spinal cord and brainstem components are not identifiable in all subjects, but when present their latencies can be used to calculate interpeak intervals; these intervals represent conduction times between different levels of the somatosensory pathways and can be used to localize the abnormality when the cortical SEPs are delayed.

In the spinal cord, the somatosensory information ascending to cerebral cortex travels in two anatomically distinct tracts: the spinothalamic tract within the anterior portion of the spinal cord and the dorsal columns within the posterior portion of the spinal cord. Most of the fibers ascending in the dorsal columns are large-diameter, rapidly conducting primary afferent neurons that ascend to the level of the dorsal column nucleus in the lower medulla before synapsing [13]. In contrast, in the spinothalamic tract there is at least one synapse around the level of root entry, which introduces a variable delay. Fiber conduction velocities that are slower and less uniform than those in the dorsal column system lead to further temporal dispersion as well as to later arrival of the afferent activity at somatosensory cortex. Because of the temporal dispersion and the longer latency of the cortical activation, activity in the spinothalamic tract does not contribute to the primary cortical SEP components that are analyzed in a clinical SEP study. Animal studies have shown that these primary cortical SEPs are mediated entirely by the dorsal columns [14]; consequently, clinical SEP studies only assess the dorsal column system [15]. Damage that is confined to the anterior portion of the spinal cord, such as an infarct in the territory of the anterior spinal artery, may leave SEPs intact yet cause major neurological deficits such as paraplegia from corticospinal tract involvement and somatosensory deficits from spinothalamic tract involvement [16–18]. Therefore, recording of normal SEPs in a patient with subjective hypesthesia does not rule out the possibility of pathology affecting the somatosensory system.

However, since the dorsal columns also carry somatosensory information to the brain, normal SEPs imply preservation of dorsal column function and would not be compatible with total anesthesia. Therefore, the presence of normal SEPs in a patient who is reporting total anesthesia in the limb(s) being tested (Fig. 30.5) is an indication that the somatosensory symptoms are not organic.

As is the case with BAEPs, if the subject maintains a degree of muscle tension, the EMG activity may be sufficient to obscure the SEPs. However, patients cannot volitionally make their SEPs abnormal (i.e., with some components delayed or absent).

Visual evoked potentials

Interpretation of VEPs is based on the P100 component, an occiput-positive component with a peak latency of approximately 100 ms that is generated in visual cortex. Longer-latency VEP components exist, but their intersubject variability makes them unsuitable for use in the assessment of a VEP study.

Although VEPs can be elicited by stroboscopic flash stimulation, pattern-reversal stimulation is preferred for clinical VEP testing because it produces VEPs with less intersubject variability than with flash stimulation [19]; the normal range is, therefore, narrower and this increases the sensitivity of the test in detecting demyelinating disease. A black-and-white checkerboard pattern is typically used to elicit VEPs. Checks subtending approximately 30' of visual angle (30 minutes of arc or half a degree) are most often used, but a variety of check sizes (ranging from 10' to 50') can be employed [20] to assess various parts of the retina. Retinal ganglion cells with receptor field dimensions similar to the check sizes are preferentially stimulated – small checks assess central vision and larger checks assess a ring of retina further away from the fovea. Overall, VEPs assess only the central 10° of the visual field [21].

Amplitudes of VEPs vary considerably across subjects because of interindividual differences in the location and orientation of primary visual cortex. A VEP study may be classified as abnormal because of absence of an obligate P100 component, latency prolongation of the P100 component (i.e., compared with latencies

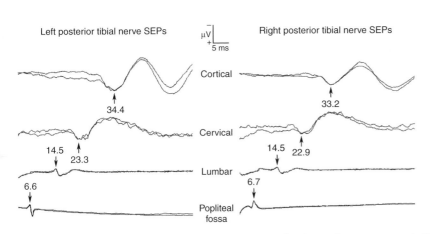

Left posterior tibial nerve SEPs   Right posterior tibial nerve SEPs

Cortical
34.4   33.2
Cervical
14.5   23.3   14.5   22.9
Lumbar
6.6   6.7
Popliteal
fossa

Fig. 30.5. Posterior tibial nerve somatosensory evoked potentials (SEPs) recorded from an 11-year-old girl who reported having repeated episodes of paraplegia and complete anesthesia in the legs; the episodes were suspected to be psychogenic. These posterior tibial nerve SEPs were recorded during one of the episodes, and they were completely normal, despite the fact that the patient reported that she could not feel the stimuli used to elicit the SEPs. Studies of the brain and of the cervical, thoracic, and lumbar spinal cord using MRI were all normal. Voltage calibration of 6 μV for the popliteal fossa waveforms and 1.5 μV for the other waveforms. Positivity is plotted as a downward deflection. The first 2 ms of each waveform was cropped off to remove the stimulus artefact. The numbers next to the arrows are the peak latencies in milliseconds.

in a control population), or because of an abnormally large interocular latency difference even if the absolute P100 latencies are within normal limits bilaterally. Visual stimulation is always delivered to one eye at a time, to permit assessment of the interocular latency differences.

In a patient with a hemianopsia, full-field stimulation may produce a normal-latency VEP that arises from stimulation of the intact hemifield. Other visual field deficits such as quadrantanopsia and sector defects are similarly compatible with a normal VEP, as long as a subset of the visual system capable of generating a normal-latency P100 component is present. If conduction is slowed rather than blocked in a subset of the visual system, this may produce a delayed VEP peak in addition to the normal-latency VEP peak, the latter arising from the unaffected visual neurons. Since a delayed peak might not be distinguishable from a normal secondary VEP component, such a study could also be interpreted as normal because of the presence of a normal-latency primary cortical VEP component. In summary, normal-appearing VEPs can be recorded in patients with disease of the visual system that is producing visual symptoms.

The presence of VEPs is evidence that visual information has reached primary visual cortex and is, therefore, in general incompatible with complete blindness. Rare exceptions are cases in which bilateral posterior hemispheric infarcts effectively disconnect primary visual cortex from the rest of the brain; pattern-reversal VEPs may be present and may even be normal in latency [22,23]. However, this pathology would also be apparent on neuroimaging studies. Rarely, clear pattern-reversal VEPs may also be present in cortically blind children with static encephalopathy, presumably caused by dysfunction which similarly prevents the rest of the brain from accessing information from primary visual cortex [24]. Flash VEPs are less specific and may be present in patients with cerebral lesions in whom pattern-reversal VEPs are absent [25,26]. In the absence of evidence of marked bilateral hemisphere dysfunction, the presence of normal pattern-reversal VEPs is evidence that the information about the visual stimulus has reached visual cortex and has, therefore, has been perceived; this would argue against a severe visual deficit. It has been reported that a visual acuity worse than 20/120 is not compatible with a well-formed VEP [26,27].

Figure 30.6 shows VEPs in a patient whose subjective visual acuity was worse than 20/120. Clear VEPs

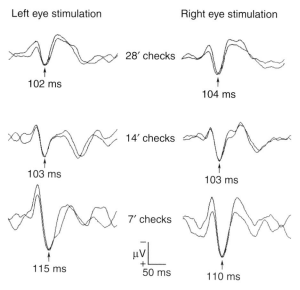

Fig. 30.6. Pattern-reversal visual evoked potentials recorded in a 45-year-old woman with thyroid ophthalmopathy who reported a progressive loss of vision in both eyes. At the time of testing, her visual acuity (on subjective testing) was 20/200 in each eye and this did not improve with pinhole correction. The P100 component latencies (shown) were all normal. The vertical gain was increased for the 7′ check stimulus condition; voltage calibration was 5 μV for the 7′ check stimulus condition and 10 μV for the other stimulus conditions. See Fig. 30.2 for plotting method.

with normal-latency P100 components were recorded to all stimulus conditions, including very small (7′) checks. There is no evidence of dysfunction within the visual system; this study suggests that the patient's reported visual loss is psychogenic. In contrast, VEPs to 14′ check stimulation of the left eye were abnormal in another patient who reported blurred vision in that eye (Fig. 30.7), indicating that he indeed did have dysfunction within the visual system anterior to the optic chiasm (i.e., optic nerve or eye) on the left. However, the presence of clear VEPs to stimulation of the left eye with all check sizes, including very small (7′) checks, suggests that his subjective visual acuity of 20/200 in the left eye most likely exaggerates the degree of true visual compromise.

During recording of pattern-reversal VEPs, the subjects must maintain visual fixation and focus on the screen on which the stimuli are presented. Therefore, by defocusing and by not paying attention to, or maintaining visual fixation on, the stimulus screen, subjects can volitionally make their VEPs abnormal or even absent. This can even be accomplished in a manner that is not apparent to the technologist performing the study [28,29].

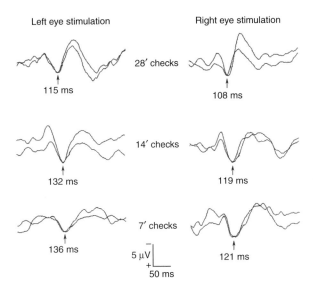

Left eye stimulation   Right eye stimulation

28' checks

115 ms   108 ms

14' checks

132 ms   119 ms

7' checks

136 ms   121 ms

5 μV

50 ms

Fig. 30.7. Pattern-reversal visual evoked potentials (VEPs) recorded in a 35-year-old man who reported blurred vision in the left eye and numbness in his hands and feet. At the time of testing, his visual acuity was 20/200 in the left eye and 20/50 in the right. Clear VEPs were recorded to all stimulus conditions, including very small (7') checks. However, the VEPs to left eye stimulation with 14' checks were abnormal; both the interocular latency difference for the 14' check stimulus condition and the absolute P100 latency to left eye stimulation with 14' checks were abnormally large. The other P100 latencies and interocular latency differences were within normal limits. See Fig. 30.2 for plotting method.

Conclusions

Abnormalities in EPs include delay and absence of components, which would reflect impairment of transmission of afferent signals in the sensory pathways. Measurement of EPs does not directly test for abnormal spontaneous firing of afferent neurons, so positive sensory phenomena (such as paresthesias) could occur without EP changes. However, abnormal spontaneous firing of afferent neurons and impairment of sensory conductions may coexist. For example, a finding of abnormal SEPs would suggest that paresthesias were most likely organic, produced by the same pathology that made the SEPs abnormal.

A sensory EP study may be normal in a patient with subjective complaints in that sensory modality if the pathology only involves part of the afferent pathways, with another part of the afferent pathways generating what appears to be normal EP, or if the pathology involves a part of the sensory system that is not assessed by the EP study. Measurement of BAEPs only assesses the auditory pathways up through the level of the mesencephalon, and SEPs and VEPs only assess

their sensory pathways through the level of primary sensory cortex. Consequently, a finding of normal sensory EPs in general does not prove that the patient's sensory complaints are psychogenic.

There are, however, limited circumstances in which EPs can be used as evidence that the patient's reported sensory deficits are psychogenic. These include (1) a clear BAEP wave V to stimulation of the "deaf" ear in a patient reporting unilateral deafness with good hearing in the other ear; (2) clear cortical SEPs to stimulation of a limb nerve at a time when the patient is reporting complete anesthesia of that limb and inability to perceive the SEP stimulus; and (3) clear pattern-reversal VEPs to stimulation of an eye with a (subjective) visual acuity worse than 20/120, if one can exclude the possibility of extensive bilateral cerebral lesions that could isolate primary visual cortex from the rest of the brain. In these circumstances, if EPs are abnormal (delayed in latency) but still present, they would suggest that there is indeed dysfunction within the sensory pathways but that the patient is exaggerating the degree of the deficit.

In subjects who maintain a high degree of muscle tension during the recording, the raw data may be sufficiently noisy as to preclude recording of interpretable EPs. This would be a technically inadequate study, not an abnormal study. Subjects cannot volitionally make their BAEP or SEP results abnormal. However, they can make pattern-reversal VEPs that appear to be abnormal, and they can do so in a manner that is not apparent to the technologist performing the study.

A finding of abnormal BAEPs or SEPs in a technically adequate study would indicate that there is dysfunction within the auditory or somatosensory pathways, respectively, and would be evidence that the patient's reported sensory deficits are organic rather than psychogenic. Abnormal VEPs should be interpreted more cautiously, since malingerers with normal visual function could volitionally make their VEP study results abnormal.

References

1. American Clinical Neurophysiology Society. Guideline 9A: guidelines on evoked potentials. *J Clin Neurophysiol* 2006;**23**:125–137.

2. Jewett DL, Williston JS. Auditory-evoked far fields averaged from the scalp of humans. *Brain* 1971;**94**:681–696.

3. Legatt AD. Evoked potentials (EPs). In Aminoff MJ, Daroff R, eds. *Encyclopedia of the Neurological Sciences.* San Diego: Elsevier Science, 2003:309–313.

4. Epstein CM, Boor DR. Principles of signal analysis and averaging. *Neurol Clin* 1988;**6**:649–656.

5. Legatt AD. Brainstem auditory evoked potentials: Methodology, interpretation, and clinical application. In Aminoff MJ, ed. *Electrodiagnosis in Clinical Neurology*, 5th edn. New York: Churchill Livingstone, 2005:489–523.

6. Legatt AD, Arezzo JC, Vaughan HG, Jr. The anatomic and physiologic bases of brain stem auditory evoked potentials. *Neurol Clin* 1988;**6**:681–704.

7. Özdamar Ö, Kraus N, Curry F. Auditory brain stem and middle latency responses in a patient with cortical deafness. *Electroencephalogr Clin Neurophysiol* 1982;**53**:224–230.

8. Evans EF, Nelson PG. On the functional relationship between the dorsal and ventral divisions of the cochlear nucleus of the cat. *Exp Brain Res* 1973;**17**:428–442.

9. Hausler R, Levine RA. Brain stem auditory evoked potentials are related to interaural time discrimination in patients with multiple sclerosis. *Brain Res* 1980;**191**:589–594.

10. Trussell LO. Synaptic mechanisms for coding timing in auditory neurons. *Annu Rev Physiol* 1999;**61**:477–496.

11. Legatt AD. Mechanisms of intraoperative brainstem auditory evoked potential changes. *J Clin Neurophysiol* 2002;**19**:396–408.

12. American Clinical Neurophysiology Society. Guideline 9D: guidelines on short-latency somatosensory evoked potentials. *J Clin Neurophysiol* 2006;**23**:168–179.

13. Davidoff RA. The dorsal columns. *Neurology* 1989;**39**:1377–1385.

14. Cusick JF, Myklebust JB, Larson SJ, Sances A, Jr. Spinal cord evaluation by cortical evoked responses. *Arch Neurol* 1979;**36**:140–143.

15. Emerson RG. Anatomic and physiologic bases of posterior tibial nerve somatosensory evoked potentials. *Neurol Clin* 1988;**6**:735–749.

16. Ben-David B, Haller G, Taylor P. Anterior spinal fusion complicated by paraplegia: a case report of a false-negative somatosensory-evoked potential. *Spine* 1987;**12**:536–539.

17. Jones SJ, Buonamassa S, Crockard HA. Two cases of quadriparesis following anterior cervical discectomy, with normal perioperative somatosensory evoked potentials. *J Neurol Neurosurg Psychiatry* 2003;**74**:273–276.

18. Zornow MH, Grafe MR, Tybor C, Swenson MR. Preservation of evoked potentials in a case of anterior spinal artery syndrome. *Electroencephalogr Clin Neurophysiol* 1990;**77**:137–139.

19. Halliday AM, Barrett G, Halliday E, Mushin J. A comparison of the flash and pattern-evoked potential in unilateral optic neuritis. *Wiss Z Ernst-Mortiz-Arndt Univ* 1979;**28**:89–95.

20. American Clinical Neurophysiology Society. Guideline 9B: guidelines on visual evoked potentials. *J Clin Neurophysiol* 2006;**23**:138–156.

21. Celesia GG. Visual evoked potentials in clinical neurology. In Aminoff MJ, ed. *Electrodiagnosis in Clinical Neurology*, 5th edn. New York: Churchill Livingstone, 2005:453–471.

22. Celesia GG, Archer CR, Kuroiwa Y, Goldfader PR. Visual function of the extrageniculo-calcarine system in man. *Arch Neurol* 1980;**37**:704–706.

23. Fera L, Bonito V, Fiorentini E, Ubiali E. VEP and EEG in cortical blindness: a case with a complicated course. *Ital J Neurol Sci* 1990;**11**:617–621.

24. Wygnanski-Jaffe T, Panton CM, Buncic JR, Westall CA. Paradoxical robust visual evoked potentials in young patients with cortical blindness. *Doc Ophthalmol* 2009;**119**:101–107.

25. Hess CW, Meienberg O, Ludin HP. Visual evoked potentials in acute occipital blindness. Diagnostic and prognostic value. *J Neurol* 1982;**227**:193–200.

26. Howard JE, Dorfman LJ. Evoked potentials in hysteria and malingering. *J Clin Neurophysiol* 1986;**3**:39–49.

27. Halliday AM, McDonald WI. Visual evoked potentials. In Stålberg E, Young RR, eds. *Clinical Neurophysiology*. London: Butterworths, 1981:228–258.

28. Tan CT, Murray NM, Sawyers D, Leonard TJ. Deliberate alteration of the visual evoked potential. *J Neurol Neurosurg Psychiatry* 1984;**47**:518–23.

29. Bumgartner J, Epstein CM. Voluntary alteration of visual evoked potentials. *Ann Neurol* 1982;**12**:475–478.

Chapter

31

Characterizing and assessing the spectrum of volition in psychogenic movement disorders

Fatta B. Nahab and Bonnie E. Levin

Introduction

Psychogenic movement disorders (PMDs) represent a constellation of symptoms and signs for which no neurological mechanism can be identified. They may present as any variety of abnormal movement phenomenologies, including tremors, jerks, dystonia, paralysis, or a gait disorder. The physiological mechanisms leading to PMDs are poorly understood, although two features are common. First, PMDs show similar physiological constraints as voluntary movements. These constraints include entrainment (the inability to generate different non-synchronous motor frequencies simultaneously in different limbs), distractibility, and in many cases a movement-related cortical potential. The second common feature among PMD cases is the report by the individual that the movements are involuntary. This apparent contradiction between the appearance of the movement as volitional and the report of the individual with PMD denying control remains a source of study and debate.

The most widely accepted hypothesis to date seeks to consolidate the patient's history of involuntary movements with the physiology by suggesting that PMD patients suffer from somatoform disorders whereby the PMD is taking place without the subject's awareness. The current description of somatoform disorders in the *Diagnostic and Statistics Manual*, 4th edn text revision (DSM-IV-TR) [1] necessitates the experience of physical or organic ailments as a result of underlying psychological or psychiatric dysfunction. The framework underlying these disorders is based on the historic supposition, originating with Freud, that repressed emotions could manifest in more socially acceptable forms as medical illness, and that such disorders had

no underlying structural cause. This viewpoint differed from earlier theories by Hippocrates, who considered such disorders as organic in nature and attributed their occurrence to the abnormal flow of blood in the uterus (since this disorder was thought to only affect women), hence the term hysteria [2].

Treatment of the underlying psychological cause (i.e., often presumed to be traumatic in origin) is hypothesized to result in resolution of the PMD [3–5]. This chapter discusses the role of volition and methods that may help to characterize the level of volition in patients with PMD.

The somatoform disorders include somatization, conversion, factitious, pain, hypochondriasis, and body dysmorphic disorders [1], representing various theoretical levels of awareness on the part of the patient, which are nearly impossible for the clinician to ascertain. Conversion disorder, by definition, requires that "the symptom or deficit is not intentionally produced or feigned," whereas DSM criteria for factitious disorder describe "the intentional production or feigning of physical or psychological symptoms or signs," usually for the purpose of gaining the attention, sympathy, or leniency of a family member or care provider [1]. A discussion of malingering, or illness deception, is also traditionally included among these various diagnoses even though it is not officially classified as a disorder in the DSM. The secondary goal of malingering is more tangible than in factitious disorder, and may include gaining formal disability status or receiving financial benefits through various means. Recently, however, both the utility and validity of this diagnostic entity in explaining the physiological mechanisms underlying PMD has been questioned [6,7]. Despite the potential

Psychogenic Movement Disorders and Other Conversion Disorders, ed. Mark Hallett, Anthony E. Lang, Joseph Jankovic, Stanley Fahn, Peter W. Halligan, Valerie Voon, and C. Robert Cloninger. Published by Cambridge University Press. © Cambridge University Press 2011.

clinical implications and the probable controversy, there is no clear research utility for differentiating the type of gain in the setting of deception (factitious versus malingering); therefore, the exclusion of both populations is strongly recommended in studies of PMD physiology [8].

Before proceeding, it is essential to define what is meant by "spectrum of volition." Although neuroscience continues to delve into the meaning and physiological mechanisms of free will and self-agency, our current understanding of this spectrum extends from a complete lack of will or agency to the opposite extreme of free will. In the setting of PMDs, abnormal movements can be thought of as originating either unconsciously without the subject's awareness or consciously with full intention, accepting that intermediate gray areas may exist in between the ends of the spectrum. A similar spectrum can be found in neurological disorders, where, for example, an individual may experience a total lack of volition when experiencing a partial seizure, with a complete inability to control or suppress the event. Conversely, a feigned disorder such as Munchausen is consciously mediated with the explicit intent to deceive for gain. Disorders representing incomplete volition include Tourette syndrome and early Huntington's disease, whereby affected individuals may report having the ability to partially control or suppress their tics or chorea, respectively [9].

Demographics of psychogenic movement disorders and their causes

Studies examining the demographics of patients with PMD highlight the broad age range (10–83 years; mean, 50) at symptom onset and slightly larger proportion of female (61%) to male cases [10]. Estimates of the prevalence of PMDs in clinical settings have not been well characterized and remain a subject of controversy: 20% of patients seen in outpatient neurology clinics have unexplained symptoms [11], 16% with functional and psychogenic symptoms [12], while psychogenic symptoms represent 5% of all inpatient neurology admissions [13]. Of 198 first-time referrals to a neurology service over a 3-month period, 69 (35%) fulfilled DSM IV-TR criteria for somatoform disorders [14]. Although 2% of patients seen in neurological practice are diagnosed with a conversion disorder [15,16], clinicians are justifiably concerned about the potential for misdiagnosis, its impact on the physician–patient relationship, and the fear of stigmatization for their

patients. Stone and colleagues reviewed the rate of "misdiagnosis" of patients who were first diagnosed with conversion disorder since the 1950s [17] and found an overall misdiagnosis rate of 8.4%, with a reduction to 4% since the 1970s. This finding suggests that overdiagnosis may not be a problem. Furthermore, there is little need for the clinician to perform exhaustive unnecessary testing for fear of missing an alternative diagnosis. Despite the high frequency of conversion disorder in non-psychiatric patients, no information is known about the comparative prevalences of conversion disorder, factitious disorder, and malingering in cases of PMD, since most if not all cases are assumed to be conversion by default.

Lacking in most discussions of the epidemiology of PMDs is the acknowledgement that a small but significant number of cases may be those of frank illness deception or feigning. There is little debate that humans have evolutionarily evolved the ability to deceive; it has been suggested that the average individual may lie as much as twice daily, or in one-quarter of interactions with others [18]. Little is known or has been studied regarding rates of illness deception. Anecdotal studies of the prevalence of malingering have estimated 1–8% of all medical cases [19,20]. Such estimates are, however, confounded by the clinician's own subjective perceptions and biases of illness deception, and a lack of any objective measures.

The challenges

Our understanding of the causes of PMD remains limited, with no cohesive framework that combines physiology with behavior and intention. We know that patients report their PMDs to be involuntary, despite demonstrating similar physiological constraints to voluntary movement. Little is also known about the relative prevalence of conversion disorder, factitious disorder, and malingering in PMDs, although the majority of cases are assumed to be conversion reactions. The development of objective methods to characterize the level of volition experienced by the subject is critical to the advancement of PMD research and for the clinician, and would help to prevent unnecessary testing, procedures, and delays in the time to treatment. One potential place to begin this process is by developing the means to detect and exclude cases of feigning.

No validated objective methods currently exist to detect illness deception. Currently, the frontline of illness detection remains the clinician. This notion of the clinician "lie-detector" is, however, fraught with problems. The principal limitation is that humans are poor at detecting deception and generally have a truth bias [21]. Furthermore, truth is typically assessed based on irrelevant factors such as personality and appearance. According to Ekman and O'Sullivan [22], this limitation is in part because we lack a refined idea of what a successful lie looks and sounds like, since we almost never receive feedback on the ones that we have been told. Our ability to build an internal model of deception is further constrained by the fact that "The best lies go undetected…' [23]. Despite the clinician's additional experience and examination skills, studies have also shown their ability to identify a lie was no better than chance [22].

Potential solutions

The interest in developing methods to reliably detect deception is common to our human history. Gaining the ability to characterize the spectrum of volition in PMDs is simply a new application of the age-old dilemma. Little is known about the prevalence of feigning in PMDs, with only rare reports in the literature documenting proven illness deception [24]. Based on this lack of data, the bulk of the research reviewed here comes from other fields, including forensics, law, and military intelligence. Many strategies have been used to detect deception. Some of the methods that have been developed include the polygraph, gesture or voice stress analysis, cognitive chronometry or reaction time measures, functional neuroimaging, and neuropsychological profiling. Most methods are based on the principle that deception requires a greater cognitive demand and may induce a cognitive or autonomic stress response. Contrary to the common perception, however, there is likely no unique signature associated with deception. This is underscored by the general inadmissibility of these methods as evidence in court and the conclusion by the National Academy of Sciences review, describing the data supporting the use of polygraph as "scant and scientifically weak" [25].

The use of methods such as functional magnetic resonance imaging (fMRI) may provide a more direct and reliable means of detecting deception compared with the previous methods that evaluate the downstream signal of the autonomic nervous system rather than the brain itself. Since the initial work by Spence *et al.* [26], there have been over 60 publications on the use of fMRI for lie detection (see [27–31] for selected examples). Findings to date have consistently shown preferential involvement of the prefrontal cortices while subjects are engaged in lying. Other regions showing greater activations during lying include the anterior cingulate, hippocampus, and the lingual gyrus. In general, lie conditions also lead to greater activations than truth, confirming the idea that lying is more cognitively demanding. Despite the promise of this new technology, there remain substantial limitations to the use of fMRI lie detection in clinical populations or otherwise. Most studies to date have not utilized ecologically valid paradigms, instead concentrating on standard forensics-based paradigms such as the Guilty Knowledge Test or by using mock crimes. The test's reliability is also currently limited, with the majority of studies demonstrating adequate sensitivity only when averaging across multiple trials and individuals. These methodological problems make it difficult to generalize outside the laboratory setting, but even if these limitations are addressed, it is still not clear how subjects with conversion disorder or self-deception differ from those with feigned illness, since inter- and intrasubject levels of awareness most likely vary over time. Finally, there remain substantial ethical concerns regarding informed consent, the legal sequelae of uncovering deception, and the ramifications for the subject, the clinician, and the researcher. Despite the promise, much work remains before this technology gains wide acceptance and use outside of research.

In contrast to the more conventional lie detection methods, the use of neuropsychological testing to assess credibility is well established. There is a sizable literature on the neuropsychological detection of feigned disorders. However, the research in this area is complex, often because it may not be possible to make clear-cut distinctions between malingering (conscious intent) and conversion disorder (lacking conscious intent). Recognizing this limitation is important since these labels are not necessarily mutually exclusive entities, with some individuals exaggerating true neurological problems [32]. In addition, demographic factors such as low educational level, ethnicity, and advanced age may impact test performance and must be taken into account in an evaluation of deception.

While there is little agreement as to which measures are most sensitive in detecting either an unconscious or a conscious attempt to deceive, there is general consensus that the best approach incorporates multiple methods. A carefully selected battery of core neuropsychological measures examining a wide range of neuropsychological abilities is necessary to test an individual's cognitive level as well as provide a metric from which to assess intraindividual consistency within and between each cognitive domain. In addition, a direct assessment of effort and response bias and a personality screen are also important. Test scores used alone are, however, often inadequate and there are times when the most useful information comes from a detailed assessment of background information, including the patient's history, and a comprehensive face-to-face interview.

There is a sound rationale for not relying solely on test scores to assess feigning. First, the detection of feigning often depends on the consistency and congruency between the neuropsychological test scores, the client's emotional presentation while relating subjective symptoms and pertinent background information, the client's motivational status, and the evidence from mood and/or personality tests. Second, it has been shown that the inclusion of collateral sources of information such as historical information improves the validity of clinical judgments that involve malingering [33]. Third, it can no longer be assumed that the subject is naive with regard to the testing material and the effects of neurological disease or brain injury on behavior. The easy access to select tests and literature on the Internet, describing classic neurological presentations of various conditions, has provided a rich resource for individuals who may be seeking secondary gain. This is particularly true for forensic cases, where attorneys will try and learn as much as possible about the neuropsychological examination [34]. In some US states, attorneys will petition the court to allow a third party (e.g., the attorney, a court reporter, or videographer) to sit in and record the neuropsychological evaluation being carried out on their client. This has been raised as a concern regarding the potential for attorneys to directly impact the evaluation process through either suggestion or frank coaching [35]. Both kinds of interference can invalidate the test findings, but the latter situation is particularly problematic for clinicians and scientists who rely on an open exchange of information pertaining to research methods and interpretation of test findings [36,37].

The types of measure used by neuropsychologists to assess feigning can generally be subdivided into two categories: questionnaires designed to assess symptom magnification and those that directly assess test-taking performance [38]. While a description of each measure and its psychometric properties is beyond the scope of

this review, it is important to select those measures that are considered to have both high sensitivity (able to detect feigning) and high specificity (yield few false positives). A recent survey of neuropsychologists [39] indicated that the five most frequently used measures to assess suboptimal effort were the Test of Memory and Malingering (TOMM), Minnesota Multiphasic Personality Inventory (MMPI-2) F-K ratio, MMPI-2 FBS, Rey-15 item test, and the California Verbal Learning Test (CVLT). Of interest, the tests rated most accurate in actually detecting response bias or reduced effort were the TOMM, Validity Indicator Profile, Victoria Symptom Validity Test, and the Computerized Assessment of Response Bias.

One approach commonly used to assess response bias is symptom validity testing, a term introduced by Pankratz [40] to refer to a technique that involves examining the specific complaint reported by the patient. The most frequent mental status complaint is memory impairment, but this technique can be applied to most symptoms. Some symptoms involving sensory and perceptual complaints do not necessarily require formal testing. When tests are required to formally evaluate a problem, many examiners prefer to use a forced choice paradigm, requiring the subject to make a decision between two options. This paradigm minimizes any opportunity to vacillate or provide "don't know" responses. By chance alone, at least 50% of the responses should be correct; scores lower than 50% raise the possibility of a subject actively avoiding the correct response. Furthermore, some forced choice tests use material that is easily recalled, where healthy normals are expected to perform close to 100%. In this situation, scores lower than 85% may indicate feigning. This approach may be particularly useful with patients presenting with movement disorder complaints.

With the above caveats in mind, we prospectively studied eight subjects with probable, clinically established, or documented PMDs based on the established Fahn and Williams criteria [41]. None of the subjects was known to have medical, legal, or financial claims pending. The goal of this study was to determine whether neuropsychological profile testing (NPT) could identify performance inconsistencies suggesting a volitional etiology to the PMD and providing corroborative evidence to the findings on neurological examination. All subjects underwent a complete neurological evaluation by a movement disorder neurologist in addition to an extensive NPT battery. The NPT battery was designed to sample a range

Table 31.1 Neuropsychological test battery administered to assess multiple cognitive domains, in addition to motivation, deception, and personality

Cognitive domain	Neuropsychological tests utilized
Premorbid functioning	North American Adult Reading Test (NAART)
Mental status	Mini-Mental State Examination (MMSE)
General fund of knowledge	WAIS-III Information
Language	Boston Naming Test (BNT) Controlled Oral Word Association Test (COWAT) Animal Fluency WAIS-III: Arithmetic, Similarities Shipley Institute of Living Scale (SHIP): Vocabulary
Memory	California Verbal Learning Test, 2nd edition (CVLT-II) Wechsler Memory Scales, 3rd edition (WMS-III): Logical Memory (LM), Verbal Paired Associates (VPA), Visual Reproduction (VR)
Visuospatial skills	WAIS-III: Block Design Rey Complex Figure Test (RCFT) Hooper Visual Orientation Test (HVOT) Judgment of Line Orientation (JLO)
Attention and executive function	WAIS-III: Digit Span Shipley Institute of Living Scale (SHIP): Abstraction Design Fluency- Fixed Response Condition Stroop Color-Word Test Trail Making Test (TMT) Wisconsin Card Sorting Test (WCST)
Fine motor skill	Grooved Pegboard Test
Motivation and malingering	Test of Memory Malingering, 2nd edition (TOMM-2) Rey 15-Item Test
Mood and affect	Beck Depression Inventory, 2nd edition (BDI-II) Beck Anxiety Inventory (BAI)
Personality inventory	Minnesota Multiphasic Personality Inventory, 2nd edition (MMPI-2)

WAIS-III, Wechsler Adult Intelligence Scale, 3rd edition.

of neuropsychological abilities including an estimate of premorbid function, general fund of knowledge, select language skills (word retrieval and verbal fluency), verbal learning and memory, visuospatial functions (visuospatial perception and visuoconstruction), fine motor skills (dominant and non-dominant hand), attention, executive functions, effort and malingering, mood, and a personality screen. Table 31.1 summarizes the tests used for each cognitive domain. Each individual was also given a formal comprehensive interview, including a detailed history, a description of current complaints and pertinent background information.

The study showed impaired motor performance across the group in both the symptomatic and unaffected limbs (see Fig. 31.1). Of note, all subjects showed normal performance on select challenging tasks such as Shipley Institute of Living Scale Abstraction scale and the Wechsler Adult Intelligence Scale (WAIS) III similarities subtests. Two subjects (S2 and S8) had performance profiles suggestive of feigning. In each case, the TOMM was below expectancy, suggesting intentional poor effort. These same two subjects showed consistently poor performance across tests of various domains and difficulties. These subjects had the lowest total scores on the Mini-Mental State Examination, scoring below dementia cutoffs (< 26), and disproportionately worse than the remaining subjects on the WAIS Arithmetic, Block Design, and Digit Span subtests; the

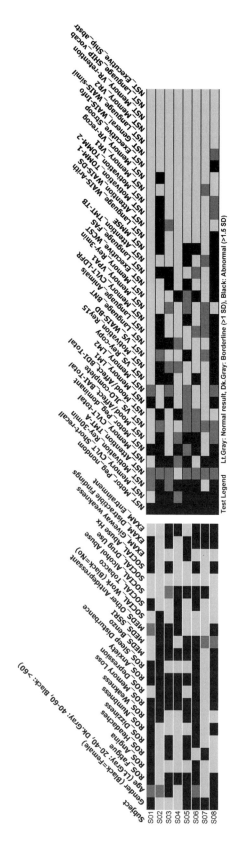

Fig. 31.1. Summary of individual clinical and neuropsychological profiles for patients with pyschogenic movement disorders. Clinical profiles provide demographic information, symptom complaints (ROS), medication history (MEDS), work history, substance abuse history (SOCIAL), and relevant neurological examination findings (EXAM). The neuropsychological profile (NST) lists test performance in ascending order of performance (worst to best) (see Table 31.1 for more details of the assessment tools used). Two patients (S2 and S8) demonstrated poor yet incongruent performance across a broad spectrum of tests, while demonstrating intact higher cognitive functions including abstraction, visuospatial memory, and verbal paired association.

Boston Naming Test; Animal Fluency; and subtests of the CVLT. However, in each case, the subject exhibited wide variability within and between individual subtests. For example, both subjects failed easier problems while successfully completing more difficult items and showed contradictory performance between tests measuring similar cognitive domains. As stated above, neither subject had any outstanding claims to differentiate them from the remainder of the group, although S2 did have long-standing permanent disability status for this disorder. These preliminary results emphasize the need to assess patients with PMD across multiple clinical and neuropsychological domains, since individual tests lack adequate sensitivity and specificity to characterize the level of volition in a particular individual. The use of NPT routinely for evaluation of PMD has been limited so far, likely because of the time and effort required on the part of both the patient and the psychologist, as well as the limited coverage of such testing by insurers and health systems. However, the information gained can provide a significant cost saving in uncertain cases as additional costly neuroimaging, laboratory studies, and physiological testing can be minimized.

Conclusions

The PMDs comprise a diverse set of neurological symptoms and signs. The physiological basis for PMD remains poorly understood, with patients reporting involuntary movements despite these movements exhibiting similar constraints to voluntary movement. The association of PMDs with the somatoform disorders emphasizes the spectrum of volition or awareness that different individuals may have, spanning from conversion disorder to frank malingering. Further epidemiological research is needed to measure the comparative prevalences of conversion disorder and feigned illness in the setting of PMDs. The development of objective methods to characterize the level of volition experienced by the subject for the purpose of excluding confounding cases of illness deception is critical to the advancement of PMD research. A wide assortment of objective measures may be implemented to assess volition and identify feigned illness, with neuropsychological testing and functional neuroimaging showing the greatest promise. Further work is needed to test the validity of such testing in the setting of PMDs; however this approach has the potential to reduce the heterogeneity in PMD research, which poses a significant problem, leading to inconsistent findings and limiting the ability to identify novel physiological impairments in this disorder. The use of objective measures to characterize volition thus offers the potential to make an earlier diagnosis, minimize unnecessary testing, minimize treatment delays, and improve overall outcomes.

References

1. American Psychiatric Association. *Diagnostic and Statistical Manual of Diseases*, 4th edn, text revision. Washington DC: American Psychiatric Press, 2000.

2. Halligan PW, Bass C, Oakley DA (eds.). *Malingering and Illness Deception*: Oxford: Oxford University Press, 2003.

3. Hinson VK, Weinstein S, Bernard B, Leurgans SE, Goetz CG. Single-blind clinical trial of psychotherapy for treatment of psychogenic movement disorders. *Parkinsonism Relat Disord* 2005;**12**:177–180.

4. Thomas M, Jankovic J. Psychogenic movement disorders: diagnosis and management. *CNS Drugs* 2004;**18**:437–452.

5. Williams DT, Ford B, Fahn S. Treatment issues in psychogenic-neuropsychiatric movement disorders. *Adv Neurol* 2005;**96**:350–363.

6. Stone J, LaFrance WC, Levenson JL, Sharpe M. Issues for DSM-5: conversion disorder. *Am J Psychiatry* 2010;**167**:626–627.

7. Nicholson TR, Stone J, Kanaan RA. Conversion disorder: a problematic diagnosis. *J Neurol Neurosurg Psychiatry* 2010; E-pub ahead of print.

8. Bass C, Halligan PW. Illness-related deception: social or psychiatric problem? *J R Soc Med* 2007;**100**:81–84.

9. Hallett M. Volitional control of movement: the physiology of free will. *Clin Neurophysiol* 2007;**118**:1179–1192.

10. Mendoza-Rodriguez A, Riveira-Rodriguez C, Castrillo-Sanz A. Psychogenic movement disorders. *Rev Neurol* 2009;**48**:S49–S55.

11. Mace CJ, Trimble MR. "Hysteria," "functional" or "psychogenic"? A survey of British neurologists' preferences. *J R Soc Med* 1991;**84**:471–475.

12. Stone J, Carson A, Duncan R, *et al.* Who is referred to neurology clinics? The diagnoses made in 3781 new patients. *Clin Neurol Neurosurg* 2010;**112**:747–751.

13. Lempert T, Dieterich M, Huppert D, Brandt T. Psychogenic disorders in neurology: frequency and clinical spectrum. *Acta Neurol Scand* 1990;**82**:335–340.

14. Fink P, Steen Hansen M, Sondergaard L. Somatoform disorders among first-time referrals to a neurology service. *Psychosomatics* 2005;**46**:540–548.

15. Binzer M, Kullgren G. Motor conversion disorder. A prospective 2- to 5-year follow-up study. *Psychosomatics* 1998;**39**:519–527.

16. Ron MA. Somatisation in neurological practice. *J Neurol Neurosurg Psychiatry* 1994;**57**:1161–1164.

17. Stone J, Smyth R, Carson A, *et al.* Systematic review of misdiagnosis of conversion symptoms and "hysteria." *BMJ* 2005;**331**:989.

18. DePaulo BM, Kashy DA, Kirkendol SE, Wyer MM, Epstein JA. Lying in everyday life. *J Pers Soc Psychol* 1996;**70**:979–995.

19. Mittenberg W, Patton C, Canyock EM, Condit DC. Base rates of malingering and symptom exaggeration. *J Clin Exp Neuropsychol* 2002;**24**:1094–1102.

20. Keiser L. *The Traumatic Neurosis*. Philadelphia, PA: Lippincott, 1968.

21. Vrij A. *Detecting Lies and Deceit: The Psychology of Lying and Implications for Professional Practice*. Chichester, UK: John Wiley, 2000.

22. Ekman P, O' Sullivan M. Who can catch a liar? *Am Psychologist* 1991;**46**:913–920.

23. Talbot M. Duped: can brain scans uncover lies? *New Yorker* 2007; July 2.

24. Kurlan R, Brin MF, Fahn S. Movement disorder in reflex sympathetic dystrophy: a case proven to be psychogenic by surveillance video monitoring. *Mov Disord* 1997;**12**:243–245.

25. Board on Behavioral Cognitive, and Sensory Sciences and Education and Committee on National Statistics. The Polygraph and Lie Detection. Washington, DC: National Academies Press, 2003.

26. Spence SA, Farrow TF, Herford AE, *et al.* Behavioural and functional anatomical correlates of deception in humans. *Neuroreport* 2001;**12**:2849–2853.

27. Gamer M, Bauermann T, Stoeter P, Vossel G. Covariations among fMRI, skin conductance, and behavioral data during processing of concealed information. *Hum Brain Mapp* 2007;**28**:1287–1301.

28. Kozel FA, Johnson KA, Mu Q, *et al.* Detecting deception using functional magnetic resonance imaging. *Biol Psychiatry* 2005;**58**:605–613.

29. Langleben DD, Loughead JW, Bilker WB, *et al.* Telling truth from lie in individual subjects with fast event-related fMRI. *Hum Brain Mapp* 2005;**26**:262–272.

30. Mohamed FB, Faro SH, Gordon NJ, *et al.* Brain mapping of deception and truth telling about an ecologically valid situation: functional MR imaging and polygraph investigation: initial experience. *Radiology* 2006;**238**:679–688.

31. Priori A, Mameli F, Cogiamanian F, *et al.* Lie-specific involvement of dorsolateral prefrontal cortex in deception. *Cereb Cortex* 2008;**18**:451–455.

32. Lezak MD, Loring DW, Howieson DB, Howieson D, Hannay HJ (eds.). *Neuropsychological Assessment*. Oxford: Oxford University Press, 2004.

33. Garb HN, Schramke CJ. Judgement research and neuropsychological assessment: a narrative review and meta-analyses. *Psychol Bull* 1996;**120**:140–153.

34. Miller RD. Hidden agendas at the law-psychiatry interface. *J Psychiatry Law* 1990;**18**:35–58.

35. Pope KS, Butcher JN, Seelen J. *The MMPI, MMPI-2 and MMPI-A in Court: A Practical Guide for Expert Witnesses and Attorneys,* 3rd edn. Washington, DC: American Psychological Association, 2006.

36. Ben-Porath YS, McCully E, Almagor M. Incremental validity of the MMPI-2 content scales in the assessment of personality and psychopathology by self-report. *J Pers Assess* 1993;**61**:557–575.

37. Berry DTR, Lamb DG, Wetter MW, Baer RA, Widiger TA. Ethical considerations in research on coached malingering. *Psychol Assess* 1994;**6**:16–17.

38. Borckardt JJ, Engum ES, Lambert EW, *et al.* Use of the CBDI to detect malingering when malingerers do their "homework." *Arch Clin Neuropsychol* 2003;**18**:57–69.

39. Sharland MJ, Gfeller JD. A survey of neuropsychologists' beliefs and practices with respect to the assessment of effort. *Arch Clin Neuropsychol* 2007;**22**:213–223.

40. Pankratz L. Symptom validity testing and symptom retraining: procedures for the assessment and treatment of functional sensory deficits. *J Consult Clin Psychol* 1979;**47**:409–410.

41. Fahn S, Williams DT. Psychogenic dystonia. *Adv Neurol* 1988;**50**:431–455.

Rating scales for psychogenic movement disorders

Christopher G. Goetz and Vanessa K. Hinson

Introduction

Psychogenic movement disorders (PMDs) can mimic the full spectrum of traditional structure-based or known chemical-based disorders [1]. They can affect normal motor function and influence specific and global activities [2]. In addition, some PMDs have distinctive movement patterns that are not typical of other disorders [3]. As a clearer understanding of PMDs emerges and treatment strategies is developed, it is important to have assessment tools to rate these movements, both in terms of their objective severity (impairment) and their impact on function (disability). Three complementary approaches can be utilized. First, scales that are adapted from other movement disorders can be applied to PMDs when the cohort studied has one type of phenomenology. This approach, however, is problematic for rating severity when different patients have different types of disorder or when individual patients have more than one type of PMD at the same time. A second approach is the use of global scales that do not monitor movement disorders individually but consider an overall severity or change score. The third option is the use of the Psychogenic Movement Disorder Rating Scale, which considers numerous movement disorder types, rates their severity, duration, and resultant impact on function and provides a single score based on objective observation.

This chapter considers strategies to evaluate and monitor the motor elements of PMDs. It does not consider the issue of the diagnostic criteria, which is treated elsewhere in this book [1–3]. Further, it does not consider the assessment methods of rating psychopathologies underlying the movements nor psychiatric comorbidities [2]. A number of physiological tests have been applied to the evaluation of psychogenic tremor, myoclonus, and other movements, but these are not considered because they are utilized as the basis for diagnosis rather than tools to assess movement impairment or disability [4].

Rating scales in psychogenic movement disorders

Given the wide array of movement disorders described under the term PMDs, descriptive categorization based on phenomenology of movements is usually implicit to reported cases or cohorts. These descriptive categorizations can help clinicians and researchers in the choice of an appropriate rating tool to assess the movement disorder severity. Reports of PMDs anchor themselves first in the standard definitions of movement disorders, including tremor, chorea, myoclonus, tics, and parkinsonism [2]. Within neurological nosology, these terms are adequately defined in textbook sources and accepted, although no free-standing phenomenology glossary has been established by such international bodies as the Movement Disorder Society (MDS). Further, in spite of accepted definitions of the various types of involuntary movement, these designations are based on movements seen in non-psychogenic conditions; consequently when the focus changes to PMDs, such definitions cannot be assumed to be automatically applicable. Further, because the movements in PMDs are often mixed in character and distinctive in themselves, some may be difficult to place firmly into a given category of movement impairment [3]. In this context, many reports of PMDs are accompanied with video or other pictorial demonstration in journals such as *Movement Disorders* [5,6]. All these issues are important considerations when a clinician or researcher chooses a rating measure to assess the severity of a PMD.

Psychogenic Movement Disorders and Other Conversion Disorders, ed. Mark Hallett, Anthony E. Lang, Joseph Jankovic, Stanley Fahn, Peter W. Halligan, Valerie Voon, and C. Robert Cloninger. Published by Cambridge University Press. © Cambridge University Press 2011.

Many scales have been developed to assess the major movement disorders, including parkinsonism, dyskinesia, tics, dystonia, and myoclonus. These instruments are often disease specific (e.g., Parkinson's disease), but sometimes, they focus on the primary phenomenology (e.g., tremor). They have been largely developed based on expert opinion, been introduced into the scientific community by authorities, and tested clinimetrically thereafter. Disease-specific scales have been utilized in other disorders that share clinical features with the core illness, for example the application of the Unified Parkinson's Disease Rating Scale (UPDRS) to patients with progressive supranuclear palsy [7,8]. In such cases, the clinimetric profile of the scale needs additional definition for the new target disorder, because reliability, validity, and factor structures of a given scale cannot be presumed to be similar when the scale is applied to new conditions.

The rating of PMDs is particularly complex, because the movements encountered fall into many possible phenomenological categories and, therefore, multiple rating scales of this type might need to be applied. This section first reviews scales that can be used to assess severity of different types of movement disorder and have been clinimetrically tested in well-defined movement disorder populations. They have the potential for serving as rating tools in PMDs as well but have not been studied clinimetrically in this group of disorders. Individual scales could be applied and tested in cohorts of patients with PMDs and a given type of psychogenic symptom, tremor, myoclonus, tics, and so on. When the cohort includes different types of movement, different scales would need to be applied, limiting statistical analyses of group effects. A second approach for rating PMDs would be to ignore the individual movements themselves and simply rate the global severity of the movements. The second section of this chapter summarizes scales that could be used in this context. Finally, the Psychogenic Movement Disorder Rating Scale (PMDRS) [9] is presented as the first composite scale that rates many different types of phenomenology simultaneously, considers their impact on task-specific activities, and provides a single measurement score that integrates objective impairment and disability.

Scales from other movement disorders

Most movement disorders have rating scales that have been developed to rate the intensity of impairment,

their disability, or a combination of these features. Impairment refers to objective severity and disability to the impact of the movement disorder on daily function. As such, the impairment score is traditionally anchored in a rater-based observational assessment of the patient at rest and during the performance of prescribed tasks (tapping fingers, speaking, walking), and the maximal severity of induced movements is rated. Often, as in the UPDRS [7] and its revision, the MDS-UPDRS [10], these ratings have a 0–4 range from normal function (0) to severe 4. Disability scores are traditionally based on patient questionnaire or interviews between rater and patient with or without caregiver input. In some cases, such as the Rush Dyskinesia Rating Scale, disability is rated by the rater after observation of tasks of daily living [11]. In the Unified Dyskinesia Rating Scale, both patient questionnaire and direct observation of the patient completing tasks (talking, drinking, dressing, and walking) make up the disability evaluation [12]. Table 32.1 summarizes several scales commonly used in movement disorders and with potential use in the study of PMDs that fit the phenomenological category captured by the scales. The table includes reference sources for the scales, but because these scales have not been applied extensively in research or clinical reports on PMDs, they are not specifically discussed further here.

Scales that assess global disease severity without specific reference to movements

In rating the severity of PMDs, a global approach can also be used, whereby the movements themselves are not categorized or rated but instead a summary score is generated based on overall function. These scales can be completed both by the rater and by the patient. One example of this rating approach is the Clinical Global Impression Severity Scale (CGI-S), which ranks disease severity from "normal", scored as 1, to "among the most extremely ill", scored as 7 [23]. This scale has been widely used in movement disorders and has the advantage that it can be used for disorders with multiple phenomenologies, such as the PMDs, because the severity rating is global rather than specifically related to any single movement phenomenon. This scale has a second component, the Change scale (CGI-C) that assesses change from an intervention or the passage of time. Again, this assessment can be completed by the rater and the patient separately. This scale ranges

Table 32.1 Scales utilized in the assessment of movement disorders based on phenomenology and specific diseases

Phenomenology	Primary applications	Example scales	Reference
Parkinsonism	Parkinson's disease	Unified Parkinson's Disease Rating Scale (UPDRS)	7
		Movement Disorder Society–UPDRS (MDS-UPDRS)	10
		Hoehn and Yahr Staging Scale	13
Tremor	Essential tremor	Clinical Tremor Rating Scale (CTRS)	14
		Unified Tremor Rating Scale (UTRS)	15
Tics	Gilles de la Tourette syndrome	Yale Global Tic Severity Scale (YGTSS)	16
		Tourette Syndrome Global Scale (TSGS)	17
Myoclonus	Post-hypoxic myoclonus	Unified Myoclonus Rating Scale	18
Dystonia	Generalized and focal dystonias	Burke–Fahn–Marsden Scale (BFMS)	19
		Toronto Western Spasmodic Torticollis Rating Scale (TWSTRS)	20
		Unified Dystonia Rating Scale (UDRS)	21
Dyskinesia	Tardive dyskinesia, levodopa-induced dyskinesia	Abnormal Involuntary Movement Scale (AIMS)	22
		UPDRS, Part IV	7
		MDS-UPDRS, Part IV	10
		Rush Dyskinesia Rating Scale (RDRS)	11
		Unified Dyskinesia Rating Scale (UDysRS)	12

from 1 to 7, with 1 assigned to "marked improvement" and 7 assigned to "very much worse." In this scale, "no change" is marked as 4. The CGI has been applied in one study of antidepressant treatment in PMDs with CGI-S and CGI-C scores monitored for global change as well as for motor change [24]. The CGI was also utilized in one open-label study of somatization disorder and its response to nafazodone [25].

The Schwab and England Activities of Daily Living ranks patient functional independence and is not restricted to any single disorder [26]. This scale ranges from 100% (completely normal) to 90% (completely independent, able to do all chores with some degree of slowness) down to 0% (completely bedridden and vegetative functions such as swallowing, bladder, and bowel functions not functioning). Some global measures that rely entirely on the patient include quality of life measures. Whereas some quality of life scales have been developed for specific disorders, such as the Parkinson's Disease Quality of Life Questionnaire-39 [27], for PMDs, more generic scales are likely to be more applicable. Examples include the Sickness Impact Profile and the 36-Item Short Form Health Survey (SF-36) [28,29]. Some authors have also used the McMaster Health Index questionnaire [30].

Rating scales specifically for psychogenic movement disorders

Two scales have been developed and tested clinimetrically for assessing the type and severity of PMDs. The first, the Video Rating Scale for Motor Conversion Symptoms (VRMC), was specifically developed for the assessment of treatment outcome in patients with motor conversion disorders, a subcategory within the larger designation of PMDs [31]. Patients are videotaped before and after treatment performing motor exercises that stress their symptoms and impairments. The number of exercises depends on the exact nature and complexity of the symptoms and, therefore, the testing paradigm is tailored to each patient. The rating scale allows for up to three different types of movement to be considered, and the selection is based on the rater's overall clinical judgment. Based on the video findings in the pre-treatment and post-treatment assessments, a CGI-C score is generated. In the case of multiple movements, the mean change score for the different movements (up to three) is the final outcome. The reliability of the instrument has a weighted kappa square coefficient of 0.89, and concurrent validity was considered satisfactory by the scale developers as shown by Spearman's correlation (−0.433) with the International Classification of Impairments, Disabilities and Handicaps subscale for physical activities (Dutch version). Specifically developed as a scale for rating response to treatment intervention, the VRMC description does not include the use of video protocol with a standard CGI-S rating.

A second scale specifically developed for the rating of psychogenic movement disorders is the PMDRS [9]. This scale is not limited to three movement types and aims to gather multiple types of information with a single overall score. Six types of information are assessed and rated: movement phenomenology, anatomical distribution, severity, duration, functional impact of movements, and incapacitation. A total score is thereby generated that crosses all types of PMDs and allows a rating for patient populations with various presentations.

During the neurological examination and observation, Part I of the PMDRS rates 10 phenomena: rest tremor, action tremor, dystonia, chorea, bradykinesia, myoclonus, tics, athetosis, ballism, and coordination in 14 body regions (upper face, lips/perioral region, jaw, tongue, neck, head, right and left shoulders, right and left upper extremities, right and left lower extremities, trunk, and other body regions). For each type of movement in each body region, a severity score is generated based on descriptive anchors ranging from 0 for none to 4 for severe. These values are then considered to generate a Global Severity score for each phenomenon. Each phenomenon is also given a Duration Factor score to describe how much of the examination involved the abnormal movement, from 0 (never), to 1 (< 25% of the examination time), and to 4 (> 75% of the examination time). A Global Incapacitation score is also generated by an assessment of the overall functional impact of each movement disorder type during the examination, ranging from 0 (none) to 4 (severe). The sum of the regional and the three Global Scores across the 10 phenomena generates the final Total Phenomenology Score (range of possibilities, 0–680). Part II focuses specifically on gait and speech and rates the severity, duration, and incapacitation for each of these target activities. These activities were chosen because of their importance to overall function and their relevance across all movement disorders. Each activity receives a 0–4 rating for the three areas, severity, duration, and incapacitation, to generate the Total Function Score (range of possibilities, 0–24). The sum

of Part I and Part II provides the final total PMDRS score (range of possibilities, 0–704).

The PMDRS has undergone clinimetric testing and has successfully demonstrated interrater reliability, construct validity, and responsiveness to therapeutic intervention [9]. It has likewise been utilized in cross-cultural analyses of PMDs [32]. In testing the scale against the more non-specific but more easily applied CGS-S, the interrater agreement was higher with the PMDRS, with Spearman correlations of 0.90 versus 0.81 [9]. The scale developers argue that the broader range of the PMDRS (a range of 0 to 704, whereas the CGI is a range of 0 to 7) provides more sensitivity for small changes. The high correlation between the two scales, however, confirms that the PMDS quantifies the global severity of PMDs and is a valid measure.

The PMDRS has been used by the scale developers as the primary outcome in a single-blind treatment protocol utilizing psychotherapy to treat PMDs [33]. A blinded observer rated patient videotapes before and after psychiatric intervention. In this study, all subjects presented with multiple movement disorder phenomena (range, 2–6; median, 3), precluding the use of any single disease-specific or phenomenon-specific scale. Total PMDRS scores significantly improved with treatment compared with baseline ($p < 0.02$).

Future perspectives

As the field of PMDs develops further rigor and as treatment studies expand, the importance of rating scales increases. Whereas the PMDRS is a first step in the development of a uniform and comprehensive movement disorder tool, it clearly needs to be tested further among researchers and clinicians other than the investigators who developed it. For studies focusing on single forms of psychogenic disorders, where the key question may be separating signs or patterns from traditional movement disorders, disease-specific scales may be more directly applicable to the research question. For example, if the patient cohort involves only tremor, even though the PMDRS will capture the behavior well and be rapidly applied because all other phenomena will be marked 0, when the question of interest focuses on differences between Parkinson's disease and psychogenic parkinsonism, a standard Parkinson's disease rating scale such as the MDS-UPDRS could be added to the PMDRS. In clinical practice, where longitudinal monitoring is the goal and global assessments are more important than specific details, the CGI may be the most practical. In all instances, matching the rating scale to the research or clinical goal of the assessment will guide physicians to the appropriate selection.

References

1. Factor S, Podskalny G, Molho E. Psychogenic movement disorders: frequency, clinical profile and characteristics. *J Neurol Neurosurg Psychiatry* 1995;**59**:406–412.

2. Williams DT, Ford B, Fahn S. Phenomenology and psychopathology related to psychogenic movement disorders. *Adv Neurol* 1995;**65**:231–257.

3. Marjama J, Troester A, Koller W. Psychogenic movement disorders. *Neurol Clin* 1995;**13**:283–297.

4. Deuschl G, Raethjen J, Kopper F, Govindan RB. The diagnosis and physiology of psychogenic tremor. InHallett M, Fahn S, Jankovic J, *et al.*, eds. *Psychogenic Movement Disorders: Neurology and Neuropsychiatry*. Philadelphia, PA: Lippincott Williams & Wilkins, 2006:265–273.

5. Hayes MW, Graham S, Heldorf P, de Moore G, Morris JG. A video review of the diagnosis of psychogenic gait: appendix and commentary. *Mov Disord* 1999;**14**:914–921.

6. Kurlan R, Brin MF, Fahn S. Movement disorder in reflex sympathetic dystrophy: a case proven to be psychogenic by surveillance video monitoring. *Mov Disord* 1997;**12**:243–245.

7. Fahn S, Elton RL, for the UPDRS Development Committee. Unified Parkinson's disease rating scale. In Fahn S, Marsden CD, Calne D, Goldstein M, eds. *Recent Developments in Parkinson's Disease*, Vol. 2, Florham Park, NJ: Macmillan Healthcare Information, 1987:153–163.

8. Cubo E, Stebbins GT, Golbe LI, *et al.* Application of the Unified Parkinson's Disease Rating Scale in progressive supranuclear palsy: factor analysis of the motor scale. *Mov Disord* 2000;**2**:276–279.

9. Hinson VK, Cubo E, Comella CL, Goetz CG, Leurgans S. Rating scale for psychogenic movement disorders: scale development and clinimetric testing. *Mov Disord* 2005;**20**:1592–1597.

10. Goetz CG, Fahn S, Martinez-Martin P, *et al.* Movement Disorder Society-sponsored revision of the Unified Parkinson's Disease Rating Scale (MDS-UPDRS): process, format, and clinimetric testing plan. *Mov Disord* 2007;**22**:41–47.

11. Goetz CG, Stebbins GT, Shale HM, *et al.* Utility of an objective dyskinesias rating scale for Parkinson's disease inter-and intrarater reliability assessment. *Mov Disord* 1994,**9**:390–394.

12. Goetz CG, Nutt JG, Stebbins . The Unified Dyskinesia Rating Scale. *Mov Disord* 2008;**23**:2398–2403.

13. Hoehn MM, Yahr MD. Parkinsonism: onset, progression, and mortality. *Neurology* 1967;**17**:427–442.

14. Fahn S, Tolosa E, Martin C. Clinical rating scale for tremor. In Jankovic J, Tolosa E. eds. *Parkinson's Disease and Movement Disorders*. Munich: Urban and Schwarzenberg, 1988:225–234.

15. Bain PG, Findley LJ, Atchison P, *et al.* Assessing tremor severity. *J Neurol Neurosurg Psychiatry* 1993;**56**:868–873.

16. Leckman JF, Riddle MA, Hardin MT. The Yale Global Tic Severity Scale: initial testing of a clinician-rated scale of tic severity. *J Am Acad Child Adolesc Psychiatry* 1989;**28**:566–573.

17. Harcherik DF, Leckman JF, Detlor J. A new instrument for clinical studies of Tourette's syndrome. *J Am Acad Child Psychiatry* 1984;**23**:153–160.

18. Frucht SJ, Leurgans SE, Hallett M, Fahn S. The Unified Myoclonus Rating Scale. *Adv Neurol* 2002;**89**:361–376.

19. Burke RE, Fahn S, Marsden CD, *et al.* Validity and reliability of a rating scale for the primary torsion dystonias. *Neurology* 1985;**35**:73–77.

20. Consky ES, Basinki A, Belle L, *et al.* The Toronto Western Spasmodic Torticollis Rating Scale (TWSTRS): assessment of validity and inter-rater reliability. *Neurology* 1990;**40**(Suppl 1):445.

21. Comella CL, Leurgans S, Chmura T, *et al.* The Unified Dystonia Rating Scale: initial concurrent validity testing with other dystonia scales. *Neurology* 1999;**52**(Suppl 2):A292.

22. Gardos G, Cole JO, Rapkin RM. Anticholinergic challenge and neuroleptic withdrawal. *Arch Gen Psychiatry* 1984;**41**:1030–1035.

23. Guy W. *ECDEU Assessment Manual for Psychopharmacology*. Washington, DC: US Government Printing Office, 1976.

24. Voon V, Lang AE. Antidepressant treatment outcomes of psychogenic movement disorder. *J Clin Psychiatry* 2005;**66**:1529–1534.

25. Menza M, Lauritano M, Allen L, *et al.* Treatment of somatization disorder with nefazodone. *Ann Clin Psychiatry* 2001;**13**:153–158.

26. Schwab JF, England AC. Projection technique for evaluating surgery in Parkinson's disease. In Billingham FH, Donaldson MC, eds. *Third Symposium on Parkinson's Disease*. Edinburgh: Livingstone, 1969:152–157.

27. Peto V, Jenkinson C, Fitzpatrick R, Greenhall R. The development and validation of a short measure of functioning and well being for individuals with Parkinson's disease. *Qual Life Res* 1995;**4**:241–248.

28. Bergner M, Bobbit RA, Pollard WE. The Sickness Impact Profile: validation of a health status measure. *Med Care* 1981;**14**:57–67.

29. Stewart AL, Hays RD, Ware JE. The MOS Short-Form General Health Survey: reliability and validity in a patient population. *Med Care* 1988;**26**:724–735.

30. Jankovic J, Vuong KD, Thomas M. Psychogenic tremor: long-term outcome. *CNS Spectr* 2006;**11**:501–508.

31. Moene FC, Spinhoven P, Hoogduin KAL, van Dyck R. A randomized controlled clinical trial on the additional effect of hypnosis in a comprehensive treatment programme for in-patients with conversion disorder of the motor type. *Psychother Psychosom* 2002;**71**:66–76.

32. Cubo E, Hinson VK, Goetz CG, *et al.* Transcultural comparison of psychogenic movement disorders. *Mov Disord* 2005;**20**:1343–1345.

33. Hinson VK, Weinstein S, Bernard B, Leurgans SE, Goetz CG. Single-blind clinical trial of psychotherapy for treatment of psychogenic movement disorders. *Parkinsonism Rel Disord* 2006;**12**:177–180.

Chapter

33

Quality of life in psychogenic disorders: the cause, not the effect

Lisa M. Shulman

Introduction

Quality of life (QoL) is the degree of well-being perceived by an individual or a group. It contains elements of impairment, disability, and handicap, but most importantly it encompasses the *subjective perception* of health and well-being. Consequently, objective assessment of QoL is not possible since QoL is *subjective by definition*. Therefore, when evaluating a person with a psychogenic disorder, the clinician may assess the level of impairment or disability associated with the disorder (e.g., intermittent tremors or severe gait disturbance), but only the patient can evaluate their quality of life.

Quality of life studies

Anderson *et al.* [1] examined QoL in 66 patients with psychogenic movement disorders (PMD) by comparing these patient ratings of health-related QoL with ratings in 704 patients with Parkinson's disease (PD). A demographics comparison of the two groups showed that the PMD group was significantly younger (49.6 years [SD,13.0] versus 65.5 years [SD,10.3]), less educated (36% versus 26% with education less than 12th grade), and less affluent (60% versus 27% with household annual income less than $50 000), and had much greater female representation (75% versus 36%). On the SF-12 Health Status Survey, both patients with PMD and those with PD reported similar levels of physical health QoL (38.9 [SD, 14.5] and 39.8 [SD, 11.6], respectively; $p = 0.19$). However, mental health QoL was worse in PMD than PD (41.6 [SD, 13.4] and 48.9 [SD, 11.0], respectively; $p < 0.001$; Fig. 33.1). These results show that patients with PMD and PD similarly described their physical health QoL as reduced by more than 1 SD. Mental health QoL was also reduced by nearly 1 SD in the PMD subjects, but the PD subjects rated their mental health QoL

in the normative range of the scale. These results show that physical health QoL is significantly reduced in both PMD and PD, but mental health QoL is only reduced in PMD. Comparing psychiatric symptoms and disability between the PMD and PD groups, the patients with PMD had greater depression, anxiety, and somatization than those with PD, but similar levels of self-reported disability (Fig. 33.1). Therefore, people with PMD report a level of physical impairment and disability that is equivalent to that reported in a progressive neurodegenerative disorder, but a greater degree of psychiatric distress.

The relationship between QoL in psychogenic non-epileptic seizures (PNES) and epilepsy has been compared in a similar manner [2,3]. Based on an epilepsy-specific QoL instrument (QOLIE89), patients with PNES reported a poorer health-related QoL than patients with epilepsy (41.0 [SD,15.6] versus 57.6 [SD, 18.2]; $p < 0.001$). The lower QoL ratings in PNES (i.e., worse) were explained by the presence of greater depression, medication adverse effects, and somatization. Again, there were more females in the PNES group. The age at onset of the seizure episodes was later among the PNES subjects; however, the number of seizures per week was greater in PNES than in epilepsy.

The similarities between these comparative studies of two different psychogenic disorders raises the question of whether PMD and PNES should really be "lumped" together, rather than "split." In order to study the similarities and differences between these two psychogenic disorders, the psychosocial and demographic profiles of 21 patients with PNES and 104 patients with PMD were compared [4]. The PNES and PMD groups reported similarly low levels of physical and mental health QoL, and similarly high levels of somatization, depression, and anxiety. Demographic data regarding age, education, marital status, and employment were

Psychogenic Movement Disorders and Other Conversion Disorders, ed. Mark Hallett, Anthony E. Lang, Joseph Jankovic, Stanley Fahn, Peter W. Halligan, Valerie Voon, and C. Robert Cloninger. Published by Cambridge University Press. © Cambridge University Press 2011.

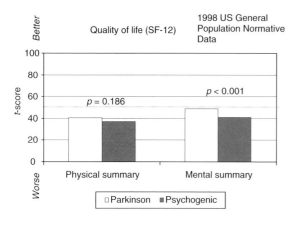

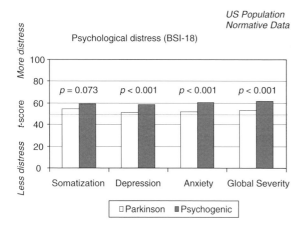

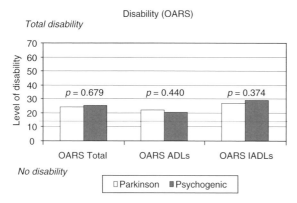

Fig. 33.1. Comparison of patient-reported quality of life (QoL), mental health, and disability in Parkinson disease and psychogenic movement disorders (PMDs). On outcome measures of health-related QoL, psychiatric symptoms, and disability, patients with PMDs reported similar levels of physical health QoL and disability but greater psychiatric comorbidity and poorer mental health QoL compared with patients with Parkinson disease. The horizontal dotted lines on each graph indicate the 50th percentile on the SF-12 Health Status Survey (SF-12) and Brief Symptom Inventory-18 (BSI-18) graphs, and the score associated with "no disability" on the Older American Resource and Services Disability Subscale (OARS) graph. ADL, activities of daily living; IADL, instrumental activities of daily living scale.

similar among these two psychogenic groups; however, the PNES patients were more likely to be female than the ones with PMD. Therefore, it is plausible that these two psychogenic disorders, which are generally studied separately, are actually a single disorder. An interesting difference in the phenomenology of the psychogenic disorders was that the patients with PNES were more likely to have episodic symptoms. This suggests that patients with more episodic symptoms are more likely to be referred to the epilepsy specialists, while patients with more continuous symptoms are referred to the movement disorders specialists, even though the quality of the movements (e.g., tremulousness, myoclonic, dystonic) may be similar.

These studies suggest that conversion disorders are characterized by reductions in QoL and disability that are commensurate with serious medical conditions, but conversion disorders are associated with a greater burden of psychiatric symptoms. Expanding on this theme, a review of literature was conducted to investigate whether other disorders characterized by medically unexplained symptoms, such as fibromyalgia and irritable bowel syndrome, share a similar profile with PMD and PNES. In fact, studies comparing fibromyalgia and rheumatoid arthritis recapitulate many of the results of the previous comparisons. Patients with fibromyalgia reported worse QoL, similar or greater levels of disability, and more psychiatric comorbidity than those with rheumatoid arthritis [5–8]. Also, when fibromyalgia was compared with complex regional pain syndrome and chronic low back pain, there was reduced QoL and greater psychological distress in fibromyalgia than in the other two disorders [9]. In yet another study, patient's ratings on two different QoL measures, the SF-36 and EQ-5D, were compared among five disorders: fibromyalgia, herniated disc, epicondylitis, osteoarthritis of the knee, and rheumatoid arthritis. This study found that QoL ratings were lower in fibromyalgia than in the other four musculoskeletal disorders [10].

Both physical and mental health QoL was also reduced in patients with irritable bowel syndrome compared with controls, and QoL was associated with symptom severity, anxiety, and hypochondriasis in the patients with irritable bowel syndrome [11]. Patients with a range of medical conditions were asked, "During the past 30 days, how many days did poor physical or mental health keep you from doing your usual activities?" The patients with irritable bowel syndrome reported an average of 15 days of disability per month – more than respondents with arthritis, diabetes, heart

Table 33.1 Comparisons of psychiatric symptoms, quality of life and disability among disorders with medically unexplained and medically explained symptoms

Features	Comparison of MUS with MES				Comparison of two MUS
	PMD versus PD[1]	PNES versus epilepsy	FM versus RA	IBS versus controls	PMD versus PNES
Psychiatric symptoms	PMD > PD	PNES > E	FM > RA	IBS > C	PMD = PNES
Mental health QoL	PMD < PD	PNES < E	FM < RA	IBS < C	PMD = PNES
Physical health QoL	PMD = PD	PNES < E	FM < RA	IBS < C	PMD = PNES
Disability	PMD = PD	–	FM ≥ RA	IBS > C	PMD = PNES

C, controls; E, epilepsy; FM; fibromyalgia; IBS, irritable bowel syndrome; MES, medically explained symptoms; MUS, medically unexplained symptoms; PD, Parkinson's disease; PMD, psychogenic movement disorder; PNES, psychogenic non-epileptic seizures; QoL, quality of life; RA, rheumatoid arthritis.

disease, stroke, or cancer. In a general comparison study of patients with medically unexplained symptoms and medically explained symptoms in primary care, the patients with medically unexplained symptoms had poorer QoL, more somatic symptoms, and greater anxiety and depression [12].

In summary, multiple comparison studies show that disorders with medically unexplained symptoms have greater psychiatric comorbidity and worse mental health QoL than disorders with medically explained symptoms, while a comparison of two psychogenic disorders (PMD and PNES) show similar levels of psychiatric comorbidity and reduced mental health QoL (Table 33.1).

Determinants of quality of life

Common predictors of QoL include disease severity and depression. Another important determinant of QoL is self-efficacy, defined as an individual's perception of their ability to successfully perform certain tasks or behaviors. Self-efficacy for self-management of disease is defined more specifically as the belief that one can carry out a behavior to achieve a desired goal related to one's health. Self-efficacy is a major determinant of human behavior and acts as a key mediator of the acquisition of the necessary skills for self-management. Lower self-efficacy in achieving desired outcomes is associated with a lower quality of life. Both cross-sectional and longitudinal studies show self-efficacy to be associated with better health outcomes and a greater sense of well-being in many chronic medical conditions. Self-efficacy has two significant features: (1) it is a pivotal mediator of human behavior, and (2) it has

been shown to be modifiable by interventions that foster self-management skills.

The relationship between QoL and fibromyalgia is highlighted by a study showing that patients with fibromyalgia perceive little personal control over their symptoms (low self-efficacy) and do not expect medical treatment to be effective; these factors were both found to be related to their QoL [13]. What role does self-efficacy play in psychogenic movement disorders? In a comparison of PMD and PD, the patients with PMD reported less self-efficacy than those with PD, even when the data were corrected for greater psychiatric symptomatology in the PMD subjects [14]. In a comparison of four movement disorders (PD, PMD, essential tremor and atypical parkinsonism), better QoL and greater self-efficacy were reported in PD and essential tremor. Conversely, worse QoL and less self-efficacy were reported in PMD and atypical parkinsonism (L. M. Shulman, unpublished data, 2009). These results suggest that a lack of confidence and control in managing one's daily activities and health may be a risk factor for excessive somatization and the emergence of psychogenic disorders. Therefore, it is plausible that interventions to improve self-efficacy may be effective in preventing or reducing symptoms of conversion disorders. These interventions might include training in problem-solving, confidence-building, decision-making, skills mastery. and reinterpretation of symptoms.

Conclusions

Identifying novel approaches to prevent and treat psychogenic disorders is important since these disorders are both highly prevalent and very difficult to manage. Carson reported that 30% of new patients (90/300) in a general neurology practice had medically unexplained symptoms, with more than half of these unimproved at 8 months of follow-up [15,16]. Stone reported that 83% of patients with psychogenic weakness or sensory loss were unimproved 12 years later, with the majority of the group developing multiple medically unexplained symptoms and disability over time [17].

In summary, a diverse group of disorders characterized by MUS are associated with the presence of greater psychiatric symptoms and disability, and poorer quality of life than commonly recognized organic disorders. The similarities in the profiles of a range of psychogenic disorders and their relationships with health-related QoL suggest that poor general well-being associated with poor self-efficacy skills may be key risk factors for the development of psychogenic conditions.

References

1. Anderson KE, Gruber-Baldini, Vaughan CG, *et al.* The impact of psychogenic movement disorders on psychiatric co-morbidity, disability and quality of life compared to Parkinson's disease. *Mov Disord* 2007;**22**:2204–2209.

2. Szaflarski JP, Hughes C, Szaflarski M, *et al.* Quality of life in psychogenic nonepileptic seizures. *Epilepsia* 2003;**44**:236–342.

3. Testa SM, Schefft BK, Szaflarski JP, Yeh HS, Privitera MD. Mood, personality, and health-related quality of life in epileptic and psychogenic seizure disorders. *Epilepsia* 2007;**48**:973–982.

4. Hopp J, Price M, Anderson KE, *et al.* Psychogenic nonepileptic seizures and psychogenic seizure disorders. *Neurology* 2009;**72**(Suppl 3):A262.

5. Tander B, Cengiz K, Alayi G, *et al.* A comparative evaluation of heatlh related quality of life and depression in patients with fibromyalgia syndrome and rheumatoid arthritis. *Rheumatol Int* 2008;**28**:859–865.

6. Birtane M, Uzunca K, Tastekin N, Tuna H. The evaluation of quality of life in fibromyalgia syndrom: a comparison with rheumatoid arthritis by using SF-36 Health Survey. *Clin Rheumatol* 2007;**26**:684.

7. Strombeck B, Ekadhl C, Manthorpe R, Wikstrom I, Jacobsson L. Health-related quality of life in primary Sjögren's syndrome. *Scand J Rheumatol* 2000;**29**:20–28.

8. Walker EA, Keegan D, Gardner G, *et al.* Factors in fibromyalgia compared with rheumatoid arthritis. I. Psychiatric diagnoses and functional disability. *Psychosom Med* 1997;**59**:565–571.

9. Verbunt JA, Pernot DH, Smeets RJ. Disability and quality of life in patients with fibromyalgia. *Health Qual Life Outcomes* 2008;**6**:8.

10. Picavet HSJ, Hoeymans N. Health related quality of life in multiple musculoskeletal disease: SF-36 and EQ-5D in the DMC3 study. *Ann Rheum Dis* 2004;**63**:723–729.

11. Rey E, Garcia-Alonso MO, Moreno-Ortega M, Alvarez-Sanches A, Diaz-Rubio M. Determinants of quality of life in irritable bowel syndrome. *J Clin Gastroenterol* 2008;**42**:1003–1009.

12. Duddu V, Husain N, Dickens C. Medically unexplained presentations and quality of life: a study of a predominantly South Asian primary care population in England. *J Psychosom Res* 2008;**65**:311–317.

13. van Wilgen CP, van Ittersum MW, Kaptein AA, van Wijhe M. Illness perceptions in patients with fibromyalgia and their relationship to quality of life and catastrophizing. *Arthritis Rheum* 2008;**58**:3618–3626.

14. Anderson KE, Gruber-Baldini, Mullins JR, *et al.* Self-efficacy: a marker for psychogenic movement disorders. *Mov Disord* 2008;**23**:S253.

15. Carson AJ, Ringbauer B, Stone J, *et al.* Do medically unexplained symptoms matter? A prospective cohort study of 300 new referrals to neurology outpatient clinics. *J Neurol Neurosurg Psychiatry* 2000;**68**:207–210.

16. Carson AJ, Best S, Postma K, *et al.* The outcome of neurology outpatients with medically unexplained symptoms: a prospective cohort study. *J Neurol Neurosurg Psychiatry* 2003;**74**:897–900.

17. Stone J, Sharpe M, Rothwell PM, Warlow CP. The 12 year prognosis of unilateral functional weakness and sensory disturbance. *J Neurol Neurosurg Psychiatry* 2003;**74**:591–596.

Chapter

34

Psychiatric testing

Karen E. Anderson

Introduction

Psychogenic movement disorders (PMDs) are known to have a high rate of comorbidity with other psychiatric disorders. Studies of patients with PMD rarely include any systematic evaluation of common psychiatric symptoms such as depressed mood, anxiety, or other conditions. One prospective study found point diagnosis of major depression to be 12%, anxiety disorder 38%, and concomitant major depression with anxiety disorder 12% in a group of patients with PMD [1]. The same group reported a lifetime diagnosis of major depression in 43% of patients with PMD, anxiety disorder in 62%, and major depression with anxiety disorder in 27%. Other work has also shown that depression and anxiety are predominant psychiatric disorders in this population [2–4]. Suicidal ideation and suicide completion have been reported in patients with PMD, underlying the severity of psychiatric comorbidity [1]. It is helpful, both for characterization of comorbid emotional symptoms and for design of future treatment studies, to have measures of emotional symptoms in PMD. Rating scales can help to separate symptoms that are caused by other psychiatric conditions from those that are purely psychogenic. This is quite useful when designing specific interventions for PMD, since improvement of PMD symptoms is not necessarily related to change in other psychiatric symptoms [5,6]. Finally, questions of malingering, an overriding and complex issue in PMD, can be addressed through use of standardized testing in patients with PMD [7].

This chapter will review the few rating scales most frequently used to date in studies of PMD, assess their utility, and will make recommendations for future work.

Psychiatric rating scales commonly used for psychogenic movement disorder studies

Structured Clinical Interview

The Structured Clinical Interview (SCID-I), which is based on the American Psychiatric Association's *Diagnostic and Statistical Manual* (DSM) has been used in several studies of PMD to assess lifetime and current axis I (major) mental illness [8,9]. Elevated prevalence of major psychiatric disorders, compared with the general population and with many neurological populations, is frequently reported from SCID data [1,10]. A shortened version of the SCID, the Mini International Neuropsychiatric Interview (MINI), has been used successfully in PMD studies to identify axis I psychopathology [11]. It should be noted that the MINI does not include diagnosis of somatoform disorders, which include PMDs; these must be diagnosed separately if the MINI is used.

Some studies have also used the SCID-II, which rates personality traits and disorders – axis II conditions [12]. The SCID-II has demonstrated high levels of psychopathology in PMD [1]. It can be administered as a patient self-report questionnaire if interviews are not feasible.

Depression rating scales

Several depression rating scales have been used in PMD studies to assess concomitant mood disorders. The Hamilton Depression Scale [13] is a common and widely used instrument that has been utilized in PMD studies [4,10,14], as has the Montgomery Asberg

Psychogenic Movement Disorders and Other Conversion Disorders, ed. Mark Hallett, Anthony E. Lang, Joseph Jankovic, Stanley Fahn, Peter W. Halligan, Valerie Voon, and C. Robert Cloninger. Published by Cambridge University Press. © Cambridge University Press 2011.

Depression Rating Scale (MADRAS [15]), which was used by Voon and Lang [11], and the Beck Depression Inventory (BDI [16]), used by Seignourel et al. [17]. Depression measures showed improvement in the treatment studies noted above.

Anxiety rating scales

The Beck Anxiety Inventory [18] has been used in PMD treatment studies [10,11]. It was used as a secondary outcome measure in a recent study of physical activity as a therapy for PMD [14]. Improvement in anxiety was found in patients with PMD who took part in a low-intensity exercise program. The State-Trait Anxiety Inventory (STAI [19]) was used in other PMD work to differentiate anxiety symptoms from core PMD symptoms [17].

Symptom Checklist-90

The Symptom Checklist-90 (SCL-90) is a self-report measure of numerous psychiatric symptoms, and is an extremely valuable screening measure. Eight subscales are included for the different categories of symptoms. The SCL-90 is available in several different languages. It has been used to demonstrate a high level of multiple psychiatric symptoms in patients with PMDs and is available in several languages [6,7,20].

Hypnosis rating scales

Hypnosis has been proposed as a treatment for PMD. The Stanford Hypnotic Susceptibility Scale (SHSS [21]) has been used in PMD work to assess hypnotizability. The SHSS measures five different hypnotic phenomena and is available in several versions, depending on the needs of a study. Moene and colleagues [6] found that SHSS score did not show a greatly increased level of hypnotizability in PMD and that SHSS score did not predict response to hypnosis in PMD. Other work by Roelofs and colleagues [20] used the SHSS, the Dissociative Experiences Scale (DES [22]), and the Dissociation Questionnaire (DIS-Q [23]) and found that patients with PMD were more responsive to hypnotic suggestions than control patients. They also showed a positive correlation between SHSS score and the number of conversion symptoms as measured on the Somatoform Dissociation Questionnaire (SDQ [24]).

Other rating scales

The General Health Questionnaire (GHQ [25]) is an assessment of overall psychological distress that gives subscale ratings of anxiety, depression, somatic symptoms, and social dysfunction. Elevated levels of psychological distress are seen on this scale in PMD [1]. Anderson et al. [26] used the Brief Symptom Inventory 18 (BSI-18 [27]) in a comparison of PMD with Parkinson's disease. The scale assesses depressed mood, anxiety, and somatization. In addition to these three subscales, the BSI-18 gives an overall rating of psychiatric symptom burden. Quality of life measures have been used in several studies, demonstrating reduced quality of life in PMD. Jankovic et al. [3] used the McMaster Health Index Questionnaire [28] and Anderson et al. used the SF-12 Health Survey [29].

Patients with PMD are often suspected of malingering. Van Beilen et al. [7] addressed this issue in patients with PMD and psychogenic paralysis. They used the Amsterdamse Korte Termijn Geheugen test (AKTG [30]), which is presented to subjects as a memory test but actually detects underachievement, indicating performance below the level expected with a cooperative subject. They also used the Structured Inventory of Malingered Symptomatology (SIMS [31]). This test is based on the concept that malingerers are not familiar with genuine symptoms and will, therefore, demonstrate bizarre and atypical symptoms that they perceive to be related to the condition they are feigning. The SIMS has five subscales, which assess intelligence, affective disorders, neurological impairment, psychosis, and declarative memory disorders. In each case, subjects are queried about highly atypical symptoms. Endorsing high levels of these symptoms is indicative of malingering. Using these measures, van Beilin et al. found that patients with psychogenic neurological disorders reported the highest levels of psychological symptoms and showed the most malingering, but patients with non-psychogenic neurological disorders also showed elevated rates of both psychiatric symptoms and malingering when compared with normal controls [7]. This study shows the value of formal assessment in challenging the assumption that presence of psychological distress and characteristics of malingering are indicative of a psychogenic condition. These characteristics may, in fact, be a marker for a patient's distress, regardless of etiology.

Studies with comprehensive psychiatric rating

The most wide ranging uses of psychiatric rating scales in patients with PMD to date have been in treatment studies. One was in a study by Hinson *et al.* [10]. The main study objective was to examine efficacy of psychotherapy for treatment of PMDs. The Hamilton Depression Scale, Beck Anxiety Inventory, Minnesota Multiphasic Personality Inventory-2 [32], Global Assessment of Function (GAF), and the SCID. In that study, the Hamilton, Beck, and GAF all improved with psychotherapy. Voon and Lang [11] used a similarly comprehensive battery of testing to assess response to antidepressant treatment in PMD, including the MINI, MADRS, Beck Anxiety Inventory, and the Clinical Global Impressions subscales Severity of Illness and Change (CGI-S and CGI-C [33]). The CGI-S and CGI-C are both clinician-rated instruments referencing change in illness relative to normal function (CGI-S) and to a patient's original symptoms (CGI-C). The study demonstrated improvement on the MADRS with antidepressant medication treatment.

Psychiatric rating scales in pathophysiological investigations

Studies focusing on understanding psychogenic pathophysiology have also used psychiatric assessments. Seignourel *et al.* [17] showed that level of depression (assessed on BDI) and anxiety (measured with STAI) did not correlate with affective startle modulation. This is useful in assuring that work focuses on the actual psychogenic cause rather than concomitant depressive or anxiety symptoms.

Future assessment considerations

It may be that psychiatric assessments focusing on measurement of mood or anxiety are not particularly sensitive to the core symptoms of PMD. Of course, assessment and treatment of comorbid depression and anxiety are important, but even when these conditions improve, it does not follow that a patient's PMD will also resolve [5,6]. Measures of coping skills and resilience may prove to be better outcome assessments for treatment studies in PMD. Work assessing coping strategies in other psychogenic conditions such as non-epileptic seizures and chronic fatigue suggests that psychogenic patients use more passive rather than active coping, in contrast to healthy controls [34,35]. Van Beilen *et al.* [7] conducted the one study of coping in PMD to date. They used the Utrechtse Coping List (UCL, [36], a 47-item questionnaire that assesses various components of coping including active problem solving, looking for distraction from the problem, avoidance, seeking social support, worrying but not being able to act, expression of emotions in reaction to a situation to work off tension, and self-reassurance. They found that patients with PMD had lower IQ and lower active coping skills compared with healthy controls, but not in comparison with patients who had non-psychogenic neurological disorders. Therefore, non-active coping was not specific to having a PMD. Rather, lack of active coping may be a feature of illness. Since this is an area open to potential modification, studies of effective interventions to retrain coping skills may benefit patients with both psychogenic and non-psychogenic disorders.

Conclusion

Little work done to date has used standard rating scales in studies of PMD. Use of standard psychiatric rating scales to assess depression, anxiety, and other psychiatric symptoms is helpful in separating out whether a treatment response results from amelioration of symptoms specific to the psychogenic condition or linked to concomitant other psychiatric conditions. Use of validated assessments can help to address clinical lore regarding PMD, such as the assumed high level of hypnotizability and high levels of malingering. Future work on assessment of coping skills and other measures of how patients deal with illness may be the most useful studies in PMD.

References

1. Feinstein A, Stergiopoulos V, Fine J, Lang AE. Psychiatric outcome in patients with a psychogenic movement disorder: a prospective study. *Neuropsychiatry Neuropsychol Behav Neurol* 2001;**14**:169–176.

2. Thomas M, Vuong KD, Jankovic J. Long-term prognosis of patients with psychogenic movement disorders. *Parkinsonism Relat Disord* 2006;**12**:382–387.

3. Jankovic J, Vuong KD, Thomas M. Psychogenic tremor: long-term outcome. *CNS Spectr* 2006;**11**:501–508.

4. Grimaldi I, Dubuc M, Kahane P, Bougerol T, Vercueil L. Anxiety and depression in psychogenic movement disorder and non-epileptic seizures: a prospective comparative study. *Rev Neurol (Paris)* 2010;**166**:515–522.

5. Kroenke K, Swindle R. Cognitive-behavioral therapy for somatization and symptom syndromes: a critical review

of controlled clinical trials. *Psychother Psychosom* 2000;**69**:205–215.

6. Moene FC, Spinhoven P, Hoogduin KA, van Dyck R. A randomised controlled clinical trial on the additional effect of hypnosis in a comprehensive treatment programme for in-patients with conversion disorder of the motor type. *Psychother Psychosom* 2002;**71**:66–76.

7. van Beilen M, Griffioen BT, Gross A, Leenders KL. Psychological assessment of malingering in psychogenic neurological disorders and non-psychogenic neurological disorders: relationship to psychopathology levels. *Eur J Neurol* 2009;**16**:1118–1123.

8. American Psychiatric Association. *Diagnostic and Statistical Manual of Diseases*, 4th edn. Washington DC: American Psychiatric Press, 1994.

9. First MB, Spitzer RL, Gibbon M, *et al. Structured Clinical Interview for Axis I DSM-IV Disorders*, patient edition (SCID-I/P, version 2.0). New York: New York State Psychiatric Institute, 1994.

10. Hinson VK, Weinstein S, Bernard B, Leurgans SE, Goetz CG. Single-blind clinical trial of psychotherapy for treatment of psychogenic movement disorders. *Parkinsonism Relat Disord* 2006;**12**:177–180.

11. Voon V, Lang AE. Antidepressant treatment outcomes of psychogenic movement disorder. *J Clin Psychiatry* 2005;**66**:1529–1534.

12. First MB, Gibbon M, Spitzer RL, *et al. Structured Clinical Interview for DSM-IV Axis II personality disorders (SCID-II)*. Washington, DC. American Psychiatric Press, 1997.

13. Hamilton M. Development of a rating scale for primary depressive illness. *Br J Soc Clin Psychol* 1967;**6**:278–296.

14. Dallocchio C, Arbasino C, Klersy C, Marchioni E. The effects of physical activity on psychogenic movement disorders. *Mov Disord* 2010;**25**:421–425.

15. Davidson J, Turnbull CD, Strickland R, Miller R, Graves K. The Montgomery–Asberg Depression Scale: reliability and validity. *Acta Psychiatr Scand* 1986;**73**:544–548.

16. Beck AT, Steer RA, Brown GK: *Manual for Beck Depression Inventory II (BDI-II)*. San Antonio, TX, Psychology Corporation, 1996.

17. Seignourel PJ, Miller K, Kellison I, *et al.* Abnormal affective startle modulation in individuals with psychogenic movement disorder. *Mov Disord* 2007;**22**:1265–1271.

18. Beck AT, Epstein N, Brown G, Steer RA. An inventory for measuring clinical anxiety: psychometric properties. *J Cons Clin Psychol* 1988;**56**:893–897.

19. Spielberger CD, Gorsuch RL, Lushene PR, Vagg PR, Jacobs AG. *Manual for the State-Trait Anxiety Inventory (Form Y)*. Palo Alto, CA: Consulting Psychologists Press, 1983.

20. Roelofs K, Hoogduin KA, Keijsers GP, *et al.* Hypnotic susceptibility in patients with conversion disorder. *J Abnorm Psychol* 2002;**111**:390–395.

21. Weitzenhoffer A, M., Higard E, R. *Stanford Hypnotic Susceptibility Scale: Forms A and B*. Palo Alto, CA: Consulting Psychologists Press, 1959.

22. Bernstein EM, Putnam FW. Development, reliability, and validity of a dissociation scale. *J Nerv Ment Dis* 1986;**174**:727–735.

23. Vanderlinden J, van Dyck R, Vandereycken W, Vertommen H. The Dissociation Questionnaire (Dis-G): development, reliability and validity of a new self-reporting Dissociation Questionnaire. *Acta Psychiatr Belg* 1994;**94**:53–54.

24. Nijenhuis ER, Spinhoven P, van Dyck R, van der Hart O, Vanderlinden J. The development and psychometric characteristics of the Somatoform Dissociation Questionnaire (SDQ-20). *J Nerv Ment Dis* 1996;**184**:688–694.

25. Goldberg DP, Hillier VF. A scaled version of the General Health Questionnaire. *Psychol Med* 1979;**9**:139–145.

26. Anderson KE, Gruber-Baldini AL, Vaughan CG, *et al.* Impact of psychogenic movement disorders versus Parkinson's on disability, quality of life, and psychopathology. *Mov Disord* 2007;**22**:2204–2209.

27. Zabora J, BrintzenhofeSzoc K, Jacobsen P, *et al.* A new psychosocial screening instrument for use with cancer patients. *Psychosomatics* 2001;**42**:241–246.

28. Chambers LW, Macdonald LA, Tugwell P, Buchanan WW, Kraag G. The McMaster Health Index Questionnaire as a measure of quality of life for patients with rheumatoid disease. *J Rheumatol* 1982;**9**:780–784.

29. Ware JE, Kosinski M, Turner-Bowker DM, Gandek B. *How to Score Version 2 of the SF-12 Health Survey*. Lincoln, RI: Quality Metric, 2002.

30. Schagen S, Schmand B, De Sterke S, Lindeboom J. Amsterdam Short Term Memory test. A new procedure for the detection of feigned memory deficits. *J Clin Exp Neuropsychol* 1997;**19**:43–51.

31. Smith GP, Burger GK. Detection of malingering: validation of the Structured Inventory of Malingered Symptomatology (SIMS). *J Am Acad Psychiatry Law* 1997;**25**:2:183–189.

32. Butcher JN, Dahlstrom WG, Graham JR, Tellegen A, KraemerB. *MMPI-2: Minnesota Multiphasic Personality Inventory-2 Manual for Administration and Scoring*. Minneapolis, MN: University of Minnesota Press, 1989.

33. Guy W. *ECDEU Assessment Manual for Psychopharmacology- Revised*. [Department of Health, Education, and Welfare publication (ADM) 76–338] Rockville, MD: National Institutes of Mental Health, 1976.

34. Goldstein LH, Drew C, Mellers J, *et al.* Dissociation, hypnotizability, coping styles and health locus of control: characteristics of pseudoseizure patients. *Seizure* 2000;**9**:314–322.

35. Nater UM, Wagner D, Solomon L. Coping styles in people with chronic fatigue syndrome identified from the general population of Wichita, KS. *J Psychosom Res* 2006;**60**:567–573.

36. Schreurs PJG, ve de Willige G, Brosschot JF, *et al. Utrecht Copinglist:UCL/De Utrechte Copinglist.* Lisse: Swetz & Zeitlinger, 1993.

Chapter

35

Diagnostic considerations for the assessment of malingering within the context of psychogenic movement disorders

Richard Rogers and Chelsea Wooley

Introduction

Psychogenic movement disorders (PMD) represent a comparatively rare but complex syndrome confronting neurologists, psychiatrists, and other healthcare providers. Given its highly varied and atypical presentation, the legitimacy of PMD presentations is sometimes questioned. This chapter outlines the current knowledge of malingering for PMD and PMD-related disorders. Potential detection strategies are identified for further investigation. Regarding the issue of feigned PMD, current data are reviewed and the perils of unwarranted extrapolations are considered.

Conceptual issues

The accurate assessment of malingered PMD is fraught with clinical challenges. For example, PMD lacks the diagnostic precision found with many mental and neurological disorders. Sharpe, a member of the DSM-V Somatoform Disorders Working Group, described the current PMD psychological factors as "virtually impossible to operationalize" [1]. As a result, PMD diagnosis lacks the clear boundaries, such as DSM-IV inclusion and exclusion criteria. When considering a PMD diagnosis, this lack of precision raises the important consideration of whether an atypical presentation represents a genuine variant of PMD or other related disorder, or a less-than-adequate effort to feign these disorders. Beyond diagnostic imprecision, PMD diagnoses include atypical presentations that are explored further in the next section.

Diagnostic challenges

The PMDs often include diagnostic characteristics that are indicative of atypical presentations and intentional distortions. Lang [2] described the atypical presentation sometimes associated with PMD (p. 35): "abrupt onset often triggered by a minor injury for which litigation is sought for a rapid progression to maximal disability." Atypical presentations also include incongruities with neurological data and inconsistencies across examinations. Intentional distortions are also implicated. According to Lang, patients with PMD can exhibit secondary gain as well as an embellishment of other disordered movements, false weakness, and false sensory complaints. Seasoned practitioners can immediately appreciate the diagnostic quandary. If genuine patients with PMD produce false symptoms, then how can they be accurately differentiated from PMD malingerers, who also produce false symptoms?

The assessment of response styles is further complicated because many presumably genuine patients with PMD perceive physicians as questioning their credibility. Stone and Sharpe [3] showed how medical explanations of PMD were interpreted by neurological patients as being accused of feigning ("putting it on") and manipulation (being able to "control symptoms"). When *psychosomatic weakness* was used as the medical explanation for PMD, 24% believed they were being accused of "putting on" their symptoms and 40% of imagining their symptoms. An important yet unexplored issue is how perceived accusations of feigning and imaginary problems affect the clinical presentations of patients with PMD and their subsequent response to treatment [4].

Practitioners face several additional diagnostic challenges in establishing valid diagnoses of PMD. This constellation of disorders is relatively rare, even in movement disorders [5] (i.e., 4.1%) and neurological settings [6] (2.2%). Rare disorders are often missed

---

Psychogenic Movement Disorders and Other Conversion Disorders, ed. Mark Hallett, Anthony E. Lang, Joseph Jankovic, Stanley Fahn, Peter W. Halligan, Valerie Voon, and C. Robert Cloninger. Published by Cambridge University Press. © Cambridge University Press 2011.

during initial medical and psychiatric evaluations, thereby adding to the diagnostic uncertainties. The diagnostic picture is further complicated by extensive comorbidity [7]. Moreover, pilot research [8] suggests substantial diagnostic disagreement between neurologists and psychiatrists, which adds a further layer of complexity to the challenging diagnosis of PMD.

The next section introduces malingering, secondary gain, and malingering domains. This overview provides the framework for clinical investigations of feigned PMDs.

Malingering and secondary gain

Malingering is characterized in DSM-IV [9] (p. 739) as "the intentional production of false or grossly exaggerated physical or psychological symptoms, motivated by external incentives." Importantly, malingering is a classification and not a formal diagnosis; therefore, it lacks requisite inclusion and exclusion criteria for establishing a disorder. Instead, it is considered to be a *condition* that is likely "the focus of clinical attention." Such conditions cover a broad range of issues, unrelated to diagnoses, including (1) academic and occupational problems, (2) religious or spiritual problems, and (3) acculturation problems.

Unfortunately, some practitioners mistake the screening indicators for malingering with formal inclusion criteria. These indicators were simply designed to raise the index of suspicion about the possibility of malingering. However, they perform poorly even at this function. When used for possible feigning, the available data suggest they are wrong four out of five times [10]. Therefore, it is essential that healthcare providers do not accept the classification of malingering in medical records at face value. Instead, they must carefully compile clinical findings to confirm or disconfirm this classification. Before examining the assessment methods, it is important to first differentiate between malingering and secondary gain.

Malingering is a clearly defined response style that must be clearly distinguished from secondary gain – a clinical construct with three disparate conceptualizations: psychodynamic, behavioral medicine, and forensic [11]. From a psychodynamic perspective, secondary gain serves intrapsychic needs to protect the patient to avoid further psychic harm. From a behavioral medicine perspective, secondary gain is conceptualized as illness behavior that is reinforced by healthcare providers and involved others. In sincere efforts to be helpful, psychosocial reinforcers unintentionally support and prolong the patient's disabled role by increasing his or her dependency on others. From a forensic perspective, monetary gain is posited as the intentional motivation for protracted disabilities. Unlike the other two models, the forensic perspective lacks a solid foundation in both theory and research. It is overly simplistic in positing an intentional motivation without carefully examining rival explanations. Moreover, it confuses possibility with probability. While it is clearly possible that a particular patient's recovery is delayed by disability payments, it cannot be simply assumed to be true. As an analogy, many healthcare providers have opportunities to overstate their services for monetary gain. It would be a terrible mistake to confuse possibility with probability and accuse medical consultants of widespread fraud.

The PMD literature occasionally confuses possibility with probability in its examination of secondary gain. For example, Factor and his colleagues [12] concluded that secondary gain was found in more than 60% of their cases. However, they sometimes equated secondary gain with simply the presence of worker's compensation claims and even unemployment benefits. The construct of secondary gain should not be applied in healthcare settings because of the divergence in its conceptualization and the grave risks of assuming what needs to be proven.

Malingerers do not engage in a monolithic effort to feign everything. Even the most unsophisticated malingerers do not attempt to fabricate every possible psychological and physical symptom. Moreover, malingerers must engage in different tasks if they are feigning PMD rather than hallucinations or memory deficits. Understanding these tasks provides insights into how malingering can be detected. Rogers [10] identified ithree broad domains of malingering common in clinical practice: mental disorders, cognitive impairment, and medical conditions. Malingerers in the domain of feigned mental disorders (e.g., simulated schizophrenia) must make a series of decisions about how to report and portray symptoms, the onset and course of the disorder, and its effects on their daily functioning. In stark contrast, malingerers in the domain of feigned cognitive impairment (e.g., simulated memory loss) have very different decisions and tasks. They must decide on areas of memory loss (e.g., personal or procedural memory), its effects on daily functioning, and how to appear credible of cognitive tests. Malingerers in the domain of medical disorders have myriad of choices.

According to Rogers [10] (p. 17), "patients can specialize in one debilitating symptom (e.g., pain), portray a constellation of common but distressing ailments (e.g., headaches, fatigue, and gastro-intestinal difficulties), or specialize in complex syndromes (e.g., fibromyalgia)." Feigned PMD would typically represent a complex syndrome, but malingerers could also add other medical conditions. A major challenge of feigned PMD is that many purported symptoms (i.e., physical movements) are directly observable by others. These movements are often difficult to sustain for extended periods. Chronic, highly observable conditions such as most feigned PMD appear far more challenging to malinger than most other disorders. We have no data on why patients would choose to feign something as difficult as PMD.

Many malingerers also experience genuine disorders. Given the complexity of PMD and its extensive comorbidity, each of the three domains must be considered for malingered and genuine pathology. Even within the same syndrome such as PMD, some symptoms may be feigned whereas others are genuinely experienced.

Assessment issues

The complexity of malingering with its different domains and diverse assessment methods poses a formidable challenge to practitioners. As an overview, this section examines the evolution in assessment methods for malingering. It also includes detection strategies that were originally developed for feigned mental disorders. However, these strategies may be adapted for the detection of feigned PMD.

Malingering

The first sustained efforts to evaluate malingering were drawn from case-based observations. As documented by Geller and his colleagues [13], the nineteenth century practitioners attempted to identify malingerers by their unusual presentation, atypical symptoms, and unexpected areas of intact functioning. Practitioners recommended interventions such as asking an individual with disorganized thoughts to repeat them; malingerers were sometimes identifiable by their superior performance (e.g., verbatim recall). The case study approach forms the first stage in assessment of malingering. Without standardized methods, however, their observations cannot be rigorously tested.

The second stage for the assessment of malingering involves the systematic examination of group differences [14]. Beginning with the Minnesota Multiphasic Personality Inventory (MMPI) in 1947, researchers investigate group differences between simulators asked to feign mental disorders and genuine patients. A comprehensive review of feigning by Rogers in 1984 [15] revealed group differences on 26 MMPI studies plus a handful of other tests. While the strength of this approach is its standardization, it was often limited by the lack of a strong conceptual framework.

As the third and current stage, Rogers [16] advocated the development of domain-specific detection strategies for the assessment of malingering. Detection strategies were defined by their conceptual basis and rigorous testing using relevant criterion groups (e.g., feigned versus genuine post-traumatic stress disorder). Their effectiveness should be cross-validated across more than one measure. Rogers [10] conducted a comprehensive review of detection strategies for two domains: feigned mental disorders and feigned cognitive impairment.

An understanding of these three stages is crucial to the emerging area of feigned PMD. The domain of feigned medical disorders is the most challenging to evaluate and lags behind the other two domains. As a complex and relatively rare syndrome, the study of genuine PMD versus feigned PMD poses a formidable challenge. As a result, very little is known about feigned PMD beyond general descriptions and the occasional case study [17,18]. Therefore, practitioners must be circumspect in their conclusions about feigned PMD and never attempt to extrapolate across domains. The next section, intended primarily for researchers, considers potential avenues for the development of detection strategies for feigned PMD.

Feigned psychogenic movement disorder and proposed detection strategies

This section provides a conceptual framework for identifying potential detection strategies for feigned PMD. Extensive research [10] has established two general categories for detection strategies: *amplified* and *unlikely*. Amplified detection strategies identify malingerers based on the *magnitude* of the symptom presentation. An example of an amplified detection strategy is symptom selectivity (e.g., more symptoms than most patients). Intuitively, amplified detection strategies should *not* be effective at distinguishing between genuine and feigned PMD. Genuine PMD with its extensive comorbidity is characterized by many symptoms and clinical features. Moreover, some embellishments are common to genuine PMD [2]. Given this intensity of symptom presentation for genuine PMD, the likely effectiveness of amplified detection strategies is called into question.

Unlikely detection strategies constitute the second general category and may represent a promising avenue for PMD malingering research. Unlikely strategies identify malingerers by merely the *presence* of highly unusual – sometimes implausible – clinical characteristics that are almost never found in genuine clinical populations. In extensive research on the Structured Interview of Reported Symptoms, 2nd edition (SIRS-2), Rogers and his colleagues [19] identified several unlikely strategies for feigned mental disorders. Even inpatients rarely report items associated with unlikely detection strategies [20].

Drawn from the other two domains of malingering, four potential detection strategies are summarized:

1. *Rare symptoms.* This strategy refers to clinical characteristics that occur very infrequently in genuine patients. Persons malingering disorders, such as feigned PMD, are unaware of which symptoms are very uncommon; their pattern of these rare characteristics almost never occurs in genuine patients. The first step in establishing rare symptoms for PMD would be a systematic examination of which clinical characteristics (common and uncommon) are unique to PMD; otherwise, comorbid features may nullify the effort of establishing the rare-symptom strategy.

2. *Improbable and absurd symptoms.* A set of inquiries can be generated about clinical characteristics that have a fantastic or preposterous quality to them. Improbable items would need to be developed and pilot-tested with PMD content (e.g., "Do you find when you try to… [a specific movement] that body temperature sometimes fluctuates by more than several degrees?"). Because patients with genuine PMD may respond idiosyncratically, improbable items must be tested rigorously to ensure their discriminability between feigned and genuine PMD.

3. *Symptom combinations.* Within the domain of feigned mental disorders, some symptoms are common by themselves but are rarely paired together. It is a very sophisticated strategy that is difficult for malingerers to detect and foil. Researchers would need to test the applicability of this detection strategy to PMD and related syndromes.

4. *Unlikely examples of intact functioning.* Drawn from case studies [13], malingerers are sometimes identified because their ability to complete certain tasks is markedly disparate with their other abilities. For medical disability cases, surveillance tapes occasionally reveal vigorous, coordinated activities (e.g., playing tennis) for a person claiming limited, painful movements.

In summary, the validation of detection strategies is the next essential step in standardizing the assessment of feigned PMD. Moreover, research is needed to test whether feigned PMD can be considered a unitary construct or whether different strategies will be needed for specific types of PMD.

The next two sections examine the role of psychological measures in the evaluation of PMD. First, we consider their effectiveness as ancillary measures for the diagnosis of PMD. This effort is focused on test patterns that may assist in establishing genuine PMD. Second, we examine the potential usefulness of these measures in differentiating between feigned and genuine PMD.

Psychological measures and psychogenic movement disorder determinations

Practitioners frequently request psychological consultations to assist in differential diagnoses. In addition to traditional tests, structured axis I and axis II interviews provide highly reliable diagnoses with standardized inquiries and concomitant ratings [21]. Current research does not focus on PMD but does include broader categories, such as somatoform disorders. Incorporating their findings, we have examined three related issues: (1) the legitimacy of somatoform and other PMD-related disorders, (2) PMD-related disorders as potential confounds to the assessment of malingering, and (3) potential indicators of feigned medical disorders.

Can psychological measures assist in establishing diagnosis of psychogenic movement disorders?

The MMPI [22] and MMPI-2 [23] represented for decades the standard psychological measure for evaluating patterns of psychopathology, including hypochondrical (scale 1) and hysterical (scale 3) features. For scale

1, Greene [24 noted (p. 131) that persons with physical illness "will endorse legitimate physical symptoms, but they will not endorse the entire gamut of vague physical symptoms;" these features may be used to manipulate or control significant others. According to Greene [24] scale 3 measures histrionic features and the denial of psychological problems. Because one-third of its items also appear on scale 1, it provides both additional coverage and some duplication of somatic symptoms. Practitioners are cautioned that these scales are frequently elevated in both normal and psychiatric populations. Therefore, their interpretation is not specific to PMD-related disorders and cannot be used for diagnostic purposes.

Several studies have been conducted on the MMPI and MMPI-2 for PMD-related disorders. Brandwin and Kewman [25] conducted a small MMPI study of 11 patients with movement disorders. Their modal profile evidenced elevated scores on scale 1, which includes many items about vague concerns of bodily functioning. All other clinical and validity scales were within normal limits. A study of conversion disorders with the MMPI-2 found no significant differences in modal profiles between patients diagnosed with conversion disorders and those with complex regional pain syndrome [26]. The modal profile for conversion disorder demonstrated an elevated scale 3 score. Finally, Wetzel and his colleagues [27] examined the MMPI-2 profiles of 39 female outpatients diagnosed with conversion disorder; their modal profiles produced elevated scales 1 and 3 scores. Two key findings were observed across these studies. First, patients with PMD-related disorders did not, on average, evidence high scores on validity scales, including scale F. Second, patterns of clinical scales are not specific to these disorders but are frequently found in other patient populations.

The Psychological Assessment Inventory (PAI [28,29], a new-generation multiscale inventory, includes a Somatic Complaints subscale that reflects psychological reactions to medical problems [29]. Of relevance to PMD-related disorders, this scale is divided into three further subscales: Conversion (SOM-C), Somatization (SOM-S), and Health Concerns (SOM-H). The SOM-C scale focuses on memory and motor dysfunctions; it is minimally related to depression and anxiety compared with the other SOM subscales [30]. The SOM-S scale covers dramatic physical symptoms and unusual sensory and motor complaints. It is useful in differentiating between somatoform disorder and PTSD. Finally, the SOM-H scale assesses preoccupation with health status and physical problems.

For structured interviews, practitioners can choose between a general axis I interview, the Anxiety Disorders Interview Schedule for DSM-IV (ADIS-IV [31]), and a focused interview, the Somatoform Disorders Schedule (SDS [32]. The ADIS-IV provides a good coverage of somatization disorder: its extensive review of symptoms systematically includes ratings of severity (e.g., mild to very severe) and relationship to known medical conditions. Several pseudoneurological symptoms are particularly relevant (i.e., movement, seizures, and sensations). In contrast, the SDS focused on pain and bodily discomfort. Because the SDS has limited coverage and validity [33] the ADIS-IV is recommended as the better measure of somatized symptoms.

For establishing PMD-related disorders, two measures, the PAI and ADIS-IV are recommended. The PAI provides useful clinical correlates for conversion and somatization, whereas the ADIS-IV affords the opportunity to examine somatic symptoms and diagnose somatization disorder.

Is the assessment of malingering confounded by psychogenic movement disorders?

In a meta-analysis of the MMPI-2 and malingering, Rogers and his colleagues [34] found that presumably genuine patients with certain diagnoses (e.g., post-traumatic stress disorder and schizophrenia) had marked elevations on feigning scales. This finding raises questions about their effectiveness.

Given the atypical and variable presentation associated with PMD, a major concern is that presumably patients with genuine PMD may be misclassified as feigning.

This subsection highlights one scale that has been tested with PMD-related disorders: the MMPI-2 Fake Bad Scale (FBS). As an important caveat, the FBS is moderately useful for the assessment of *feigned mental disorders*; however, its effectiveness has not been tested for *feigned PMD*.

The FBS [35] was designed to evaluate feigning in disability cases of distress and functional impairment following an injury. Greiffenstein *et al.* [36] examined data from 1049 patients from different groups (e.g., psychiatric, traumatic brain injury, and medical disorders) relevant to PMD-related disorders. They included inpatient epilepsy and a mixed neurological sample. They found that an FBS score of ≥ 30 almost never misclassified (false positive rate of 0.003) genuine patients irrespective of their diagnoses

Measures of feigned cognitive impairment have not been extensively tested with samples of PMD-related disorders. Two promising measures are the Word Memory Test (WMT [37]) and the "b" test [38]. The WMT has been tested in very large samples of disability cases with a range of diagnostic categories [36]; it is used with some success in measuring effort for patients with epilepsy and patients with psychogenic non-epileptic seizures [39]. The "b" test has not been evaluated as extensively but its criterion groups do include both head injury and stroke.

In summary, the best available data indicate that the FBS is unlikely to be confounded by PMD-related disorders. Therefore, we would recommend its use for the assessment of feigned mental disorders when PMD is suspected or diagnosed.

What are the potential indicators of feigned medical disorders?

Despite extensive literature searches, we have found no clinical studies that examine feigned PMD via psychological measures. Practitioners must view with frank skepticism any claims by psychologists or other clinicians that their testing *confirms*, or even *supports*, feigned or malingered PMD.

Only a handful of studies examine broad categories, such somatic feigning. For example, Larrabee [40] examined somatic malingering on the MMPI and MMPI-2 with 12 patients. Importantly, somatic malingerers had elevated scores on the FBS but not on other feigning scales. Clinical profiles had marked elevations on scales 1 and 3. While encouraging, the study suffered from a small sample and limited comparison group. A meta-analysis by Nelson *et al.* [41] suggested that the FBS could be used with a range of conditions including chronic pain. Despite its strengths, the FBS should only be viewed as an initial screen for possible feigning of somatic problems. Its scores should not be seen as direct, or even indirect, evidence of feigned PMD.

The recently published MMPI-2-RF [42] includes a specific scale for somatic feigning (Fs-r scale) using 16 items described as "uncommon medical complaints." Its lax criterion for item selection (i.e., being reported by less than 25% of genuine patients) is unlikely to be effective when applied to a rare and complex syndrome, such as PMD. If this is correct, Fs-r may misclassify

genuine PMD as somatic feigning. A second problem is that Fs-r correlates very highly with scales for feigned mental disorders; it raises an important question about whether the Fs-r can be used specifically for somatic feigning, With an SEM of 8 T points in clinical populations [43], only extreme elevations are likely to be useful, even for non-specific interpretations (e.g., "possible feigning of either somatic or psychiatric symptoms").

Future directions can include the use of other psychological measures such as the Health Problems Exaggeration subscale from the PSI [44] or psychophysiological methods. Regarding the latter, initial work has investigated patterns of brain activation in assessing the genuineness of paralysis [45]. However, such efforts have yet to be refined sufficiently for use in clinical practice.

Conclusions

The dictum of *primum non nocere* should be closely heeded in applying our general assessment methods to the complex and rare syndrome of PMD, whether its presentation is genuine or feigned. Without extensive validation of systematic differences between genuine and feigned PMD, the likelihood of misclassifications is substantial. Accurate classification is further complicated by the varying presentations of genuine PMD and its extensive comorbidity. Detection strategies provide a useful starting place for clinical investigations of questionable PMD presentations. Assessment methods for somatoform disorders (e.g., ADIS-IV and PAI), provide useful and reliable methods of assessing broader categories of somatoform disorders that can be evaluated across time and collateral sources. Additionally, the FBS may be helpful in signaling the need for further assessment of questionable PMD. Still, practitioners fully aware of their weaknesses may view these measures as a first, small, step in standardizing their investigations of questionable PMD.

References

1. Sharpe M. Somatoform disorders and DSM-IV. In *Proceedings of the 2nd International Conference on Psychogenic Movement Disorders and Other Conversion Disorders*, Washington, DC, April 2009.

2. Lang AE. General overview of psychogenic movement disorders: Epidemiology, diagnosis, and prognosis. In Hallett M, Fahn S, Jankovic J, *et al.*, eds. *Psychogenic Movement Disorders: Neurology and Neuropsychiatry*. Philadelphia, PA: Lippincott Williams & Wilkins, 2006:35–41.

3. Stone J, Sharpe M. Functional paralysis and sensory disturbance. In Hallett M, Fahn S, Jankovic J, *et al.*, eds. *Psychogenic Movement Disorders: Neurology and Neuropsychiatry*. Philadelphia, PA: Lippincott Williams & Wilkins, 2006:88–111.

4. Stone J. Presenting the diagnosis In *Proceedings of the 2nd International Conference on Psychogenic Movement Disorders and Other Conversion Disorders*, Washington, DC, April 2009.

5. Thomas M, Banuelas PA, Vuong KD, Jankovic J. Long-term prognosis of psychogenic movement disorders. In Hallett M, Fahn S, Jankovic J, *et al.*, eds. *Psychogenic Movement Disorders: Neurology and Neuropsychiatry*. Philadelphia, PA: Lippincott Williams & Wilkins, 2006:344–345.

6. Baez-Torres S, Galvez-Jimenez M. Psychogenic movement disorders: Is there a changing frequency and clinical profile? In Hallett M, Fahn S, Jankovic J, *et al.*, eds. *Psychogenic Movement Disorders: Neurology and Neuropsychiatry*. Philadelphia, PA: Lippincott Williams & Wilkins, 2006:83.

7. Thomas M, Jankovic J. Psychogenic movement disorders: diagnosis and management. *CNS Drugs* 2004;**18**:437–452.

8. Savard G, Panisset M. Simultaneous examination of patients by neurologist and psychiatrist provides clues for the diagnosis of psychogenic movement disorder. In Hallett M, Fahn S, Jankovic J, *et al.*, eds. *Psychogenic Movement Disorders: Neurology and Neuropsychiatry*. Philadelphia, PA: Lippincott Williams & Wilkins, 2006:339.

9. American Psychiatric Association. *Diagnostic and Statistical Manual of Diseases*, 4th edn, text revision. Washington DC: American Psychiatric Press, 2000.

10. Rogers R. Detection strategies for malingering and defensiveness. In Rogers R, ed. *Clinical Assessment of Malingering and Deception,* 3rd edn. Boston, MA: Guilford Press, 2008:14–35.

11. Rogers R, Reinhardt V. Conceptualization and assessment of secondary gain. In Koocher GP, Norcross JC, Hill SS, eds. *Psychologist's Desk Reference*. New York: Oxford University Press, 1998:57–62.

12. Factor S, Podskalny G, Molho E. Psychogenic movement disorders: frequency, clinical profile, and characteristics. *J Neurol Neurosurg Psychiatry* 1995;**59**:406–412.

13. Geller JL, Erlen J, Kaye NS, Fisher WH. Feigned insanity in nineteenth-century America: tactics, trials, and truth. *Behav Sci Law* 1990;**8**:3–26.

14. Rogers R, Correa AA. Determinations of malingering: evolution from case-based methods to detection strategies. *Psychiatry Psychol Law* 2008;**15**:213–223.

15. Rogers R. Towards an empirical model of malingering and deception. *Behav Sci Law* 1984;**2**:93–111.

16. Rogers R. Current status of clinical methods. In Rogers R, ed. *Clinical Assessment of Malingering and Deception*, 3rd edn. Boston, MA: Guilford Press, 2008:373–397.

17. Kapfhammer H, Rothenhäusler H. Malingering/Münchausen: factitious and somatoform disorders in neurology and clinical medicine. In Hallett M, Fahn S, Jankovic J, *et al.*, eds. *Psychogenic Movement Disorders: Neurology and Neuropsychiatry*. Philadelphia, PA: Lippincott Williams & Wilkins, 2006:154–162.

18. Nowak D, Fink G. Psychogenic movement disorders: aetiology, phenomenology, neuroanatomical correlates and therapeutic approaches. *Neuroimage* 2009;**47**:1015–1025.

19. Rogers R, Sewell KW, Gillard N. *Structured Interview of Reported Symptoms-2 (SIRS-2) and Professional Manual*. Odessa, FL: Psychological Assessment Resources, 2010.

20. Rogers R, Payne JW, Correa AA, Gillard ND, Ross CA. A study of the SIRS with severely traumatized patients. *J Personality Assess* 2009;**91**:429–438.

21. Rogers R. *Handbook of Diagnostic and Structured Interviewing*. New York: Guilford Press, 2001.

22. Hathaway SR, McKinley JC. A Multiphasic Personality Schedule (Minnesota): I. Construction of the schedule. *J Psychol* 1940;**10**:249–254.

23. Butcher JN, Dahlstrom WG, Graham JR, Tellegen A, Kaemmer B. *MMPI-2: Manual for Administration and Scoring*. Minneapolis, MN: University of Minnesota Press, 1989.

24. Greene RL. *The MMPI-2: An Interpretive Manual,* 2nd edn. Needham Heights, MA: Allyn & Bacon, 2000.

25. Brandwin MA, Kewman DG. MMPI indicators of treatment response to spinal epidural stimulation in patients with chronic pain and patients with movement disorders. *Psychol Rep* 1982;**51**:1059–1064.

26. Shiri S, Tsenter J, Livai R, Schwartz I, Vatine J. Similarities between the psychological profiles of complex regional pain syndrome and conversion disorder patients. *J Clin Psychol Med Settings* 2003;**10**:193–199.

27. Wetzel RD, Brim J, Guze SB, *et al.* MMPI screening scales for somatization disorder. *Psychol Rep* 1999;**85**:341–348.

28. Morey LC. *The Personality Inventory: Professional Manual*. Odessa, FL: Psychological Assessment Resources, 1991.

29. Morey LC. *Essentials of PAI Assessment*. New York: John Wiley, 2003.

30. Morey LC. *An Interpretive Guide to the Personality Assessment Inventory*. Odessa, FL: Psychological Assessment Resources, 1997.

31. Brown TA, DiNardo P, Barlow DH. *Anxiety Disorders Interview Schedule Adult Version (ADIS-IV): Client Interview Schedule*. New York: Oxford University Press, 2004.

32. Janca A, Burke JD, Isaac M, *et al.* The World Health Organization Somatoform Disorders Schedule: a preliminary report on design and reliability. *Eur Psychiatry* 1995;**10:**373–378.

33. Phillips KA, Fallon B. Somatoform and factitious disorders and malingering measures. In Rush JA, Jr., First MB, Blacker D, eds. *Handbook of Psychiatric Measures*. Washington, DC: American Psychiatric Press, 2005:591–616.

34. Rogers R, Sewell KW, Martin MA, Vitacco MJ. Detection of feigned mental disorders: a meta-analysis of the MMPI-2 and malingering. *Assessment* 2003;**10:**160–177.

35. Lees-Haley PR, English LT, Glenn WJ. A fake bad scale on the MMPI-2 for personal-injury claimants. *Psychol Rep* 1991;**68:**203–210.

36. Greiffenstein MF, Fox D, Lees-Haley PR. The MMPI-2 Fake Bad Scale in detection of noncredible claims. In Boone KB, ed. *Assessment of Feigned Cognitive Impairment*. New York: Guilford Press, 2007:210–235.

37. Green P. *Green's Word Memory Test for Microsoft Windows*. Edmonton, Alberta: Greens Publishing, 2003.

38. Boone KB, Lu P, Sherman D, *et al.* Validation of a new technique to detect malingering of cognitive symptoms: The b Test. *Arch Clin Neuropsychol* 2000;**15:**227–241.

39. Williamson DJ, Dran DL, Strong ES. Symptom validity tests in the epilepsy clinic. In Boone KB, ed. *Assessment of Feigned Cognitive Impairment*. New York: Guilford Press, 2007:346–365.

40. Larrabee GJ. Somatic malingering on the MMPI and MMPI-2 in litigating subjects. *Clin Neuropsychologist* 1998;**12:**179–188.

41. Nelson NW, Sweet JJ, Demakis GJ. Meta-analysis of the MMPI-2 Fake Bad Scale: Utility and forensic practice. *Clin Neuropsychol* 2006;**20:**39–58.

42. Ben-Porath YS, Tellegen A. *Minesota Multiphasic Personality Inventory-2 Restructured Form (MMPI-2-RF)*. San Antonio, TX: Pearson Assessments, 2008.

43. Tellegen A, Ben-Porath YS. *Minnesota Multiphasic Personality Inventory-2 Restructured Form: Technical Manual*. Minneapolis, MN: University of Minnesota Press, 2008.

44. Lanyon RI. Assessing the misrepresentation of health problems. *J Person Assess* 2003;**81:**1–10.

45. Oakley DA, Ward NS, Halligan PW, Frackowiak SJ. Differential brain activations for malingered and subjectively "real" paralysis. In Halligan PW, Bass C, Oakley DA, eds. *Malingering and Illness Deception*. Oxford: Oxford University Press, 2003: 267–284.

Chapter

36

Prognosis in patients with psychogenic motor disorders

Christopher Bass

Introduction

This chapter focuses on adult presentations of psychogenic movement disorders (PMDs). The evidence suggests that a diagnosis of a motor conversion disorder or PMD is stable over time when detailed investigations are carried out to exclude the presence of neurological disease [1].

The prevalence of PMDs is similar to that of multiple sclerosis. Indeed, studies suggest a burden of disability associated with chronic functional movement disorders that is far higher than a typical practicing psychiatrist might suspect or than is reflected in standard textbooks of psychiatry or clinical neurology (50 per 100 000 for cases of conversion disorder known to health services at any one time, with perhaps twice that number affected over a 1–2 year period [2]). Sadly the resources assigned to the treatment of these patients are scarce, which may be one of the many factors that contribute to the relatively poor prognosis in this group of disorders.

The PMDs are a heterogeneous group of disorders, which include the following:

- functional weakness of limbs
- movement disorders of non-organic base
- abnormal movements in patients with complex regional pain syndrome type I or what used to be called reflex sympathetic dystrophy [3]
- abnormal movements/paresis after various injuries or surgical procedures [4].

Various aspects of prognosis will be considered: the outcome of the index symptom[s], the development of neurological and psychiatric disorder over time, and factors that predict prognosis. The prognosis of PMDs is further complicated by the need for the diagnosis to be confirmed by a neurologist; how this initial diagnosis is established and then communicated in a sensitive fashion to the patient may influence many factors that have a bearing on outcome, including the patient's capacity to engage effectively in treatment.

Early follow-up studies

One of the earliest studies is that of Ljungberg [5], who followed up 381 patients for over 15 years. Patients were recruited from both neurological and psychiatric settings, and patients presented with a variety of symptoms. Ljungberg's key finding, which has been reinforced by a recent systematic review (R. Ruddy, A. House, and L. Madeley, unpublished data), was that when recovery occurred it tended to happen early, usually during the first year of the illness (62% became symptom free). In general, the majority of patients obtaining marked or complete improvement do so in the first year but there are smaller numbers who can show improvement beyond that time.

Ljundberg's study was followed by the much-publicized work of Slater in 1965 [6]. Slater followed up 85 patients seen in the 1950s at the National Hospital for Nervous Diseases in London. The surprising finding was that 60% of the patients had acquired a neurological diagnosis at follow-up that, in the view of Slater, could have explained the original symptoms. Only 19 patients were symptom free at follow-up, 12 had died, and 40 were totally or partially disabled. Slater concluded that hysteria was "a fertile source of clinical error ... not only a delusion but a snare." Although influential for about 30 years, it has become evident that this study was flawed. More recent studies have refuted Slater's findings, and rates of misdiagnosis in conversion disorder have been shown to be low [7,8].

Psychogenic Movement Disorders and Other Conversion Disorders, ed. Mark Hallett, Anthony E. Lang, Joseph Jankovic, Stanley Fahn, Peter W. Halligan, Valerie Voon, and C. Robert Cloninger. Published by Cambridge University Press. © Cambridge University Press 2011.

Table 36.1 Summary of follow-up studies carried out on conversion disorders between 1998 and 2010

Study	No. patients (No. followed up)	Mean follow-up (years)	Axis I diagnosis (mental illness) (%)	Axis II diagnosis (personality disorder) (%)	Outcome/disability at follow-up
Crimlisk et al.,1998 [7], UK	73 (64)	6.0	75	45	50% had either retired on ill health grounds or sick leave
Binzer and Kullgren, 1998 [10], Sweden	30 (30)	3.8	33	50	13 (43%) not working at one year; only 3 (10%) unchanged or worse
Feinstein et al., 2001 [11], Canada	88 (42)	3.2	95	45	Persistence of abnormal movements in > 90,: 57% disabled, 75% unemployed
Stone et al., 2003 [12], UK	60 (56)	12.5 (median)	–	–	83% report weakness or sensory symptoms; 30% medically retired
Jankovic et al., 2006 [13], USA	517 (228)	3.4	–	–	56% reported improvement
Sharpe et al., 2010 [14], UK	1144 (716)	1.0	–	–	67% reported poor outcome (rated unchanged, worse or much worse)

Recent follow-up studies

Advances in clinical diagnosis, in particular imaging, allow for the safe detection of neurological disease in its early stages. In addition, advances in molecular genetics have made it possible to classify as organic conditions hitherto thought to be hysterical (e.g., certain types of dystonia). The widespread use of standardized psychiatric diagnostic criteria is also likely to have had an impact on the detection of psychiatric morbidity [1]. A good example of a recent follow-up study that failed to detect any covert organic neurological disease was reported by Carson et al. [9]. In this study, over half the patients who presented to neurologists with symptoms that were rated as largely or completely medically unexplained had not improved 8 months later. Significantly, in no case was a disease explanation for the original presenting symptoms subsequently identified.

A survey of follow-up studies carried out since 1998 revealed that, in general, the prognosis is poor, with over half the patients reporting symptoms and functional impairments, and many not being able to work. A typical finding is that a significant number of patients are left with chronic symptoms after a long follow-up period of about 6 years, with 52% reporting ongoing symptoms [7]. A summary of the main studies carried out since 1998 is shown in Table 36.1.

A systematic survey of outcomes and prognostic factors in PMDs (R. Ruddy, A. House, and L. Madeley, unpublished data) took a narrative review and identified 2501 references in 2007, of which 34 were included in the review (although only 16 of these discussed prognostic factors). Studies were grouped according to setting (psychiatry or neurology) and length of follow-up to consider potential relationships with outcome tables. Studies were ranked by duration of follow-up and separated into four groups: < 6 months, 0.51–3 years, 3.1–7 years, and > 7 years. Table 36.2 shows the weighted mean percentage recovery for the four follow-up periods. The findings suggest that approximately 40% fully recover within the first 6 months, with perhaps a further 20% making a recovery later (over 7 years) in follow-up. This is a tentative finding, as the standard deviations were large. Many of the longer-term studies lost large numbers in follow-up and many did not have face-to-face contact with the research team.

The data reveal that although the number of people completely recovering varied, there was a significant

Table 36.2 Recovery and chronic symptom rates for different durations of follow-up

Grouped duration of follow-up (years)	No. studies	Total sample population	Weighted complete recovery (% [SD])	Weighted % chronic symptoms of conversion disorder (SD)
< 0.5	7	655	40 (29)	30 (23)
0.51–3	5	232	50 (24)	20 (3)
3.1–7	11	631	33 (25)	36 (17)
> 7	10	918	63 (20)	25 (11)

Unpublished data from R. Ruddy, A. House, and L. Madeley.

proportion left with chronic symptoms even with a long follow-up period, with some patients described as having chronic conversion disorder or somatization disorder.

A recent example of this poor outcome was reported by Crimlisk et al. [15], who interviewed patients on average 6 years after their original admission to the National Hospital for Neurology and Neurosurgery in London. Psychiatrists saw 75% of the patients and treatment was initiated in 60% of these. Despite this, during the 6-year follow up, many patients were subsequently referred to neurologists and other specialists, but subsequent psychiatric referral once the patient had been discharged from hospital was rare. Many (61%) changed their primary care clinician after discharge from the hospital and a disproportionate number of re-referrals were made by primary care clinicians who had known their patients for less than 6 months. Psychological attribution of symptoms was rare and did not appear to be related to the pattern of referrals. Only 14% were in psychiatric care at follow-up. The poor outcomes in this study may relate to the long duration of symptoms often necessary to warrant a referral to a tertiary care center specializing in functional motor disorders.

The potential for iatrogenic harm in these patients appears to be limitless, as was confirmed in a series of chronically disabled patients with conversion disorders referred to either the liaison psychiatry or the neurological disability service in a general hospital for assessment [16]. These patients use considerable healthcare resources, are often unemployed, and receive welfare benefits.

The *setting* in which patients are seen may influence outcome, with psychiatric settings being associated with more positive results. In the systematic survey of outcomes and prognostic factors described above, five out of eight studies in psychiatric settings record recovery rates of more than 50% compared with three out

of ten in neurology. In the remaining 14 studies with different hospital settings only six recorded a recovery rate of 50% or more.

In the most recently published follow-up study of a large consecutive series of neurology outpatients after 1 year, outcomes of "unchanged", "worse," or "much worse" were reported by two-thirds. Patients' beliefs (expectation of non-recovery)], non-attribution of symptoms to psychological factors, and the receipt of illness-related financial benefits were strong independent baseline predictors of this [14]. Together, these factors predicted 13% of the variance in outcome. The authors concluded that illness beliefs and financial benefits are more useful in predicting poor outcome than the number of symptoms, disability, and distress. As research studies on prognostic factors begin to address more complex variables, such as illness beliefs and expectations, illness-related financial benefits, antecedent life events, and difficulties with sick role potential, our knowledge of predictive factors in these complex disorders should become more meaningful.

Patients with psychogenic dystonia

A group of patients has been described who are characterized by fixed dystonia (which includes patients fulfilling criteria for CRPS-I [3]) as well as for psychogenic dystonia. The majority of these have symptoms affecting the limbs, particularly the foot, and trauma is often a precipitating factor. A diagnosis of a somatoform disorder can usually be established, but in a proportion conclusive features of a somatoform disorder or psychogenic disorder cannot be found, and the diagnosis remains open to question [17]. The disorder has also been described in adolescents, when it is often associated with significant psychological morbidity [18]. Two additional factors are pertinent. First, as trauma is so often a cause, litigation not infrequently lurks in the background. Second, very rare instances of malingering, as revealed by covert video surveillance, have also been reported [3].

Follow-up data in these patients is scarce, but recent evidence suggests that the outcome is poor. Ibrahim *et al.* [19] followed 41 patients with fixed dystonia after a mean of 7.6 years and found that 31% had worsened, 46% were the same, and 23% had improved; in the improved group 6% had major remissions. Patients with CRPS at baseline had a worse outcome. The authors concluded that the prognosis was poor, with improvement in less than a quarter, and the emergence of new neuropsychiatric features in some.

Other relevant factors influencing outcome

Many factors can influence prognosis, including the type and duration of the motor symptom, coexisting psychiatric morbidity, and availability and stage of commencing treatment. It would be foolish not to consider the role that society, and the legal and welfare system in particular, can play in perpetuating symptoms. Iatrogenic factors will also play a role but are very difficult to quantify in research.

Feinstein *et al.* [11] reported a very poor outcome after a mean period of 3.2 years, with a persistence of abnormal movements in more than 90% of subjects. They found that prevalence rates of mental illness in excess of those found in the general population plus high rates of personality disorder (45% of the sample), as well as a lack of psychological mindedness, characterized the outcome and contributed to the poor long-term prognosis. Binzer and Kullgren [10] also found poor outcome to be associated with the presence of personality disorder.

In the survey mentioned above, younger age was the only factor related to the individual found to influence outcome. With regard to social circumstances, a change in marital status, good family functioning, and the elimination of a stressor has a positive effect on outcome, whereas receiving benefits and pending litigation claims had a negative influence. This is an interesting result because, despite widespread belief that secondary gain in the form of family functioning, benefits, or litigation is important in the maintenance of conversion disorder, only two studies found evidence of this, the recent finding of Sharpe *et al.* [14] being an example.

There was a consensus from nine papers used in the survey that a shorter duration of symptoms was a

positive prognostic factor. Some authors have focused on specific symptoms; for example, Stone *et al.* [12] found that sensory symptoms alone, compared with motor symptoms or a combination, were associated with a better outcome.

Examination of treatment factors revealed that compliance with the treatment regimen was a positive prognostic factor while negative factors were use of non-psychotropic medication and dissatisfaction with the clinician. There is no consensus about the impact on outcome of comorbid psychiatric disorder, but negative prognostic conditions were personality disorder and somatic disease, whereas raised anxiety levels were found to be a positive factor [13,20].

Conclusions

In terms of prognostic indicators in those with PMDs, younger age and shorter duration of symptoms are the only factors found to influence outcome in a favourable direction. The fact that a short duration of symptoms is a positive prognostic factor suggests that early treatment is probably indicated, with the awareness that some people may require long-term follow-up. Any intervention will need to be multimodal and should probably involve a psychiatrist. There is a consensus that the intervention should be directed towards the cause of the disorder. More recent research findings also suggest that both illness beliefs and the receipt of disability payments may have an important bearing on prognosis, and that future outcome studies should incorporate these measures.

References

1. Ron M. The prognosis of hysteria/somatisation disorder. In Halligan P, Bass C, Marshall J, eds. *Contemporary Approaches to the Study of Hysteria: Clinical and Theoretical Perspectives*. Oxford: Oxford University Press, 2001:271–282.

2. Akagi H, House A. The epidemiology of hysterical conversion. In Halligan P, Bass C, Marshall J, eds. *Contemporary Approaches to the Study of Hysteria: Clinical and Theoretical Perspectives*. Oxford: Oxford University Press, 2001:73–87.

3. Verdugo R, Ochoa J. Abnormal movements in complex regional pain syndrome: assessment of their nature *Muscle Nerve* 2000;**23**:198–205.

4. Stone J, Carson J, Aditya H, *et al.* The role of physical injury in motor and sensory conversion symptoms: a systematic and narrative review. *J Psychosom Res* 2009;**66**:383–390.

5. Ljungberg L. Hysteria: a clinical, prognostic and genetic study. *Acta Psychiatr Neurol Scand* 1957;**32**(Suppl 112):1–162.

6. Slater E. Diagnosis of hysteria. *BMJ* 1965;**1**:1395–1399.

7. Crimlisk H, Bhatia K, Cope H, *et al*. Slater revisited: 6 year follow up of patients with medically unexplained motor symptoms. *BMJ* 1998;**316**:582–586.

8. Stone J, Smyth R, Carson A, *et al*. Systematic review of misdiagnosis of conversion symptoms and "hysteria." *BMJ* 2005;**331**:989.

9. Carson A, Best S, Postma K, *et al*. The outcome of neurology outpatients with medically unexplained symptoms: a prospective cohort study. *J Neurol Neurosurg Psychiatry* 2003:**74**:897–900.

10. Binzer M, Kullgren G. Motor conversion disorder. A prospective 2- to 5-year follow up study. *Psychosomatics* 1998;**39**:519–527.

11. Feinstein A, Stergiopoulos V, Fine J Lang A. Psychiatric outcome in patients with a psychogenic movement disorder. *Neuropsych Neuropsychol Behav Neurol* 2001;**14**:169–176.

12. Stone J, Sharpe M, Rothwell P, Warlow C. The 12-year prognosis of unilateral functional weakness and sensory disturbance. *J Neurol Neurosurg Psychiatry* 2003;**74**:591–596.

13. Jankovic J, Vuong K, Thomas M. Psychogenic tremor: long-term outcome. *CNS Spectr* 2006;**11**:501–508.

14. Sharpe M, Stone J, Hibberd C, *et al*. Neurology outpatients with symptoms unexplained by disease: illness beliefs and financial benefits predict one-year outcome. *Psychol Med* 2010;**40**:689–698.

15. Crimlisk H, Bhatia K, Cope H, *et al*. Patterns of referral in patients with medically unexplained motor symptoms. *J Psychosom Res* 2000;**49**:217–219.

16. Allanson J, Bass C, Wade D. Characteristics of patients with severe disability and medically unexplained neurological symptoms: a pilot study. *J Neurol Neurosurg Psychiatry* 2002;**73**:307–309.

17. Schrag A, Trimble M, Quinn N, Bhatia K. The syndrome of fixed dystonia: an evaluation of 103 cases. *Brain* 2004;**127**:2360–2372.

18. Majumdar A, Lopez-Casas J, Poo P, *et al*. Syndrome of fixed dystonia in adolescents: short term outcome in 4 cases. *Eur J Paed Neurol* 2008;**30**:1–7.

19. Ibrahim N, Marino D, van den Warrenburg B, *et al*. The prognosis of fixed dystonia: a follow up study. *Parkinsonism Relat Disord* 2009;**15**:592–597.

20. Mace C, Trimble M. Ten-year prognosis of conversion disorder. *BMJ* 1996;**169**:282–288.

Chapter 37

Psychogenic movement disorders: explaining the diagnosis

Jon Stone, Alan J. Carson, and Michael Sharpe

Introduction

There are many difficulties in the delivery of a diagnosis of psychogenic movement disorder (PMD) or other conversion disorder. A common scenario is the patient who becomes angry when their "neurological work-up" is negative and they are offered no diagnosis. Alternatively, patients often feel upset because they equate "psychogenic" with being "mad" or "faking it."

Recent data from a survey of 519 members of the Movement Disorder Society has shown how important the issue of explanation is in patients with PMD [1]. "Acceptance of the diagnosis" was the runaway winner among 11 factors rated by neurologists as being likely to predict patient outcome, and "educating the patient" was the second most effective perceived treatment (after "avoiding iatrogenic harm"). The same study also revealed wide variation in the terms used by neurologists both with each other and with patients. For example, 83% of neurologists use the term "psychogenic movement disorder" with their colleagues, but only 59% use it with patients. Conversely, only 10% use the term "stress-related" with colleagues, whereas 67% use it with patients; only 34% of neurologists actually use the DSM-IV term "conversion disorder" among themselves (Fig. 37.1).

The debate about what to tell the patient is closely related to the discussion about the ways in which doctors conceive of the problem of "psychogenic" symptoms. This chapter will largely avoid a discussion of the merits of different theoretical concepts and concentrate on practicalities:

- why patients and doctors find this such a difficult problem

- the current evidence regarding the outcome of different explanations
- the different options available to the doctor in presenting a diagnosis
- whether there is a "one size fits all" approach in initial and subsequent explanations.

Why is this such a difficult clinical problem?

The patients' perspective

The difficulties that arise in giving a psychological diagnosis for a physical symptom are fairly unique within medicine. There is a significant chance that the patient, with a paralysis or tremor for example, will be upset by this diagnosis for a number of potential reasons.

The patient thinks the doctor may be implying that they are doing it on purpose

The thought that the doctor may be implying that the patient is "doing it on purpose" may make the patient upset because

- they feel very strongly that they are not doing it on purpose
- they had been secretly concerned that they did have some degree of control of their symptoms – perhaps they were aware that it seemed to get worse when they thought about it – and this suggests a possible explanation which they do not wish to confront themselves.

Psychogenic Movement Disorders and Other Conversion Disorders, ed. Mark Hallett, Anthony E. Lang, Joseph Jankovic, Stanley Fahn, Peter W. Halligan, Valerie Voon, and C. Robert Cloninger. Published by Cambridge University Press. © Cambridge University Press 2011.

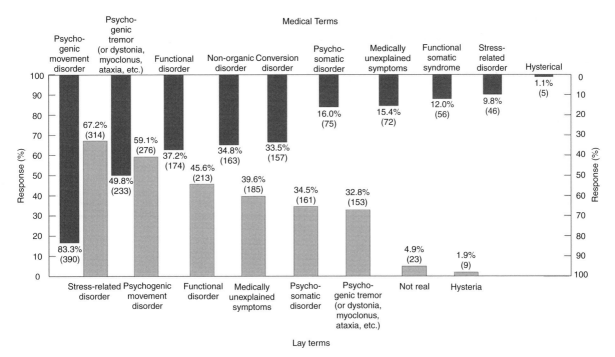

Fig. 37.1. Preferred "medical"and "lay" terms used by 519 respondents to the Movement Disorder Society survey on psychogenic movement disorders when respondents were asked to rate their "top three." [1] (reproduced by permission of John Wiley and Sons)

The patient wonders or is concerned that the doctor has missed a more "sinister" neurological disease causing their symptoms

Patients may have read about alternative explanations such as Parkinson's disease or multiple sclerosis. While they may be upset to have those diagnoses too, patients sometimes express disappointment that they have not been given a disease diagnosis [2]. The presence of psychogenic chorea in patients with a family history of Huntington's disease, convinced that they have the disease, illustrates this [3]. A disease diagnosis such as multiple sclerosis comes with guaranteed public recognition and perceived benefits for support or treatment (although these have often not been thought through by the patient). They may also feel that they have not been given a diagnosis at all and are still in diagnostic limbo [4].

The patient feels very strongly that they do not have a psychological problem

There is accumulating evidence to back up the common clinical experience that patients with conversion symptoms frequently feel strongly that their symptoms do not have a psychological cause (Table 37.1).

For example Kapfhammer *et al.* [5] found in a sample of 103 patients with conversion disorder that 78 (76%) believed there was a somatic cause, 15 (15%) thought there was a psychological cause, and only 7 (7%) thought stress was the main cause. Other studies have shown that patients with conversion symptoms are even less likely to consider that psychological factors might be involved than patients who actually have a comparable disease [7,8,10,11]. Studies comparing illness beliefs of patients with chronic fatigue syndrome or multiple sclerosis [12], or patients with fibromyalgia or rheumatoid arthritis, have shown that the experience of the patient with a somatoform disorder is remarkably similar to a patient with a corresponding organic disease: they have the same physical experience and cannot understand why it appears to be dismissed as psychological.

The patient shares the general public's negative ideas about psychosomatic disorders

All mental health problems suffer from the problem of societal stigma. This is particularly the case for psychogenic disorders. Two of our own studies of general neurology outpatients looked at patients' perceptions of different labels for symptoms [13,14]. We found that

Table 37.1 Studies examining illness beliefs in patients with conversion symptoms show that only a minority endorse psychological causation, and often less so than disease controls

Study	Patients (No.)	Findings
Kapfhammer *et al.*, 1992 [5]	Motor/non-epileptic attacks (103)	76% believed there was a somatic cause, 15% thought there was a psychological cause, and only 7% thought stress was the main cause
Ewald *et al.*, 1994 [6]	Neurology inpatient somatizers (40) versus disease controls (60)	36% of neurology inpatients with conversion symptoms thought psychological factors were of importance versus 76% of neurology inpatients with disease
Bibzer *et al.* 1998 [7], Binzer 1999 [8]	Paralysis (30) versus disease controls (30)	Patients with conversion had greater disease conviction (IBQ) and a more external locus of control than controls with disease
Crimlisk *et al.*, 2000 [9]	Weakness/movement disorder (64)	5% thought that psychological factors were important, 22% thought psychological factors had played a part (e.g., stress), 73% thought psychological factors irrelevant
Stone *et al.*, 2003 [10]	Non-epileptic attacks (20) versus epilepsy (20)	Patients with non-epileptic attacks had greater disease conviction (IBQ) and a more external locus of control than controls with epilepsy
Stone *et al.*, 2010 [11]	Weakness (107) versus disease controls (85)	24% thought that stress was a potential factor versus 56% of neurological controls

IBQ, Illness Behavior Questionnaire.

words like psychosomatic or hysterical, when used to describe paralysis or blackouts, were often equated with words like "mad" or "imagining symptoms" (Tables 37.2 and 37.3). In addition, a study of the word "psychosomatic," as used in UK and US newspapers, showed that it was used in a negative way in 34% of articles [15]. In our experience, some patients with conversion symptoms have especially sensitive views about mental health problems, because of the views of someone in their family or because a family member does have mental health problems.

The patient (or family member) are secretly concerned that there was a psychological problem and this diagnosis confirms their worst fears

In particular, some patients who have experienced childhood abuse may secretly wonder if this is relevant to their symptoms but be terrified to consider the possibility as they view this as something that cannot be changed.

There can be great difficulties in giving a diagnosis of motor neuron disease or terminal cancer to a patient, but the patient's truthfulness, their state of mind, or their willingness to believe the doctor is not usually at stake. If a patient with cancer is concerned that the diagnosis is wrong, they are usually desperately wondering if perhaps the diagnosis is not as bad as the doctor thinks.

The doctor's perspective

The doctor's difficulties in this process mirror those of the patient but also reflect more generally on the uncertainty about how to classify and think about these disorders: are these symptoms really purely "psychogenic" or is it "conversion"? How important are biological factors and how do they alter our view of these disorders?

The neurologist is uninterested in diagnosing or treating what they perceive as a psychological disorder

Conversion disorder is defined currently as a psychiatric disorder not a neurological one. Many neurologists may feel their role is simply to look for neurological disease. When it is not present, they may feel that it is not their job to diagnose and treat a patient with a psychiatric disorder and that they should simply do nothing or refer to a psychiatrist.

The neurologist may not know what they think themselves about this area

Conversion disorders are not an area that has been highlighted as important in neurological training programs or research agendas. As a consequence, neurologists may feel that they do not know what to do with the patient (and neither does anybody else).

Table 37.2 Percentage responses among 86 new neurology outpatients to the question, "If you had leg weakness, your tests were normal, and a doctor said you had "X" would he be suggesting that you were Y (or had Y)."

Diagnoses (X)	Connotations (Y) (% response)					Offence score (%)[a]	The "number needed to offend" (95% CI)[b]
	Putting it on (yes)	Mad (yes)	Imagining symptoms (yes)	Medical condition (no)	Good reason to be off sick from work (no)		
Symptoms all in the mind	83	31	87	66	70	93	2 (2–2)
Hysterical weakness	45	24	45	33	42	50	2 (2–3)
Medically unexplained weakness	24	12	31	37	41	42	3 (2–4)
Psychosomatic weakness	24	12	40	21	28	35	3 (3–4)
Depression-associated weakness	21	7	20	15	28	31	4 (3–5)
Stress-related weakness	9	3	14	14	23	19	6 (4–9)
Chronic fatigue	9	1	10	19	14	14	8 (5–13)
Functional weakness	7	2	8	8	20	12	9 (5–16)
Stroke	2	5	5	6	12	12	9 (5–16)
Multiple sclerosis	0	1	3	3	8	2	43 (13–∞)

CI, confidence interval.
[a] Proportion of patients who responded "yes" to one or more of the three questions: "putting it on," "mad," or "imagining symptoms."
[b] Calculated based on the offence score: the number of patients who would have to be given this diagnostic label before one patient is "offended."
Source: Reproduced from Stone *et al.*, 2002 [13], with permission of BMJ publications.)

One of our studies found that the more the patients' symptoms were unexplained by disease the more neurologists found the patient difficult to help (Fig. 37.2) [16].

If neurologists are uncertain themselves what kind of problem they are dealing with, it is perhaps not surprising that they have difficulty communicating the diagnosis even when they are interested or sympathetic to the problem.

The doctor is wondering if the patients is "doing it on purpose"

For PMDs and other conversion disorders, the question of whether the patients is "doing it on purpose" is a particularly important issue, even compared with other somatoform disorders. Kanaan and colleagues have found evidence for the persistence of these thoughts in neurologists [17,18]. There are several simple reasons for this.

- Conversion disorder is a disorder of voluntary function. Patients have symptoms which, therefore, can be voluntarily mimicked.
- Unlike, chronic fatigue syndrome or fibromyalgia for example, patients with PMDs are diagnosed on the basis of inconsistency. Their symptoms can be demonstrably made to improve temporarily. For example, Hoover's sign makes psychogenic hip extension weakness transiently strong or distraction can transiently improve a psychogenic tremor.

Table 37.3 Percentage responses among 102 new neurology outpatients to the question "If you had blackouts, your tests were normal and a doctor said you had X would he be suggesting that you were Y (or had Y)"

Diagnoses (X)	Connotations (Y) (% response)						Offence score (% [95% CI])[a]
	Putting it on (yes)	Doctor doesn't know what it is (yes)	Mad (yes)	Medical condition (no)	Imagining symptoms (yes)	A good reason to be off sick from work (no)	
Symptoms all in the mind	74	55	29	70	70	67	89 (82–94)
Hysterical seizures	38	34	12	32	30	55	48 (38–58)
Pseudoseizures	29	25	6	23	21	46	33 (24–43)
Psychogenic Seizures	22	17	5	10	16	27	26 (18–36)
Non-epileptic attack disorder	17	21	2	15	17	38	22 (15–32)
Tonic–clonic seizures	8	10	3	8	6	31	12 (6–20)
Stress-related seizures	6	18	0	10	5	21	8 (3–15)
Functional seizures	3	7	0	5	4	30	6 (2–12)
Grand mal seizures	4	4	3	5	3	28	5 (2–11)
Epilepsy	0	0	0	1	0	31	0 (0–4)

CI, confidence interval (calculated by exact Clopper–Pearson method).
[a] Proportion of patients who responded "yes" to one or more of the three questions: "putting it on," "mad," or "imagining symptoms."
Source: Reproduced from Stone *et al.*, 2003 [14], with permission of BMJ publications.)

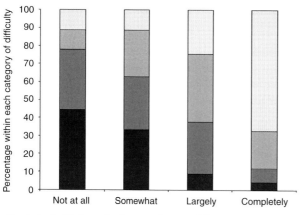

To what extent is the patient's presenting complaint explained by organic disease?

Fig. 37.2. Neurologists' perceptions of difficulty by "organicity" of presenting complaint (*n* = 299), indicating that they find patients with symptoms unexplained by disease more difficult to help. (Taken from Carson *et al.*, 2004 [16], with permission of BMJ publications.)

- The methods available to discriminate a psychogenic problem from an "organic" problem do not distinguish a conversion symptom from a factitious symptom.
- The psychological model of conversion symptoms is understood by most doctors, but this is usually held in parallel with a "deception" model in which the doctor remains concerned that the patient may be "doing it on purpose" [17]. The persistence of an untestable criterion in the DSM IV definition of conversion disorder in which the doctor is asked to be confident that the patient is "not feigning" serves to accentuate this. Such a criterion is not applied to other psychiatric disorders.

The doctor is reluctant to make a "psychogenic" diagnosis

Doctors may be reluctant to make a diagnosis of PMD and other conversion disorders, for a number of reasons:

- an awareness that psychogenic neurological symptoms, and movement disorders especially, are hard to diagnose and require lots of experience
- studies suggesting high rates of misdiagnosis from the 1960s [19]
- the way in which some conditions such as task-specific dystonia were erroneously reformulated as psychogenic by psychodynamic theory
- a perception that erroneously labeling a symptom as psychogenic when it is organic is worse than erroneously labeling something as organic when it is psychogenic [18]
- a perception that patients given this diagnosis may react badly, with letters of complaint.

Does good communication of the diagnosis affect clinical outcome?

Intuitively, a good explanation of the diagnosis which leaves the patients with a feeling that their doctor believes them, that they do not need any more investigations, and that they can get better would seem to be an important objective. The evidence to support this for conversion symptoms is rather slim and relies on prognostic studies.

In a study of patients with psychogenic tremor, the perceived effectiveness of treatment by the physician (something that perhaps correlates with overall satisfaction) was the best predictor of outcome in a logistic model [20]. In a retrospective study of 84 patients with non-epileptic attacks, 20% reacted angrily to the diagnosis, 40% were confused, and 21% were relieved [21]. Two-thirds agreed with the diagnosis. Anger ($p < 0.002$) and confusion ($p < 0.002$) correlated with ongoing seizures at follow-up. Relief at the diagnosis ($p < 0.0001$) related to good outcome. Other studies of non-epileptic attacks have found that patients who believed the diagnosis [22] or had a comprehensive approach to explanation and treatment [23] had a better outcome.

These data do not tell us whether the things that go wrong in the initial explanation are predominantly to do with the patient's response and how much may be entirely preventable on the doctor's side. Some patients may be angry whatever is said.

In a primary care study, Salmon and colleagues looked at the perceptions of 228 patients with "somatization disorders" toward the explanation offered by their primary care physician [24]. Their perceptions divided into three categories. The first was one of rejection (e.g., the symptoms are imaginary, etc.); the second was collusion (e.g., the doctors just agreed that it was a particular diagnosis, for example fibromyalgia or myalgic encephalomyelitis, but did not seem to really know much about it), and the third was "empowering." In this last, more successful consultation the primary care physician typically gave the patients a tangible mechanism for their symptoms, removed blame from the patients but at the same time phrased the problem in a way that allowed more for self-management.

In addition, qualitative studies have looked at this issue in small numbers of patients with conversion symptoms. In the study of 18 patients with conversion symptoms by Nettleton et al. [25], the patients were aware that their illnesses were viewed as "imagined" or "faking it," something that made them feel as if their illness was not legitimate. Another common theme in this and other studies is the report from patients that they felt in diagnostic limbo [4].

What are the options for presenting the diagnosis?

There are a large variety of ways in which a PMD or other conversion disorder can be explained to a patient. Before discussing the various options available, we summarize the components of a constructive explanation where there is less debate.

Core components of the explanation

1. Explain what they do have: options discussed below

2. Explain how you have made the diagnosis: show the patient their Hoover's sign, or dissociative seizure video

3. Explain what they don't have: "You do not have MS, epilepsy, etc."

4. Indicate that you believe them: "I do not think you are imagining/making up your symptoms/mad"

5. Emphasize that it is common: "I see lots of patients with similar symptoms"

6. Emphasize reversibility: "Because your brain is not damaged you have the potential to get better"

7. Emphasize that self-help is a key part of getting better: "This is not your fault but there are things you can do to help it get better"

8. Introduce the role of depression/anxiety: "If you have been feeling low/worried that will tend to make the symptoms even worse"

9. Use written information: send the patient their clinic letter, give them a leaflet or website

10. Stop any drugs that indicate a disease diagnosis: for example stop the anticonvulsant in someone with non-epileptic attacks

11. Suggesting antidepressants: "'So-called' antidepressants often help these symptoms even in patients who are not feeling depressed. They are not addictive"

12. Making the psychiatric referral: "I don't think you're mad but Dr. X has a lot of experience and interest in helping people like you to manage and overcome your symptoms. Are you willing to overcome any misgivings about their specialty to try to get better?"

13. Involve the family/friends: explain it all to them as well.

This shopping list of less controversial elements indicates that there is probably a consensus regarding many parts of the consultation with patients with conversion disorder [26,27]. In particular, a recent study has gathered some evidence for the first time that written information can be provided in an acceptable way to patients with non-epileptic attacks [28]. There is, however, still debate around the core explanation of the symptoms that the clinician (usually the neurologist) uses during the initial consultation. Even if steps 2–10

above go well, there is still a point at which the patient will ask, "So what do I have doctor?". The options for answering this question can be simplified into three main options.

1. Explanation of the symptoms as psychologically based

2. Explanation of the symptoms as a disorder of nervous system functioning

3. Explanation of the symptoms as not explained, "I don't know."

Straight away, one can see that these explanations are not necessarily contradictory. The first is primarily an explanation of (at least part of) the etiology; the second is more about mechanism. They could be used together either at the same time or sequenced together in additional consultations. Nonetheless, it is perhaps useful to look at the "pros and cons" of these different explanations.

In thinking through this issue, it is also important to ask who is giving these explanations. Is it the neurologist who has made the diagnosis? Does it matter how interested or experienced they are in the problem? Is there such a thing as a "one size fits all" explanation? Is a doctor's general manner and the way he or she delivers the explanation more important than the precise language used? Since there are a variety of views about the etiology of these symptoms, there are bound to be differences in how people express a view to the patient about them.

The psychological explanation

The psychological explanation may take different forms ranging from an upfront explanation of conversion disorder or psychogenic disorders to descriptions of somatization or a description of how "stress" can affect the brain. For example

> You have a psychogenic movement disorder. Your movements are a physical manifestation of stress or emotions in your body. When you get low, upset, or stressed there are a number of changes in the body that can produce unpleasant physical symptoms, for instance when people get frightened they often feel sick. This is the kind of problem that is causing your tremor.

The potential advantages of the psychological explanation

This may hasten the patient's acceptance and referral for psychological treatment aimed at improvement.

A referral to a psychologist or psychiatrist will be concordant with this explanation. As described above, approximately one-quarter of patients with conversion symptoms will have already come to the conclusion that their symptoms are at least partly psychologically mediated anyway.

Helping the patient make links between their physical symptoms and emotions. If no one suggests the possibility of a link between emotions and physical symptoms, then perhaps the patient will not think of it themselves.

There is no room for confusion regarding the possibility of disease. The patient is being told explicitly that they have a mental health problem.

They may find it easier to access information about their condition. Current descriptions of these conditions are largely based on psychological theory. This explanation will, therefore, accord with what they find on the Internet.

Patients with a negative reaction to a "psychological" explanation. These patients may have a poor outcome regardless of what is said to them.

The potential disadvantages of the psychological explanation

Narrowing of the etiological discussion. In giving a purely psychological explanation, the doctor may be wrong. A broader biopsychosocial model of these symptoms may be more correct than a purely "psychogenic" explanation. Studies using functional imaging [29] and neurophysiology [30] are providing more support for the role of biological factors.

An increased likelihood that the patient will be concerned that the doctor thinks they are crazy or imagining the symptoms. For the reasons described above.

An increased likelihood that the patient will be concerned that the doctor thinks they are feigning symptoms. For the reasons described above.

Deterioration of doctor–patient relationship. As a consequence of the first two points, the patient may be inclined to disbelieve other less controversial aspects of the consultation, such as the absence of disease or the possibility for recovery, and may be less willing to share information with their family or employers. This kind of explanation also makes it harder to share clinic letters without potentially angry replies from patients.

Summary

The psychological model of explanation, in which physical symptoms are re-attributed to psychological causes, remains popular [31]. A large trial of "reattribution" in primary care for patients with generally milder somatic symptoms showed that it was possible to train doctors in this method, and it generally made them more confident in dealing with the patients, but it did not affect patient outcome [32].

The functional/mechanistic explanation

In the functional/mechanistic approach, the patient is given an explanation of the *mechanism* of the symptoms, without necessarily straying into *why* they have them. These kinds of explanation may revolve around functional changes in the nervous system, for example,

> You have functional paralysis, that is a condition where there is a problem with the function of your nervous system, even though it is not damaged.

Dissociation, a concept which is at once both psychological and neurological can be used in a similar way,

> You have dissociative attacks; when you have your attacks you are going in to a trance like state, a bit like someone who has been hypnotized.

The potential advantages of the functional explanation

A decreased likelihood that the patient will be concerned that the doctor thinks they are crazy or imagining the symptoms. For the reasons described above.

A decreased likelihood that the patient will be concerned that the doctor thinks they are feigning symptoms. For the reasons described above.

In explaining the mechanism of the symptoms the door is left open to multiple potential causes. The use of a "functional" paradigm does not assume any particular etiology and is an equally good fit for biological explanations. Although some doctors may be convinced that they know the "psychogenic" etiology of their patients symptoms [18], others may feel that a biopsychosocial model is appropriate and be very uncertain as to why the patient has the symptoms. At a time when we have so much yet to find out about the neural correlates of these symptoms, this is an approach which is potentially more scientifically accurate and "future-proof." A functional explanation shifts the discussion from "Is it physical or psychological?" to "Is it structural or functional?" (although this can be seen to be a disadvantage too, see below) As in migraine, multiple sclerosis, or motor neuron disease, the diagnostic label is not a description of the etiology, it is a description of the problem.

Easier to use metaphors. For example, a patient with a PMD can be told that they have a "software problem, not a hardware problem," or that the problem is "like a piano that is out of tune." Patients with non-epileptic attacks have a "short circuit."

A better fit with potential reversibility. A problem that is psychological may be viewed by some patients as irreversible, particularly if it is formulated as having its roots in childhood. By contrast, it is possible to see that something that is "not functioning but is not damaged" has the potential to function again.

Not a reinvention of the wheel. This kind of explanation is not new. It was commonplace at the end of the nineteenth century as the term "functional nervous disorder." This was at a time when psychological theories were emerging for "hysteria," but had not yet achieved their later dominance.

The potential disadvantages of the functional explanation

Delay in appreciating psychological factors psychological treatment. Just because a patient is happier with the explanation they have been given does not mean that they will have a better outcome. It is possible that a more mechanistic explanation delays or prevents appropriate psychiatric treatment. If a doctor uses a functional explanation simply as a euphemism for a psychogenic explanation the patient may feel deceived at a later date.

Increased likelihood that the patient interprets the diagnosis as an organic disease. The patient may believe they do have neurological damage, which could impair rehabilitation. This problem has recently been rehearsed in relation to whether dissociative/non-epileptic/psychogenic episodes resembling epilepsy should be called "seizures" [33] or "attacks" [34], with an advocate of "attacks" suggesting the word too strongly implies epilepsy.

Too much political correctness. Some authors have suggested that it is taking political correctness too far to take the patients' views of the labels into account [35]. One argument is that such views are likely to change over time anyway, for example if the terms become incorporated into the media in a negative way [36].

Too wide a term. For some, the term "functional" is simply too wide. All symptoms whether caused or not by disease must be arising from disordered nervous function. Migraine, dystonia, and epilepsy, in particular, could all be said to be functional nervous disorders, and indeed they were considered as such in the nineteenth century. For some doctors, this regrouping would not be a problem, for others it would be. The term dissociative can also suffer from a loose definition. Many patients with conversion disorder have no specific dissociative symptoms other than the neurological symptom they present with.

Saying "I don't know"

Many doctors believe that patients with conversion symptoms are looking primarily for reassurance that they do not have a disease. Often offering this reassurance is insufficient. The patient has symptoms and they want an explanation for them. Doctors, however, may feel that it is easier simply to say "I don't know" or "I can't explain this on the basis of neurological disease" even when they recognize the nature of the symptoms [37]. They may not even feel it is their job to diagnose anything else.

A randomised trial by Thomas [38] in primary care found that patients who received a positive explanation regarding their unexplained symptoms had a much better outcome at 2 weeks (64%) than those who had been told "I cannot be certain what the matter is with you" (39%).

One can make an argument that since we do not know that much about why people do get conversion disorder, we should stick with an apparently neutral term like "medically unexplained symptoms." While this may appear theoretically sound, it actually promotes dualistic thinking and in clinical practice it is highly problematic. Not only does this term imply that we have no idea *why* the patient has their symptoms, it suggests that we are unable to reliably diagnose their condition either – we have no idea *what* is wrong with them. Clearly, for most neurological disease – motor

Table 37.4 Potential short- and long-term consequences of different explanations for psychogenic movement disorders and other conversion disorders

	Short-term outcome	Longer-term outcome
Psychological explanation	Less acceptable	Greater understanding?
Functional explanation	More acceptable	Less understanding?
Functional explanation first then introduction of psychological factors later	More acceptable	Greater understanding?
Tailored explanation: default position is a functional explanation but some patients may have psychological factors introduced at the first consultation whereas this occurs much later for others	Even more acceptable?	Even greater understanding?

neuron disease, multiple sclerosis, migraine – we do not really know *why* people get them but we can nonetheless recognize them at the bedside and can treat accordingly with varying degrees of success. In this sense, patients with conversion symptoms are no different. A recent consensus paper from a group of authors active in research in this area also concluded that the term "medically unexplained symptoms" could no longer be recommended (although they also failed to come up with an alternative!) [39].

Combining models of explanation: having your cake and eating it

As alluded to above, unless you are planning to see the patient only once, then a stark choice between psychological explanation and a functional explanation does not have to be made. In practice, there are many patients who are so hostile to the introduction of psychological factors, even as a contributory factor, at the first interview that it is easier to use the functional model.

However, things may be different at subsequent appointments. In our own experience, many such patients, after realizing that their symptoms are being taken seriously (and particularly when they receive their clinic letter or other self-help material), often spontaneously want to discuss relevant psychosocial factors that they themselves introduce as potentially relevant. These can be incorporated into a biopsychosocial model of the problem.

Furthermore, there are patients for whom psychological factors can be introduced at the first consultation without any difficulty (perhaps one-quarter). It can be relatively easy to identify these patients by simply asking them what they think is the cause of their symptoms during assessment. In practice, therefore,

the explanation can be tailored to the patient but with the default position being a mechanistic explanation. This probably represents the best solution of all. Table 37.4 summarizes this.

Simon Wessely [2] has discussed the ethics of the clinical dilemma of presenting a psychological or more mechanistic model to patients with somatic symptoms, pointing out that it may be unethical to give a patient an unacceptable diagnosis that makes them less likely to receive or engage in treatment. However, is it unethical to give a diagnosis which may not completely reflect the truth as the doctor sees it (for example if they view the symptoms as purely psychogenic)? He concludes that the "aim of telling is to get the patient better."

Finally, the maxim "it aint what you say, it's the way that you say it" may have particular relevance in this area. A doctor who says all the "right" things but is not really interested or sympathetic to the problem may be less effective than an empathic doctor who says all the "wrong" things. Doctors who have negative attitudes to patients with unexplained symptoms certainly find patients with somatic symptoms more difficult to deal with [40].

Investigations and reassurance

A topic that is sometimes missed out in this discussion of explaining diagnoses to patients is the issue of investigations. Investigations may be necessary, but physicians often fail to realize how harmful investigations can be to patients with conversion symptoms. They prolong the sense of diagnostic limbo mentioned above, tend to increase health anxiety and lack of confidence in the physician, and may turn up incidental abnormalities that cause further anxiety.

These are good arguments to suggest that when investigations are required they should be done as quickly as possible and with prior counseling. A randomized trial of patients with chest pain showed that pre-investigation counseling not only improved levels of reassurance once the test was normal but also improved symptomatic outcome [41]. If a patient has suspected conversion symptoms, at the bedside the physician can explain that they believe the tests will be normal and they are simply being thorough.

Sometimes doctors do tests specifically to reassure patients. But the reassurance provided by negative investigations can be overestimated. A study of patients with dyspepsia showed that patients with low levels of health anxiety *were* reassured by negative endoscopy but those with high levels of health anxiety were only reassured for a very short time, on average, less than a week [42]. This is in keeping with the concept that patients with severe health anxiety get addicted to reassurance, which has increasingly shorter duration of effect the longer their illness persists. Another study of neuroimaging for tension headache found that it reduced worry for several months on average, but at 1 year, the patients were no more reassured than those patients who had not been scanned [43].

Some other awkward questions

Finally there are some other "awkward questions" that may arise during an initial explanation and are worth mentioning here

"*Do I qualify for a wheelchair doctor?*" Some doctors may take the view that walking aids or wheelchairs should be prohibited in patients with functional disorders. There is no evidence here. Our own view is that there is no correct answer. Some patients undoubtedly do worse with walking aids or a wheelchair. In others, however, the increased independence can boost morale and be part of rehabilitation.

"*Can you sign my work incapacity form?*" There are often similar concerns here from health professionals. While some patients appear to slide rather easily into a "benefit lifestyle," others do not. There is no good evidence that the situation is any different for conversion disorder than it is in multiple sclerosis, for example, where some patients (in the UK at least), appear to obtain disability benefits at a stage when they could still work.

"*What should I tell my family/friends/employer?*" Announcing at work that you have a psychogenic or functional movement disorder is likely to be met with confusion. It seems reasonable to make efforts to inform and educate close family and friends about the diagnosis. For insurance companies and official organizations, the patient may need to know about official terminology for their condition such as conversion disorder. For "nosey parkers" at work, it may be helpful to advise the patient to tell them simply that they have a "tremor" or "blackouts", and are under hospital care.

Conclusions

The effective presentation of the diagnosis of PMDs and other conversion disorders is generally regarded as a crucial step in treatment. The reasons why giving the diagnosis can be difficult are numerous and relate to factors in the patient, in the doctor, and in society. Appreciation of these reasons and how they vary in individual patients allows greater confidence in navigating the diagnostic consultation.

On the question of whether a "psychological" or a "functional" explanation is best, there are arguments both for and against. These reflect debate generally about how to conceive of these disorders. It may not be necessary, however, to choose between these approaches, but instead they may both be useful at different times in the same patient, depending on the beliefs of the doctor and of the patient. Saying "I don't know" or "it's medically unexplained" is generally regarded as unhelpful.

Many elements of what can be usefully said to patients, such as explaining the positive features that have allowed the diagnosis to be made, are not particularly subject to debate. It appears particularly important for the diagnosis to be delivered without any judgmental or perjorative connotations. Ultimately, the attitude of the physician may play as important a role as the words he or she chooses to use with the patient.

Appendix: some sources of self-help for patients

Functional/dissociative neurological symptoms: free self help website for patients written by J. Stone www.neurosymptoms.org

Non-epileptic attacks: self-help material is improving on the web, e.g.,
www.nonepilepticattacks.info
www.neadtrust.co.uk

References

1. Espay AJ, Goldenhar LM, Voon V, *et al.* Opinions and clinical practices related to diagnosing and managing patients with psychogenic movement disorders: an international survey of Movement Disorder Society members. *Mov Disord* 2009;**24**:1366–1374.

2. Wessely S. To tell or not to tell? The problem of medically unexplained symptoms. In Zeman A, Emmanuel L, eds. *Ethical Dilemmas in Neurology.* London: WB Saunders, 2000:41–53.

3. Fekete R, Jankovic J. Psychogenic chorea associated with family history of Huntington disease. *Mov Disord* 2010;**25**:503–504.

4. Thompson R, Isaac CL, Rowse G, Tooth CL, Reuber M. What is it like to receive a diagnosis of nonepileptic seizures? *Epilepsy Behav* 2009;**14**:508–515.

5. Kapfhammer HP, Dobmeier P, Mayer C, Rothenhausler HB. Konversionssyndrome in der Neurologie: Eine psyhopathologische und psychodynamische Differenzierung in Konversionsstörung, Somatisierungstörung und artifizielle Störung. *Psychother Psychosom Med Psychol* 1998;**48**:463–474.

6. Ewald H, Rogne T, Ewald K, Fink P. Somatization in patients newly admitted to a neurological department. *Acta Psychiatr Scand* 1994;**89**:174–179.

7. Binzer M, Eisemann M, Kullgren G. Illness behavior in the acute phase of motor disability in neurological disease and in conversion disorder: a comparative study. *J Psychosom Res* 1998;**44**:657–666.

8. Binzer M. Hopelessness and locus of control in patients with motor conversion disorder. *Nord J Psychiatry* 1999;**53**:37–40.

9. Crimlisk HL, Bhatia KP, Cope H, *et al.* Patterns of referral in patients with medically unexplained motor symptoms. *J Psychosom Res* 2000;**49**:217–219.

10. Stone J, Binzer M, Sharpe M. Illness beliefs and locus of control: a comparison of patients with pseudoseizures and epilepsy. *J Psychosom Res* 2004;**57**:541–547.

11. Stone J, Warlow C, Sharpe M. The symptom of functional weakness: a controlled study of 107 patients. *Brain* 2010;**133**:1537–1551.

12. Trigwell P, Hatcher S, Johnson M, Stanley P, House A. "Abnormal" illness behaviour in chronic fatigue syndrome and multiple sclerosis. *BMJ* 1995;**311**:15–18.

13. Stone J, Wojcik W, Durrance D, *et al.* What should we say to patients with symptoms unexplained by disease? The "number needed to offend." *BMJ* 2002;**325**:1449–1450.

14. Stone J, Campbell K, Sharma N, *et al.* What should we call pseudoseizures? The patient's perspective. *Seizure* 2003;**12**:568–572.

15. Stone J, Colyer M, Feltbower S, Carson A, Sharpe M. "Psychosomatic": a systematic review of its meaning in newspaper articles. *Psychosomatics* 2004;**45**:287–290.

16. Carson AJ, Stone J, Warlow C, Sharpe M. Patients whom neurologists find difficult to help. *J Neurol Neurosurg Psychiatry* 2004;**75**:1776–1778.

17. Kanaan R, Armstrong D, Barnes P, Wessely S. In the psychiatrist's chair: how neurologists understand conversion disorder. *Brain* 2009;**132**:2889–2896.

18. Kanaan R, Armstrong D, Wessely S. Limits to truth-telling: neurologists' communication in conversion disorder. *Patient Educ Couns* 2009;**77**:296–301.

19. Slater ET. Diagnosis of "hysteria." *BMJ* 1965;**i**:1395–1399.

20. Jankovic J, Vuong KD, Thomas M. Psychogenic tremor: long-term outcome. *CNS Spectr* 2006;**11**:501–508.

21. Carton S, Thompson PJ, Duncan JS. Non-epileptic seizures: patients' understanding and reaction to the diagnosis and impact on outcome. *Seizure* 2003;**12**:287–294.

22. Ettinger AB, Dhoon A, Weisbrot DM, Devinsky O. Predictive factors for outcome of nonepileptic seizures after diagnosis. *J Neuropsychiatry Clin Neurosci* 1999;**11**:458–463.

23. Meierkord H, Will B, Fish D, Shorvon S. The clinical features and prognosis of pseudoseizures diagnosed using video-EEG telemetry. *Neurology* 1991;**41**:1643–1646.

24. Salmon P, Peters S, Stanley I. Patients' perceptions of medical explanations for somatisation disorders: qualitative analysis. *BMJ* 1999;**318**:372–376.

25. Nettleton S, Watt I, O' Malley L, Duffey P. Enigmatic illness: narratives of patients who live with medically unexplained symptoms. *Social Theory Health* 2004;**2**:47–66.

26. Shen W, Bowman ES, Markand ON. Presenting the diagnosis of pseudoseizure. *Neurology* 1990;**40**:756–759.

27. Creed F, Guthrie E. Techniques for interviewing the somatising patient. *Br J Psychiatry* 1993;**162**:467–471.

28. Hall-Patch L, Brown R, House A, *et al.* Acceptability and effectiveness of a strategy for the communication of the diagnosis of psychogenic nonepileptic seizures. *Epilepsia* 2010;**51**:70–78.

29. Vuilleumier P, Chicherio C, Assal F, *et al.* Functional neuroanatomical correlates of hysterical sensorimotor loss. *Brain* 2001;**124**:1077–1090.

30. Espay AJ, Morgante F, Purzner J, *et al*. Cortical and spinal abnormalities in psychogenic dystonia. *Ann Neurol* 2006;**59**:825–834.

31. Fink P, Rosendal M, Toft T. Assessment and treatment of functional disorders in general practice: the extended reattribution and management model: an advanced educational program for nonpsychiatric doctors. *Psychosomatics* 2002;**43**:93–131.

32. Morriss R, Dowrick C, Salmon P, *et al*. Cluster randomised controlled trial of training practices in reattribution for medically unexplained symptoms. *Br J Psychiatry* 2007;**191**:536–542.

33. LaFrance WC, Jr. Psychogenic nonepileptic "seizures" or "attacks"? It's not just semantics: seizures. *Neurology* 2010;**75**:87–88.

34. Benbadis SR. Psychogenic nonepileptic "seizures" or "attacks"? It's not just semantics: attacks. *Neurology* 2010;**75**:84–86.

35. Starcevic V. Somatoform disorders and DSM-V: conceptual and political issues in the debate. *Psychosomatics* 2006;**47**:277–281.

36. Page LA, Wessely S. Medically unexplained symptoms: exacerbating factors in the doctor-patient encounter. *J R Soc Med* 2003;**96**:223–227.

37. Friedman JH, LaFrance WC, Jr. Psychogenic disorders: the need to speak plainly. *Arch Neurol* 2010;**67**:753–755.

38. Thomas KB. General practice consultations: is there any point in being positive? *BMJ* 1987;**294**:1200–1202.

39. Creed F, Guthrie E, Fink P, *et al*. Is there a better term than "medically unexplained symptoms"? *J Psychosom Res* 2010;**68**:5–8.

40. Jackson JL, Kroenke K. Difficult patient encounters in the ambulatory clinic: clinical predictors and outcomes. *Arch Intern Med* 1999;**159**:1069–1075.

41. Petrie KJ, Muller JT, Schirmbeck F, *et al*. Effect of providing information about normal test results on patients' reassurance: randomised controlled trial. *BMJ* 2007;**334**:352.

42. Lucock MP, Morley S, White C, Peake MD. Responses of consecutive patients to reassurance after gastroscopy: results of self administered questionnaire survey. *BMJ* 1997;**315**:572–575.

43. Howard L, Wessely S, Leese M, Page L, McCrone P, Husain K, *et al*. Are investigations anxiolytic or anxiogenic? A randomised controlled trial of neuroimaging to provide reassurance in chronic daily headache. *J Neurol Neurosurg Psychiatry* 2005;**76**:1558–1564.

Chapter 38

Patterns of practice: report of the Movement Disorder Society questionnaire

Alberto J. Espay and Anthony E. Lang

Introduction

Little is known about neurologists' acquisition and delivery of diagnoses of psychogenic movement disorder (PMDs), extent of testing, use of ancillary services, or treatment and long-term follow-up practices. Physician-related factors such as training and gender, patient-related factors such as type of movement disorder and degree of disability, and ecological factors such as type of practice and medicolegal environment may introduce substantial variability in practice behaviors.

This chapter discusses the main findings from a recently conducted survey of experts on how they make, communicate, and manage a diagnosis of PMD. Several key knowledge gaps in opinions and clinical practices were identified prior to the development of the survey (Table 38.1). The 22-item questionnaire probing diagnostic and management issues in PMD was completed by 519 members of the Movement Disorder Society. The full report has been published in *Movement Disorders* [1]. The survey and related supplementary material can be found in the online version of the same issue. Methodological details regarding the construction, dissemination, and analysis of the questionnaire and the respondent demographics are available in that publication and will not be addressed here.

Clinical practices in the diagnosis of psychogenic movement disorders

Emotional disturbance and obvious psychiatric disturbance were needed by only 18% and 8%, respectively, of neurologists when making the diagnosis of PMD. The "essential or absolutely necessary" findings to establish a clinically definite diagnosis of PMD for 70% of respondents was incongruity with a classical movement disorder and presence of psychogenic signs on neurological examination (Fig. 38.1). Respondents reported using suggestion (guiding or encouraging a change in the movement) sometimes (34%), often (30%), or always (17%) to document and diagnose PMD; however, almost as many said they would never (51%) or rarely (24%) use placebo (using an inert intravenous or oral drug to resolve or worsen a movement) to do so. Excessive loss of function or disability relative to examination findings was "very predictive" (45%) or "extremely predictive" (16%) of a PMD diagnosis. This observation correlated with extensive normal or inconclusive neurological investigations and the presence of other medically unexplained symptoms in predicting a PMD diagnosis. By comparison, extremes of age were "very influential" for a non-PMD diagnosis, which also correlated with lack of non-physiological findings, little or no employment disruption, and normal social or personal function.

Just over half of neurologists (51.3%) requested standard neurological investigations to exclude organic causes in patients already fulfilling criteria for clinically definite PMD (with no other unexplained clinical features) before informing the patients of the diagnosis. This practice was associated with shorter fellowship training and fewer patients with PMD seen per month but not with type or years of postresidency practice. The reduction of diagnostic certainty from clinically definite to clinically probable did not substantially influence this behavior, although the percentage of neurologists that disclosed the diagnosis without standard investigations fell from almost 20% to 2% (Fig. 38.2). That is, "probable" PMD was treated as an organic disorder

Psychogenic Movement Disorders and Other Conversion Disorders, ed. Mark Hallett, Anthony E. Lang, Joseph Jankovic, Stanley Fahn, Peter W. Halligan, Valerie Voon, and C. Robert Cloninger. Published by Cambridge University Press. © Cambridge University Press 2011.

Table 38.1 Knowledge gaps in opinion and clinical practices used to develop survey

Area	Questions of import
On diagnosis	Is the diagnosis of PMD made by movement disorders neurologists achieved by exclusion (ruling out other diseases) or inclusion (applying diagnostic criteria)?
	How is the diagnosis of PMD delivered by the movement disorders neurologist?
	What history and examination findings do movement disorders neurologists consider predictive of the diagnosis of PMD and of a diagnosis *other* than PMD?
On management and prognosis	What is the role of movement disorders neurologists in the management of PMD?
	What history and examination findings do movement disorders neurologists consider of prognostic significance in PMD?
	What is the perception of efficacy in PMD of various treatment options by movement disorders neurologists?
	What are the main limitations to the management of PMD by movement disorders neurologists?
On terminology	What are the preferred lay and medical terminologies used by movement disorders neurologists to refer to PMD?

PMD, psychogenic movement disorder.

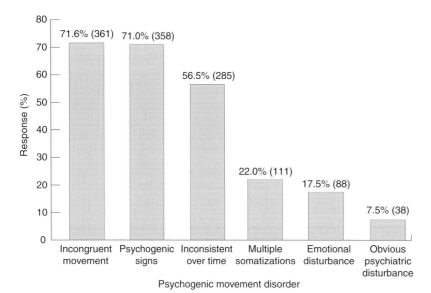

Fig. 38.1. Findings believed "essential or absolutely necessary" for a clinically definite diagnosis of a psychogenic movement disorder. (From Espay *et al.*, 2009 [1], with permission from John Wiley and Sons.)

until proven otherwise by the overwhelming majority of movement disorders neurologists.

An electrophysiology laboratory was not available to one-quarter of all respondents (24%) to confirm the myoclonus or tremor forms of PMD; an additional 9% did not believe it useful for this purpose. For the remaining two-thirds with access to electrophysiology testing, most used it only to confirm the diagnosis when clinical examination alone was insufficient (i.e., in uncertain cases); almost 40% said they never or rarely use the test results to explain the diagnosis to the patient while 21% said they used it often or always.

Differences between countries

Compared with other countries, US respondents more frequently inform patients of the definite diagnosis at the initial evaluation without requesting neurological investigations (30% in the USA versus 15% elsewhere; $p < 0.001$). Also US respondents regarded the following factors as "somewhat," "very," or "extremely" predictive of PMD, to a significantly greater extent than in other countries: ongoing litigation, spontaneous remissions/cures, non-physiological deficits, and history of mental health problems or psychological stressors.

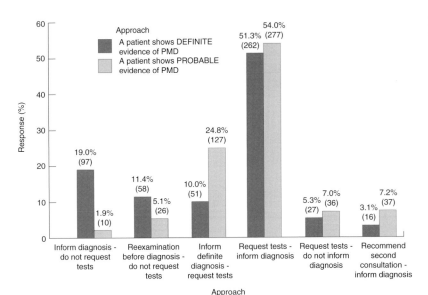

Fig. 38.2. Approach to delivering the diagnosis in clinically definite (black bars) and clinically probable (gray bars) psychogenic movement disorder (PMD). (From Espay *et al.*, 2009 [1], with permission from John Wiley and Sons.)

Clinical practices in the management of psychogenic movement disorders

Two-thirds of respondents referred patients with PMD to a psychiatrist or mental health specialist while also providing personal follow-up. This pattern of referral and personal follow-up was more common among younger respondents and academic clinician researchers. Of interest, 50% of respondents reported that psychiatrists, psychologists, or rehabilitation specialists "sometimes" (35%) or "often" (14%) questioned the neurologist's original diagnosis and recommended the neurological basis for the disorder be reconsidered.

Avoiding iatrogenic harm (46%) and educating the patient (29%) were the only two management modalities believed to be "very" or "extremely effective" by approximately one-third or more of respondents (Table 38.2). A majority of respondents ranked pharmacological treatment and alternative or complementary therapies as "mostly not effective" or "not at all effective."

Cultural beliefs about psychological illnesses (40%), ongoing litigation (37%), and availability of referral services (33%), "often" or "always" limited the ability to manage patients. The largest consensus for "never" affecting PMD management was for physician reimbursement (50%) and insurability of patients with PMD (42%) (Table 38.3).

Acceptance of the diagnosis by the patient was the only variable endorsed as "extremely important" (60%) in predicting a favorable prognosis. Identification and management of psychological stressors (54%) and concurrent psychiatric disorders (55%) were rated as "very important." (Table 38.4).

Differences between countries

Educating the patient about PMD was the only strategy showing a country-based difference, being perceived as more effective by US respondents than by non-US respondents. Compared with non-US respondents, US respondents significantly believed that reimbursement, insurability, availability of referral services, ongoing litigation by the patient, and potential for litigation involvement of the physician "often" or "always" affected physicians' ability to treat and manage patients with PMD. Also, a larger percentage of US respondents believed that the absence of ongoing litigation as well as the identification and management of psychological stressors and associated psychiatric disorders were important for predicting a favorable prognosis.

Terminology

Although "psychogenic movement disorder" was the preferred medical term (84%), other terminologies were variably endorsed by respondents (see Fig. 37.1, p. 255).

Discussion

Expert opinions and practices regarding diagnosis and management of patients with PMD differed

Table 38.2 Perceived effectiveness of specific treatment strategies

Strategy	Response (%)				
	Not effective	Mostly not effective	Somewhat effective	Very effective	Extremely effective
Avoiding iatrogenic harm			34.4	30.5	
Educating the patient			51.1	23.9	
Psychotherapy with antidepressant/anxiolytic treatment			60.7	20.1	
Rehabilitation services (physiotherapy, biofeedback, etc.)			58.4	19.2	
Psychotherapy without antidepressant/anxiolytic treatment		23.1	63.1		
Alternative or complementary medicine		42.8	34.1		
Pharmacological treatment of specific movement impairment	30.8	52.4			

Factors are listed in descending order of rated effectiveness. Percentages represent the two most frequently chosen levels of efficacy per treatment category.
Source: Adapted from Espay *et al.*, 2009 [1].

Table 38.3 Limitations to being able to manage patients with psychogenic movement disorders

Limitation to management	Response (%)				
	Never	Rarely	Sometimes	Often	Always
Cultural beliefs about psychological illnesses			34.2	35.7	
Ongoing litigation related to the PMD			35.5	29.4	
Availability of referral services			32.9	27.1	
Potential for your involvement in litigation		34.7	26.2		
Insurability of PMD	41.6	28.1			
Physician reimbursement	50.3	22.8			

PMD, psychogenic movement disorder.
Factors are listed in descending order of rated effectiveness. Percentages represent the two most frequently chosen levels of efficacy per treatment category.
Source: Adapted from Espay *et al.*, 2009 [1].

among neurologists with movement disorder expertise. Some of the discrepancies were partly accounted for by length of training (e.g., investigations prior to diagnosis), type of practice (e.g., referral pattern to psychiatrists or mental health specialists), and country, but they also reflected absence of uniform practice guidelines. Part of the difficulty in establishing the diagnosis comes from the findings that some features typically associated with recognized movement disorders may be seen in patients with otherwise definite PMD (e.g., geste antagoniste) [2]; classic diagnostic electrophysiological findings may be lacking (e.g., psychogenic tremor may not always be associated with complete coherence or may not show changes in response to tests of distraction) [3], and *overt* psychiatric problems are often absent [4]. In addition, neurologists show limited reliance on neurophysiological methods to make or confirm the PMD diagnosis, largely an indication of lack of experience with or availability of electrophysiology.

Table 38.4 Importance of various factors in predicting a better prognosis for psychogenic movement disorders

Factor	Response (%)				
	Not important	**Mostly not important**	**Somewhat important**	**Very important**	**Extremely important**
Acceptance of diagnosis by patient				31.7	59.9
Identification and management of concurrent psychiatric disorder				54.5	30.7
Identification and management of psychological stressors				53.9	30.3
Supportive social network				47.2	25.2
A short latency period between onset of symptoms and diagnosis				49.8	23.4
Absence of ongoing litigation			32	40.0	
Less extensive disability			36.9	44.0	
Paroxysmal rather than persistent or fixed movement disorders			44.8	33.5	
Younger age when developing the movement disorder			45.8	26.0	
Type of movement (e.g., tremor or chorea versus dystonia or ataxia)		37.7	35.8		
Pharmacological treatment of specific movement impairment		38.0	31.3		

Factors are listed in descending order of rated effectiveness. Percentages represent the two most frequently chosen levels of importance for putative predictors of favorable prognosis.
Source: Adapted from Espay *et al.*, 2009 [1].

Challenges in reaching a diagnosis of a psychogenic movement disorder

Despite efforts at making "definite" PMD a diagnosis of inclusion by following previously published diagnostic criteria [5–7], a majority of respondents confirmed the diagnosis only after excluding a range of organic neurological conditions. Only one-fifth of respondents acted on the clinical diagnostic criteria and informed the patients of the definite PMD diagnosis during the initial assessment without requesting additional investigations. Importantly, the frequency with which neurologists requested standard neurological investigations was similar for clinically definite and probable categories of PMD, suggesting that the level of diagnostic certainty does not alter the exclusionary manner in which this diagnosis is predominantly made. This behavior may in part be explained by the lasting influence of seminal papers on PMD, which stated that "the emphasis of the evaluation rests upon excluding organic lesions that might mimic the presenting symptoms …

Negative studies can strengthen the certainty of the psychogenic diagnosis and reassure the patient that a possible organic lesion has not been overlooked" [5,6].

There may be a number of other reasons neurologists request standard neurological investigations despite a clinically definite PMD diagnosis. At a basic level, PMD was recognized as occurring together with an organic movement or general neurological disorder in approximately 5–10% of patients by a substantial majority of respondents to the survey, in line with prior reports [8,9]. Some respondents viewed themselves as taking patients' symptoms "seriously" by ordering a battery of tests in order to fully "placate" those determined to find an organic basis for their symptoms and minimize their "doctor shopping." However, a recent controlled study found that patients with chronic daily headache who underwent an MRI scan 1 year earlier were equally "worried" (as measured by the Hospital Anxiety and Depression Scale) as those not offered this investigation [10]. Against this, these patients had lower utilization of additional medical resources (with resulting lower medical costs), likely in part mediated by a reduction of referrals [10]. Finally, there exist conflicting views on the use of suggestibility and placebo in diagnosing PMD. A recent review suggested that, as transient improvements can be seen in organic movement disorders with placebo therapies, "a diagnosis of a PMD should not be made on the basis of the presence of a placebo response alone" [11] (presumably referring to a transient response). Yet the original classification of "documented PMD," was reserved for movements "relieved by psychotherapy, suggestion, or *placebo* [author's italic], or spontaneous symptom resolution when the patient feels unobserved" [6]. Here, the necessary response should be profound and more persistent than transitory. While 81% felt that response to suggestion was useful in making a diagnosis, placebo itself, as a diagnostic tool, was not endorsed by most respondents in this survey. Although we believe that a complete resolution of a movement disorder in response to placebo is highly supportive of a diagnosis of PMD, this approach may not be widely used because of ethical (and litigation) concerns rather than its lack of utility.

Country of practice had some impact on opinions of respondents about diagnosis. A positive psychiatric history and spontaneous remissions and cures were considered strong predictors of PMD diagnosis among US respondents but not among those from other countries. Similarly, ongoing litigation was held as predictive of a PMD diagnosis in the USA whereas it was not predictive for non-US respondents. These differences may relate to various factors such as delivery and availability of services for mental healthcare, differences in each healthcare system, litigation environment, training-related factors, and cultural issues.

Challenges in the management and prognosis of psychogenic movement disorder

Up to half of respondents found that psychiatrists often (14%) or sometimes (35%) questioned the diagnosis and recommended that it be reconsidered. This may be because of the requirement for a psychological stressor for the diagnosis of conversion disorder in the *Diagnostic and Statistical Manual of Mental Disorders*, 4th edition (DSM-IV) [12]. The DSM-IV also fails to mention the presence of positive physical signs in the form of psychogenic signs as supportive of the diagnosis.

A better prognosis for PMD was strongly predicted by the acceptance of the diagnosis by the patient. Indeed, acceptance of diagnosis is a critical turning point in the psychotherapeutic management of these patients [13] and the inability to acknowledge the psychological nature of this condition has been found to be a strong predictor of the persistence of abnormal movements and unemployment [14]. As such, it is likely that any efforts made towards encouraging patients to fully embrace the diagnosis and "take the lead" in the subsequent identification of psychological stressors and mental and physical rehabilitation will greatly improve the prognosis.

Although two-thirds of neurologists surveyed provided personal follow-up for patients with PMD, lack of controlled clinical trials examining the effect of specific treatment modalities have limited the creation of management guidelines on which to base the practice. What little high-level evidence exists comes from psychodynamic therapies (e.g., cognitive behavioral therapy [15], hypnosis [16]), which are not directly applicable by neurologists. Other interventions without accepted efficacy for treatment of PMD, such as acupuncture [17], may be viewed as "placebo." This background may have resulted in respondents endorsing as "very" or "extremely effective" only two interventions: education about psychogenic disorders and avoidance of potentially harmful pharmacotherapy. Psychotherapy with or without antidepressant or anxiolytic treatment and rehabilitation services were rated as "somewhat effective" and, importantly, pharmacological treatment directed at the specific type of movement disorder was rated as "mostly not effective" or "not at all effective."

Conclusions: suggested next steps

Limitations notwithstanding (mainly, a survey response rate that may not be fully representative of the entire community of experts and our inability to fully interpret differences in diagnostic and therapeutic behaviors between countries), the opinions and clinical practices summarized above highlight the need to foster research that may assist in the eventual creation of diagnostic and management guidelines. A number of challenges to the diagnosis and treatment of PMD are identified and need addressing (Table 38.5). In planning further steps in the understanding and treatment of PMD, the following areas require greater focus: (1) an effort, perhaps driven by the Movement Disorder Society, to encourage a positive rather than exclusionary

Table 38.5 Challenges to the diagnosis and management of psychogenic movement disorders

Challenges	Recommendations, possible solutions
In diagnosis	
Defining PMD as "not real" or "faked"	Admit movements are real and assume them as neurological but discuss their psychological or stress-related roots
"I probably order more tests than I should but a psychogenic overlay can limit examination" "Traditional neurological movement disorders are characterized by lots of stress, placebo response, and high rates of psychiatric comorbidity"	In the setting of probable or possible categories of PMD (corresponding to "psychogenic overlay," "psychiatric comorbidity"), act on the assumption that the movements have organic basis until proven otherwise
Placebo: "fear of litigation is primary reason placebos are not used, major barrier to diagnosis." Placebo response is also present in organic disease	Placebo ethics and potential diagnostic usefulness need to be studied; validation, sensitivity, and specificity in PMD will be needed
In management	
Psychiatrists are widely seen as unhelpful or even obstructive to the treatment of patients with PMD when overt psychopathology is absent, and they assume the sole role of psychopharmacologists	Education of psychiatrists on PMD is critical to success of future treatment
Perception of intractability and poor prognosis of PMD	Emphasize the positive: not necessarily progressive or disabling and potentially reversible with full commitment and appropriate psychological and rehabilitation therapy and management of stress-related inductors
Diagnostic tests when delivering a diagnosis of definite PMD	Decisiveness by the diagnosing neurologist in clinically definite cases increases the likelihood of improved outcomes

PMD, psychogenic movement disorder.

diagnosis for PMD; (2) removing the requirement of psychological stressors from the upcoming DSM-V criteria for conversion disorders; (3) establishing PMD as a complex neurobehavioral disorder for which neurologists have a primary role in establishing the diagnosis and coordinating management; (4) examining the therapeutic value in PMD of interventions without currently accepted efficacy such as acupuncture, yoga, or meditation; and (5) exploring the functional and biochemical brain abnormalities that underlie specific PMD behaviors, receiving belated attention in other psychogenic disorders [18–20] and their potential role as surrogate markers to measure the success of future therapeutic efforts.

Acknowledgements

Linda Goldenhar, Valerie Voon, Anette Schrag, and Noël Burton co-authored the survey report published in *Movement Disorders*. Joseph Jankovic, Guenther Deuschl, Christopher Goetz, Mark Hallett, Stanley Fahn, and Stephen Reich served as external reviewers to ensure content and face validity of the survey. Mary Kemper, medical editor, and Martha Headworth, medical illustrator, of the UC Neuroscience Institute assisted in the editing and figure design for this manuscript.

References

1. Espay AJ, Goldenhar LM, Voon V, *et al*. Opinions and clinical practices related to diagnosing and managing patients with psychogenic movement disorders: an international survey of Movement Disorder Society members. *Mov Disord* 2009;**24**:1366–1374.

2. Munhoz RP, Lang AE. Gestes antagonistes in psychogenic dystonia. *Mov Disord* 2004;**19**:331–332.

3. Hung SW, Molnar GF, Ashby P, *et al*. Electrophysiologic testing in psychogenic tremor: Does it always help? In Hallett M, Fahn S, Jankovic J, *et al.*, eds. *Psychogenic Movement Disorders: Neurology and Neuropsychiatry*. Philadelphia, PA: Lippincott Williams & Wilkins, 2006:334–335.

4. Schrag A, Lang AE. Psychogenic movement disorders. *Curr Opin Neurol* 2005;**18**:399–404.

5. Fahn S, Williams DT. Psychogenic dystonia. *Adv Neurol* 1988;**50**:431–455.

6. Williams DT, Ford B, Fahn S. Phenomenology and psychopathology related to psychogenic movement disorders. In Weiner WJ, Lang AE, eds. *Behavioral Neurology of Movement Disorders*. New York: Raven Press, 1995:231–257.

7. Gupta A, Lang AE. Psychogenic movement disorders. *Curr Opin Neurol* 2009;**22**:430–436.

8. Ranawaya R, Riley D, Lang A. Psychogenic dyskinesias in patients with organic movement disorders. *Mov Disord* 1990;**5**:127–133.

9. Stone J, Smyth R, Carson A, *et al*. Systematic review of misdiagnosis of conversion symptoms and "hysteria." *BMJ* 2005;**331**:989.

10. Howard L, Wessely S, Leese M, *et al*. Are investigations anxiolytic or anxiogenic? A randomised controlled trial of neuroimaging to provide reassurance in chronic daily headache. *J Neurol Neurosurg Psychiatry* 2005;**76**:1558–1564.

11. Hinson VK, Haren WB. Psychogenic movement disorders. *Lancet Neurol* 2006;**5**:695–700.

12. American Psychiatry Association. *Diagnostic and Statistical Manual of Mental Disorders*, 4th edn. Washington, DC: American Psychiatric Press, 1994.

13. Hinson VK, Weinstein S, Bernard B, Leurgans SE, Goetz CG. Single-blind clinical trial of psychotherapy for treatment of psychogenic movement disorders. *Parkinsonism Relat Disord* 2006;**12**:177–180.

14. Feinstein A, Stergiopoulos V, Fine J, Lang AE. Psychiatric outcome in patients with a psychogenic movement disorder: a prospective study. *Neuropsychiatry Neuropsychol Behav Neurol* 2001;**14**:169–176.

15. Speckens AE, van Hemert AM, Spinhoven P, *et al*. Cognitive behavioural therapy for medically unexplained physical symptoms: a randomised controlled trial. *BMJ* 1995;**311**:1328–1332.

16. Moene FC, Spinhoven P, Hoogduin KA, van Dyck R. A randomised controlled clinical trial on the additional effect of hypnosis in a comprehensive treatment programme for in-patients with conversion disorder of the motor type. *Psychother Psychosom* 2002;**71**:66–76.

17. Van Nuenen BF, Wohlgemuth M, Wong *et al*. Acupuncture for psychogenic movement disorders: treatment or diagnostic tool? *Mov Disord* 2007;**22**:1353–1355.

18. Vuilleumier P. Hysterical conversion and brain function. *Prog Brain Res* 2005;**150**:309–329.

19. Mailis-Gagnon A, Giannoylis I, Downar J, *et al*. Altered central somatosensory processing in chronic pain patients with "hysterical" anesthesia. *Neurology* 2003;**60**:1501–1507.

20. Ghaffar O, Staines WR, Feinstein A. Unexplained neurologic symptoms: an fMRI study of sensory conversion disorder. *Neurology* 2006;**67**:2036–2038.

Chapter

39

Psychotherapy for psychogenic movement disorders

Michael Sharpe, Jon Stone, and Alan J. Carson

Introduction

There is a long history of using psychotherapy to treat patients who have conditions thought be to psychogenic. This chapter considers the rationale and also the evidence to support the use of psychotherapy in the treatment of psychogenic movement disorders (PMD) and associated conditions. What is meant by psychotherapy and PMD will be defined before reviewing the evidence for the efficacy of psychotherapy in PMD and associated conditions and considering how we should best treat these patients. Finally, suggestions are made for how future treatment research should be directed.

Definitions

Psychotherapy

"Psychotherapy," "psychological treatment," "psychological intervention," and "talking treatments" are overlapping terms which tend to be used interchangeably. While the term "psychotherapy" is most often used to describe traditional treatments such as psychodynamic psychotherapy and the other terms to describe more modern treatments such as cognitive behavioral therapy (CBT), this chapter will use the term psychotherapy to refer to all these treatments.

What is it about a treatment that makes it psychotherapy? The answer to this question is less obvious than it may first appear. Most people would agree that CBT is a form of psychotherapy and that surgery is not. However, between these extremes it may not be so clear; homeopathy, on the one hand, is physical treatment acting largely through a psychologically mediated placebo response while, on the other hand, an apparently psychological treatment such

as persuading a person to exercise acts by a physical mechanism. Therefore, in order to be clearer about what we mean by psychotherapy we will consider which features of a treatment qualify it as psychotherapy. One or more of a number might and these are listed in Table 39.1.

Therefore, it can be seen that treatment can be judged to be psychotherapy on a number of different criteria. The point is that the range of treatments that can be considered as wholly or partially psychotherapeutic is wide. For the purpose of this chapter, psychotherapy will be defined as a treatment that has a predominantly psychological *content* irrespective of its hypothesized action, the nature of the desired outcome, or the method of its delivery. The specific treatments considered as psychotherapies are:

- psychodynamic psychotherapy
- behavior therapy (including strategic behavior therapy and paradoxical intention)
- cognitive therapy
- CBT
- hypnosis
- education advice and suggestion by verbal, written, or other means
- the physician–patient relationship.

Psychodynamic psychotherapy

Psychodynamic psychotherapy developed from Freudian psychoanalysis has developed into a number of different forms over the last 100 years. The term "psychodynamic" refers to the psychological forces that influence the function of the mind, especially emotions. The relationship between the therapist and the patient and the relationship of the patient's current symptoms to previous, often unconscious, memories

Psychogenic Movement Disorders and Other Conversion Disorders, ed. Mark Hallett, Anthony E. Lang, Joseph Jankovic, Stanley Fahn, Peter W. Halligan, Valerie Voon, and C. Robert Cloninger. Published by Cambridge University Press. © Cambridge University Press 2011.

Table 39.1 Characteristics of treatment, one or more of which may lead it to be considered a psychotherapy

Content	There is a large psychological component to the intervention such as relaxation, education, or hypnosis
Proposed mechanism of action	The mechanism of action is hypothesized to be psychological, such as a change in belief or behavior
Target outcome(s)	The intervention affects a psychological outcome (whether psychogenic movement disorders are psychological is a moot point)
Method of delivery	Interventions given in the form of talking are generally regarded as psychotherapy; however, the term may also apply to interventions delivered by computer, written materials, or other methods

of events and relationships, including those from childhood, are central. The aim is to achieve understanding of the psychological origin of the symptoms (including sometimes their symbolic nature), with the assumption that this understanding will lead to their resolution. Therapy sessions are generally given as an outpatient, last an hour, and may continue over many months, although modern versions are typically briefer. It requires the patient to accept that their symptoms are psychological in origin and to be willing to talk about their psychological life to a therapist.

Behavior therapy

Behavior therapy developed in relation to psychological learning theory in the 1950s. The focus of treatment is on the patient's observable behavior rather than their internal psychological world. Therapy aims to relieve symptoms by changes in behavior. Changes in behavior can be brought about in different ways: one is by changing the patient's environment, such as by not responding to their requests for reassurance; the other is more collaborative by persuading the patient to behave differently, such as by ceasing to avoid certain situations. Therapy is usually brief and given as an outpatient. It may also be integrated into inpatient and outpatient rehabilitation programs. It does not require the patient to accept that their symptoms are psychological in origin, merely to be able to change their behavior and maintain that change.

Cognitive therapy

Cognitive therapy was developed in the 1960s by Aaron Beck, a psychodynamic psychotherapist, who observed the importance of the patient's current thoughts (cognitions) in the perpetuation of symptoms (originally of depression). These cognitions can be automatic responses to situations that the patient is only dimly aware of, such as the recurrent thought "I am going to

shake" in a social situation. Emotion and behavior are seen as being driven by cognitions; the person with the aforementioned automatic thought will feel anxious and avoid these situations. Cognitive therapy aims to help the patient to be more aware of their cognitions and to practice ways of changing them. Therapy usually lasts several months and is given as an outpatient. It requires the patient to accept that their thoughts may perpetuate their symptoms but not necessarily that the symptoms are originally psychogenic in origin.

Cognitive behavior therapy

The CBT approach is an amalgam of cognitive and behavior therapy. The content is based on cognitive therapy with an emphasis on change in behavior. As well as 1-hour sessions in which the patient and therapist discuss the patient's symptoms, thoughts, emotions, and behavior, the patient is also required to keep written records of these and to carry out "homework" in which they observe the effects of changing their behavior. The aim is to collaboratively achieve changes in thought and action that result in relief of the symptoms. The development of CBT has led to a pragmatic, clearly specified, widely used, and extensively evaluated form of psychotherapy. It is used as a generic term for a wide range of techniques. As with cognitive and behavior therapies, it requires the patient to accept that their thoughts and behaviors may perpetuate their symptoms, but not necessarily that the symptoms are originally psychogenic in origin.

Other specific therapies that have been evaluated as treatments for conversion disorder

Strategic behavior therapy. This is an interesting, though ethically questionable, form of behavior therapy whereby one aims to improve the patient's symptoms by influencing the contingencies of non-recovery. Specifically, the patient is told that failure to recover would indicate that their illness was psychogenic (an outcome that is assumed to be psychologically unacceptable), whereas recovery would indicate that it has been a genuine illness.

Paradoxical intention. The paradox is that the patient is told that they can get better by intentionally making the symptoms worse. The theory is that by overcoming the fear of the symptoms, the avoidance and anxiety that causes them is reduced and the sense of control increased. It is best suited to symptoms of variable intensity such as non-epileptic attacks.

Hypnosis. Hypnosis involves the induction of an altered state of consciousness. In this so-called hypnotic state, the therapist may seek to obtain information from the patient about the origin of the symptom that was otherwise not available, encourage changes in behavior, or, specifically in PMD, to enable the patient to gain control over a movement disorder. The encouragement to regain normal function is often called "suggestion." Hypnosis has a long history, although its efficacy remains controversial. It requires that the patient is willing to be hypnotized, but not that they explicitly accept a conscious cause for their symptoms.

Abreaction. While not clearly a psychotherapy, abreaction involves the use of psychological techniques in conjunction with the administration of sedative agents such as benzodiazepines or barbiturates to induce an altered brain state similar to that in hypnosis. Similar techniques to those used in hypnosis have been described. In addition, "emotional catharsis" was at one time a popular reason for abreaction. More specifically in PMD, sedation can be used in psychogenic dystonia not only to look for contractures but in a psychotherapeutic sense to demonstrate to the patient that their apparently fixed posture is potentially reversible [1].

Education, advice and self help

Although not usually regarded as psychotherapy, the provision of information and advice about symptoms (including information supporting the possibility of recovery) meets our definition of psychotherapy. It may be of particular benefit in conditions such as PMD that are not well understood by patients. In addition, the techniques of psychotherapies such as CBT can be described to patients in simple form using a verbal, written, or computerized delivery, and the patient is thereby given the means of self-help. Assistance to use such self-help materials is called guided or supported self-help.

The physician–patient relationship

Finally, we must not neglect the most widely used form of psychotherapy: interactions between doctors and patients. The use of the doctor–patient relationship to treat patients by instilling hope and a communication of caring has always been a part of medicine and indeed is an important aspect of the ubiquitous so-called "placebo effect." It has also long included what we now regard as simple psychotherapeutic and behavioral techniques included in modern CBT [2]. Indeed, one potential danger of describing apparently esoteric psychotherapies is that it may undermine physicians' confidence in regarding their medical consultations as opportunities for simple psychotherapy.

Psychogenic movement disorders

By PMD, we refer to symptoms imitating the "organic" movement disorders – tremor, myoclonus, chorea, dystonia, and gait disorder – but considered not to be organically based. However, the boundaries of PMD are unclear and a large proportion of the various symptoms seen by neurologists are similarly considered "non-organic" or "medically unexplained" [3,4]. For example, does the reduced movement seen in "psychogenic" weakness make it potentially a PMD? Are the abnormal movements seen during non-epileptic attacks an intermittent PMD with associated amnesia? Does the psychiatric diagnosis of conversion disorder describe many similar patients? We propose that because there is so little evidence available about PMD narrowly defined it is worth considering the evidence relevant to this broader group of similar conditions.

All these conditions have in common the assumption that they are psychogenic. However, it is important that we remember that psychogenesis is only an assumption, and that the fundamental causes of these disorders remain unknown [2].

Evidence for the efficacy of psychotherapy in psychogenic movement disorders

At first glance, psychotherapy would seem to be a logical choice of treatment for conditions assumed

Table 39.2 Randomized controlled trials of psychotherapy for psychogenic movement disorders and conversion disorders

Disorder	Treatments evaluated	No. participants	Outcome	Ref.
Motor conversion disorder	Hypnosis versus waiting list	44	Better with hypnosis	Moene *et al.*, 2003 [8]
Motor conversion disorder	Rehabilitation plus hypnosis versus rehabilitation alone	45	No additional benefit of hypnosis	Moene *et al.*, 2002 [9]
Non-epileptic seizures	CBT versus medical care	66	Better with CBT	Goldstein *et al.*, 2010 [10]
Non-epileptic seizures (acute)	Paradoxical intention (prescribing the symptom) versus diazepam	30	Better with paradoxical intention	Ataoglu *et al.*, 2003 [11]

CBT, cognitive behavioral therapy.

to be psychogenic. However, as the analysis above has suggested this assumption may be too simplistic. Psychotherapies, such as hypnosis, can influence non-psychogenic conditions, such as surgically induced pain [5]. Similarly, non-psychotherapeutic treatments such as brain surgery can influence clearly psychological conditions, such as depression [6]. Two important implications are, first, that treatments considered for PMD should not be restricted to psychotherapies, and, second, that although listed as criteria for PMD it should not necessarily be concluded that a PMD is psychogenic because it responds to psychotherapy. At present, the criteria for PMD contains "response to psychotherapy" as evidence of a definite PMD [7]. Perhaps this is not a correct assumption.

Notwithstanding this broader analysis, the available evidence for the efficacy of psychotherapy as we have defined it for PMD and associated disorders will be considered. While the best evidence of efficacy is that from randomized clinical trials, we are not aware of any published randomized trials solely of PMD. The published randomized trials of psychotherapies for conversion disorder, which includes patients with PMD, are listed in Table 39.2.

As we can see from the table, the trial evidence is limited to patients described as having mixed type of motor conversion disorder and non-epileptic seizures. The trials are also small and none has been replicated. We will, however, consider them in more detail.

Trials in conversion disorder

There have been two randomized trials of treatment for patients suffering from motor conversion disorder. The first trial randomized 44 outpatients to either

hypnosis or waiting list [8]. The patients had a variety of complaints, including weakness, tremor, and gait and coordination problems. The hypnosis was given in 10 weekly outpatient sessions and included both the exploration of traumatic memories associated with the symptoms and the encouragement of functional recovery. The patients allocated to hypnotherapy were much better in terms of both symptoms and general functioning at the 3-month outcome. In a second trial from the same group, similar patients were randomized to receive either general psychologically informed rehabilitation plus sessions of hypnotherapy or rehabilitation plus a similar number of general counseling sessions. In this trial, no specific effect of hypnotherapy was apparent, but the majority of patients in both groups improved. This was a tough test for hypnosis and should not lead to its rejection as a treatment. However, it does also point to the benefits of non-specific factors in a comprehensive treatment approach.

There have been a large number of publications of non-randomized evaluation of psychotherapy for patients with conditions described as conversion disorder, mostly with limb weakness. Almost all are reports of a small case series of patients selected in order to illustrate a treatment and, consequently, of very limited value in evaluating efficacy [12–22]. In the only evaluation of psychotherapy in PMD, Hinson et al. [22] evaluated a psychodynamic intervention in only nine patients.

Several larger case series of various other psychotherapies have also been reported. One tested so-called strategic behavior therapy (see above) as a treatment for patients who had not improved with behavior therapy and reported a high success rate in patients with more chronic conditions [23]. Another described a varied outcome in a large series of patients (220) who had received inpatient rehabilitative treatment in Germany. The authors commented on the problem of getting these patients to accept a psychological explanation of their symptoms [24]. This is a useful reminder of a major issue in providing psychotherapy for such patients.

Other treatments that have been reported as potentially useful include simple biofeedback [21] and the use of sedation with thiopentonal sodium to facilitate return of movement [25]. Studies of abreaction in conversion disorder have generally been of poor quality but this does not exclude the possibility of benefit [26].

Trials in non-epileptic seizures

Two randomized trials of treatment have been reported and both utlized forms of CBT. The first from Korea was described as being of paradoxical intention (see above) compared with drug treatment with diazepam. Patients in the paradoxical intention group were admitted to hospital and encouraged to imagine situations that might bring on their seizure twice daily for 3 weeks. Patients in the diazepam group were given this drug as outpatients. Almost all of patients allocated to paradoxical intervention (93%) were reported to be symptom free at 6 weeks compared with 60% of those given diazepam. The findings are interesting but clearly hard to interpret [11].

The second trial was of a more typical form of CBT [10]. The therapy included helping the patient to gain an understanding of the psychological nature of the attacks, to use relaxation when they felt an attack coming on, and to provide encouragement to overcome avoidance of situations associated with the attacks [27]. The trial randomized 66 patients to receive either CBT or standard medical care. The 3-month outcome in terms of seizure frequency and social functioning was much better with CBT. These results are promising. The trial was, however, small and the amount of attention the patients received was not matched between groups. Replication is required.

There are also a number of published case series of treatments for non-epileptic attacks [28]. As well as case series of CBT [29], there is a description of a series of patients treated with psychodynamic psychotherapy (see above) in a large group of 63 patients, most of whom had non-epileptic attacks [30]. Another was a retrospective case series of inpatient rehabilitation (which included behavior therapy) that reported a

good initial response rate but frequent relapse after discharge [31]. This reminds us of the need for long-term follow-up of patients.

Summary of trial results

There have been no published randomized trials of the efficacy on psychotherapy for PMD. There is some evidence for the use of hypnosis in patients described as having conversion disorder (which include some patients with PMD), although this is equivocal as it had efficacy in a randomized trial comparing with a waiting list but was not effective when tested in more demanding design. Despite clinical reports of its value, there is no randomized control trial evidence to enable us to evaluate psychodynamic psychotherapy in PMD. There are numerous case series that are generally supportive of a variety of psychotherapies and which emphasize the challenges of persuading patients that their symptoms are psychogenic. Drawing the net wider, there is some evidence for the efficacy of CBT in the associated condition of non-epileptic seizures. If we draw the net even wider and consider evidence of efficacy of psychotherapy in related conditions, there is a larger body of randomized controlled trial evidence for other physical symptoms unexplained by disease, so-called somatoform disorders. In a review of all randomized controlled trials for somatoform disorders, CBT was seen to be effective in 11 of 13 published studies [32,33]. Randomized controlled trials of short-term psychodynamic therapy have also shown promising results for irritable bowel syndrome and chronic pain [34].

How should patients be treated?

The harsh reality is that there is inadequate high-quality research evidence to tell us the place of psychotherapy in the management of patients with PMD. Clearly, we need to get a balance between therapeutic nihilism on the one hand, and the over-enthusiastic application of non-evidence-based treatment on the other. Taking the evidence for the treatment of other physical symptoms unexplained by disease, the following guidelines for "good practice" might be proposed (see Chapter 37).

Establish and use a positive therapeutic relationship

A positive therapeutic relationship is the basis of all psychotherapy, if not all effective medical practice. It is based on the non-specific aspects of all psychotherapy, as described by Frank [35], which includes an intense confiding relationship plus a plausible rationale for understanding and treating the problem.

Provide a plausible explanation of the condition that the patient can accept

Providing a plausible explanation starts with a name. There is evidence that some names, such as hysteria or psychosomatic, are likely not to be accepted by, and consequently rejected by, the patient [36]. The advantages and disadvantages of describing symptoms as "psychological", "functional," or "unexplained" are described in Chapter 37. In that chapter important elements of explanation are proposed, such as sharing the reasoning behind the diagnosis (e.g., showing the patient how their tremor disappears with distraction or how their leg weakness improves with Hoover's sign); explaining why they do not have the corresponding neurological condition; emphasizing that this is common, that you believe the patient, and that their condition is potentially reversible. Written information or a website (e.g., www.neurosymptoms.org) may also be useful. Our own preference is to tell the patient that they have a functional tremor or functional gait disorder that is a result of changes in nervous system functioning and then to go on to explain that correcting this dysfunction should include addressing psychological factors [37].

Encourage a return to normal activity

A return to normal activity may be achieved by verbal encouragement, explanation of the importance of this in normalizing brain functioning, and maybe supplementing it by the application of general physical rehabilitation.

Use of a specific psychotherapy

Although the amount of evidence is small, given the evidence for the efficacy of CBT in other physical symptoms unexplained by disease, this is probably the treatment of choice. It must, however, be given by a therapist who is able to work with patients whose complaints are predominantly physical, rather than psychological.

Other treatments

Finally, there is a potential role for other more controversial treatments. These would include hypnosis, abreaction, and paradoxical intention. The use of strategic behavioral therapy may be considered by many to be unethical.

Examples of using cognitive behavioral therapy in specific ways for psychogenic movement disorders

Having emphasized the importance of evidence, we also recognize that in the clinic it is not enough to tell the patient "there is not enough evidence to treat you." So this section includes some comments about simple CBT-based techniques that we have found useful in treating patients with PMD. In particular, we find it helpful to ask patients to experiment with the same kind of distraction techniques that neurologists might use in order to help the patients to better understand and potentially modulate their PMD. Some examples are given.

- Patients with psychogenic tremor can often be shown how a fast (3 Hz) copied rhythmical tapping movement or ballistic movements of their good hand can abolish tremor in their affected hand. Success in this behavioral task can be used as cognitive evidence of the potential reversibility of their condition.
- Patients with dystonic postures commonly report that their hand or leg feels more "normal" in the "abnormal" position. Behavioral experiments with transient straightening of the limb (if possible) can be used to explore why they may have both a physiological and emotional reaction to the limb being in a "normal" position (e.g., brain pathways being altered to make normal feel abnormal, which need to be retrained).
- Patients with jerky myoclonic type movements are often stimulus sensitive to noise, light, or touch (e.g., with tendon hammer). This gives an opportunity for triggering movement under predictable circumstances when the patient can learn cognitive techniques (such as relaxation or distraction) to gain more control.
- Patients with gait disorder can try out experiments of walking backwards or even running (if their gait is better in these situations).
- When PMD is intermittent, we look hard for panic or dissociative symptoms prior to onset, as in non-epileptic attacks, which may be amenable to a standard CBT approach for panic.

Table 39.3 Design requirements of future trials of psychotherapy for psychogenic movement disorders

Trial component	Requirement
Patients	An adequate number of patients willing to take part
	Patients who represent a clinical population
	A sample which is adequately homogeneous in terms of symptoms and chronicity
Randomization	Randomization adequately conducted with allocation concealment
Treatment condition	Clearly defined and manualized
	Compared with an appropriate comparison treatment
	Quality assurance to ensure they are delivered as specified
Comparison condition	Carefully designed and matched for non-specific aspects of treatment
Outcomes	Clinically meaningful outcome measures
	Valid and reliable, preferably with blind ratings (such as blind rating videotapes)
	Long-term follow-ups
Analysis	Intention-to-treat analyses
	Analysis that addresses therapists' defects, such as clustering

Summary

A positive approach to the patient with PMD is essential, despite the dearth of evidence for specific therapies. It is important to optimize the clinical consultation by providing a positive and acceptable diagnosis and a good explanation to the patient; additional information can be provided by means of further consultations, a leaflet, or a website. If appropriate, the normalization of behavior can be encouraged, with the provision of rehabilitation. Other medical and psychiatric conditions such as depression and panic should, of course, be treated. Above all, clinicians must be vigilant to the possibility of iatrogenic harm arising from excessive and inappropriate investigation and medical treatment.

Future research

Treatments

We all hope that, in the future, robust and effective new treatments for PMD will emerge. We already have a number of candidate treatments, which arguably only need to be developed and evaluated in well-conducted randomized trials.

We propose that for a treatment to merit further evaluation it should (1) have preliminary evidence for its efficacy, (2) be a treatment that is practically testable in a clinical trial, and (3) plausibly be deliverable in routine clinical practice. In applying these criteria, we suggest the following as the top three candidate treatments.

1. Use of a psychotherapeutically enhanced neurological consultation. A consultation which pays careful attention to the relationship between the physician and patient and to the information given encapsulates many of the key aspects of psychotherapy. There is some evidence for its value in medically unexplained symptoms in general [38] but it has not been adequately evaluated for PMD.

2. Cognitive behavior therapy of a form specifically tailored to the patient with PMD and given according to a manual is a strong candidate for further evaluation in PMD.

3. Given the requirement for deliverability in practice, we also think it will be important to evaluate brief forms of psychotherapy, such as CBT-based self-help, that can be given in book or computerized form.

In addition to these top three candidates, others which may merit further evaluation include comprehensive inpatient rehabilitation, including psychotherapeutic ingredients as above; psychodynamic psychotherapy that is brief and delivered according to a manual; and hypnosis given according to a manual.

Trials

As well as strong candidate treatments, future trials will require to be of robust design. In particular, they will need to meet the requirements listed in Table 39.3.

Conclusions

While, on the one hand, the simplistic notion that a psychological condition requires a psychological treatment is naive, on the other hand, there is good reason to think that psychotherapy (treatment with a psychological content) is an important component of the management of patients with PMD. However, the scientific evidence available to support the efficacy of these treatments is limited, and there is a pressing need to continue to develop and evaluate psychotherapies for these neglected patients. We should, however, not allow a focus on psychotherapy to lead us to neglect simple psychotherapeutic aspects of the medical consultation or to justify forcing patients to make strong assumptions about the nature of their symptoms.

This is a potentially exciting time for research into the treatments of PMD, as there are several candidate treatments ripe for development and evaluation in a new generation of rigorously conducted randomized controlled trials. We look forward to much needed progress in the field.

References

1. Garofalo ML. The diagnosis and treatment of hysterical paralyses by the intravenous administration of pentothal sodium: case reports 1942. *Conn Med* 1992;**56**:159–160.

2. Sharpe M, Carson AJ. "Unexplained" somatic symptoms, functional syndromes, and somatization: do we need a paradigm shift? *Ann Intern Med* 2001;**134**(9 Suppl 2):926–930.

3. Carson AJ, Ringbauer B, Stone J, *et al*. Do medically unexplained symptoms matter? A prospective cohort study of 300 new referrals to neurology outpatient clinics. *J Neurol Neurosurg Psychiatry* 2000;**68**:207–210.

4. Stone J, Carson A, Duncan R, *et al*. Symptoms "unexplained by organic disease" in 1144 new neurology out-patients: how often does the diagnosis change at follow-up? *Brain* 2009;**132**:2878–2888.

5. Lang EV, Benotsch EG, Fick LJ, *et al*. Adjunctive non-pharmacological analgesia for invasive medical procedures: a randomised trial. *Lancet* 2000;**355**:1486–1490.

6. Leiphart JW, Valone FH. Stereotactic lesions for the treatment of psychiatric disorders. *J Neurosurg* 2010;**113**:1204–1211.

7. Williams DT, Ford B, Fahn S. Phenomenology and psychopathology related to psychogenic movement disorders. *Adv Neurol* 1995;**65**:231–257.

8. Moene FC, Spinhoven P, Hoogduin KA, van Dyck R. A randomized controlled clinical trial of a hypnosis-based treatment for patients with conversion disorder, motor type. *Int J Clin Exp Hypn* 2003;**51**:29–50.

9. Moene FC, Spinhoven P, Hoogduin KA, van Dyck R. A randomised controlled clinical trial on the additional effect of hypnosis in a comprehensive treatment programme for in-patients with conversion disorder of the motor type. *Psychother Psychosom* 2002;**71**:66–76.

10. Goldstein LH, Chalder T, Chigwedere C, *et al*. Cognitive-behavioral therapy for psychogenic nonepileptic seizures: a pilot RCT. *Neurology* 2010;**74**:1986–1994.

11. Ataoglu A, Ozcetin A, Icmeli C, Ozbulut O. Paradoxical therapy in conversion reaction. *J Korean Med Sci* 2003;**18**:581–584.

12. Teasell RW, Shapiro AP. Strategic-behavioral intervention in the treatment of chronic nonorganic motor disorders. *Am J Phys Med Rehabil* 1994;**73**:44–50.

13. Speed J. Behavioral management of conversion disorder: retrospective study. *Arch Phys Med Rehabil* 1996;**77**:147–154.

14. Behr J. The role of physiotherapy in the recovery of patients with conversion disorder. *Physiotherapy Canada* 1996;**48**:197–202.

15. Watanabe TK, O' Dell MW, Togliatti TJ. Diagnosis and rehabilitation strategies for patients with hysterical hemiparesis: a report of four cases. *Arch Phys Med Rehabil* 1998;**79**:709–714.

16. Withrington RH, Wynn Parry CB. Rehabilitation of conversion paralysis. *J Bone Joint Surg* 1985;**67**:635–637.

17. Silver FW. Management of conversion disorder. *Am J Phys Med Rehabil* 1996;**75**:134–140.

18. Daie N, Witztum E. Short-term strategic treatment in traumatic conversion reactions. *Am J Psychother* 1991;**45**:335–347.

19. Weiser HI. Motor sensory dysfunction of upper limb due to conversion syndrome. *Arch Phys Med Rehabil* 1976;**57**:17–19.

20. Delargy MA, Peatfield RC, Burt AA. Successful rehabilitation in conversion paralysis. *BMJ* 1986;**292**:1730–1731.

21. Fishbain DA, Goldberg M, Khalil TM, *et al*. The utility of electromyographic biofeedback in the treatment of conversion paralysis. *Am J Psychiatry* 1988;**145**:1572–1575.

22. Hinson VK, Weinstein S, Bernard B, Leurgans SE, Goetz CG. Single-blind clinical trial of psychotherapy for treatment of psychogenic movement disorders. *Parkinsonism Relat Disord* 2006;**12**:177–180.

23. Shapiro AP, Teasell RW. Behavioural interventions in the rehabilitation of acute v. chronic non-organic (conversion/factitious) motor disorders. *Br J Psychiatry* 2004;**185**:140–146.

24. Krull F, Schifferdecker M. Inpatient treatment of conversion disorder: a clinical investigation of outcome. *Psychother Psychosom* 1990;**53**:161–165.

25. White A, Corbin DO, Coope B. The use of thiopentone in the treatment of non-organic locomotor disorders. *J Psychosom Res* 1988;**32**:249–253.

26. Poole NA, Wuerz A, Agrawal N. Abreaction for conversion disorder: systematic review with meta-analysis. *Br J Psychiatry* 2010;**197**:91–95.

27. Goldstein LH, Deale AC, Mitchell-O' Malley SJ, Toone BK, Mellers JD. An evaluation of cognitive behavioral therapy as a treatment for dissociative seizures: a pilot study. *Cogn Behav Neurol* 2004;**17**:41–49.

28. LaFrance WC, Jr. Psychogenic nonepileptic seizures. *Curr Opin Neurol* 2008;**21**:195–201.

29. LaFrance WC, Jr., Miller IW, Ryan CE, *et al.* Cognitive behavioral therapy for psychogenic nonepileptic seizures. *Epilepsy Behav* 2009;**14**:591–596.

30. Reuber M, Burness C, Howlett S, Brazier J, Grunewald R. Tailored psychotherapy for patients with functional neurological symptoms: a pilot study. *J Psychosom Res* 2007;**63**:625–632.

31. Betts T, Boden S. Diagnosis, management and prognosis of a group of 128 patients with non-epileptic attack disorder. Part 1. *Seizure* 1992;**1**:19–26.

32. Kroenke K. Efficacy of treatment for somatoform disorders: a review of randomized controlled trials. *Psychosom Med* 2007;**69**:881–888.

33. Kroenke K, Swindle R. Cognitive-behavioral therapy for somatization and symptom syndromes: a critical review of controlled clinical trials. *Psychother Psychosom* 2000;**69**:205–215.

34. Abbass A, Kisely S, Kroenke K. Short-term psychodynamic psychotherapy for somatic disorders. Systematic review and meta-analysis of clinical trials. *Psychother Psychosom* 2009;**78**:265–274.

35. Frank JD. Therapeutic factors in psychotherapy. *Am J Psychother* 1971;**25**:350–361.

36. Stone J, Wojcik W, Durrance D, *et al.* What should we say to patients with symptoms unexplained by disease? The "number needed to offend." *BMJ* 2002;**325**:1449–1450.

37. Stone J, Carson A, Sharpe M. Functional symptoms and signs in neurology: assessment and diagnosis. *J Neurol Neurosurg Psychiatry* 2005;**76**(Suppl 1):i2–i12.

38. Price JR. Managing physical symptoms: the clinical assessment as treatment. *J Psychosom Res* 2000;**48**:1–10.

40

Pharmacotherapy

Kevin J. Black and Bonnie Applewhite

The evidence base for treatment of psychogenic movement disorder

The key question in determining the evidence base for treatment of psychogenic movement disorder (PMD) is nosology. To illustrate this point, a literature search of PubMed for the phrase "Psychogenic Movement Disorder" yielded 38 articles, with only three treatment studies. None of these was randomized and only one was rater-blind. By contrast, a search on the same date for the medical subject heading "Somatoform Disorders" – limiting PubMed to articles for which this is a major focus of the article, and further limiting that result to controlled trials – still returned 153 citations, including 16 reviews and six systematic meta-analyses from the Cochrane collaboration. Numerous additional articles report clinical trials in typical movement disorders. Therefore, if PMD is a distinct diagnostic entity, there is almost no evidence to guide therapy; if, however, it is really a minor variation of established psychiatric illnesses (or, for that matter, of typical movement disorders), the evidence base for treatment is rather solid.

Given this central role of nosology in determining the evidence base for treatment, this chapter very briefly reviews the nosological status of PMD. To lead with the conclusion, there is substantial work to do. Since there is no consistent pathology for some common movement disorders (e.g., most adult-onset dystonia), validation of the PMD diagnosis must be clinical. Robins and Guze [1] discussed one commonly accepted approach to diagnostic validation that requires data on clinical description, delimitation from other disorders, follow-up study (including treatment response), family study, and laboratory studies. For the diagnosis of PMD, there have been few data in any of these areas. The most important concern for using the diagnosis of PMD to guide treatment is with "delimitation from other disorders." For example, there are very limited data to demonstrate that psychogenic dystonia is meaningfully and consistently different from DSM-IV-defined conversion disorder, or for that matter from non-epileptic seizures or even from typical dystonia.

Longitudinal course and treatment outcome are additional areas needing much more research to determine whether PMD is a valid diagnosis. Placebo response is one example; dramatic response to placebo or to psychotherapy was proposed as a criterion indicating PMD [2]. Hunter et al. [3], for example, diagnosed nine patients with psychogenic parkinsonism in large part based on the improvement in parkinsonism after a single dose of carbidopa ("marked or moderate" improvement in three patients and "mild improvement" in six). Unfortunately, placebo improvement is also common in idiopathic Parkinson's disease, and its mechanism is even known to involve dopamine release [4]. In other words, there is better evidence for a placebo response in Lewy body Parkinson's disease than in psychogenic parkinsonism! Similarly, although all five children in one study with "documented PMD" (Fahn–Williams criteria [2]) remitted completely after psychotherapy or suggestion, some with "organic" movement disorders also remitted [5]. Nevertheless, sometimes clinical hunches pay off. Despite the unproven nature and theoretical weakness of the placebo test for Parkinson's disease described above, convincing the patients that they did not have Parkinson's disease seemed to cure them, as six of the nine had no symptoms at follow-up [3].

Therefore, despite the clear potential advantages, current data are inadequate to demonstrate that one in fact gains additional information about prognosis or

Psychogenic Movement Disorders and Other Conversion Disorders, ed. Mark Hallett, Anthony E. Lang, Joseph Jankovic, Stanley Fahn, Peter W. Halligan, Valerie Voon, and C. Robert Cloninger. Published by Cambridge University Press. © Cambridge University Press 2011.

treatment response by diagnosing "psychogenic movement disorder" as opposed to "conversion symptom" or "atypical action tremor." We would argue that until a new diagnosis (PMD) has been shown to add value to existing diagnoses, it is not clinically useful. The field should not move beyond the data. Ideally, diagnostic criteria should be guided by data, and until those data are available the proposed diagnosis should be recognized as useful primarily for research.

For the purposes of this chapter there are two main practical concerns. For patients whose signs do not faithfully mimic a typical movement disorder and have features of conversion or somatization, we do not yet know whether PMD requires separate treatment studies from conversion disorder, somatization disorder, or other medically unexplained symptoms. For patients with typical clinical phenomenology but with worrisome features such as prominent personality disorder, onset after a psychological stressor, or prominent placebo response, we do not yet know whether PMD requires separate treatment studies from the typical movement disorder. A third practical implication for patient care comes from observing the birth of other diagnoses that are not helpful (like chronic fatigue syndrome or multiple personality disorder) [6,7]. A newly proposed diagnosis (like PMD) can distract the patient and doctor from diagnoses with firmer prognostic or treatment implications (such as somatization disorder).

Fortunately, as this volume attests, research on nosological questions is beginning to move forward, and many of the questions about the diagnostic validity of PMD may be adequately addressed in the near future.

Research on treatment of psychogenic movement disorders per se

Hinson et al. [8] reported the first treatment study in PMD according to Fahn–Williams criteria [2] to use blind outcome assessments: a rater-blind study of psychodynamic psychotherapy. This and other studies of psychotherapeutic and other treatments for PMD are reviewed in separate chapters in this volume and in the review by Hinson and Haren [9]. There are few pharmacotherapy studies in PMD and no large randomized placebo-controlled trial (RCT).

The largest published treatment study specifically directed at PMD is an open case series by Voon and Lang [10]. This 2005 study included only patients with PMD according to Fahn and Williams criteria, but excluded symptoms "that were… elaboration of… underlying primary neurologic disorder." Fifteen patients were studied after excluding four with dystonia and four who refused treatment; 35% had a current major depressive episode and 53% were diagnosed with an anxiety disorder. For 12 patients (78%), the first study visit was their first encounter with a psychiatrist. All patients were told that PMD was not a neurological disease and that the effect of the proposed treatment on their motor symptoms was not known. Initial treatment included either citalopram or paroxetine 10 mg daily with titration upwards to 40 mg daily as needed. If a patient did not respond to 4 weeks at 40 mg daily, the treatment was changed to venlafaxine 37.5–300 mg daily. Clinical assessments occurred before and approximately 3 months after initiation of treatment.

Diagnosis and treatment response divided the 15 patients into two groups. Ten participants demonstrated a single conversion symptom. All 10 had a current or prior depressive episode or anxiety disorder, and the treatment was effective: seven reported complete remission of symptoms and one other patient reported "marked" improvement. The other five subjects were diagnosed with somatization disorder (two), factitious disorder or malingering (two), and hypochondriasis (one); only two of these five met criteria for major depression or an anxiety disorder, and none improved with treatment.

This study provides valuable data. Conservative conclusions include the following. First, psychiatric diagnosis matters: somatization disorder and factitious disorder identify patients who are resistant to treatment, whereas patients with a single, non-intentional pseudoneurological symptom have a better prognosis. Second, patients with a history of depression or anxiety may improve with adequate antidepressant treatment, including improvement in the motor signs. It is worth noting that these conclusions do not require a new diagnosis; one could simply tell the patient, "your symptoms are quite atypical; this is not a recognized neurological disease; but the fact that you've been depressed in the past may mean that you are likely to improve with an antidepressant even if you're not especially depressed now." It is also worth noting that the specificity of these results is not clear, as there is limited prospective data on the benefit of antidepressant therapy on typical movement disorders.

Rotstein and colleagues [11] treated nine children with documented PMD, nine with clinically established

PMD, and one with probable PMD (Fahn–Williams criteria). Follow-up was available in 11 of the 19. Of this 11, nine had "significant improvement after combined psychotherapy, physiotherapy, and pharmacotherapy." However, children may differ from adults with PMD in several important ways, including treatment resistance. For example, in one study 38 of 42 adults with PMD still had the abnormal movements an average of 3.2 years after diagnosis [12].

Other relevant treatment studies

Most of the evidence on treatment of PMD, and all of the RCT evidence, comes from other treatment studies on somatoform disorders, that is, studies not specifically directed at PMD. Given the paucity of treatment research specifically on PMD, such studies constitute the primary evidence base for treatment. In this literature cognitive behavioral therapy (CBT) and other behavioral interventions show robust and often superior treatment effects, but this chapter will focus on pharmacotherapy. Kroenke [13] identified 34 RCTs in somatoform disorders including short- and long-term trials of antidepressant medication and other treatments. The five antidepressant trials enrolled a median of 149 subjects each; all of these trials were of less than 6 months in duration. Four of the antidepressant trials were in "lower threshold somatization disorder," and three of these showed clear benefit for the antidepressant. Sumathipala reached similar conclusions in his review [14].

Numerous controlled studies report treatment data in patients with "functional" or medically unexplained symptoms, including back pain, chronic fatigue, fibromyalgia, chronic pelvic pain, and many others [15–17]. In the absence of classic depressive symptomatology, 94 RCTs demonstrated marked improvement of medically unexplained symptoms with antidepressant therapy, with a number needed to treat of only four [18]. Similarly, non-epileptic seizures responded significantly better to sertraline than to placebo in an RCT [19]. Sulpiride but not haloperidol appeared effective in a RCT of conversion disorder [20].

Somatization disorder is the prototypical somatoform illness, yet it is defined as chronic and has been considered to have a poor response to treatment. Nevertheless, an open study suggested benefit for nefazodone [21], and a RCT in a form fruste, called "multisomatoform disorder," showed significant efficacy for escitalopram [22]. A three-way crossover study of chronic fatigue demonstrated greater benefit for mirtazapine than for placebo, although CBT was more effective [23].

Non-specific management

Non-specific elements of treatment are also important. At our movement disorders center, this includes an atheoretical, rehabilitative approach to diagnosis and management of patients. This approach is not novel but it is consistent with long-standing sensible suggestions [24,25].

We attempt to separate patients who might be diagnosed with PMD at other centers into those who clearly do not have a typical movement disorder, and those whose signs resemble a typical movement disorder but who have some unusual features. We prefer the term "atypical" for such patients in preference to "psychogenic," thus avoiding speculation on etiology and diagnostic validity [26]. We first tell these patients that we've seen many people with a similar presentation. We emphasize that not having various neurological diseases is good news. We convey the principal diagnosis and what it means in lay terms. Occasionally that diagnosis is tentative. If asked what causes their symptoms, we may reply that no one knows for sure, but we know what will likely happen with them over time and that we have had good outcomes taking care of similar patients. We often tell patients with a single conversion symptom that most people in their shoes recover, and (if relevant) that these symptoms will likely disappear as suddenly or unpredictably as they appeared.

We encourage treating depression and anxiety if present, regardless of whether the movements are typical. If somatization disorder can be diagnosed, we inform the patient of the diagnosis, provide relevant education on its implications, and attempt to work with other physicians involved in the patient's care to avoid iatrogenic injury. If signs vary with suggestion, distraction, or entrainment, we point out that this proves there is residual neurological function *and* that behavioral interventions can modify their symptoms. Since most movement disorders worsen with stress, we encourage practical psychotherapy as a non-specific rehabilitative treatment. Finally, we encourage returning to full activity despite any persistent motor symptoms, and attempt to address any psychosocial problems discovered during the evaluation.

We recognize that RCTs are required to determine whether any treatment (including this approach) is effective. Nevertheless, we believe this approach side-steps many of the issues that render patients hesitant to accept a diagnosis of psychogenic movements or to impute their symptoms to psychological stressors. It also allows the skeptical doctor to refrain from endorsing unproven or untestable theories of symptom causation or treatment response (such as those represented by the word "psychogenic").

Conclusions

In summary, the extent of the treatment literature on PMD depends on whether it differs from other diagnoses; only a few studies have targeted PMD, but numerous well-executed treatment studies are probably relevant. These show clear benefits primarily for antidepressants on a variety of somatoform presentations ranging from single functional symptoms to somatization disorder. Some evidence (and common sense) suggests that if patients with PMD have current or past major depression or anxiety, their movements may be more likely to improve with antidepressant medication. By contrast, diagnoses of somatization disorder, malingering, factitious disorder, or hypochondriasis may portend a less optimistic outcome. Further treatment research is needed and may clarify how best to diagnose and manage patients with unusual movements.

References

1. Robins E, Guze SB. Establishment of diagnostic validity in psychiatric illness: its application to schizophrenia. *Am J Psychiatry* 1970;**126**:983–987.

2. Fahn S, Williams DT. Psychogenic dystonia. *Adv Neurol* 1988;**50**:431–455.

3. Hunter C, Adam O, Jankovic J. Psychogenic parkinsonism: use of placebo. In *Proceedings of the 2nd International Conference on Psychogenic Movement Disorders*, Washington, DC, 2009:93–94.

4. de la Fuente-Fernandez R, Stoessl AJ. The placebo effect in Parkinson's disease. *Trends Neurosci* 2002;**25**:302–306.

5. Ahmed MA, Martinez A, Yee A, Cahill D, Besag FM. Psychogenic and organic movement disorders in children. *Dev Med Child Neurol* 2008;**50**:300–304.

6. Price RK, North CS, Wessely S, Fraser VJ. Estimating the prevalence of chronic fatigue syndrome and associated symptoms in the community. *Public Health Rep* 1992;**107**:514–522.

7. North CS, Ryall J-EM, Ricci DA, Wetzel RD. *Multiple Personalities, Multiple Disorders: Psychiatric Classification and Media Influence*. New York: Oxford University Press, 1993.

8. Hinson VK, Weinstein S, Bernard B, Leurgans SE, Goetz CG. Single-blind clinical trial of psychotherapy for treatment of psychogenic movement disorders. *Parkinsonism Relat Disord* 2006;**12**:177–180.

9. Hinson VK, Haren WB. Psychogenic movement disorders. *Lancet Neurol* 2006;**5**:695–700.

10. Voon V, Lang AE. Antidepressant treatment outcomes of psychogenic movement disorder. *J Clin Psychiatry* 2005;**66**:1529–1534.

11. Rotstein M, Pearson T, Williams DT, Frucht S. Psychogenic movement disorders in children and adolescents. In *Proceedings of the 2nd International Conference on Psychogenic Movement Disorders*, Washington, DC, 2009:92.

12. Feinstein A, Stergiopoulos V, Fine J, Lang AE. Psychiatric outcome in patients with a psychogenic movement disorder: a prospective study. *Neuropsychiatry Neuropsychol Behav Neurol* 2001;**14**:169–176.

13. Kroenke K. Efficacy of treatment for somatoform disorders: a review of randomized controlled trials. *Psychosom Med* 2007;**69**:881–888.

14. Sumathipala A. What is the evidence for the efficacy of treatments for somatoform disorders? A critical review of previous intervention studies. *Psychosom Med* 2007;**69**:889–900.

15. Henningsen P, Zipfel S, Herzog W. Management of functional somatic syndromes. *Lancet* 2007;**369**:946–955.

16. Hatcher S, Arroll B. Assessment and management of medically unexplained symptoms. *BMJ* 2008;**336**:1124–1128.

17. Hauser W, Bernardy K, Uceyler N, Sommer C. Treatment of fibromyalgia syndrome with antidepressants: a meta-analysis. *JAMA* 2009;**301**:198–209.

18. O' Malley PG, Jackson JL, Santoro J, *et al.* Antidepressant therapy for unexplained symptoms and symptom syndromes. *J Fam Pract* 1999;**48**:980–990.

19. LaFrance WC, Keitner GI, Papandonatos GD, *et al.* Pilot pharmacologic randomized controlled trial for psychogenic nonepileptic seizures. *Neurology* 2010;**75**:1166–1173.

20. Rampello L, Raffaele R, Nicoletti G, *et al.* Hysterical neurosis of the conversion type: therapeutic activity of neuroleptics with different hyperprolactinemic potency. *Neuropsychobiology* 1996;**33**:186–188.

21. Menza M, Lauritano M, Allen L, *et al.* Treatment of somatization disorder with nefazodone: a

prospective, open-label study. *Ann Clin Psychiatry* 2001;**13**:153–158.

22. Muller JE, Wentzel I, Koen L, *et al.* Escitalopram in the treatment of multisomatoform disorder: a double-blind, placebo-controlled trial. *Int Clin Psychopharmacol* 2008;**23**:43–48.

23. Stubhaug B, Lie SA, Ursin H, Eriksen HR. Cognitive-behavioural therapy v. mirtazapine for chronic fatigue and neurasthenia: randomised placebo-controlled trial. *Br J Psychiatry* 2008;**192**:217–223.

24. Brenner C, Friedman AP, Merritt HH. Psychiatric syndromes in patients with organic brain disease. 1. Diseases of the basal ganglia. *AmJPsychiatry* 1947;**103**:733–737.

25. Guze SB, Brown OL. Psychiatric disease and functional dysphonia and aphonia. *Arch Otolaryngol* 1962;**76**:84–87.

26. Tibbetts RW. Spasmodic torticollis. *J Psychosom Res* 1971;**15**:461–469.

Suggestion

Irving Kirsch

41

Introduction

"Suggestion" is a broad term denoting a variety of different phenomena. *Merriam-Webster's Medical Dictionary* (2007) defines suggestion as "the process by which a physical or mental state is influenced by a thought or idea." The term is most closely associated with hypnosis, a culturally defined situation in which a person designated as a "hypnotist" gives suggestions to a person designated as a "subject" for alterations in subjective experience and overt behavior [1]. Hypnotic suggestions can produce alterations in the perceived voluntary control of movement and in perception. Most people can experience some of the effects of suggestion on movement, but profound perceptual alterations seem to be limited to highly suggestible subjects.

Other domains in which suggestion is a prominent feature include the placebo effect and memory suggestibility. The placebo effect refers to changes in subjective and/or physical states induced by the belief that one is receiving a physically active medical treatment [2]. Physically inactive treatments, such as inert pills and sham surgery, have been found to produce substantial effects, particularly in mood disorders and in pain perception. In some cases, the alterations are so great that it is difficult to demonstrate an effect with the active treatment for which it is serving as a control.

The effects of suggestion on memory retrieval are most pernicious in legal and therapeutic contexts. In the legal context, eye witness testimony can be influenced by relatively subtle forms of suggestion [3]. For example, asking how fast a car was going when it *smashed* into another car leads witnesses to remember the car going faster than when they are asked how fast it was going when it *hit* the other car. A less subtle form of suggestion on memory involves the provision of misleading information after an event has been witnessed. The misinformation effect is the distortion of an episodic memory by inaccurate subsequent information. Suggestion can do more than distort memories. Intensively suggestive procedures can lead to the formation of memories for events that have never happened. This phenomenon makes it difficult to determine whether supposedly repressed memories recovered in therapy refer to events that have actually occurred [4].

Hypnosis, the placebo effect, and memory suggestibility involve overlapping processes. For one thing, they are all forms of suggestion. That is, they all involve changes in experience that are induced by thoughts or ideas. For another, two of them can be involved in the same phenomenon. For example, hypnosis can be used as a way of retrieving memories and can exacerbate the misinformation effect [5]; it can also be used as a means of eliciting placebo effects without deception [6], and placebos can affect memory processes [7]. Although hypnosis, placebo effects, and memory suggestions are related, they are also distinguishably different phenomena. Hypnosis, for example, involves suggestions for experiences that are palpably contrary to what the subject knows to be true, with no attempt to convince them otherwise. Conversely, placebos and memory suggestions aim to convince the person that the world is (or was) different than it really is. Placebo pills are given in the guise of chemically active medications, and memory suggestions produce mistaken beliefs about past events.

The distinction between these different types of suggestion is reinforced by the finding that they are only weakly correlated with each other, at best [8]. Moreover, whereas hypnotic suggestibility is a highly stable trait, responsiveness to placebo is not. The test–retest reliability of measures of hypnotic responsiveness is as high as 0.75 over a 25-year interval, and different

Psychogenic Movement Disorders and Other Conversion Disorders, ed. Mark Hallett, Anthony E. Lang, Joseph Jankovic, Stanley Fahn, Peter W. Halligan, Valerie Voon, and C. Robert Cloninger. Published by Cambridge University Press. © Cambridge University Press 2011.

measures of the construct are highly correlated [9,10]. In contrast, placebo responding is highly unstable. In one study, two different placebo analgesic creams, differing only in name, were administered twice each, and a pain stimulus was administered to treated (by placebo) and untreated body locations [11]. Although test–retest correlations for the placebo effect when the placebo bore the same name were substantial (0.60 and 0.77), when the name of the placebo was changed, the correlation was rendered non-significant.

Of the various types of suggestion, hypnotic suggestion is the most relevant to understanding movement disorders and, in particular, conversion disorders and will be the focus of the remainder of this chapter.

Hypnotic suggestion

Historically, conversion disorders constituted a subset of the broader category of hysteria, which also included dissociative disorders. The subsequent separation of these into unlinked entities may have been a mistake, as they are most likely the result of underlying common processes. One indication of this is the degree to which symptoms of conversion and dissociative disorders go in and out of fashion. Glove anesthesia was fairly common in Western Europe at the end of the nineteenth century, but later went out of style when it became known that it was physiologically nonsensical. Similarly, dissociative identity disorder (formerly multiple personality disorder) was fashionable during the nineteenth century and all but disappeared during the first half of the twentieth century, only to return with a vengeance after being popularized in books and films such as *The Three Faces of Eve* and *Sybil*.

The phenomenon of hypnotic suggestion provides further evidence of the commonality between conversion and dissociative disorders, as well as hints as to the psychological mechanisms by which their symptoms are produced. A list of typical hypnotic suggestions resembles a catalogue of symptoms of these disorders. Indeed, tests of hypnotic suggestibility (aka hypnotizability) are measures of the number of conversion and dissociative symptoms a person can experience and display in response to verbal requests. Measures of hypnotic suggestibility are reliably correlated with the belief that one can experience hypnotic suggestions and with a trait called fantasy proneness, which is a tendency to engage in vivid fantasies, both as a child and as an adult [12]. Hypnotic suggestibility also seems to have a genetic component [13], and patients with

psychogenic movement disorders show particularly high hypnotic suggestibility scores [14].

Conventionally, there are three broad classifications of hypnotic suggestions: ideomotor, challenge, and cognitive. An arguably more useful classification scheme divides these suggestions into four types: motor production, motor inhibition, cognitive production, and cognitive inhibition. Motor production or ideomotor suggestions are requests to experience normally voluntary movements as automatic or involuntary occurrences. For example, subjects might be told "your arm is feeling lighter and lighter and is lifting into the air." Motor inhibition suggestions are requests for partial paralysis, such as "your arm is becoming rigid like an iron rod, so rigid that you cannot bend it." When moderately or highly suggestible people are given this suggestion and then asked to bend their arm, they report that they cannot bend it, and, in fact, the arm does not bend. Cognitive production suggestions are requests for sensory hallucinations, like seeing a non-existent cat or hearing a non-existent voice. Cognitive inhibition suggestions ask the subject to not see, hear, feel, or remember something. The clinically important phenomenon of hypnotic pain control is an example of a cognitive inhibition suggestion.

There are two notable differences between hypnotic suggestions on the one hand and conversion and dissociative symptoms on the other. The first difference is that hypnotic suggestions are ego-syntonic. Hypnotized subjects experience suggested effects because they want to, and it is easy for them to stop responding to the suggestions whenever they wish. Ideomotor suggestions are experienced as automatic, but they are not involuntary in the sense of being against the subject's will. Indeed, experiencing suggestions requires cognitive effort and is rendered more difficult by competing cognitive tasks [15]. The second difference is that the ability to respond to suggestion is very widespread, particularly for motor suggestions [16]. Approximately 80% of the population are capable of producing simple ideomotor movements that they experience as automatic, and 50% are able to experience motor inhibitions [16]. The ability to experience cognitive suggestions is much rarer, with figures ranging from 10 to 20% depending on the specific suggestion.

Psychological mechanisms

At this point, we know more about how responses to hypnotic suggestions are not produced than we do about how they are produced. In particular, we know that they are not a result of simple compliance with demand characteristics, and they are not a result of the induction of a hypnotic state.

Compliance

There are two reasons for suspecting that hypnotic responses might simply result from intentional compliance and that hypnotized subjects do not really experience the suggested phenomena that they display behaviorally and that they report experiencing. First, some of the responses seem rather exceptional. People report seeing things that are not there, hearing nonexistent sounds, failing to see things on which their eyes are focused, not being able to remember selected things and then easily remembering them as soon as an appropriate signal is given, and so on. The incredibility of hypnotic phenomena is enhanced by stage hypnosis, in which volunteers seem to believe that they are on a spaceship heading towards Mars or that they have been transformed into famous rock singers.

A second reason for suspecting compliance is that hypnotic responses are very easy to fake. One method of testing whether subjects might simply be complying with experimental demand is by using the real–simulator experimental design developed by Martin Orne [17]. In the real–simulator design, low-suggestible individuals are asked by an experimenter to pretend to be highly suggestible and to fool a second experimenter who will not be told which of the participants are pretested high suggestibles and which are low suggestibles who have been instructed to fake. In most studies using this design, no significant differences are found between highly suggestible subjects and simulators, and experimenters with many years of experience in the field are incapable of distinguishing which is which.

Nevertheless, there are behavioral and physiological data demonstrating that hypnotically suggested responses reflect genuine alterations in experience, rather than simple compliance. The first set of studies reporting behavioral data that directly address the issue of compliance used a variant of the real–simulator design in which highly suggestible subjects and low-suggestible simulators were asked to listen to a recorded hypnotic induction and suggestions twice, once with an experimenter present and once on their own without the presence of the experimenter [18,19]. What the participants did not know was that there was a hidden camera recording their behavior when the experimenter was not present. When the simulators thought they were alone, they stopped pretending to be hypnotized. Instead of responding to suggestion, they scratched their arms, read magazines, and engaged in other behaviors that were inappropriate to the role of hypnotized subject. In contrast, the highly suggestible subjects continued to respond to suggestion when the experimenter was absent, petting hallucinated kittens, swatting at hallucinated mosquitoes, and grimacing when tasting hallucinated lemons.

A second set of studies involves the use of suggestion to modulate cognitive processes that are generally thought to be automatic and thus beyond topdown control. The first of these studies was conducted by Amir Raz and his colleagues on the Stroop effect [20]. In its classical form, the Stroop effect involves asking people to identify the color in which a word is printed [21]. The word may be the name of the color in which it is printed or it may be the name of a different color. The Stroop effect is the finding that people are slower in identifying the color in which a word is printed when the word and the color are incongruent (e.g., when the word "red" is printed in green ink) than they are when the word and the color are congruent (e.g., the word "red" printed in red ink). The standard explanation of the Stroop effect is that reading words in one's native language becomes an automatic process, which then interferes with the color naming task. Raz and colleagues were able to reduce the Stroop effect substantially by giving highly suggestible subjects the suggestion that the words would appear as meaningless symbols, gibberish, like characters written in a foreign language [20].

Subsequently, Christina Iani and her colleagues demonstrated a similar effect of suggestion on the flanker compatibility effect [22]. Like the Stroop effect, the flanker compatibility effect involves the slowing down of responses through cognitive conflict [23]. Three letters are presented on a computer screen, with the center target letter being either the same as (e.g., TTT) or different from (e.g., FTF) the two flanking letters. The flanker compatibility task consists of the finding that people take longer to identify the center letter when the flanking distracters differ from the target. Iani and colleagues were able to reduce the flanker compatibility effect by giving subjects a suggestion to see the central letter as blurred, less luminous, and further away than the other letters. As the flanker compatibility effect, like the Stroop effect, is considered to be automatic, the presumption is that participants would not be able to reduce it without the subjective experience generated by the suggestion.

Physiological data contradicting the simple compliance hypothesis consist of changes in activation in brain regions associated with suggested experiences. For example, Rainville and colleagues gave hypnotized subjects suggestions aimed at reducing the unpleasantness of noxious stimuli, following which positron emission tomography (PET) revealed significant changes in pain-evoked activity in the anterior cingulate cortex [24]. In another PET study, suggestions to perceive color in gray scale stimuli led to bilateral changes in regions of the brain that are associated with the perception of color [25]. These suggestion-related changes in brain activity are interpreted as indicating that the subjects have experienced the subjective phenomena that they report.

Finally, a word about stage hypnosis is warranted. The phenomenon of stage hypnosis, although overlapping with clinical and experimental hypnosis, differs from these in some important ways. Most important to the current discussion, stage hypnosis involves a considerable degree of social compliance. The aim of stage hypnotists is to put on an entertaining show. How this is accomplished is of minor importance. Stage hypnotists sometimes bring ringers with them, in case they fail to find sufficiently convincing or entertaining subjects among the audience. They invariably select people who comply behaviorally to come up on stage and dismiss those whose responses are not as good as others. The presence of an audience and their prior responsiveness puts considerable pressure on subjects to comply with suggestions whether they experience them or not. The result, according to many participants in these shows, is a mix of altered experience and intentional acting, with the boundaries not always being clear.

Hypnosis

Because responses to hypnotic suggestions occur after a hypnotic induction, and because they seem so different from normal experience, the general presumption is that the induced hypnotic state (sometimes referred to as a "trance" state) is among the causal factors in producing responses to suggestion. There is, however, abundant experimental evidence that hypnotic responses, including the most unusual and difficult responses, can be produced without the induction of hypnosis. The first research demonstrating this was reported by the renown learning theorist Clark Hull in

1933 [26]. The strategy of Hull's studies was to administer the same suggestions with and without the induction of hypnosis. His finding was that all of the effects of hypnotic suggestion could be reproduced when the same suggestions were given without inducing hypnosis. Hull's findings have since been replicated in diverse laboratories spanning a period of more than a half a century [27]. In the most recent of these studies [12], for example, participants were asked to close their eyes and imagine a series of typical hypnotic suggestions (e.g., automatic movements, movement inhibition, and hallucinations), but there was no mention of hypnosis and no hypnotic induction was administered. Then the participants were told that the same suggestions would be given again, but this time they would first be hypnotized to see what the effect of hypnosis might be on their ability to experience them. The consistent findings of these studies are that the effect of a hypnotic induction is merely to amplify the suggestion effect to a relatively small degree and that the hypnotic and non-hypnotic responding are highly correlated, with correlations rivaling the test–retest correlations of the scales by means of which responsiveness is measured. Furthermore, the ability to respond to suggestion without hypnosis has been found even for the most difficult suggestions, including modulation of the Stroop effect and the production of altered color perception [28,29].

There are two ways of interpreting these data. Hull's interpretation was that the effects of the hypnotic state is quantitative rather than qualitative, as it is limited to enhancing responsiveness to suggestions that can also be experienced – albeit to a slightly lesser degree – without hypnosis. Beginning in the 1960s, some hypnosis scholars argued that the idea of a hypnotic state could be dispensed with altogether [30,31]. The enhanced responsiveness displayed following an induction might be caused by enhanced motivation and expectancies for responding. Indeed, motivation and response expectancy are among the very few correlates of hypnotic responding [12]. The debate between these two opposing views remains inconclusive, but one thing is clear: a hypnotic state is not a prerequisite for the experience of hypnotic suggestions. Even the most difficult hypnotic suggestions can be experienced without the induction of hypnosis [28,29].

What, then, is the hypnotic state? Two recent functional magnetic resonance imaging studies converge in indicating that it may involve reduction in activity in areas that have been identified as the "default mode," a network that is normally active during rest periods between tasks [32,33]. Reductions in default mode activity typically occur when people actively engage in a goal-directed cognitive task, rather than merely letting their minds wander passively. This suggests that the so-called hypnotic state is a normal state of focused attention, in which subjects suspend spontaneous non-goal-directed cognitive activity in preparation for what might be required by anticipated suggestions.

The lack of necessity of a hypnotic state for the production of responses to suggestion highlights the relevance of hypnotic phenomena to conversion and dissociative disorders. Patients suffering from these conditions have not been hypnotized, but they display behavior that is topographically identical to the symptoms of these disorders. It seems reasonable to hypothesize that similar mechanisms may be involved in the production of these behaviors through direct suggestion and its occurrence as psychological symptoms. If this is true, research into the mechanisms underlying response to suggestion might shed light on the mechanisms by which conversion and dissociative symptoms are produced by patients.

References

1. Kihlstrom JF. Hypnosis. *Annu Rev Psychol* 1985;**36**:385–418.

2. Kirsch I. Placebo: The role of expectancies in the generation and alleviation of illness. In Halligan P, Mansel A, eds. *The Power of Belief: Psychosocial Influence on Illness, Disability and Medicine*. Oxford: Oxford University Press, 2006:55–67.

3. Loftus EF. *Eyewitness Testimony*. Cambridge, MA: Harvard University Press, 1996.

4. Mazzoni G. Naturally occurring and suggestion-dependent memory distortions: the convergence of disparate research traditions. *Eur Psychologist* 2002;**7**:17–30.

5. Scoboria A, Mazzoni G, Kirsch I, Milling LS. Immediate and persisting effects of misleading questions and hypnosis on memory reports. *J Exp Psychol Appl* 2002;**8**:26–32.

6. Kirsch I. Clinical hypnosis as a nondeceptive placebo: empirically derived techniques. *Am J Clin Hypnosis* 1994;**37**:95–106.

7. Parker S, Garry M, Engle RW, Harper DN, Clifasefi SL. Psychotropic placebos reduce the misinformation effect by increasing monitoring at test'. *Memory* 2008;**16**:410–419.

8. Baker SL, Kirsch I. Hypnotic and placebo analgesia: Order effects and the placebo label. *Contemp Hypnosis* 1993;**10**:117–126.

9. Council JR. Measures of hypnotic responding. In Kirsch I, Antonio C, Cardeña E, Amigó S, eds. *Clinical Hypnosis and Self Regulation: Cognitive Behavioral Perspectives*. Washington, DC: American Psychological Association, 1998:119–140.

10. Piccione C, Hilgard ER, Zimbardo PG. On the degree of stability of measured hypnotizability over a 25-year period. *J Person Soc Psychol* 1989;**56**:289–295.

11. Whalley B, Hyland ME, Kirsch I. Consistency of the placebo effect. *J Psychosom Res* 2008;**64**:537–541.

12. Braffman W, Kirsch I. Imaginative suggestibility and hypnotizability: an empirical analysis. *J Person Soc Psychol* 1999;**77**:578–587.

13. Morgan A, Hilgard E, Davert E. The heritability of hypnotic susceptibility of twins: a preliminary report. *Behav Genet* 1970;**1**:213–224.

14. Frischholz E, Lipman L, Braun B, Sachs R. Psychopathology, hypnotizability, and dissociation. *Am J Psychiatry* 1992;**149**:1521–1525.

15. Kirsch I, Burgess CA, Braffman W. Attentional resources in hypnotic responding. *Int J Clin Exp Hypnosis* 1999;**47**:175–191.

16. Kirsch I, Silva CE, Comey G, Reed S. A spectral analysis of cognitive and personality variables in hypnosis: empirical disconfirmation of the two-factor model of hypnotic responding. *J Person Soc Psychol* 1995;**69**:167–175.

17. Orne MT. The nature of hypnosis: artifact and essence. *J Abnorm Psychol* 1959;**58**:277–299.

18. Perugini EM, Kirsch I, Allen ST, *et al*. Surreptitious observation of responses to hypnotically suggested hallucinations: a test of the compliance hypothesis. *Int J Clin Exp Hypnosis* 1998;**46**:191–203.

19. Kirsch I, Silva CE, Carone JE, Johnston JD, Simon B. The surreptitious observation design: an experimental paradigm for distinguishing artifact from essence in hypnosis. *J Abnorm Psychol* 1989;**98**:132–136.

20. Raz A, Shapiro T, Fan J, Posner MI. Hypnotic suggestion and the modulation of Stroop interference. *Arch Gen Psychiatry* 2002;**59**:1155–1161.

21. Stroop JR. Studies of interference in serial verbal reactions. *J Exp Psychol* 1935;**18**:643–661.

22. Iani C, Ricci F, Gherri E, Rubichi S. Hypnotic suggestion modulates cognitive conflict: the case of the flanker compatibility effect. *Psychol Sci* 2006;**17**:721–727.

23. Eriksen BA, Eriksen CW. Effects of noise letters upon the identification of a target letter in a nonsearch task. *Percept Psychophys* 1974;**16**:143–149.

24. Rainville P, Duncan GH, Price DD, Carrier B, Bushnell CM. Pain affect encoded in human anterior cingulate but not somatosensory cortex. *Science* 1997;**277**:968–971.

25. Kosslyn SM, Thompson WL, Costantini-Ferrando MF, Alpert NM, Spiegel D. Hypnotic visual illusion alters color processing in the brain. *Am J Psychiatry* 2000;**157**:1279–1284.

26. Hull CL. *Hypnosis and Suggestibility: An Experimental Approach*. New York: Appleton-Century Crofts, 1933.

27. Kirsch I, Mazzoni G, Montgomery GH. Remembrance of hypnosis past. *Am J Clin Hypnosis* 2007;**49**:171–178.

28. Raz A, Kirsch I, Pollard J, Nitkin-Kaner Y. Suggestion reduces the Stroop effect. *Psychol Sci* 2006;**17**:91–95.

29. Mazzoni G, Rotriquenz E, Carvalho C, *et al.* Suggested visual hallucinations in and out of hypnosis. *Conscious Cogn* 2009;**18**:494–499.

30. Barber TX. *Hypnosis: A Scientific Approach*. New York: Van Nostrand Reinhold, 1969.

31. Sarbin TR, Coe WC. *Hypnosis: A Social Psychological Analysis of Influence Communication*. New York: Holt, Rinehart & Winston, 1972.

32. McGeown WG, Mazzoni G, Venneri A, Kirsch I. Hypnotic induction decreases anterior default mode activity. *Conscious Cogn* 2009;**18**:848–855.

33. Oakley DA. Hypnosis, trance and suggestion: Evidence from neuroimaging. In Nash MR, Barnier A, eds. *Oxford Handbook of Hypnosis*. Oxford: Oxford University Press, 2008:365–92.

Chapter

42

Treating psychogenic movement disorders with suggestion

Michel C. F. Shamy

Introduction

The appropriate role of the placebo in randomized-controlled trials is a subject of much debate in contemporary medical ethics [1]. By comparison, the notion of prescribing placebos as therapy receives little attention. Supposedly, the case is closed: the treatment of patients with placebos, or with other means of suggestion (namely hypnosis and persuasion), is not ethically justifiable because "they can cause patient harm, undermine trust in the medical profession, destroy any possibility of a therapeutic alliance" and above all diminish patient autonomy [2]. However, a recent survey found that 45% of academic physicians in the Chicago area reported using placebos in clinical practice, and 88% felt that their use should not be prohibited. The authors of this study concluded that "a growing number of physicians believe in a mind–body connection… our physician respondents generally believed that placebos have therapeutic effects" [3].

Suggestion is the voluntary use by the physician of techniques that introduce into the patient's mind a belief or expectation that he or she will be healed. Persuasion, hypnosis, and placebo are all forms of suggestion in that they act via "meaning responses." As Daniel Moerman explains, conversations, procedures, and medications can have effects that are the consequences not of the entities themselves but rather of their meanings, as interpreted by the patient [4]. In this chapter, I contend that the tools of suggestion have a legitimate ethical justification in the treatment of psychogenic movement disorders (PMDs). First of all, suggestion engages the pathophysiology of psychogenic disease. Second, evidence from a variety of sources (anecdote, expert opinion, randomized controlled trials [RCTs], and meta-analysis) supports the efficacy of suggestion in this patient population. Finally, the major objections to the use of suggestion – that it impairs patient autonomy and threatens the doctor–patient relationship – are flawed and represent a prioritization of values secondary to the goal of medicine: providing care to patients.

The PMDs are prevalent, often debilitating, and suboptimally treated. The duration of psychogenic symptoms before the initiation of treatment is one of the most important predictors of prognosis [5]. Therefore, suggestion would be most appropriately used in the course of the initial neurological assessment, be it in the clinic or the emergency department. Once the diagnosis of a PMD is established by an experienced practitioner, this physician could present a suggestion, for example, "Whenever your symptom occurs, rub your elbow and this will alleviate the attack." He or she could also apply a tuning fork to the affected body part, or administer a placebo medication.

Therapeutic suggestion must be undertaken with recognition of its limitations. It may not always work, nor are its effects guaranteed to last indefinitely. Moreover, the underlying psychopathology associated with a patient's PMD will not be healed by suggestion: psychotherapy, physical therapy, and medications may be required. Because any patient may respond to suggestion, it cannot be relied upon as a specific diagnostic test for psychogenic disorders. For example, patients with idiopathic Parkinson's disease are known to demonstrate a robust placebo response [6]. Furthermore, declaring to patients that they will or they may receive a placebo often negates the intervention's effects, because most people understand placebos as inert substances. In our modern conception, suggestion induces an active therapy within a psychosocial context [7].

Psychogenic Movement Disorders and Other Conversion Disorders, ed. Mark Hallett, Anthony E. Lang, Joseph Jankovic, Stanley Fahn, Peter W. Halligan, Valerie Voon, and C. Robert Cloninger. Published by Cambridge University Press. © Cambridge University Press 2011.

Philosophy, physiology, and pathology

The exact nature of PMDs remains controversial. This is reflected in the variety of terms we use to identify them: hysteria, conversion, functional, inorganic, atypical, fake. By definition, these patients' symptoms do not fit the patterns and parameters that the medical profession has developed to define discrete illnesses. Yet we believe that these patients are not lying and that their symptoms are real. If we agree that PMDs are not consciously feigned, then they must arise from the organ that causes movement disorders, namely the brain. Simply put, they are incompletely understood brain diseases, not that different from most conditions neurologists treat.

What makes PMDs unique is their association with psychiatric pathology. Elucidating the relationship between brain and mind remains one of humanity's greatest challenges. Dualism, the notion that the mind and brain are completely separate, still has its champions in medicine. However, the profession appears to be moving closer to a general acceptance of a specific set of philosophical positions: that the mind is a product of the body, and that the mind can also act on the body. One strong proponent of this perspective is the philosopher John Searle, who explains that "all mental phenomena whether conscious or unconscious, visual or auditory, pains, tickles, itches, thoughts, indeed all of our mental life, are caused by processes going on in the brain." He goes on to clarify that "the mind and the body interact, but they are not two different things, since mental phenomena just are features of the brain" [8].

Many experts conceptualize PMDs as the unconscious conversion of psychopathology into neurological symptoms. We can explain this process as the translation of a cognitive state (fear, grief, worry) into a physical state (tremor, dystonia, weakness). The PMDs likely represent one tip of a spectrum of conditions in which patients "think with the body," turning psychic stresses into physical disease [9]. Irritable bowel syndrome, chronic fatigue syndrome, and fibromyalgia may all be related to PMDs. One could posit the formation of a pathological connection between the brain regions integral to cognitive and emotional functioning and other symptom-producing functional units. In this way, suggestion and psychogenic illness are two edges of the same sword: they both arise from the representation of a mental state as an altered physical experience. Indeed, Diederich and Goetz [6] conceptualized the power of suggestion as a "top-down" dissemination of expectation and reward onto other neurological systems, recalling our description of the pathology of psychogenic disease.

Imaging studies of suggestion and psychogenic disorders point to a common anatomical substrate: the dorsolateral prefrontal cortex and anterior cingulate gyrus. Both placebo and hypnosis have been shown to activate these areas [10]. The consistent involvement of these regions across various "meaning responses" illustrates the mechanistic similarity of the various forms of suggestion. Interestingly, so-called "active" medications such as the selective serotonin reuptake inhibitors and opioid analgesics have also been shown to stimulate these regions. The reverse of the placebo effect is called the "nocebo effect," in which disease states are induced through negative suggestion: this phenomenon has been explained as the dissemination of a heightened anxiety state, mirroring our conception of psychogenic disease. Not surprisingly, the nocebo effect has also been linked to the anterior cingulate and dorsolateral prefrontal cortices [7]. Based on their study of patients with psychogenic hemianesthesia, Ghaffar et al. [11] have proposed that hyperactivity in the dorsolateral prefrontal cortex and anterior cingulate gyrus can initiate hypoactivity in other cortical regions, thereby producing psychogenic symptoms. Furthermore, the effects of suggestion (both positive and negative) have been shown to impact motor, mood, endocrinological, and immunological systems. For example, placebo has been shown to induce clinical improvements as well as changes in dopaminergic transmission, as documented by positron emission tomography, in patients with Parkinson's disease [7].

The idea that PMDs and suggestion should share an underlying mechanism or anatomical substrate is not new: Charcot and Freud described psychogenic disease states as a form of autosuggestion [12]. More recent theories use the term "autohypnosis" to explain the pathological dissociation, or self-fragmentation, at the root of psychogenic disease. Charcot also popularized the notion, which remains widely held, that patients afflicted with psychogenic diseases are particularly sensitive to suggestion [13]. Therefore, a century-old conceptualization of the mind–body connection, as well as cutting edge neuroscience, link PMDs with suggestion. Information from history, philosophy, and physiology argues that suggestion could be an effective treatment for PMDs, and the evidence agrees.

The evidence for suggestion

The efficacy of a treatment is key to its ethical justification. Multiple forms of data, including anecdote, expert opinion, RCTs, and meta-analysis, support the treatment of PMDs with suggestion. Here we encounter a paradox: although suggestion is widely criticized, many physicians continue to use it and to study it. Medical ethics is largely concerned with establishing the standards by which we practice, and that standard clearly includes suggestion.

Anecdote is often considered the weakest form of medical evidence, but it can be a "compelling, convenient and efficient vehicle for conveying information and modifying behavior" [14]. Anecdote distills the doctor–patient experience into a concise narrative, focusing on the human story at its foundation. Tales of the healing powers of senior neurologists are passed on by the residents and students who follow them; one particularly good example comes from McGill University in Montréal, Canada. A middle-aged woman, diagnosed years before with a psychogenic tremor affecting the right hand, presented with a renewed tremor. The neurologist asked her whether she had continued to clench her fist around her thumb whenever her symptoms arose; this was the suggestion he had originally offered her, with great success. She nodded vociferously and showed him how she had attempted to abort her periodic tremor. The neurologist immediately noted that she was enclosing her fingers with the thumb on the outside. "Ah ha!" he exclaimed. Once she began to close her fingers around her thumb and not underneath it, her symptoms remitted again.

Many years of such patient encounters form the basis of expert opinion. In a variety of texts, neurologists and psychiatrists describe the use of suggestion in the management of psychogenic illness. One eminent neurologist states that suggestion is, and should be, used in diagnosis and treatment [15]. Another advocates the strategic application of tuning forks to relieve symptoms [16]. A psychiatrist describes how "patients can be taught the procedure and can use the technique to occasionally resolve or more frequently modulate their disorder" [13]. An informal survey of audience members at the *Psychogenic Movement Disorders Conference* from which this book is derived found that well over 50% of participants had witnessed the efficacy of suggestion in treating PMDs.

As a bridge to the discussion of RCTs and meta-analyses in this arena, another expert deserves citation.

Dr. A. L. Cochrane, the British physician whose work in epidemiology and public policy laid the foundation for the rise of evidence-based medicine, supported the use of placebo. In his 1972 monograph *Effectiveness and Efficiency*, Dr. Cochrane wrote (p. 31): "The effect of placebos has been shown by RCTs to be very large. Their use in the correct place is to be encouraged. What is inefficient is the use of relatively expensive drugs as placebos. It is a pity some enterprising drug company does not produce a wide range of cheap, brightly colored, non-toxic placebos" [17]. Today we recognize that placebos represent only one aspect of the "meaning response," and we appreciate the influence of individual, cultural, and situational factors [18]. Since Dr. Henry K. Beecher coined the term "placebo" in 1955, many RCTs have employed placebo arms, and patients in these placebo arms have consistently improved. To review all these studies is beyond the scope of this chapter.

A recent meta-analysis reviewed 21 RCTs in which hypnosis was compared with no treatment for a variety of psychosomatic illnesses including PMDs. Overall, 65% of patients who received hypnosis improved, while 36% of patients improved without intervention [19]. Multiple hypnotic strategies were used, with symptom-oriented suggestions being the most common. No correlation was found between the number of sessions and the outcome, indicating that suggestion in the form of hypnosis is effective in the management of psychogenic illness, even when applied temporarily and when focused on the symptomatic manifestations of patients' underlying neuropsychopathology. This is exactly the intervention we have been discussing all along.

Understanding autonomy

Why would an effective treatment be considered unethical? Contemporary medical students are taught the principalist approach to ethics, which frames all debate in terms of four key concepts: autonomy, beneficence, non-maleficence, and justice. Principalism evolved from the merger of two traditional schools of ethical thought (namely, consequentialism and deontology) to become the dominant ideology of medical ethics in our time. For most principalists, respecting patient autonomy is the core rule of medical practice. To do anything else is to be "paternalistic," supposedly recalling an era in which doctors made decisions for their patients, or even against their patients' wills. The main argument against suggestion comes from principalists who contend that its use would contradict the principle of autonomy by employing deception and by impairing informed consent. Critics contend that this would degrade the doctor–patient relationship [1].

However, principalism is not the only lens through which to view medical ethics. A new approach entitled "asymmetric paternalism" advocates protecting patients who are prone to irrational decisions from their own poor choices in matters of health [20]. Another important perspective is the ethics of care, also called feminist or maternal ethics. This paradigm, developed by Carol Gilligan and Susan Sherwin among others, emphasizes "feminine" values such as caring, relationships, and community over so-called "masculine" values such as autonomy, independence, and separation. Particularity and partiality are favored over universality and objectivity [21].

A strong argument can be made that the feminist emphasis on caring most closely resembles the basic philosophy of medicine, and as such my arguments are allied with this school of thought. I take issue with the primacy of autonomy in medical ethics, not because patient autonomy is bad, but because the goal of medicine is to care for patients, not to enhance their autonomy. Because autonomy can be defined as the ability of an individual to live his or her life to the fullest extent that he or she desires, the treatment of disease necessarily increases autonomy. However, this occurs as an indirect consequence of, rather than as the primary goal of, medical care. Using suggestion to help patients afflicted with PMDs would, therefore, enhance patient autonomy.

The concept of patient autonomy is often used to refer to respect for patients' choices. In his textbook *Doing Right*, bioethicist Dr. Phil Hébert lists three questions that should be asked when considering an ethical conundrum. The first and foremost of these is "What does the patient want?" [2]. By seeking medical attention, patients desire care and maybe even cure; by providing them with our best efforts to reach said cure, I would argue that we are respecting their autonomy. Moreover, physicians are not obliged to follow patient requests regardless of their medical validity. A patient experiencing chest pain as part of a panic attack would not, and should not, be granted a coronary artery bypass no matter how much he or she demands it. Patients' wishes are not their doctors' absolute directives.

Some authors hold that suggestion diminishes autonomy because it is deceitful to patients [1].

Deception is the act of making someone believe something that is not true. If a physician suggests to a patient that doing X may cure Y, and the suggestion does indeed relieve the symptom, then the patient was not deceived. That the therapeutic power of the intervention comes from the patient's interpretation of it, rather than from the intervention itself, makes the result no less real and no less truthful. As Dr. Peter Lichtenberg [22] has described (p. 551), the physician is simply engaging the mind–body continuum from a different direction than usual.

> In the case of the placebo, this effect transpires in a top down direction, from a level of greater to lesser complexity, from the level of the person to that of the organ system, organ or cell. In contrast, a medical treatment works in a bottom up direction, from lesser to greater complexity – for example, when the manipulation of a neurotransmitter system affects cognitive function or the person's wellbeing.

Many physicians believe that patients with psychogenic disease are "fakers" and that suggestion is a means of "tricking" them out of their lies. From this viewpoint, suggestion would certainly be deceptive. But accepting the modern theory of psychogenic disease (that it arises from unconscious processes and is associated with pathological changes in brain function) and of suggestion (that it can induce beneficial changes in brain function) defeats this objection. The treatment works to relieve the disease by engaging the fundamental interaction of body and mind, which is the cause of the disease.

The idea of consent is another important concept related to patient autonomy. Dr. Hébert explains that patients have the right to receive medical information and to refuse medical treatment. He argues that we should respect their autonomy as rational actors, free to make choices based on informed consent [2]. Dr. Hébert would hold that suggestion violates informed consent because the therapeutic act is conducted without first gaining the patient's permission. However, I contend that suggestion does not violate informed consent. Suggestion in the form of persuasion, on the one hand, evolves organically from the doctor–patient relationship; physicians cannot be expected to ask their patients' permission to be charismatic, compassionate, or convincing. By visiting their doctors in the first place, patients have implicitly accepted the healing powers of this relationship. On the other hand, suggestion in the form of hypnosis cannot occur without explicit patient approval. As practitioners of hypnosis explain, no post-hypnotic suggestion can be accepted by a patient unless he or she wants to follow the terms of that suggestion.

Complete disclosure from doctor to patient is often described as a prerequisite for informed consent. When patients question their physicians about the mechanism of action of suggestion, their doctors should answer honestly and confidently: "this treatment works through various networks in the brain, the particulars of which no one fully understands." This explanation can only be termed incomplete by those who disbelieve the physiological basis of suggestion. Patients rarely appreciate the molecular mechanisms of their treatments, and we do not consider this to be non-disclosure. However, some patient may be unwilling or unable to accept the neuropsychiatric etiology of their symptoms, particularly at the time of initial assessment. If the physician feels that full disclosure may harm the doctor–patient relationship, then he or she may elect for graduated disclosure: first name the symptom (tremor, dystonia, etc.) without divulging its etiology, then later address the underlying psychopathology. Although many ethicists recognize graduated consent as a valid approach to patient education, some critics may object to its use in the context of suggestion.

However, informed consent is not an absolute. Medicine has become so complex in recent years that even a physician with expertise in one discipline will not comprehend the nuances of clinical decisions in another. As the hematologist and philosopher Alfred Tauber explains, the notion of autonomous consent is "a conceit. Patients cannot fully exercise autonomy simply for the reason that they lack the training and knowledge to make the complex decisions required today in the setting of a highly technical and obscure science" [23]. Patients should not be consciously excluded from the decision-making process, but the explicit goal of medicine is not to have patients decide, rather it is to provide care to those patients. When a patient's well-being is dependent upon a procedure whose success may require graduated disclosure, I contend that this is a valid trade-off.

The doctor–patient relationship

Rejecting the false notions of absolute consent and the perfectly autonomous patient reveals the true nature of the doctor–patient relationship. Principalist medical ethics is dominated by the language of contract, which imagines the doctor–patient encounter as a meeting of equal and autonomous parties. Trust must be imposed externally on these independent agents because each is considered to be acting in his or her own best interest. Principalists would argue that anything less than complete disclosure violates that trust [1]. In contrast, feminist ethicists imagine the parent–child dynamic as a model for the doctor–patient relationship: trust develops between doctor and patient because the patient knows that the doctor is acting with the patient's best interests at heart. Providing treatment to a patient afflicted by a PMD, with suggestion or with any other effective technique, fulfills our obligation to care and thereby validates our patients' trust. When physicians are awoken in the middle of the night to answer the cries of their patients, are they driven by a sense of contractual obligation? Residents cite the "mother test" as a guide to clinical practice: "If that patient were my mother, what would I want the resident on call to do?" There is a familial bond between doctors and their patients that exemplifies the best of human society.

Some critics of suggestion worry that its use would endanger not just the trust between one doctor and one patient, but between all doctors and all patients [1]. If patients were to find out that doctors were using suggestion, they might be less likely to seek medical attention, to be open and forthcoming with personal information, or to follow physicians' treatment plans. This argument assumes that patients would find out about the use of suggestion and would be upset at its use, neither of which is guaranteed. Offering a successful therapy is extremely beneficial in establishing a therapeutic alliance between doctor and patient. Moreover, this critique presumes that physicians' responsibilities to future patients and to society at large supersede their responsibilities to the patient in the examining room. The physician's over-arching moral imperative is to treat that patient: the very language that describes the patient encounter, "Mr. X *presents* with…," grounds the relationship firmly in the here and now. There is little justification to deny treatment to a suffering patient in the present because of the effect such therapy may have on hypothetical, future patients.

Conclusions

The Greek word for suffering, *pathos*, is at the root of our word, the *patient*. In this chapter, I have advocated the use of suggestion in the treatment of patients afflicted with PMDs. In the age of evidence-based medicine, physicians are expected to cite reasons for their clinical decisions. Randomized controlled trials are excellent sources of information with which to construct a rationale; so too are history, theory, anecdote, and opinion. Data from all these areas coalesce to form a convincing argument in favor of the use of suggestion. Perhaps most importantly, our modern understanding of the pathophysiology of PMDs mirrors our conception of the therapeutic effect of suggestion. The traditional ethical objections to its use, namely that suggestion erodes patient autonomy and the doctor–patient relationship, fall away when each is examined thoroughly and from the perspective of an ethics of care.

Two broader concepts underlie these arguments and the first of these concerns how doctors think. Argumentation is the basis for moral as well as for medical reasoning. Evidence is used to support argument; it can never replace argument. Therefore, mastering clinical evidence is useless without understanding its meaning. And meaning is specific to every patient and to every clinical situation. Hence the importance of narrative.

The second concept integral to this discussion concerns the ethical structure through which we analyze our clinical decisions. As the psychiatrist Dr. Tony Hope wrote [24] (p. 2), "Much emphasis during my training was put on the importance of using scientific evidence in clinical decision-making. Little thought was given to justifying, or even noticing, the ethical assumptions that lay behind the decisions." Modern interpretations of the four pillars of bioethics may inadvertently encourage a formulaic approach to resolving ethical conflicts. Contemporary principalism has focused our attention on patient autonomy, while losing sight of the caring nature of the doctor–patient relationship. To reveal the truth of what we do and why we do it, and to challenge our principles and our practices, is at the heart of the study of medical ethics and is key to the practice of ethical medicine.

Acknowledgements

A version of this chapter appeared under the title "The Treatment of Psychogenic Movement Disorders with Suggestion is Ethically Justified' in the journal *Movement* Disorders (2010;**25**:260–264). I would like to recognize Drs. Ross Upshur, Mark Fedyk, and Anthony E. Lang for their assistance and guidance in the revision of this document. I would like to thank the Royal College of Physicians and Surgeons of Canada for their financial support through the 2008 K. J. R. Wightman Award for Resident Scholarship in Ethics.

References

1. Bok S. Ethical issues in the use of placebo in medical practice and clinical trials. In Guess HA, Kleinman A, Kusek JW, Engel LW, eds. *The Science of Placebo*. London: BMJ Books, 2002:54–74.

2. Hébert PC. *Doing Right: A Practical Guide to Ethics for Medical Trainees and Physicians*. Oxford: Oxford University Press, 1995.

3. Sherman R, Hickner J. Academic physicians use placebos in clinical practice and believe in the mind-body connection. *J Gen Int Med* 2008;**23**:7–10.

4. Moerman D. The meaning response and the ethics of avoiding placebos. *Eval Health Prof* 2002;**25**:399–409.

5. Lang AE. General overview of psychogenic movement disorders: epidemiology, diagnosis, and prognosis. In Hallett M, Fahn S, Jankovic J, *et al.*, eds. *Psychogenic Movement Disorders: Neurology and Neuropsychiatry*. Philadelphia, PA: Lippincott Williams & Wilkins, 2006:35–41.

6. Diederich NJ, Goetz CG. The placebo treatments in neurosciences: New insights from clinical and neuroimaging studies. *Neurology* 2008;**71**:677–684.

7. Benedetti F. *Placebo Effects: Understanding the Mechanisms in Health and Disease*. Oxford: Oxford University Press, 2009.

8. Searle J. *Minds, Brains and Science*. Cambridge, MI: Harvard University Press, 1984.

9. Ovsiew F. An overview of the psychiatric approach to conversion disorder. In Hallett M, Fahn S, Jankovic J, *et al.*, eds. *Psychogenic Movement Disorders: Neurology and Neuropsychiatry*. Philadelphia, PA: Lippincott Williams & Wilkins, 2006:115–121.

10. Benedetti F, Mayberg H, Wager TD, Stohler CS, Zubieta J-K. Neurobiological mechanisms of the placebo effect. *J Neurosci* 2005;**25**;45:10390–10402.

11. Ghaffar O, Staines WR, Feinstein A. Unexplained neurologic symptoms: an fMRI study of sensory conversion disorder. *Neurology* 2006;**67**:2036–2038.

12. Tomlinson WC. Freud and psychogenic movement disorders. In Hallett M, Fahn S, Jankovic J, *et al.*, eds. *Psychogenic Movement Disorders: Neurology and Neuropsychiatry*. Philadelphia, PA: Lippincott Williams & Wilkins, 2006:14–19.

13. Barry JJ. Hypnosis and psychogenic movement disorders. In Hallett M, Fahn S, Jankovic J, *et al.*, eds. *Psychogenic Movement Disorders: Neurology and Neuropsychiatry*. Philadelphia, PA: Lippincott Williams & Wilkins, 2006:241–248.

14. Enkin WM, Jadad AR. Using anecdotal information in evidence-based health care: Heresy or necessity? *Ann Oncol* 1998;**9**:963–966.

15. Fahn S. The history of psychogenic movement disorders. In Hallett M, Fahn S, Jankovic J, *et al.*, eds. *Psychogenic Movement Disorders: Neurology and Neuropsychiatry*. Philadelphia, PA: Lippincott Williams & Wilkins, 2006:24–32.

16. Jankovic J, Cloninger CR, Fahn S, *et al.* Therapeutic approaches to psychogenic movement disorders. In Hallett M, Fahn S, Jankovic J, *et al.*, eds. *Psychogenic Movement Disorders: Neurology and Neuropsychiatry*. Philadelphia, PA: Lippincott Williams & Wilkins, 2006:323–328.

17. Cochrane AL. *Effectiveness and Efficiency: Random Reflections on Health Services*. London: Nuffield Provincial Hospitals Trust, 1972.

18. Kleinman A, Guess HA, Wilentz JS. An overview. In Guess HA, Kleinman A, Kusek JW, Engel LW, eds. *The Science of Placebo*. London: BMJ Books, 2002:1–32.

19. Flammer E, Alladin A. The efficacy of hypnotherapy in the treatment of psychosomatic disorders: meta-analytical evidence. *Int J Clin Exp Hyp* 2007;**55**:251–274.

20. Loewenstein G. Asymmetric paternalism to improve health behaviors. *JAMA* 2007;**298**:2415–2417.

21. Tong R, Williams N. Feminist ethics. In Zalta EN, ed. *The Stanford Encyclopedia of Philosophy*. Stanford, CA: Center for the Study of Language and Information, Stanford University, 2006, http://plato.stanford.edu/archives/spr2008/entries/feminism-ethics (accessed 12 May 2011).

22. Lichtenberg P, Heresco-Levy U, Nitzan U. The ethics of the placebo in clinical practice. *J Med Ethics* 2004;**30**:551–554.

23. Tauber AI. *Confessions of a Medicine Man: An Essay in Popular Philosophy*. Cambridge, MI: MIT Press, 1999.

24. Hope T. *Medical Ethics: A Very Short Introduction*. Oxford: Oxford University Press, 2004.

Inpatient therapy: trying to transcend pathological dissociation, dependence, and disability

Daniel T. Williams, Nika Dyakina, Prudence Fisher,
Joseph Graber, and Stanley Fahn

Introduction

In recent years, there has been a growing understanding of the neuroanatomical and neurophysiological correlates of psychogenic movement disorders (PMDs) and related neuropsychiatric conditions [1– 4]. One way of understanding the implications of these studies is that they support the role of "dissociative mechanisms" in generating conversion symptoms; that is, symptoms mediated by voluntary musculature may nevertheless occur without conscious awareness of the patient. This development has coincided with an ongoing struggle to reformulate psychiatric diagnostic criteria for the relevant psychiatric categories to conceptualize these disorders for purposes of psychiatric intervention [5,6]. There has been growing interest in defining and refining the clinical practices generally used in diagnosing and managing this group of patients [7– 9]. Yet, despite these areas of progress, pessimism persists in the PMD literature regarding the prognosis for patients with these disorders, together with a paucity of systematic studies of treatment interventions [10–14].

Does some of the prevailing pessimism regarding the prognosis for these disorders derive from the triage effect, in that the most difficult and treatment-resistant cases tending to come to the tertiary care centers from which these pessimistic clinical impressions emerge? That question needs to be considered in the context of the wide variety of treatment strategies employed in different settings and the difficulty, therefore, of generating conclusions about treatment results.

In the broader domain of somatoform disorders not restricted to PMDs, the literature is more sanguine. Kroenke reviewed 34 randomized clinical trials of somatoform disorders, involving 3922 patients and a number of different treatment modalities [15]. In this review, cognitive behavioral therapy manifested convincing evidence of efficacy, proving beneficial for at least one treatment outcome in 11 of 13 trials. Four of five trials evaluating antidepressants versus placebo were positive. Three of four trials examining the impact of the mental health practitioner simply providing a psychiatric consultation letter to the primary care physician were positive in terms of improved functional status in the patients. Only 2 of the 34 trials involved inpatient treatment; one was positive and the other negative in outcome. The majority of these 34 studies evaluated a single treatment intervention in comparison with usual care, a wait list, or a placebo control group.

Why consider inpatient treatment for patients with psychogenic movement disorders?

As reflected in the above review, most patients with PMD and other somatoform disorders are directed to an outpatient setting for psychiatric evaluation and treatment once the presumptive diagnosis of a PMD or other conversion disorder has been made by the neurologist or primary care physician. This, indeed, is favored by the current "managed care model" in the USA that seeks to minimize time in hospital. However, the diagnosis of a somatoform disorder may be first entertained when the patient is admitted to an inpatient medical service for evaluation and treatment of undiagnosed, disabling symptoms. Prompt discharge without adequate diagnostic clarification for the patient and family, and without establishment of an acceptable, coordinated treatment plan, can be counterproductive. The patient may feel dismissed by an inadequately understood or a flippantly conveyed psychiatric referral, with consequent resistance to appropriate treatment and the prolongation of the course of illness.

There are also times when a consulting neurologist may appropriately conclude, at either initial hospital consultation or initial office visit, that while a PMD is indeed the most likely diagnosis, the patient is unlikely to accept this diagnosis and the associated recommended treatment without a more intensive, integrated evaluation, which can more effectively be done in an inpatient setting. Many such patients, when simply given a referral to a psychiatrist, never proceed to make an initial appointment. It has been the impression of our movement disorder group at Columbia University Medical Center (CUMC) that an inpatient admission for selected patients has enabled us to afford a transformative therapeutic opportunity to some of them, who, by reasons of geography or other limitations of access or receptivity to integrated diagnosis and treatment, would not otherwise have achieved symptomatic remission. Using a "multidisciplinary diagnostic and treatment approach," such patients have been seen intensively in hospital by the admitting neurologist, the consulting psychiatrist, and a physical therapist, together with supportive nursing care. Such hospitalization serves several functions. It removes the patient from environmental influences that were contributory to symptom formation and perpetuation, while also allowing the patient to be evaluated more thoroughly in a supportive environment. Further, bringing in the psychiatrist as a routine member of the evaluation and treatment team makes it difficult for the patient to decline this intervention and allows for the development of a therapeutic alliance while multiple diagnostic and treatment strategies are ongoing, assuring the patient that no organic factors are overlooked.

A few days into the admission, with our diagnostic impressions further clarified, we arrange a conjoint debriefing session with the patient, neurologist, and psychiatrist (as well as the physical therapist when feasible), to supportively present to the patient (and sometimes also an authorized family member) our diagnostic impressions and treatment recommendations. If neurological workup was negative and disclosed a substantial somatoform component, this is supportively reviewed, together with a more favorable prognosis for recovery than would apply with a degenerative neurological

disorder. We explain that stress of various types can contribute to physiological perturbations that generate clear physical symptoms outside the patient's awareness and despite the absence of discernible structural lesions on the available diagnostic tests. Citing commonly encountered clinical examples of how stress can activate the symptoms of hypertension, peptic ulcer disease, and asthma (also via mechanisms frequently outside the patient's awareness) facilitates patient recognition of the plausibility and relevance of this conceptual model. A treatment plan is then outlined, tailored to the needs of the individual patient. This treatment plan, generally including psychotherapy, pharmacotherapy, and physical therapy, is started in the hospital in an effort to achieve as much symptomatic improvement as possible before discharge, with the intention of it continuing on an outpatient basis as needed. A follow-up appointment is recommended with both the neurologist and the psychiatrist, to assure the patient and family that both domains are being monitored in an effort to achieve optimal symptom resolution.

While there are substantial expenditures and associated insurance hurdles to be confronted regarding hospital-based intervention, for those patients who are not otherwise effectively engaged in treatment, the cost of chronic care for years of unremitted somatoform disorder far outweigh the cost of a hospital admission for 1 to 2 weeks, which in our experience is sometimes dramatically transformative in "jump-starting treatment" for these patients.

Follow-up study of patients treated on an inpatient neurology service

In an effort to retrospectively evaluate our inpatient treatment experience with patients with PMD, a follow-up study (approved by the institutional review board) was conducted in which we attempted to contact all such patients who had been treated by our movement disorder group at CUMC over the previous 10 years, as well as all patients who had come to us for consultation and treatment after inpatient neurological evaluation and treatment at other medical centers. The neurological evaluation and treatment at our medical center was done by one of six attending movement disorder neurologists together with an assigned movement disorder fellow. The psychiatric evaluation and treatment for all patients in the study was done by a senior attending psychiatrist (DTW) working consultatively with the movement disorder group, assisted by a psychiatry fellow on the consultation-liaison service. The format of inpatient consultation at CUMC was as outlined above, with duration of inpatient stay for the majority ranging from 5 to 14 days. Further details on the collaborative diagnostic and treatment program, involving neurology, psychiatry, and physical therapy services, are available [16,17].

Methods

Patients were contacted by mail, soliciting their participation in the study, explaining its purpose and indicating that the follow-up interview could be done either by telephone or in person at CUMC, with the interviews conducted by an independent psychiatrist (ND), utilizing a semi-structured questionnaire. The patients were offered a nominal cash honorarium for their participation. One parent of adolescent patients was interviewed either instead of or in addition to the adolescent patient, at the parent's and adolescent's discretion. A chart review of participating patients was conducted by the inpatient treating psychiatrist, using an extraction form to delineate demographic characteristics, symptom histories, neurological and psychiatric diagnoses, modalities of treatment used, and responses to treatment, particularly the extent of symptomatic improvement during the hospital stay. The follow-up questionnaire by the independent evaluating psychiatrist similarly evaluated the degree of symptomatic improvement as well as the level of functioning at follow-up, the extent of intervening treatment, intervening life events, and patient judgments about the quality and impact of the treatment experience. Primary outcome variables of interest were degrees of symptomatic improvement at the end of inpatient treatment and at follow-up. Additional variables of interest were the quality of life as perceived by the patients at follow-up, the level of functioning (work, school, or homecare) of the patients at follow-up, the level of "insight" achieved regarding the role of stress and psychological factors contributing to their physical symptoms, as well as their views on the roles of the various treatment components in influencing their response to treatment.

Demographics

We succeeded in contacting and interviewing 28 patients, representing 33% of the total number of 83 patients seen who met the study's inclusion criteria. Of these, 14 were hospitalized at CUMC and 14 at other hospitals. The 14 treated at other hospitals were seen by our group and treated exclusively as outpatients with the same general approach of multimodal collaborative treatment as provided in follow-up to patients hospitalized at CUMC. Namely, follow-up treatment involved primarily psychiatric intervention, with neurological and physical therapy ancillary support as needed. The mean length of stay of CUMC patients in hospital was 9.4 days (range, 3–19); the mean length of stay of other hospitalized patients was 7.7 days (range, 2–24). There was a predominance of females (20 of 28). The mean age of the total sample was 38.1 years (SD, 19.1); the age range was from 11 to 72 years. Marital status included 8 single, 18 married, and 2 divorced/separated. Religious backgrounds included 10 Catholic, 8 Protestant, and 10 Jewish.

Results

Neurological features on initial hospital evaluation

Presenting neurological symptoms on admission (some patients had more than one) included balance and gait problems (16), tremor (14), seizures (13), tics (6), and dystonia (5). (None of our study patients was recruited from the Comprehensive Epilepsy Center at CUMC, so seizures in this group were either a secondary symptom or epilepsy had already been ruled out at time of referral to us.) Most of the study patients had at least one hospitalization for PMD symptoms prior to the index admission that brought them to our treatment team, with a range of prior admissions: 5 with none, 12 with one prior admission, 9 with two or three prior admissions, and 2 with four prior admissions. The duration of PMD symptoms in our study patients prior to establishment of a PMD diagnosis involved a mean of 3.1 years (SD, 3.8), with a range of 1 month to 13 years. After initial neurological evaluation by our movement disorder neurologists, the level of confidence regarding the PMD diagnosis [18] was probable for 3, clinically established for 12, and documented for 13.

Psychiatric features on initial hospital evaluation

Psychiatric diagnosis was established for patients admitted to our CUMC inpatient service based on unstructured but detailed psychiatric interview of roughly 7 hours in duration during the first 5 days of admission. Outpatients coming to us from other hospitals, who were not admitted, were seen for an initial 90-minute diagnostic interview, with recommendation for weekly follow-up for at least 4 weeks or until a clear diagnosis and stable treatment plan could be established. Based on this assessment, the following psychiatric diagnoses were delineated (DSM-IV-TR) [19].

Axis I (primary psychiatric diagnosis):

   A. Somatizing diagnoses: 26 with somatoform disorder, 2 with factitious disorder, and 0 with malingering.

   B. Comorbid diagnoses: 10 with depressive disorders, 9 with anxiety disorders, 4 with alcohol and substance abuse, 3 with psychological factors affecting a medical condition, and 3 with post-traumatic stress disorder.

Axis II (personality disorders):

   Cluster A (schizoid): None

   Cluster B (unstable, externalizing): 12 ([subtypes were: 8 histrionic, 2 borderline, and 2 narcissistic)

   Cluster C (internalizing): 4 dependent

   Not Otherwise Specified (mixed): 5.

Axis III (coexisting medical conditions): the vast majority of patients reported coexisting medical conditions, most of which were not independently evaluated by us. These were sufficiently numerous and diverse as to not warrant categorization here.

Axis IV (psychosocial stressors): all patients in the study were able in the course of extended evaluation to define significant stressors that were interpreted as relevant to the development of their PMD symptoms. In terms of proximate stressors that were seen as "triggering" the PMD symptoms, these were perceived as both physical (primary) and psychological (secondary) in 13 patients, and as primarily psychological in 15 patients. In terms of remote or proximate stressors involving histories of abuse, these were categorized as follows: 7 child abuse only, 3 child or adult physical abuse, 5 child or adult sexual abuse, and 6 child or adult emotional abuse.

Axis V (global assessment of function): this describes relative psychiatric impairment on a scale of 100 (fully functional) to 0 (totally incapacitated and requiring constant attendance/supervision). These scores ranged from 40 to 85 at the time of initial consultation with our group, with the vast majority (20) having scores between 55 and 65, which describes a range of moderately severe functional impairments.

Because of the attention generally given to the potential role of secondary gain factors as frequently contributing to somatoform symptoms, we evaluated the presence of postulated secondary gains based on the extended psychiatric evaluation, covering the patient's personal, social, educational, family, and work histories. The postulated secondary gain factors included avoiding school (for children and adolescents) (5), avoiding work (6), financial compensation (4), escaping abuse (1), and expressing indirect protest regarding a family problem (12).

Treatment during inpatient admission

In addition to the general treatment parameters described above, the following treatment characteristics bear mention. The patients were seen daily by the movement disorder fellow and attending neurologist, who performed regular neurological examinations, while reinforcing our consensus diagnostic formulation and encouraging each patient to cooperate and participate fully in all aspects of the treatment program, including the psychotherapy, pharmacotherapy, and physical therapy. This neurological validation of what the treatment team saw as the essential ingredients in the treatment seemed valuable in gaining patient acceptance. Physical therapy took place Monday through Friday, with a specifically formulated intervention geared to the patients' specific symptoms.

Psychiatric treatment took place Monday through Friday, with sessions of 60 to 90 minutes involving primarily individual therapy, but sometimes also conjoint family therapy, in an individually tailored format, as described elsewhere [17]. Psychotropic medication was used in all patients, again individualized and most commonly targeted to coexisting anxiety or depression. The neurologist was important in validating this recommendation, generally at the time of the conjoint diagnostic debriefing. The metaphor of "reprogramming software malfunctions in the brain" once we had established that there was "no structural hardware malfunction" seemed helpful to many patients. The rationale for the medication was explained supportively not only in terms of anti-anxiety and antidepressant effects, but also in terms of the effects on central nervous system neurotransmitters that influence both motion and emotion in subtle and complex ways. It is recognized that this strategy includes both specific psychotropic medication effects and non-specific effects of optimism-engendering suggestion, as is the case in all use of such agents.

Global improvement at time of discharge from index hospitalization

Global assessment of improvement was based on a composite assessment of both PMD symptoms and associated psychiatric symptoms as evaluated by both the treating neurologist and the treating psychiatrist at the time of hospital discharge. Ratings based on the chart review included symptoms totally resolved, markedly improved, moderately improved, mildly improved, unchanged, mildly worse, moderately worse, or markedly worse. Global assessment of clinical status at time of hospital discharge included unchanged in 2 (7%), mildly improved in 18 (65%), moderately improved in 4 (18%), and markedly improved in 4 (14%). It should be recalled that 50% of our sample came to us after prior hospitalization elsewhere, so that these patients' status at time of the most recent hospital discharge, based on review of the referring records and our own initial assessment, would be expected to be less than optimal.

Follow-up patient characteristics

There was a variable duration of time after the index hospitalization to follow-up interview for our patients, and substantial variability regarding the extent to which patients followed recommendations for follow-up treatment after leaving the hospital. The mean duration of time since hospital discharge to follow-up in our study was 3.9 years (SD, 3.2), with a range of 6 months to 10 years.

Follow-up treatment characteristics

In this study, 23 of the 28 patients had follow-up outpatient treatment with the senior attending psychiatrist in this study (DTW). The recommended format, when possible, was to start with weekly outpatient visits and then taper frequency with symptomatic improvement. Some patients whose symptoms remitted completely were able to discontinue psychiatric treatment (5), while some continued in formats ranging from monthly visits to visits every 6 months. The frequency of visits by time of follow-up for those with less than complete remission of symptoms was highly variable (from monthly to discontinued).

Global self-assessment of movement disorder symptom status at follow-up

Based on the follow-up interview by the independent evaluating psychiatrist using the above noted 8-point global assessment scale, patients' self-assessment of follow-up global status regarding the symptoms that had prompted the index hospitalization included presenting symptoms totally resolved in 10 (36%), markedly better in 7 (25%), moderately better in 4 (14%), mildly better in

0, unchanged in 2 (7%), slightly worse in 1 (4%), moderately worse in 2 (7%), and markedly worse in 1 (4%).

Level of function at follow-up

Patient self-report of level of function included full time employee, student, or homemaker in 15 (54%); part-time employee, student, or homemaker in 4 (14%); and disabled or collecting disability payments in 9 (32%).

Quality of life at follow-up

Based on the follow-up interview by the independent evaluating psychiatrist using a 7-point quality of life scale, patient self-assessment at follow-up included markedly improved in 15 (54%), moderately improved in 5 (18%), mildly improved in 2 (7%), no change in 1 (3.5%), slightly worse in 2 (7%), moderately worse in 2 (7%), and markedly worse in 1 (3.5%).

Patients' perceptions of inpatient treatment

The following were felt by the patients at follow-up to have been significant positive influences on their inpatient treatment during the index hospitalization: neurologist in 15 (54%), psychiatrist in 14 (50%), physical therapist in 8 (29%), nursing staff in 18 (64%), and medication in 5 (18%).

Patients' perceptions of outpatient follow-up treatment

The following were felt by the patients at follow-up to have been significant positive influences on their outpatient treatment following the index hospitalization: neurologist or primary care physician in 14 (50%), psychiatrist in 24 (86%), physical therapist in 4 (14%), medication in 19 (68%), other psychotherapist in 2 (7%), and hypnosis in 2 (7%). Other factors reported by patients to have been helpful included family therapy, family support, religious support, change of medication, volunteering to help others, Bible study, Alcoholics Anonymous, and patient resilience.

Discussion

There are many limitations inherent in our retrospective review of our treatment experience with patients with PMDs who had inpatient treatment. First, the small sample size is likely non-representative of the total sample, as patients who followed recommendations for follow-up treatment and those who responded more favorably to such treatment would seem to be more likely to respond to a letter soliciting their participation in a follow-up study. Second, the absence of a control group makes it difficult to know to what extent the improvement observed in our patients represented a specific response to treatment intervention. Third, since half of our sample consisted of patients treated at a variety of hospitals other than our own, with different treatment approaches that are clearly not standardized, it is difficult to equate them with our inpatients in terms of their response to inpatient treatment. What is of more interest, actually, is the response of the combined group to follow-up outpatient treatment, which clearly helped to consolidate and enhance clinical improvement of many of the patients who made partial gains during their hospital stay. We believe it was the intensive experience of organizing an integrated diagnostic and treatment plan based on a team approach that helped to bridge the divide inherent in the dissociative propensity of patients with somatoform disorders and that accounts for the relatively favorable subsequent treatment response of the majority of patients in our follow-up outpatient treatment.

As noted above, our group's inpatient treatment approach with multimodal intervention involves neurological and psychiatric assessment to supportively assure the patient of the diagnosis, followed by combined psychotherapy, pharmacotherapy, and physical therapy. This approach evolved based on empirical experience of many patients initially rejecting the diagnosis of PMD if it was simply presented by the consulting neurologist and associated with a referral to a psychiatrist, whom such patients often failed to contact. Admitting the patient for this multimodal treatment program seemed to substantially enhance the yield of positive responders to such intervention. The current follow-up study has a similar spectrum of clinical improvement as an earlier series that we reviewed [21], although our current study benefited from a structured follow-up interview by an independent rater. However, we cannot at this time confidently delineate which components of the multimodal treatment are most specifically helpful.

With so many patient variables to potentially evaluate in a relatively small sample size, it is difficult to define factors that predict outcome. It continues to be our impression, based on cumulative clinical experience, that the probability of a favorable response to treatment in PMD patients is influenced by a number of features:

- the establishment of a therapeutic rapport with the patient and family, based on a thorough initial assessment, thus reassuring the patient that all relevant neurological and psychological issues have been addressed

- the provision of a palatable neuropsychiatric conceptualization of stress-induced illness as the basis of the diagnosis and treatment of the medical condition; this requires an individual approach, based on the intellectual capacities as well as emotional and cultural predilections of the patient and family, and if conducted effectively safeguards the patient's self-esteem and provides hope for an acceptable route of recovery

- the severity and chronicity of contributory stressors as well as the nature and severity of patient and family psychopathology

- the nature of the patient's intrinsic recuperative capacities, motivation, and external support

- the effectiveness of the treatment plan formulation and the capacity for its sustained implementation.

Over time, particularly as hospital admissions have become more restricted by insurance limitations, the neurologists in our movement disorder group have modified the format of presentation of treatment options to the patient at the initial diagnostic consultation. A synthetic "neuropsychiatric" perspective is still utilized when the neurologist conveys the preliminary diagnosis of PMD in supportive terms, emphasizing the role of stress in contributing to many clearly physical disorders, often outside the patient's awareness. Our cumulative experience has suggested that some patients with PMD are indeed effectively treatable on an outpatient basis, as is reflected in the previous review of randomized controlled trials for somatoform disorders generally. The recommendation for psychiatric consultation with a psychiatrist experienced in treating these disorders is predicated by the neurologist on the premise that stress is playing a contributory role in the genesis of the symptoms. Many patients do accept this recommendation, with the understanding that the psychiatrist will share his diagnostic impressions and recommendations with the neurologist by way of a written report that will also be sent to the patient and the patient's primary care physician with patient authorization. Only if circumstances after this psychiatric consultation seem to warrant admission to the inpatient neurology service will arrangements for insurance clearance for inpatient admission be pursued.

Examples of considerations warranting admission under these circumstances include chronic, intractable PMD or other somatoform symptoms that have been resistant to adequate trials of outpatient psychiatric treatment, the patient's inability to absorb or accept a neuropsychiatric formulation as a basis for outpatient psychiatric treatment, or a pathological home or work environment that mandates treatment in a more structured and supportive setting. Our strong preference for admission to the neurology rather than the psychiatry service is based on the much greater acceptance of this setting by patients with PMD; the greater ease of integrating the neurology, physical therapy, and psychiatric treatment in that setting; and the fact that these patients usually do not meet current criteria for acute psychiatric unit admission. There is an advantage to being able to maintain continuity of care after discharge from the type of integrated treatment described here, particularly by the psychiatrist and neurologist. When this is not possible, a report with detailed delineation of the diagnostic formulation and treatment recommendations, with a copy to both the patient and the subsequent treating clinicians, is highly desirable.

While there is evidence that a more prolonged period of integrated treatment than the format of 1 to 2 weeks outlined here may generate a higher yield of symptomatic improvement by time of discharge [21], contemporary health insurance constraints regarding duration of hospital stay suggest to us that the intermediate but still intensive treatment format outlined here has merit in effectively engaging patients with PMD who might otherwise not be effectively treated.

Conclusions

As in other diagnostic categories in neurology and psychiatry, patients with PMDs and other conversion disorders present with a variety of levels of severity, chronicity, and comorbidity, as well as with a broad spectrum of intrinsic resilience, history of life adversity, and levels of external support. As with any other category of disorder, there is a requirement to individualize treatment and provide more intensive intervention for those patients where it is needed in order to reverse a course that will otherwise lead to a perpetuation of dependence and disability. It is our clinical impression, based on the experience reviewed here, that inpatient treatment that integrates a palatable and effective route for these patients to jump-start a move to recovery is worthy of further systematic study to refine and enhance the potentially effective ingredients.

Acknowledgements

The authors are appreciative of the clinical contributions of Drs. Bair Ford, Steven Frucht, Paul Greene, Pietro Mazzoni, Cheryl Waters, Elizabeth Haberfeld, and Michael Rotstein. We were aided by the support of the Neuropsychiatry Gift Fund at the CUMC in providing honoraria that made the follow-up study possible.

References

1. De Lange FP, Roelofs K, Toni I. Motor imagery: a window into the mechanisms and alterations of the motor system. *Cortex* 2008;**44**:494–506.

2. Nowak DA, Fink GR. Psychogenic movement disorders: aetiology, phenomenology, neuroanatomical correlates and therapeutic approaches. *Brain Body Med* 2009;**47**:1015–1025.

3. Voon V, Brezing C, Gallea C, *et al*. Emotional stimuli and motor conversion disorder. *Brain* 2010;**133**:1526–1536.

4. Rowe JB. Conversion disorder: understanding the pathogenic links between emotion and motor systems in the brain. *Brain* 2010;**133**:1295–1297.

5. Fava GA, Wise TN. Issues for DSM-V: psychological factors affecting either identified or feared medical conditions: a solution for somatoform disorders. *Am J Psychiatry* 2007;**164**:1002–1003.

6. Stone J, LaFrance WC, Levenson JL, Sharpe M. Issues for DSM V: conversion disorder. *Am J Psychiatry* 2010;**167**:626–627.

7. Kumru H, Begeman M, Valls-Sole J. Dual task interference in psychogenic tremor. *Mov Disord* 2007;**22**:2077–2082.

8. Voon V, Lang AE, Hallett. Diagnosing psychogenic movement disorders: which criteria should be used in clinical practice? *Nat Clin Pract Neurol* 2007;**3**:134–135.

9. Espay AJ, Goldenhar LM, Voon V, *et al*. Opinions and clinical practices related to diagnosing and managing patients with psychogenic movement disorders: an international survey of Movement Disorder Society members. *Mov Disord* 2009;**24**:1366–1374.

10. Sudarsky L. Psychogenic gait disorders. *Semin Neurol* 2006;**26**:351–356.

11. Bhatia KP, Schneider SA. Psychogenic tremor and related disorders. *J Neurol* 2007;**254**:569–574.

12. McKeon A, Ahlskog JE, Bower JH, Josephs KA. Psychogenic tremor: long term prognosis in patients with electrophysiologically- confirmed disease. *Mov Disord* 2009;**24**:72–76.

13. Peckham EL, Hallett M. Psychogenic movement disorders. *Neurol Clin* 2009;**27**:801–819.

14. Gupta A, Lang AE. Psychogenic movement disorders. *Curr Opin Neurol* 2009:**22**:430–436.

15. Kroenke K. Efficacy of treatment for somatoform disorders. In Dimsdale JE, Xin Y, Kleinman A, *et al.*, eds. *Somatic Presentations of Mental Disorders: Refining the Research Agenda for DSM-V*. Arlington, VA: American Psychiatric Association, 2009:143–164.

16. Williams DT, Fallon B, Harding K. Somatoform disorders. In Rowland LP, Pedley T, eds. *Merritt's Neurology*, 12th edn. Philadelphia, Lippincott Williams & Wilkins, 2010:1069–1075.

17. Williams DT, Harding KJ. Somatoform disorders. In Kompoliti K, Verhagen Metman L, eds. *Encyclopedia of Movement Disorders*. Oxford: Academic Press, 2010:121–127.

18. Fahn S, Williams D. Psychogenic dystonia. *Adv Neurol* 1988;**50**:431–455.

19. American Psychiatric Association. *Diagnostic and Statistical Manual of Diseases*, 4th edn, text revision. Washington DC: American Psychiatric Press, 2000.

20. Williams DT, Ford B, Fahn S. Phenomenology and psychopathology related to psychogenic movement disorders, In Weiner WJ, Lang AE, eds. *Behavioral Neurology of Movement Disorders*. New York: Raven Press, 1995:231–257.

21. Rosebush P, Mazurek M. The treatment of conversion disorder. In In Hallett M, Fahn S, Jankovic J, *et al.*, eds. *Psychogenic Movement Disorders: Neurology and Neuropsychiatry*. Philadelphia, PA: Lippincott Williams & Wilkins, 2006:289–301.

Appendix: Psychogenic movement disorders video legends

Video prepared by Anthony E. Lang and Mark Hallett

Except in selected stated examples, all cases were submitted by Guenther Deuschl, Stanley Fahn, Mark Hallett, Joseph Jankovic, Anthony Lang, and Philip Thompson.

All patients shown as having psychogenic movement disorders had clinically definite [1] psychogenic movement disorders, often with additional confirming historical or clinical features not shown on the videotapes.

A. Psychogenic tremor

Section editor: Guenther Deuschl

See also mixed myoclonus and tremor in the myoclonus videos and the tremor in psychogenic parkinson videos as well as several other videos.

1. Clinical presentations

a. Unilateral hand tremor

Tremor 1. Patient presenting with a unilateral rest, postural, and kinetic hand tremor. The frequency of the tremor changes depending on the maneuvers which are performed. This can be seen when the patient changes the motor task.

Tremor 2. Young man complaining of a spontaneous tremor in the left arm which worsens during any kind of arm and hand movement. Clinically a co-contraction tremor is seen. The tremor is most prominent when he moves the fist and the co-contraction of antagonists can be seen. Tremor is not present when the patient relaxes his hand. Slow build-up of the tremor amplitude can be seen following co-contraction. Palpating the muscles or testing for wrist rigidity discloses the co-contraction.

b. Bilateral tremors of the upper extremity

Tremor 3. Tremor of all extremities, most pronounced in the right arm and both legs. The tremor is seen during rest and posture. Tremor frequency changes when the arm is stretched out. When the patient is holding both arms in a flexed position against gravity, the tremor moves to the left arm and gets even worse than on the right side. Movements with the right leg change the frequency of the hand tremor. Movements with the left leg are accompanied by a low-frequency tremor of this leg, which is different from the frequency during the earlier maintained rest position.

Tremor 4. Bilateral forceful tremor with different "entrainment" maneuvers. At rest, the frequency fluctuations can already be seen. When pouring he maintains the tremor rhythm by high effort co-contraction. While performing repetitive finger movements with the left hand or the left leg, the tremor rhythm in the hands fluctuates.

c. Leg tremors

Tremor 5. Dystonic foot position with a co-contraction tremor of various frequencies. The foot is held in a pronated position and the patient complains about pain. The tremor is irregular in this foot position and co-contraction of the muscles is apparent. There are no signs of complex regional pain syndrome (reflex sympathetic dystrophy).

Tremor 6. Bilateral proximal leg tremor brought out by raising the legs from the floor. Tremor frequency changes dramatically with tapping maneuver (partially entraining).

d. Stance tremors

Tremor 7. Same patient as in Tremor 3 showing a psychogenic tremor during stance and walking. While getting up from the chair, the knees show a slow frequency inwards–outwards movement. The patient walks cautiously as if he has balance problems, but he balances nicely on one leg while the other moves irregularly when lifted off the floor.

e. Trunkal tremor

Tremor 8. Middle-aged woman presenting with a sudden-onset tremor. Low-frequency anterior–posterior movement of the trunk is seen during standing. While walking, this movement continues at about the same frequency, but gets more inconsistent. In addition, there is a slow rhythmic movement of the arms at approximately double the frequency. The tremor ceases when the physician places his hand on the patient's head.

f. Psychogenic orthostatic tremor

Tremor 9. Video shows a proximal leg tremor on standing that subsides when the patient leans against the table, similar to organic orthostatic tremor. The frequency of this tremor, however, was 6–7 Hz, and it was variably distractible with tapping tasks. (Courtesy of Dr. Michael Angel.)

2. Clinical tests in the evaluation of possible psychogenic tremors

a. Contrasting features during daily activities and clinical assessment: variability of tremor (inconsistent features) particularly in different situations (rest/intention)

Tremor 10. The young woman shows a distal tremor on the left side as long as her hands are freely moving and she has no tasks to perform. As soon as she performs tasks with her left hand the tremor moves from the distal hand to the proximal shoulder and trunk bilaterally. The pouring maneuver is performed better than one would have expected.

b. Tremor during distracting maneuvers

Tremor 11. Patient with rest tremor of the left hand showing distractibility with both mental and physical tasks.

c. Entrainment

Tremor 12. The patient has a relatively rapid tremor of the right hand. When asked to tap with the left hand at a much slower frequency, the tremor of the right hand slows and exactly matches the movements of the left hand (entrains). In the second part of the video, both hands are outstretched and show the psychogenic tremor; when asked to tap, the tremor disappears and is replaced by the tapping rhythm.

Tremor 13. Two patients are shown who demonstrate the spectrum of entrainment. The entrainment is more subtle in the first patient than in the second.

d. Co-contraction sign

Tremor 14. Prominent co-contraction is evident in the right arm on passive movement by the investigator.

e. Pause of tremor with ballistic movement

Tremor 15. Ballistic movement test in a young man with psychogenic tremor in the right hand. He is asked to make quick movements of the left arm. With each movement, there is a transient pause in the right hand tremor. (Courtesy of Dr. D. Haubenberger.)

Tremor 16. Patient with essential tremor showing mild mirroring but no pause in tremor in the right hand in response to ballistic movement of the left hand. (Courtesy of Dr. D. Haubenberger.)

B. Psychogenic dystonia

Section editor: Stanley Fahn (with assistance from Drs. Michael Rotstein and Toni Pearson)

a. Blepharospasm

Dystonia 1. The video shows initially normal eye opening and normal blink rate during the first visit. There is intermittent left eye closure, triggered by physical examination and reading. During the second visit, symptoms are provoked by reading silently and relieved by reading aloud (note: organic blepharospasm also often improves with speaking out loud). The short-term fluctuating presence and unilateral nature of the symptoms are not typically seen in patients with blepharospasm. Several other videos also show blepharospasm and other eyelid disturbances.

b. Lower face (see also Dystonia 18)

Dystonia 2. The video shows an asymmetrical lower face posture at rest, with downward and lateral displacement of the left lower lip. The abnormal posture is variably present at rest and is distractible with voluntary facial movements and attempts to speak. There are additional false neurological signs, including bilateral pseudoptosis, intermittent jerking, and psychogenic gait.

Dystonia 3. Patient shows variable lower facial dystonia. Initially right lower facial pulling is triggered by turning the head to the right. Later, pulling to the left side is triggered by turning of the head to the left. There are additional movements of the head seen later in the video.

Dystonia 4. Patient with left lower facial dystonia and right eyelid involvement.

c. Oromandibular (plus additional cranial and generalized involvement)

Dystonia 5. The video demonstrates the patient's typical paroxysmal episode. There are neck, face, jaw, mouth, and trunk spasms that are variable in duration and pattern. Speech is inconsistent: sometimes it is normal, sometimes slow and dysarthric. The end of the video shows the patient after the episode.

d. Cervical

Dystonia 6. The video contains three segments. The first shows the patient's initial office visit, in which she demonstrates tightness and limited mobility of the mouth and jaw when speaking. There is intermittent posturing of the neck, which is variable in direction (sometimes turned or tilted to the left, sometimes to the right, sometimes extended). On examination, she has a full active and passive range of motion of the neck. She was hospitalized 1 month later for 10 days of physical and psychotherapy. The second video segment shows her symptoms on the day of admission: limited mobility of the jaw, and retrocollis that is worse during walking. The final video segment, 7 days later, shows marked improvement.

e. Arm

Dystonia 7. The first part of the video shows the patient at her initial office visit 3 weeks after the onset of symptoms, with variable flexion of the left elbow and fingers and very limited movement. She uses the right hand to passively move the left arm. Her arm is held flexed against the trunk while walking. She was hospitalized, and the final segment of the video shows marked improvement of her symptoms the next day during a session with a physical therapist. Active and passive

movements of the arm are almost normal, and there is no arm posturing during walking.

Dystonia 8. Video demonstrates left arm and leg dystonia. As the patient mentions, at other times she has similar posturing on the right side. Note how psychogenic dystonia often persists and is non-distractible despite the patient conversing and performing a variety of actions with her opposite hand. (Courtesy Dr. William Weiner.)

f. Trunk

Dystonia 9. The video demonstrates the patient's typical paroxysmal episode: intermittent twisting postures of the trunk, neck, limbs, and face, which are variable and inconsistent in lateralization (right/left) and pattern (flexion/extension).

g. Leg

Dystonia 10. The video demonstrates right foot posturing (in-toeing, inversion, plantarflexion) at rest. The gait is stiff and awkward, with bilateral in-toeing, extended legs, and a rigid trunk and arm posture. The right foot posture is briefly distractible when she is asked to try to stand with feet together. Several false neurological signs are also found on her examination, including right wrist and hip give-way weakness accompanied by exaggerated effort and facial grimacing. See Gait 7 and Gait 21 for other patients with dystonic leg postures interfering with walking.

h. Fixed leg dystonia

Dystonia 11. The video shows a fixed, plantar-flexed, in-turned posture of the left ankle. There is good passive range of movement of the toes; however, the patient has almost no voluntary toe movement. Passive range of movement of the ankle is extremely limited during the office visit. During examination under anesthesia, there is a full passive range of motion of the ankle, demonstrating that the fixed posture when awake is not attributable to a contracture. See Dystonia 16 for an example of fixed dystonia resulting from organic brain disease.

i. Post-traumatic dystonia

Dystonia 12. The video demonstrates a fixed, inverted posture of the left foot with prominent disuse atrophy of the calf muscles. There is severe hyperesthesia, and no active or passive movement. There is normal spontaneous gesturing with the left hand; however, when her arms are examined she develops left hand tremor, slowness, and posturing of the fingers.

Dystonia 13. Patient presenting with fixed right lateral head posturing ("post-traumatic painful torticollis"). The patient had had complete remissions in the past with amytal. His most recent recurrence of tonic lateral neck tilt and shoulder elevation was accompanied by dystonic posturing in the right hand and severe abduction of the hips. When the patient attempts to lift the head from the shoulder he develops shaking of the head. When the examiner attempts to adduct the hips the patient develops prominent abduction/adduction hip tremor. See Dystonia 17 for an example of a similar neck posturing (not fixed) resulting from an organic dystonia.

j. Complex regional pain syndrome type I (previously called reflex sympathetic dystrophy)

Dystonia 14. The video shows head tilt and mild lateral flexion of the trunk to the left. The thumb, third, and fourth fingers of the left hand are inconsistently held in a flexed posture and left hand movements are slow and effortful. The left leg is swollen and the skin appears discolored and mottled, which is characteristic of complex regional pain syndrome. The leg is flexed at the knee and there is almost no voluntary movement.

k. Suggestible dystonia which moves around the body

Dystonia 15. Suggestibility in a patient with psychogenic dystonia and tremor. Upon being asked to move the abnormal posture to different parts of the body, it moves to that body part. She has the sense that she can "direct" the involuntary movement. She does not feel that she has control of tremor, but it both comes and goes when requested by the physician.

l. Organic dystonias potentially misdiagnosed as psychogenic

Dystonia 16. Fixed dystonia of the left hand secondary to a Rasmussen-like encephalitis.

Dystonia 17. Patient with idiopathic cervical and axial dystonia showing response to geste

antagoniste (sensory trick) and resolution of the dystonia on lying flat on the floor. (Courtesy Dr. John Morris.)

Dystonia 18 (psychogenic). Patient (to contrast with Dystonia 17) with psychogenic cranial–cervical dystonia responsive to a geste antagoniste. (Previously published by Munhoz and Lang [2].)

C. Psychogenic myoclonus
Section editor: Mark Hallett

a. Infrequent jerks

Myoclonus 1. Psychogenic myoclonus with synchronous jerking of the shoulders (sometimes "hung up" or sustained), often in association with a facial movement. The patient also has abdominal movements that are even more sustained.

b. Frequent body jerks

Myoclonus 2. Very frequent psychogenic myoclonus involving much of the body with a variety of violent movements. In addition, there is some underlying abnormal posturing of the trunk and neck. When asked to turn her body, there is a brief period of distractibility and cessation of the jerks.

Myoclonus 3. Frequent jerks involving the upper and lower body accentuated by mental stress and triggered by testing reflexes (latency is long, within voluntary reaction time) and with tuning fork.

c. Trunkal jerks

Myoclonus 4. Jerky movements are somewhat complex and not simple. (Video provided by M. Hallett, from Fahn and Jankovic [3], with permission.)

Myoclonus 5. Paroxysmal repetitive trunkal jerks triggered by standing up (initial segment) and the pull test. Both events are aborted by squeezing the base of the neck; it had been suggested to the patient earlier in the examination that this could be a method of relieving the symptoms.

d. Pelvic thrusts

Myoclonus 6. Patient shows trunk and pelvic jerks. Loud sound triggers the jerks while lying down (looking like startle).

e. Mixed myoclonus and tremor

Myoclonus 7. The patient has mixed myoclonus and tremor. Some suggestibility is apparent in that the movement sometimes starts and stops on request.

Myoclonus 8. The patient has mixed myoclonus and tremor. The patient appears quite distressed by the movements. The patient is undergoing physiological studies with electroencephalography and electromyography.

f. Sensory evoked myoclonus

Myoclonus 9. Myoclonus induced by median and peroneal nerve stimulation. (Courtesy Dr. Robert Chen.)

Myoclonus 10. Patient with psychogenic tremor as well as myoclonus. The myoclonus can be precipitated by pressing on select body parts. Additionally, the myoclonus is triggered by positioning the arms in only a specific posture directly in front of the patient.

Myoclonus 11. Psychogenic myoclonus precipitated by auditory and somatosensory stimulation.

Myoclonus 12. Psychogenic myoclonus of the left arm precipitated by a variety of somatosensory stimuli in many places on the body. It also is present in an anticipatory manner when the tendon hammer is stopped short of contact.

Myoclonus 13. Psychogenic myoclonus with axial movements of neck and trunk, often accompanied by movements of the arms. The myoclonus has an appearance similar to startle, which is how the patient described it. Auditory stimuli also provoke the myoclonus.

D. Psychogenic parkinsonism

Section editor: Anthony Lang

a. Tremor

Parkinson 1. Psychogenic tremor present at rest, with posture, and during action. The tremor persists during the performance of mental arithmetic but subsides with other distraction. With suggestion, tremor in the leg develops and hand tremor initially subsides, but then recurs with further suggestion.

Parkinson 2. Psychogenic tremor present at rest, with posture, and during action. Tremor is largely synchronous in the arms and is variably present in the trunk. Tremor frequency varies considerably, increasing with action. Tremor subsides with distraction (tongue movement).

Parkinson 3. Psychogenic tremor present at rest, with posture, and during action. The amplitude of the tremor is approximately the same in all three of these. Tremor persists during the performance of side-to-side tongue movements; however, the tongue movements are performed extremely poorly and slowly despite the complete absence of dysarthria or other abnormalities of orolingual function. Tremor interferes with drinking and writing; the disturbances of these functions are unusual for organic tremors, particularly drawing a "wavy line" and spiral – the patient repeatedly taps the pen on the page at the tremor frequency to complete the spiral.

Parkinson 4. Psychogenic tremor present at rest, with posture, and during action. The tremor entrains to slow side-to-side tongue movements. The tremor is distractible, subsiding each time the patient touches the target with the opposite hand.

b. "Bradykinesia" in psychogenic parkinsonism

Parkinson 5. Rapid repetitive and alternating movements are performed irregularly and somewhat slowly (particularly on the left) but without demonstrating the classical fatiguing of amplitude and speed seen in organic bradykinesia.

Parkinson 6. Abnormal performance on the right side is accompanied by head and body rocking movements, emphasizing the difficulty the patient has in performing the task. Manual tasks are variably performed but generally lack typical fatiguing.

Parkinson 7. Extreme slowness seen in attempting to touch the thumb to the individual fingers, accompanied by a fast action tremor on the right. The degree of slowness on this simple task is completely inconsistent with the patient's relatively normal performance of unbuttoning and buttoning his shirt.

Parkinson 8. Psychogenic parkinsonism with extreme slowness accompanied by a sense of great effort.

Parkinson 9. Long video demonstrating multiple aspects of psychogenic bradykinesia. There is marked but variable slowness in the performance of most manual and foot tasks. The patient gets "hung up" in approaching the target on the finger to nose task. She is barely able to lift the foot from the floor or perform tapping movements but easily "wiggles" her foot back into her shoe. There is marked difficulty arising from a chair. Writing is only slightly slowed; however, she has profound difficulties with drawing a spiral, demonstrating extreme slowness and arrests.

Parkinson 10. This patient was treated with transcutaneous electrical nerve stimulation with the electrodes placed on the abdomen. Without stimulation, he shows extreme slowness and difficulty in all activities including arising from a chair and walking. Shortly after turning the stimulator on all motor functions markedly improve. Within seconds of turning the stimulator off, he again becomes extremely slow and freezes.

c. Postural instability on the pull test (the pattern of stepping back may not differ from that seen in organic parkinsonism)

Parkinson 11. The patient tends to fall with minimal postural displacement. Despite complete lack of arm swing while walking (see Parkinson 14) and resistance to passive movement on testing tone, the patient has normal tone and arm swing when the trunk is rotated back and forth while the patient is standing.

Parkinson 12. The patient is pulled off balance with minimal displacement including a brief touch of the shoulders with the fingers by the examiner.

Parkinson 13. Retropulsion, but no falling, in response to varying (sometimes firm) postural displacements.

d. Gait (see also Gait 12)

Parkinson 14. Difficulty arising from a chair. Gait is slow, with short strides and lack of arm swing. When asked to walk quickly the patient seems to become stiffer and retains a short stride with the arms held stiffly at the sides. Asked to run, the arms remain held stiffly at the sides.

Parkinson 15. Gait is slow and shuffling with lack of arm swing; arms are held slightly abducted from the sides. When asked to take big strides the gait deteriorates further, becoming even slower with the feet sliding across the floor rather than being lifted. Running causes increased shuffling of the legs with occasional freezing.

Parkinson 16. Complete lack of right arm swing while walking and running. However, when the trunk is quickly rotated passively the right arm swings

normally and equally to the left, and on the pull test both arms lift from the sides quickly and equally. Contrast this video with Parkinson 20 (patients with Parkinson's disease).

Parkinson 17. Extremely slow antalgic gait in a patient with psychogenic parkinsonism following minor injury.

e. Other features

Parkinson 18. This patient's spontaneous speech shows little or no difficulty; this contrasts strikingly with the performance on formal speech testing at the end of the video. While talking, he shows normal spontaneous movements in the hands (this contrasts with his complaints and difficulties performing formal manual tasks on examination; see Parkinson 5). There is a variable resting tremor in the left arm and right leg, which shows distractibility later in the video.

Parkinson 19. Speech is very slow, hesitant, and "stuttering," with an additional "baby-talk" quality. The patient demonstrates a prominent psychogenic tremor in the right arm. She has marked difficulty arising from the chair and has an extremely slow, abnormal gait, with in-turning of the feet, unsteadiness, and dragging the feet across the floor.

Parkinson 20. Two patients with true Parkinson's disease, the first milder than the second. Patients show the typical discrepancy between reduced arm swing on walking and more normal swing while running. While running, the arm is usually held more flexed in front of the patient and swings much more actively; this is particularly seen in the more mildly affected first patient, who has normal swing while running. These patients also show the typical responses to passive rotational movement of the trunk and the pull test (contrast these to the patients with psychogenic parkinsonism; see Parkinson 11 and Parkinson 16).

E. Psychogenic gaits

Section editor: Joseph Jankovic

These cases show a wide variety of psychogenic gaits that are often difficult to categorize. These gaits are often very "energy inefficient."

Gait 1. The patient exhibits paroxysmal episodes of shaking in his legs while sitting or standing. The leg tremor is markedly distractable and disappears when running. The gait is quite bizarre.

Gait 2. Video shows coordinated, tic-like, self-injurious movements in upper extremities, and inability to perform the bicycle movement. She has a halting, wide-based gait, with marked "effort," dystonic posture of right foot, and flexion–adduction of arms. She bends down "to stabilize" herself.

Gait 3. Video shows whole-body jerks and a bouncy, wide-based gait. She requires assistance and has to touch the wall to support herself.

Gait 4. The patient has a somewhat infantile speech pattern, flinging movements of her arms, and a halting, bizarre gait.

Gait 5. Video shows high-stepping, irregular, bizarre gait. She has difficulty performing tandem gait, claiming her legs are "shaking really bad." She was able to perform the bicycle motion at the beginning but not later (inconsistent performance).

Gait 6. The patient has a very irregular gait requiring a great deal of effort to walk and perform bicycle motion.

Gait 7. The patient has fixed dystonia of both feet, with passive resistance when the examiner attempts to correct the dystonic inversion. She has a "labored" gait requiring a walker.

Gait 8. Stiff, bouncing, gait with "la belle indifference" despite slow collapse to the floor. From the sitting position, she has a dramatic fall to the floor with a psychogenic non-epileptic seizure, dystonic arching ("arc en circ"), and stuttering speech. With reassurance she is able to get up and walk and march.

Gait 9. A "pseudo-scissoring" gait with crossing of the legs when walking.

Gait 10. The patient is able to move her legs normally and effortlessly while seated. Upon standing, she develops a bizarre gait, characterized by tapping the ball of her right foot twice with each step including walking backward but this resolves briefly as she returns to the sitting position.

Gait 11. Elderly woman with cautious gait secondary to fear of falling following a previous fall. Her gait is slow, deliberate, and cautious, but she is able to walk better with simple reassurance. Subsequently, she markedly improved with gait training designed to help her regain her confidence in walking. A cautious gait is generally not categorized as psychogenic. See also Gait 26.

Gait 12. Psychogenic parkinsonism manifested by short-steppage, "shuffling" gait (she stomps her feet on the floor rather than typical shuffling) and freezing exacerbated when instructed to walk faster. She has intermittent right hand tremor. She has a dramatic fall during the "pull test."

Gait 13. The patient's high-amplitude synchronous leg tremor is markedly distractible. She has a bouncy gait that markedly improves with running and minimal support by holding on to examiner's finger. All her symptoms essentially resolved 30 minutes after placebo (carbidopa) challenge.

Gait 14. This woman was previously diagnosed with levodopa-responsive cerebellar ataxia. After levodopa was withdrawn for 46 hours, her wide-based gait markedly deteriorated (segment 1) but improved dramatically within 30 minutes after carbidopa (placebo) (segment 2). Her ability to arise from the chair also markedly improved.

Gait 15. Patient with sudden onset of right leg tremor and posturing of the foot interfering with her gait; she markedly improved with saline (placebo) injection into her right calf.

Gait 16. Patient with dramatic falls and great deal of effort, requiring assistance with ambulation (which is seen only briefly). He has whole-body shaking and repetitive flinging movements of his left arm.

Gait 17. Patient with bizarre slow gait and "freezing." She tends to hold her center of gravity posteriorly.

Gait 18. The patient shows a halting, unsteady gait with "walking on thin ice" characteristics. She falls slowly and carefully without injury following a pull test.

Gait 19. A "pseudo-scissoring," waddling gait with in-turning of the feet, which worsens on attempted running. Suggestion with squeezing of the neck completely relieves the gait disturbance.

Gait 20. Classical "astasia–abasia" with markedly bizarre gait and inability to ambulate for more than a few steps.

Gait 21. "Dystonic" in-turning of the feet walking forwards but normal foot posture while walking backwards, supportive of the original misdiagnosis of organic dystonia. One day later after intensive physical therapy and psychotherapy the gait is normal.

Gait 22. Psychogenic gait with a feature that might be called a "freezing gait." The patient's foot seems to stick to the floor periodically.

Gait 23. Knee buckling only seen when the patient is asked to walk quickly.

Organic gaits potentially confused with psychogenic

Gait 24. Young-onset Parkinson's disease with a very unusual diphasic dyskinetic gait disturbance. Later in the video, the patient is shown after his medications have worn off. (Courtesy Dr. John Nutt.)

Gait 25. Parkinson's disease with dyskinetic gait involving ballistic-like left leg movements during the swing phase. (Courtesy Dr. John Morris.)

Gait 26. Patient with established orthostatic tremor with a very cautious insecure gait, preferring to hold on to walls and objects. Her gait improves when she is asked to march even while turning. These symptoms relate to the marked unsteady feeling that many patients with orthostatic tremor experience if they stand still and which this patient also experienced even when slowing down to turn around.

Gait 27. Patient with neuroacanthocytosis with a very unusual gait, probably the result of a mixture of obsessive-compulsive behavior, dystonia, and chorea.

F. Miscellaneous psychogenic movement disorders

Section editor: Philip Thompson

Misc 1. Paroxysmal trunk spasms only on lying down.

Misc 2. Spasms converting to an "arc en circ" and subsequently to a psychogenic non-epileptic seizure triggered by an external sensory stimulus to a specific site on the patient's back.

Misc 3. Spontaneous generalized jerks and vocalizations.

Misc 4. Paroxysmal tremor, dystonia, and ballistic movements of the arm precipitated by movement or external stimulation, with normal motor function between events.

Misc 5. Labored, slow dysarthric speech brought out when patient is discussing an emotional topic but normalization occurring when discussing other topics.

Misc 6. Psychogenic stuttering speech associated with flinging myoclonic arm movement and swaying of her trunk on walking. (Courtesy Dr. John Morris.)

Misc 7. Psychogenic palatal tremor/myoclonus. The palatal movement can be monitored with movements of the throat. Note that tapping with either hand entrains the movements. (Previously published by Pirio *et al.* [4].)

Misc 8. Psychogenic tremor and ataxia. The dysmetric movements are rather wild and often in wide circles. Briefly she has much more normal coordination when wiping her hands together. Distraction sometimes reduces the tremor. This is seen near the end of the segment where tapping with the left hand reduces the tremor of the right hand.

Misc 9. Psychogenic convergence spasm.

Misc 10. Psychogenic stiff-person syndrome. The patient has painful axial and leg spasms. Prior to the segment showing the patient walking, she had been given a great deal of suggestion, which reduced the tone in the legs allowing her to walk (this was not possible earlier), but she remains very symptomatic.

Misc 11. Psychogenic chorea in which the patient exhibits choreiform movements during the interview, which abruptly stop during performance of visual tasks. She can protrude her tongue for 10 seconds. Her difficulty with tandem gait is suggestive of astasia–abasia (Previously published by Fekete and Janovic [5].)

Misc 12. Psychogenic camptocormia; the patient shows camptocormia that is relieved by raising his arms above his head. Subsequent "muscle pulling and pain" in the abdomen and back causes him to resume the 90 degree flexed posture. There is a variable tremor in the hands that is also likely psychogenic. (Previously published by Skidmore *et al.* [6].)

References

1. Williams DT, Ford B, Fahn S. Phenomenology and psychopathology related to psychogenic movement disorders. *Adv Neurol* 1995;65:231–258.

2. Munhoz RP, Lang AE. Gestes antagonistes in psychogenic dystonia. *Mov Disord* 2004;19:331–332.

3. Fahn S, Jankovic J. *Principles and Practice of Movement Disorders.* Philadelphia, PA: Churchill Livingstone, 2007.

4. Pirio RS, Mari Z, Matsuhashi M, Hallett M. Psychogenic palatal tremor. *Mov Disord* 2006; 21:274–276.

5. Fekete R, Jankovic J. Psychogenic chorea associated with family history of Huntington Disease. *Mov Disord* 2010; 25:503–504.

6. Skidmore F, Anderson K, Fram D, Weiner W. Psychogenic camptocormia. *Mov Disord* 2007;22:1974–1975.

Index